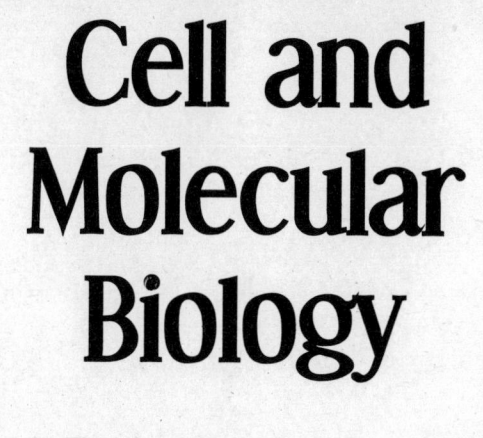

Cell and Molecular Biology

Contents

Contents

Preface

The emerging trends in contemporary sciences, particularly in molecular biology and recombinant DNA technology, have revolutionized the cell biology in regard to the understanding of the cell structure, function and organizational activities. In fact, by now it is a well established and acceptable fact that a cell is the basic unit of life that constitutes the foundation of life sciences, and biology in particular. An algorithm of advancements has taken place in cell biology during the last few decades owing to the merger of cytological, genetical, biochemical and molecular researches which in an integrative format defined and offered an opportunity of better understanding. The present book targets both undergraduate and postgraduate students covering most widely accepted current syllabus of cell biology which is included in various competitive examination also. Though there are a number of textbooks on this subject available, it was thought that it would be worthwhile to develop an acquaintance of students with conceivable and effective infusion of modern concepts in the best possible trivial and lucid language. This attempt is motivated by our age long teaching and research experience wherein it was constantly realized that the importance of the subject as well as its understanding should be introduced to the students in a way so that they opt and study the subject by choice and inseminate the contents with confidence. This book contains 13 chapters representing the core of the subject. They include evolution of biological diversity, chemical basis of life, the cell, cell receptors and cell signaling, genetics and genes, their replication and expression, cell cycle, recombinant DNA technology and genetic engineering, tissue culture, basic immunology, and lastly the biophysical chemistry. Attempts have also been made to introduce the principles of instrumentation used in cell biology, particularly covering the instruments which are used in recent techniques. It is apparent that all the recent advances are difficult to cover due to fast moving and developing subject, still the efforts have been directed to cover and introduce many of the recent concepts. We are sure that they will be highly useful to the students. We are confident that students and teachers will be benefited by the contents of this volume. Also, the book shall acquire a central place as a valuable addition in the universities, colleges and institutions. It will provide a modest opening with the introduction of the subject to a beginner, an interesting refresher for a biologist, and a guide to the basic concepts for the researcher.

We are pleased to put on record our special thanks to the students, our colleagues and researchers who motivated us to take up this very unique venture. We are thankful to our young enthusiastic scholars, namely Jinu John, Siddhartha Singh, Rishi Paliwal, Abhinav Mehta and Shivani Paliwal who contributed with their maiden ideas and existing requirements which assisted us in selecting the paradigms/concepts to be the part of this book. The authors are thankful to their family members for their continual encouragements and all sorts of help during the preparation of the manuscript. We are thankful to CBS Publishers & Distributors, New Delhi, especially Mr. Satish Jain, for his nice and excellent support in the publication. Readers are requested to provide us with the feedback on the book pointing out technical, factual and typographical mistakes, if any, and also to support us with their constructive criticism which will help in improving the book to a perfect state when it comes in its next edition.

S.P. Vyas
A. Mehta

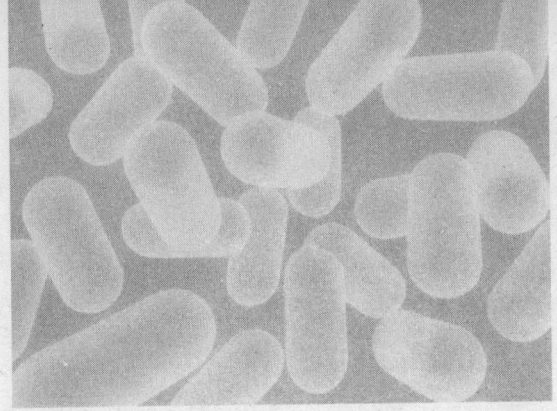

Hard cover   ISBN: 978-81-239-1957-7
Soft cover   ISBN: 978-81-239-1965-2

Cell and
Molecular Biology

ISBN: 978-81-239-1957-7

First Edition: 2011

Published by Satish Kumar Jain and produced by Vinod K. Jain for

CBS Publishers & Distributors Pvt Ltd
CBS Plaza, 4819/XI, Prahlad Street, 24 Ansari Road, Daryaganj, New Delhi 110 002, India
Website: www.cbspd.com
Ph: 23289259, 23266861/67   Fax: +91-11-23243014   e-mail: delhi@cbspd.com
                                                            cbspubs@vsnl.com
                                                            cbspubs@airtelmail.in

Branches

- Bengaluru: Seema House 2975, 17th Cross, K.R. Road,
  Banasankari 2nd Stage, Bengaluru 560 070, Karnataka
  Ph: +91-80-26771678/79   Fax: +91-80-26771680   e-mail: bangalore@cbspd.com

- Pune: Bhuruk Prestige, Sr. No. 52/12/2+1+3/2 Narhe, Haveli
  (Near Katraj-Dehu Road Bypass), Pune 411 051, Maharashtra
  Ph: 020-32404169   e-mail: pune@cbspd.com

- Kochi: 36/14 Kalluvilakam, Lissie Hospital Road,
  Kochi 682 018, Kerala
  Ph: +91-484-4059061-65   Fax: +91-484-4059065   e-mail: cochin@cbspd.com

- Chennai: 20, West Park Road, Shenoy Nagar,
  Chennai 600 030, Tamil Nadu
  Ph: +91-44-26260666, 26208620 Fax: +91-44-45530020   e-mail: chennai@cbspd.com

Printed at: India Binding House, Noida, UP

Cell and Molecular Biology

SP Vyas

M Pharm PhD Post doc (University of London)

Professor
Department of Pharmaceutical Sciences
Dr HS Gour Central University
Sagar, MP

A Mehta

MSc PhD Post doc (Czech Republic)

Department of Botany
Dr HS Gour Central University
Sagar, MP

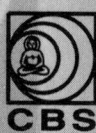

CBS

CBS Publishers & Distributors Pvt Ltd

New Delhi • Bengaluru • Pune • Kochi • Chennai

CHAPTER 1

Evolution of Life

- Origin of life
- Theories of Special Creation
- Theory of Spontaneous Generation
- Modern Theory of Origin of Life
- Lamarckism
  - Use and Disuse of Parts
  - Inheritance of Acquired Characters
- Theory of Continuity of Germplasm
- Darwinism
- Neo-Darwinism
- The First Living Cell

"Life is the sum of the distinguishing phenomena of organisms, especially metabolism, growth, reproduction, and adaptation to environment."

The origin of universe and the evolution of life is a matter of debate as old as human civilization. This search by man resulted in many theories and stories. This is because cosmogony (the study of the origin of the universe) is an area where science and theology meet. According to Hindu mythology the universe and all its inclusions are made up of five elements 'Panchabhuta', earth, water, air, fire and sky, similarly old Chinese concept of five primary elements, water, wood, fire, soil, and gold. The other prevalent theory is the Divine creation. Still science is on the way to reveal these secretes. Though, there are several theories, none of them enabled to explain well, when it comes to the origin of the universe. The "Big Bang" Theory" and its related Inflation Universe Theories are today's dominant scientific conjectures. According to these interrelated notions, the universe was created between 13 and 20 billion years ago from the random, cosmic explosion (or expansion) of a subatomic ball that hurled space, time, matter and energy in all directions. The renowned British astronomer Sir Fred Hoyle, who is accredited with first coining the term "the Big Bang" during a BBC radio broadcast in 1950. Everything - the whole universe came from an initial speck of infinite density. This speck (existing outside of space and time) appeared from no where, for no reason, only to explode (start expanding) all of a sudden. Over a period of approximately 10 billion years, this newly created space, time, matter and energy evolved into remarkably-designed and fully-functional stars, galaxies and planets, including our earth.

1.1. Origin of Life

The origin of life is supposed to be occurred by four steps, emergence of bio-molecules, emergence of organized molecular systems, emergence of self-replicating molecular systems and emergence of natural selection. Evolutionary theory appears to have seven distinct and inter related phases.

1.1.1. Cosmic: The development of space, time, matter and energy from nothing or some-how "exploded" (or expanded) from essentially nothing in the sudden "big bang" that was the birth of our universe.

1.1.2. Stellar: The development of complex stars came from the chaotic first elements. Since the big bang is thought to have produced only Hydrogen, Helium and a variety of subatomic particles, these elements must have somehow condensed into stars through some sort of evolutionary process.

1.1.3. Chemical: According to general thought, the chemical elements produced by the Big Bang were Hydrogen and Helium (and possibly Lithium). As a result of the incredible heat and pressure within stars, these original elements subsequently somehow evolved into the other naturally occurring chemical elements, which we observe today.

1.1.4. Planetary: The development of planetary systems evolved from swirling elements. The complex chemical elements thought to have evolved within ancient stars were somehow ejected, possibly at the violent deaths of stellar life cycles, releasing great clouds of swirling compounds. These clouds of chemical elements somehow formed finely-tuned solar systems, including our own.

1.1.5. Organic: It is the development of organic life from inorganic matter (a rock). The theory says that the planet Earth began as a molten mass of matter a few billions years ago. Later it cooled off into solid, dry rock. Then, it rained on the rocks for millions of years, forming great oceans. Eventually, this "prebiotic rock soup" (water + rock) came alive and formed the first self-replicating organic systems.

1.1.6. Macro: It is the development of one kind of life from a totally different kind of life. All living creatures are thought to share a common ancestor: a relatively "simple" single-celled organism, which evolved from inorganic matter (so-called, "rock soup"). Essentially, the birds and the bananas, the fishes and the flowers, are all genetically related.

1.1.7. Micro: It deals with the development of variations within the same kind of life. Micro Evolution is the variation and variety of traits expressed in sexually compatible "kinds" of organisms. Examples include the differences between various kinds of horses, dogs, cats, etc. This "variation within a kind" is what Darwin observed in the mid-18th century.

1.2. Theories of Special Creation

According to this theory the life is a spiritual entity which was created by supernatural power "God". In the chapter on Genesis in Holy Bible, the universe was created in six natural days.

1.3. Theory of Spontaneous Generation

This theory states that some life forms arose spontaneously from non-living matter. Theory of spontaneous generation was first disproved in 1668 by Francesco Redi, an Italian physician and poet. At that time, it was widely held that maggots arose spontaneously in rotting meat. Redi believed that maggots developed from eggs laid by flies. To test his hypothesis, he set out meat in a variety of flasks, some open to the air, some sealed completely, and others covered with gauze. As he had expected, maggots appeared only in the open flasks in which the flies could reach the meat and lay their eggs.

The theory of spontaneous generation was finally laid to rest in 1859 by French chemist, Louis Pasteur. He boiled meat broth in a flask, heated the neck of the flask in a flame until it became pliable, and bent it into the shape of 'S'. Air could enter the flask, but airborne microorganisms could not, they would settle by gravity in the neck. As Pasteur had expected, no microorganisms grew. When Pasteur tilted the flask so that the broth reached the lowest point in the neck, where any airborne particles would have settled, the broth rapidly became cloudy with life. Pasteur had both refuted the theory of spontaneous generation and convincingly demonstrated that microorganisms are everywhere - even in the air.

1.4. Modern Theory of Origin of Life

Scientific explanation for the origin of life was first given by Russian scientist I. A. Oparin in his book "Origin of life". According to him the planets were formed as a result of fragmentation of sun. The temperature was high about 5000–6000°C; the carbon elements existed in the form of carbon, cyanogens and methane. After that the atmosphere contained water vapors, ammonia and methane which were formed as result of inter reaction of protoplasmic elements. As the earth cooled down molecules of water liquefied to form water in which along with methane and ammonia, minerals were present in dissolved state. Later by inter reaction sugars, organic acids, proteins and nucleic acids were formed by polymerization. During various mechanisms some microscopic colloidal particles developed in the ocean water. These particles had the properties of protoplasm. Oparin considered these particles as living molecules from which the primary organisms could have developed.

The chemical basis of origin of life was proved experimentally by Stanley Miller and Harold Urey in 1953. This was the first experiment to test the Oparin-Haldane theory about the evolution of prebiotic chemicals and the origin of life on Earth (Fig. 1.1).

A mixture of methane, ammonia, hydrogen and water vapor to simulate the version of Earth's primitive, reducing atmosphere proposed by Oparin, was introduced into a 5-liter flask and energized by an electrical discharge apparatus to represent ultraviolet radiation from the sun. The products were allowed to condense and collect in a lower flask which modeled a body of water on the Earth's surface. Heat supplied to this flask recycled the water vapor just as water evaporates from lakes and seas, before moving into the atmosphere and condensing again as rain. After a day of continuous operation, Miller and Urey found a thin layer of hydrocarbons on the surface of the water. After about a week of operation, a dark brown scum was collected in the lower flask and was found to contain several types of amino acids, including glycine and alanine, together with sugars, tars, and various other unidentified organic chemicals.

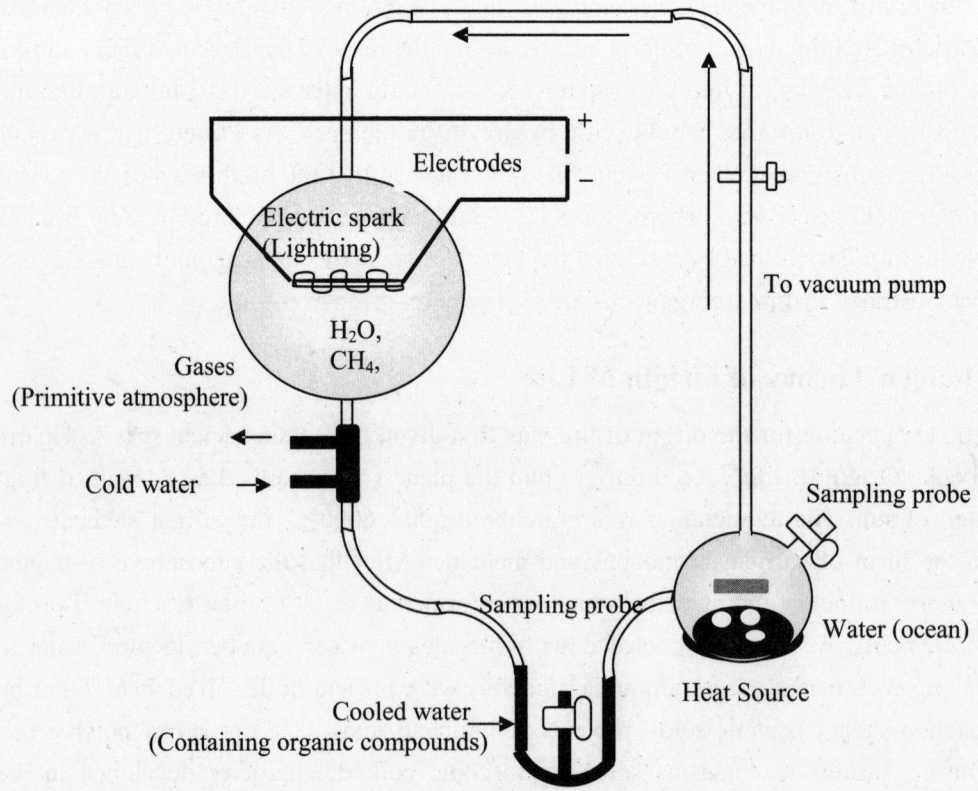

Figure 1.1: Miller-Urey apparatus

Which molecule came first, Protein, RNA or DNA? All metabolisms depend on enzymes and, until recently, every enzyme has turned out to be a protein. But proteins are synthesized from information encoded in DNA and translated into mRNA. So here is a chicken-and-egg dilemma. The synthesis of DNA and RNA requires proteins. Initial theories hypothesized that the first living thing was a protein. This assumption seemed reasonable at the time because many of the building blocks of proteins, amino acids, are easily synthesized under plausible prebiotic conditions, as proteins regulate and control almost all of the activities necessary for life. The living protein theory quickly gained widespread acceptance, but soon scientists realized that there was a major flaw with the protein theory. Proteins can not self replicate, so the first living protein would not be able to reproduce itself, and without replication there can be no natural selection; therefore, the first living protein would have no way to evolve. This led to the emergence of the RNA theory. This theory gained substantial momentum when it was found that just like proteins, some RNA molecules can catalyze chemical reactions. Today, the most popular theory involves a self replicating pre-RNA molecule. The discovery of enzymatic RNA called ribozymes supports this theory.

In principle, the minimal functions of life might have begun with RNA and only later proteins take over as catalytic machinery of metabolism and then DNA takes over as the repository of the genetic code. These evidences support this notion of an original "RNA world". Many of the cofactors that play critical roles in the functioning of life are based on ribose i.e. ATP, NAD, etc. In the cell, all deoxyribonucleotides are synthesized from ribonucleotide precursors and many bacteria control the transcription and/or translation of certain genes with RNA molecules and not protein molecules.

Evolution is the process by which all living things have developed from primitive organisms through progressive changes, which include the most advanced animals and plants. The occurrence of evolution is a scientific fact but exactly how it occurs is still a matter of debate. According to biologists, living things evolved as a result of long changes shaped by physical and chemical processes.

The most direct proof of evolution is furnished by the science of paleontology or the study of life in the past through fossil remains or impressions, usually in rock. Additional evidence comes from comparative studies of living animals and plants, including their structure (comparative anatomy), biochemistry, embryology, and geographical distribution. Approximately 2 million different species of organisms are now exist, but it is estimated that at least 99.9 percent of the species that have ever lived are now extinct and that some 2 billion species might have evolved during the past 600 million years. Different theories which have been proposed to explain the evolution are discussed in this chapter.

1.5. Lamarckism

The theory of evolution as put forth by French biologist Lamarck has come to be known as Lamarckism. This theory has two salient features:

1.5.1. Use and Disuse of Parts

According to Lamarck, continuous use of a part results in its well-development, while disuse of a part over a long period of time results in to its degeneration. For example, giraffes were forced to extend their necks and stretch their legs to reach higher vegetation over a period of time. This resulted in every generation having a little longer neck and legs than the previous one. Webbed feet in aquatic birds are thought to have developed due to constant spreading of toes and the stretching of the skin between. Flatfish thought to have developed its shape due to lying on their sides in shallow water.

1.5.2. Inheritance of Acquired Characters

According to Lamarck, the characters that an organism acquired due to a change in their environment such as long neck, webbed feet, flat bodies, etc. were passed on to the next generation. In this way, evolution from simpler to complex forms took place. However, this theory was not widely accepted as it is known that acquired characters are only phenotypic changes and not genotypic. Though giraffe, aquatic birds and flatfish do show that evolution has occurred, where as Lamarckism does not provide a satisfactory answer to the mystery of evolution.

1.6. Theory of Continuity of Germplasm

This was proposed by Weismann, who did not agree with Lamarck's theory of inheritance of acquired characters. To prove his point, he cut off the tails of many successive generations of mice. This resulted in forced disuse of the tail. According to the theory of use and disuse, the tails should have become progressively shorter. But, this did not happen. According to Weismann, the changes affected only the somatic (vegetative) cells and did not affect the germ cells or the gametes. Only the changes that affect the germ cells and the germplasm (the collection of genes) could be inherited by successive generations.

1.7. Darwinism

Evolution is a revolutionary concept that took the human world by surprise, when it was first proposed by Darwin almost 150 years ago, encountering a heavy amount of criticism and speculation that hasn't been able to deny the feasibility of this process taking place. The theory of natural selection was put forth by Charles Darwin in his book 'On the Origin of Species by Means of Natural Selection', co-authored by Alfred Russel Wallace. According to

Darwin, nature has its own way of selecting the best from the available species for continuation of life.

The mechanism of natural selection works as individuals of a species produce more offspring than necessary to replace themselves, which results in competition and struggle for existence among the individuals. Within the species itself there is variation that results in minor differences between the individuals. Thus in the struggle for existence only the ones those adapted the environmental variation could survive. In this manner nature ensures the survival of the fittest.

1.8. Neo-Darwinism

The theory put forth by Darwin and Wallace gained wide acceptance. However, in the light of modern evidences, it was slightly modified and called the neo-Darwinism. In neo-Darwinism, organic evolution is considered to be by natural selection of inherited characters. The neo-Darwinism utilizes the evidences from various fields such as genetics, palaeontology, molecular biology, ecology and ethology (study of behavior).

Changes occur in living organisms that serve to increase their adaptability, or potential for survival and reproduction, in the face of changing environments. Evolution apparently has no built-in direction or foreordained purpose. A given kind of organism may evolve only when it occurs in a variety of forms differing in hereditary characteristics, or traits that are passed from parent to offspring. Purely by chance, some varieties prove to be ill adapted to their current environment and thus disappear, whereas others prove to be adaptive, and their numbers increase. The elimination of the unfit, or the "survival of the fittest," is known as natural selection because it is nature that discards or favors a particular variant. Basically, evolution takes place only when natural selection operates on a population of organisms containing diverse inheritable forms.

1.9. The First Living Cell

During the initial degassing stage of the earth, which resulted in the formation of the atmosphere and hydrosphere, prebiotic C-H-N-O-P-S compounds became rapidly discharged along the same channels, where lower-melting material is presently moving upward. As a function of temperature gradients within the rock formation, a series of organic fronts developed with organic compounds. Since minerals could act as catalysts or as templates in the course of this development, a wide spectrum of new compounds were generated, many of which were eventually released to the hydrosphere and atmosphere. A proto-biosphere was then formed in which minerals, emulsions, and water-soluble compounds coexisted. This type of substrate is considered the starting material for the generation of the first living cell.

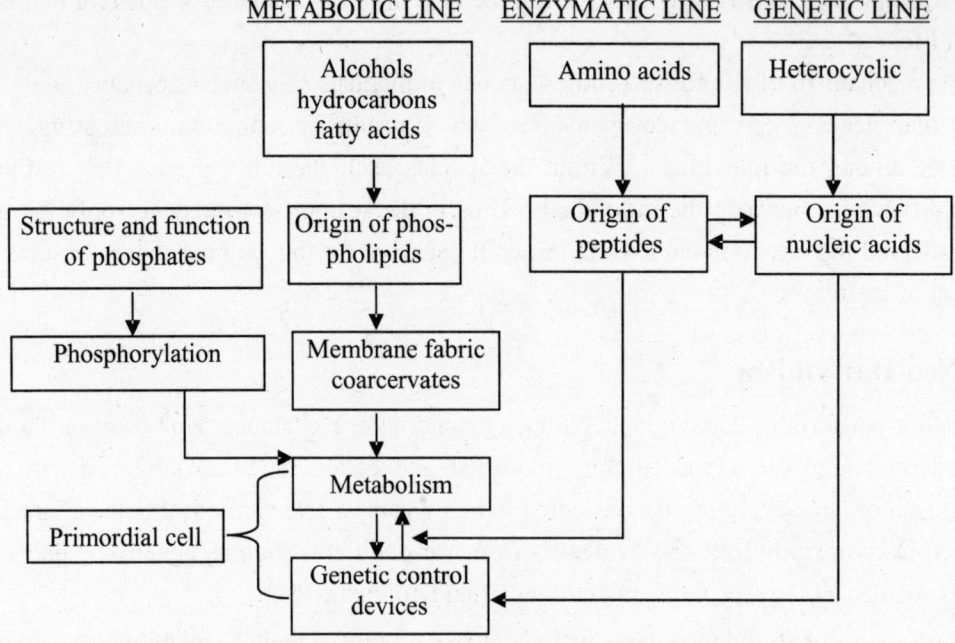

Figure 1.2: Principal events for the creation of a primordial cell

Cell is the basic building block of all living organisms. To protect the integrity and maintain the function, the cellular inclusions must be separated from its surroundings. This function is provided by the plasma membrane, which is made up of a double layer of phospholipids. They are only permeable to small, uncharged molecules like H_2O, CO_2, and O_2. Specialized transmembrane transporters are needed for ions, hydrophilic and charged organic molecules (e.g., amino acids and nucleotides) to pass into and out of the cell.

The first beings were probably much like coacervates. As a group, these bacteria are called heterotrophic anaerobes, because there was virtually no oxygen in the atmosphere at that time. The fossils of some these oldest known forms of life have been found in Australian rocks dating back 3.5 billion years (Fig. 1.2).

To create energy, these early bacteria probably consumed naturally occurring amino acids. Amino acids, sugars, and other organic compounds formed spontaneously in the atmosphere then dissolved in liquid water. Upon digesting these molecules, early bacteria produced methane and carbon dioxide as waste products. Fermenting bacteria would be an example from today of what these early creatures might have been like. Bacteria take the sugars and produce alcohol and carbon dioxide gas as waste products. In the early earth, the alcohol and carbon dioxide became part of the natural environment.

Over a very long time, gradual changes in the earliest cells gave rise to new life forms (Fig. 1.3). These new cells were very different from the earlier heterotrophs because they were able to get their energy from a new source - the sun, the origin of autotrophs, meaning "self-feeders". The autotrophic bacteria were able to feed themselves by using the energy of the Sun and they were no longer dependent on the same limited food supply as their ancestors were able to flourish. Over millions of years of evolution, photosynthetic bacteria eventually gave rise to modern day plants.

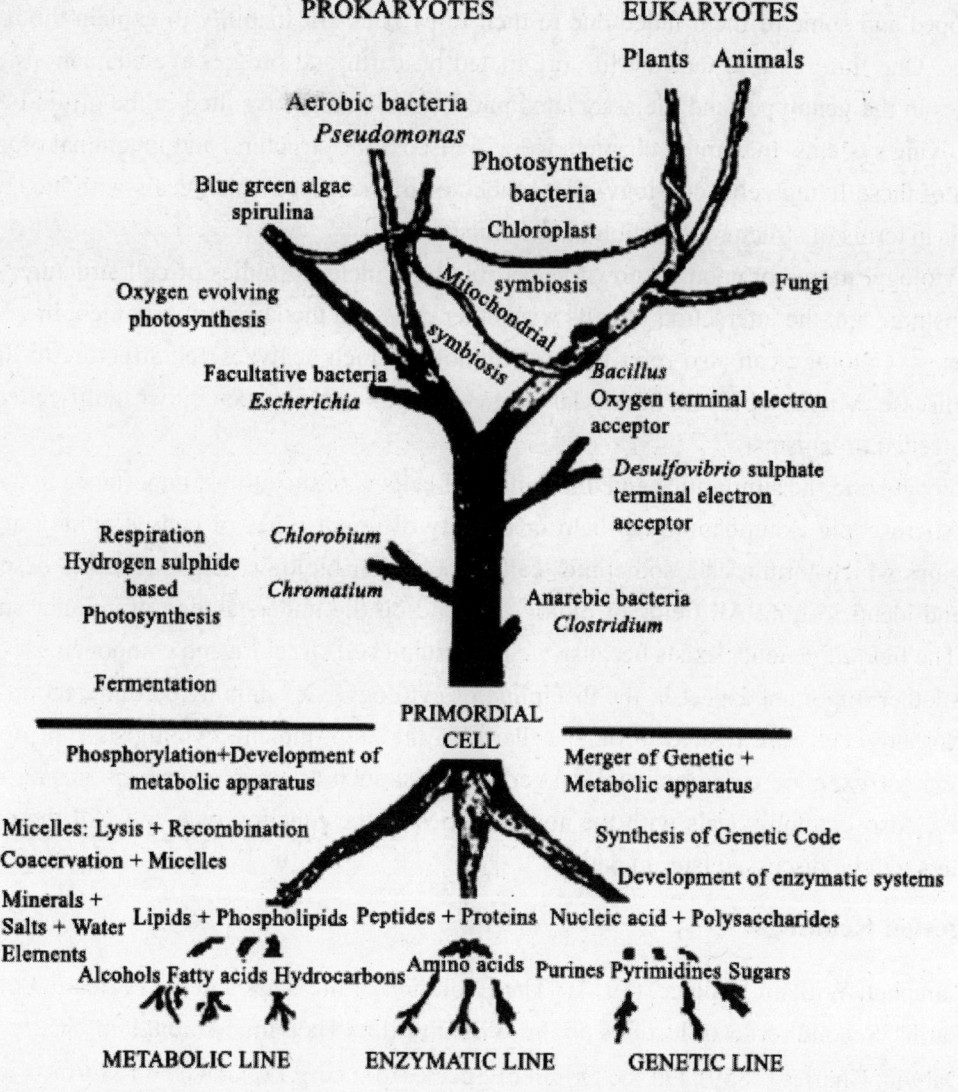

Figure 1.3: Composite evolutionary tree (schematic) summarizing the principal steps in chemical and biological evolution

The origin and evolution of man has been the most attractive and complicated problem for the man himself since the time immemorial. Religion had shed impressions such as man had been created by God until the last century when Charles Darwin was able to put forward his theory of evolution of organic world. There are convincing evidences to support the evolutionary origin of human from common ancestors of other anthropoids such as Chimpanzee and Gorilla. The evidences include similarities in morphological, physiological and embryonic features.

The search for the scientific basis of evolution of life is still going on. Many theories are developed and some of them faded due to their draw backs or inability to explain the basic science. One thing is true that the life originated on earth and progressive adaptations and changes in the genotypes and the associated phenotypic changes resulted in the origin of diverse living systems. In coming chapters we will discuss the structural and functional organization of these living cells, cytology- that branch of life science, which deals with the study of cells in terms of structure, function and chemistry.

Cytology, more commonly known as cell biology, include studies of cell structure, cell composition, and the interaction of cells with other cells and the larger environment in which they exist. Cytology can also refer to cytopathology, which analyzes cell structure to diagnose disease. Microscopic and molecular studies of cells can focus on either multi-celled or single-celled organisms.

Recognizing the similarities and differences of cells is of the utmost importance in cytology. Microscopic examination can help in identify different types of cells. Looking at the molecules which form a cell, sometimes called molecular biology, helps in further description and identification. All fields of biology depend on the understanding of cellular structure. The field of genetics exists because we understand cell structure and components.

Another important aspect in the discipline of cytology is examining cell interaction. By studying how cells are related to other cells or to the environment, cytologists can predict problems or examine environmental dangers to cells, such as toxic or cancer-causing substances. Also cytology deals with the abnormalities in the function of a cell. All these parameters will be discussed later in detail.

Suggested Readings

- Campbell William Wallace. (1914) "The Evolution of the Stars and the Formation of the Earth". Second series of lectures on the William Ellery Hale foundation, Pop. Sci.
- Darwin, Charles (1859). On the Origin of Species (1st ed.). London: John Murray.
- Gould, S.J. (2002). The Structure of Evolutionary Theory. Cambridge: Belknap Press
- Mayr, E. (2001). What Evolution Is. New York: Basic Books.

Biodiversity

"Oh, the beauty of the nature!! The pleasure of walking through it, enjoying the smells of the flowers and the wild; watching the insects flitting about and listening to the birds chirp - how we all love it and wish to return to it again and again. It is this biodiversity that we have to protect and take care of in order to enjoy the joy of it all by us and the coming generation" .(J. John)

About 3.9 billion years ago, the energy from heat, lightning, or radioactive elements caused the formation of complex proteins and nucleic acids into strands of replicating genetic code. These molecules then organized and evolved to form the first simple forms of life. Prokaryote cells, the ancestors, are very simple, containing few specialized cellular structures and their DNA is not surrounded by a membranous envelope. The more complex cells of animals and plants, known as eukaryotes, first showed up about 2.1 billion year ago. Eukaryotes have a membrane-bound nucleus and many specialized structures located within their cell boundary. By 680 million years ago, eukaryotic cells began to organize themselves into multicellular organisms. Starting at about 570 million years ago an enormous diversification of multicellular life occurred, which is known as the Cambrian explosion. In this period all the life forms are supposed to be originated. Thus, gradually the earth filled with a wide variety of living organisms.

Biodiversity is the variety and differences among living organisms from all sources, including terrestrial, marine, and other aquatic ecosystems and the ecological complexes of which they are a part. This includes genetic diversity within and between species and of ecosystems. Thus, in essence, biodiversity represents all life. India is one of the mega biodiversity centers of the world and has two of the world's 18 'biodiversity hotspots' located in the Western Ghats and in the Eastern Himalayas (Myers 1999). The forest cover in these areas is very dense and diverse which incredible biodiversity.

More than a million, species of living organisms have been discovered and described so far and a large number of them are yet to be discovered. The scientific practice of identifying, naming and grouping of living organisms is called classification. The branche of biology that deals with classification is called taxonomy or systematics. Taxonomy (from Greek *taxis* meaning arrangement or division and *nomos* meaning law), as the name indicates, it deals with describing and naming organisms while systematics deals with grouping and arranging the described taxa into a hierarchical classification. Scientists involved in this task, called taxonomists, estimate that there may be around 30 million species of living organisms of which the known number of species forms a very small percentage. The vast number of plant and animal species that have been identified and described, exhibit a great deal of variation in their form, structure, mode of life and various other aspects. Unless, the plants and animals are divided into discrete groups based on the differences and similarities between them, it becomes practically impossible to study them.

A hierarchy is an arrangement of items, in which the items are represented as being above or below or at the same level as one another. Taxonomy is one of the most conventionally hierarchical kinds of knowledge, placing all living beings in a nested structure of divisions related to their probable evolutionary descent. Most evolutionary biologists assert a hierarchy extending from the level of the specimen, to the species of which it is a member, outward to further successive levels of genus, family, order, class, phylum, and kingdom.

2.1. Advantages of Biological Classification

It makes the study of living organisms convenient by helping in the specific identification of any given organism. The study of a few representatives from each distinct group helps us to integrate the idea of life as a whole, since it reveals the relationships among various groups of organisms. Also, it provides information about plants and animals, which occur in specific geographical regions and provides the evolutionary relationship by establishing the gradually increasing complexity of form and structure in different groups of organisms.

2.1.1. Artificial System of Classification

Classification of living organisms is probably as old as human civilization. Organisms have been grouped on different basis at different periods of time. The earliest classification was probably on the basis of utility to man. Plants and animals were classified on different basis such as edible and non-edible ones, useful and harmful ones and so on. Through out the history there are several attempts made to classify living organisms by many ancient philosophers in Greek and India. Charaka, ancient Indian sage who lived in the first century A.D., had listed about 340 plant types and about 200 animal types in his treatise 'Charaka Samhitha'. Another ancient sage, Parashara in his treatise 'Vrikshayurveda' divided plants into several "ganas" (families) based on their characters. The description of characters for these ganas, given by Parashara, is very close to modern taxonomy. Aristotle, the famous Greek philosopher (384 to 322 B.C.) had identified different types of plants and animals and described some organisms under an intermediate group indicating that such organisms could be placed neither under plants nor under animals. He tried to classify the organisms on the basis of their form and habitat. This type of ancient classification systems that are based mainly on superficial characteristics are described as artificial systems of classification.

The artificial system of classification has several drawbacks like it is based on superficial characters and do not reflect the natural relationships. The system does not reflect the evolutionary relationships amongst the organisms. Closely related organisms have been placed in different groups because of the differences in their habitat, feeding habits, etc. and many unrelated organisms are placed in the same group on the basis of their habitats such as whales and fishes in the same group.

2.1.2. Natural System of Classification

Development of science and advent of the microscope in the 17th century opened up a new world for scientists looking for more and more details about different groups of organisms. It resulted in the investigation of various aspects of life such as mode of reproduction, pattern of development, etc. As a result, more and more similarities and differences started emerging between the different groups in both plants and animals. This led to a more systematic and scientific approach to classification, which is now known as the natural system of classification.

The natural system of classification has specific advantages over the artificial system of classification. It avoids the heterogeneous grouping of unrelated organisms and places only related groups of organisms together. It indicates the natural relationships among organisms and provides a clear view on the evolutionary pattern.

The initial attempt towards a natural system of classification came from an English biologist, John Ray (1627–1705). He identified a large number of plants and animals based on natural relationships among themselves and classified them into specific groups. He was probably the first biologist to have developed the modern concept of a species. He described the species as an assemblage of individuals derived from similar parents and having the ability to pass on their characteristics to the subsequent generations. He published a three-volume compendium - 'Historia Generalis Plantarum' in which he has given a detailed description of over 18,000 types of plants.

Carolus Linnaeus (1707–1778), Swedish biologist, classified living organisms into two kingdoms, the plant kingdom and the animal kingdom. He made an attempt to classify living organisms in to two kingdoms-the plant kingdom and the animal kingdom. He divided each of these kingdoms into smaller groups called classes. Each class was split into orders. Each order was divided into genera and each genus into many species. Each of these groups was formed on the basis of certain specific morphological features. He recorded nearly 6,000 species of plants in his book 'Species Plantarum' published in 1753. He listed more than 4,300 species of animals. He has given detailed system of his classification in another book 'Systema Naturae'. His system of classification provided a firm basis for modern taxonomy.

Another significant contribution from Linnaeus is the system of binomial nomenclature. He proposed the idea of giving a scientific name consisting of two words - the first word describing the name of the genus and the second word describing the name of the species. This system has found universal acceptance since such a system helped to avoid confusion created by vernacular names given to the plants or animals. Binomial nomenclature fits within the larger framework of taxonomy, the science of categorizing living organisms and assigning traits to them to understand the links and differences between them. The scientific name of an organism could be understood by scientists all over the world and considered as its definitive name. Because of these significant contributions Linnaeus is known as the Father of Modern Taxonomy.

The binomial aspect of this system means that each organism is given two names, a 'generic name,' which is called the genus (pl. genera) and a 'specific name,' the species. When written, a scientific name is always either italicized, or if hand-written, underlined. The genus is capitalized and the species name is in lower case. For example, the proper format for the scientific name of humans is *Homo sapiens*.

2.2. Taxonomy

The science of taxonomy and systematics involves the classification of organisms according to evolutionary relationships; how closely they are related to each other. Before scientists were able to use DNA sequencing to examine evolutionary relationships, organisms were classified based on physical similarities and differences. Modern systematics combines data from many sources, including: the fossil record, comparative homologies (similarity of structures due to shared ancestry), and comparative sequencing of nucleic acids (DNA and RNA) among organisms.

2.2.1. Evolutionary Taxonomy

It is based on the fossil materials collected from the field. In constructing a hierarchy, a traditional and very flexible combination of criteria was used. Firstly, morphological resemblance and then phylogenetic relationships, the way in which the animals actually related to each other, in terms of the recency of a common ancestor (as far as could be determined). The order of succession in the rock record (biostratigraphy) and the geographical distribution may play an important part in deciding these relationships. This practical approach, which takes all factors into consideration, has long been the basis of palaeontological classification, and is still seen as the best method by many.

2.2.2. Numerical Taxonomy

Evolutionary method has limitations like uncertainties and subjectivity of classification by observation, along with the preservation of the fossil record. To avoid this, numerical taxonomists attempt to use quantified observations of the animal in an attempt to decide on natural groupings. They consider that if enough characteristics are measured, and computed, then represented by the use of 'cluster scatters' (a form of graph) followed by the distance between clusters can be used as a measure of their differences. However, although useful in some instances, the operator still needs to (subjectively) choose how best to analyze the measurements taken, and possibly give greater precedence (weight) to certain more-important characteristics again, a subjective choice. Thus, numerical taxonomy is not as objective as it may first appear.

2.3. Taxonomic Categories

Through, in this system, organisms are hierarchically classified into increasingly specific groupings. The seven basic taxonomic categories are: Kingdom, Phylum, Class, Order, Family, Genus and Species; kingdom being the broadest category, while species being the most specific. It can be easily remembered by the mnemonic sentence "King Philip came over for green soup".

Species: It is the fundamental unit of taxonomy. This is a group of very similar individuals that typically have similar anatomical characteristics and have the potential to interbreed freely, to produce fertile offspring - but cannot interbreed successfully with individuals from other species. A mule, for example, is not a distinct species. It is an infertile hybrid of a male donkey (*Equus asinus*) and a female horse (*Equus caballus*). There are, as ever, exceptions where the rule breaks down, especially in the plant Kingdom. However, in the majority of cases, interbreeding of species does not produce fertile offspring.

Genus: The generic name refers to the genus, which is a group of species that are fairly closely related - such as the genus *Equus* which includes several species, such as the *Equus caballus*, *Equus asinus* and *Equus zebra* (domestic horse, wild ass and zebra respectively). 'Genus' is the taxonomic classification lower than 'family' and higher than 'species'. In other words, genus is a more general taxonomic category than the species.

Family: Genera are grouped into families, which are major groups of generally similar organisms; such as Felidae, which includes all cat-like animals from domestic cat to wild lynx to tiger to cheetah to jaguar to snow leopard. Family names always end in the letters "ae", but are not printed in any special way.

Order: Families are grouped into orders, whose individuals may vary in many ways; such as the order of Carnivora - which includes cats, dogs and weasels. Orders begin with a capital and usually end in "a" - but not always.

Class: The class is a major division within the Kingdom, and forms the basis on which most fossil study is based. For example, the phylum Molluscas contains 4 classes: the Gastropoda, Cephalopoda, Pelecypoda and Scaphopoda.

Phylum: Classes are grouped into phyla (the plural of phylum), and phyla into Kingdoms. Within the Kingdom Animalia, the most common phyla are:

- Arthropoda (e.g. insects)
- Mollusca (e.g. snails)
- Chordata (e.g. fishes, amphibians, reptiles, birds, mammals)
- Platyhelminthes (e.g. tapeworms)
- Nematoda (i.e. unsegmented worms)
- Annelida (i.e. segmented worms)
- Cnidaria and Ctenophora (e.g. jellyfish)
- Echinodermata (e.g. starfish)
- Porifera (e.g. sponges)

Kingdom: Living organisms are subdivided into 5 major kingdoms

Monera : Prokaryotes (i.e., without a nucleus) Unicellular and colonial, including the true bacteria (eubacteria) and cyanobacteria (blue-green algae) [~10,000 species].

Protista : Unicellular protozoans and unicellular and multicellular (macroscopic) algae with 9 + 2 cilia and flagella (called undulipodia[~250,000 species]).

Fungi : Haploid and dikaryotic (binucleate) cells, multicellular, generally heterotrophic, without cilia and eukaryotic (9 + 2) flagella (undulipodia) [~100,000 species].

Planta : Haplo-diploid life cycles, mostly autotrophic, retain embryo within female sex organ on parent plant [~250,000 species].

Animala : Multicellular animals, without cell walls and without photosynthetic pigments, form diploid blastula [~1,000,000 species].

2.4. Domains and Kingdoms of Life

In 1990 American molecular biologist Carl Woese proposed a new category, called a Domain, further highest level: Archaea, Bacteria, and Eukaryota. Archaea are a group of organisms that are adapted to live in extreme habitats like thermal volcanic vents, saline pools, and hot springs (Fig. 2.1). Though, they are quite similar in appearance to bacteria, molecular studies have shown that they are biochemically and genetically very different. Bacteria are simple single-celled organisms that generally lack chlorophyll (an exception is cyanobacteria). Bacteria generally obtain energy for survival by breakdown organic matter through fermentation and respiration. They are generally heterotrophic. Bacteria such as cyanobacteria and those belonging to the genus *Rhizobium* play an important role in the fixing of atmospheric nitrogen.

Eukaryota are organisms that have a eukaryote type of cell. This group of life includes the four primary kingdoms: Protista, Fungi, Plantae (plants) and Animalia (animals). Kingdom Protista is made up of single celled organisms and some of their simple multi-cellular

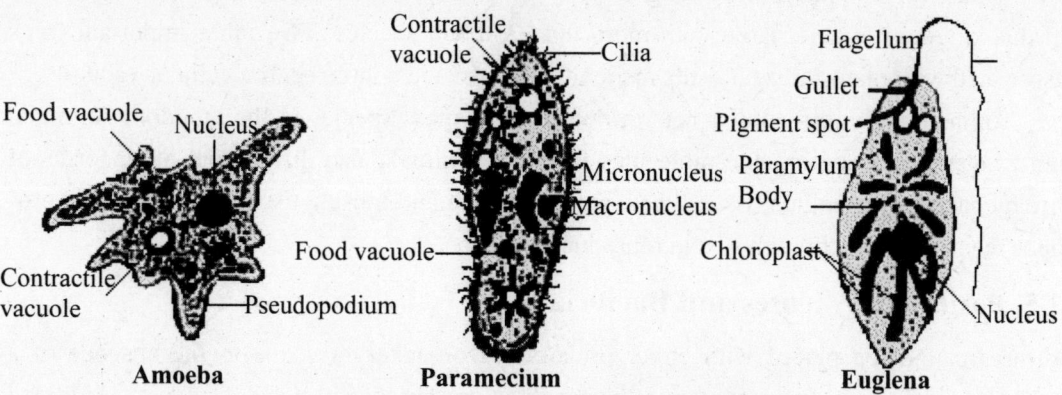

Figure 2.1: Members of kingdom Protista

close relatives. Some examples of unicellular protists include dinoflagellates, amoebas, paramecium, diatoms, and volvox. Slime molds, brown, red and green algae like *Ulva* are typical examples of multi-cellular forms of protests (Fig. 2.1).

According to recent estimation there are about 1.5 million different species of fungi exist in our planet. Most of these life-forms are multi-cellular. The biologists at large have grouped the fungi with plants. However, investigations of this life-form indicate that fungi are quite different from other eukaryotes in terms of feeding strategies, physiological organization, reproduction and growth. Many species of fungi are heterotrophic decomposers or they live in symbiosis with another species. Lichens are good examples of this type of biotic relationship (Fig. 2.2). Lichens involve the symbiotic relationship between a fungus and a photosynthetic alga.

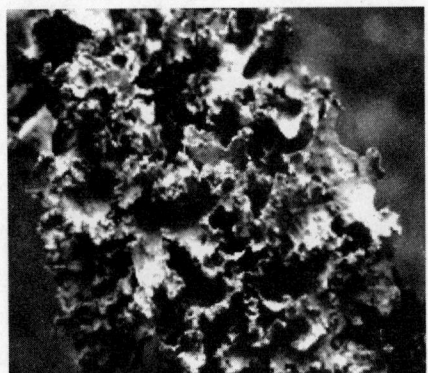 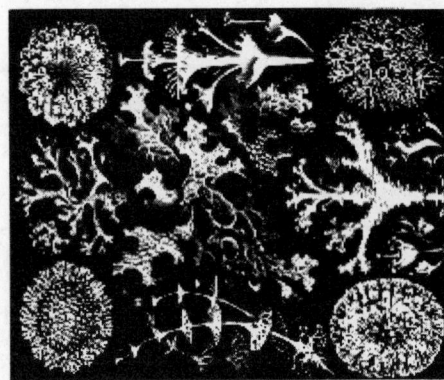

Figure 2.2: Lichenes

The kingdom Plantae is composed of multi-cellular photosynthetic organisms that can convert inorganic elements, with the help of the sun's energy into organic compounds. Plantae includes all land plants, including mosses, ferns, conifers, and flowering plants. Diversity in this kingdom is quite large with more than 250,000 species. Two other important traits associated with plants are cell walls made of cellulose and a large central cellular vacuole.

Animals are multi-cellular heterotrophic eukaryotes. Species in the kingdom Animalia must ingest produced organic molecules for food. Animals also differ from other forms of life by having two unique tissue types: nervous tissue and muscle tissue. Most animals produce their offspring through sexual reproduction.

2.5. Position of Viruses and Bacteria

Viruses cannot be placed with either prokaryotes or eukaryotes due to the absence of a cellular organization, hence it remains as unsolved mysteries in biology. They are considered as intermediate between living and non-living systems. Viruses are active and show reproduction only inside the host cell and are inactive in free state. They may even be purified and crystallized like chemical substances. Viruses have a genetic material represented by either DNA or RNA, surrounded by a protein sheath. Viruses reproduce by using the metabolic machinery and raw materials of the host cell. It is because of these peculiarities that viruses do not fit into any of the five kingdoms of life.

The bacterial cell has a cell wall like other plant cells. However, most bacteria show flagella which are used for locomotion. Some bacteria are autotrophic while most of them cannot prepare their own food. They have prokaryotic cells which lack a definite nucleus and cytoplasmic (membrane-bound) organelles. They also do not have a mitotic apparatus and do not exhibit meiosis. In view of these features, some of which they share with blue green algae, it is imminent that bacteria are to be given a separate taxonomic status. The five-kingdom classification has given a justification to bacteria by placing them in a separate kingdom called Monera (Fig. 2.3).

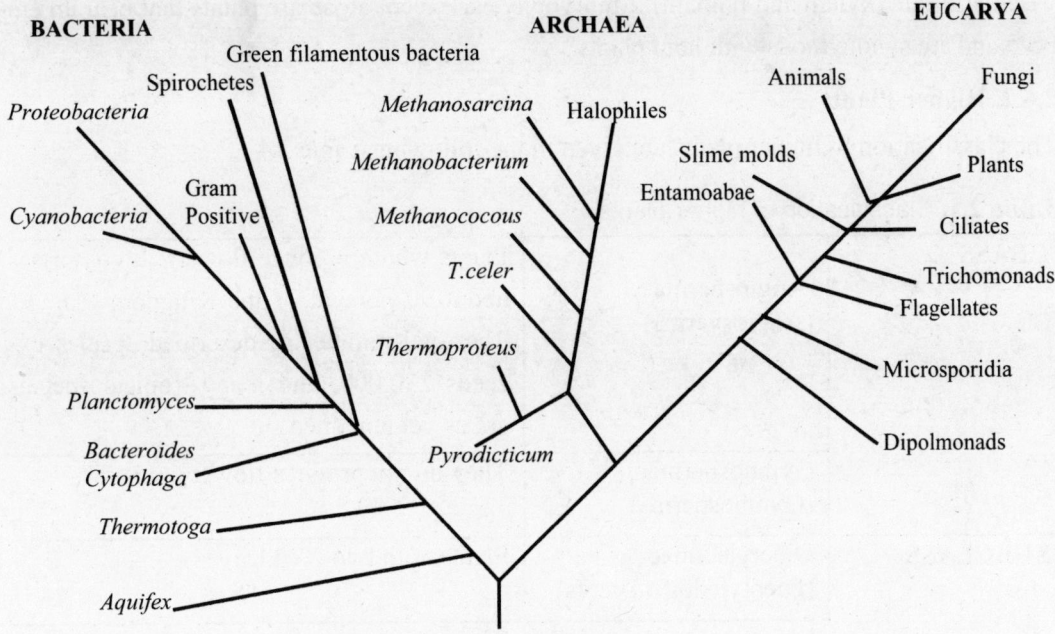

Figure 2.3: The Phylogenetic tree

2.6. Classification of Plants

The plant kingdom includes nonvascular and vascular plants. Nonvascular plants lack a water-conducting system of tubular cells called xylem tissue, and do not have true roots, stems and leaves. Like algae and fungi, the plant body of some nonvascular plants is often called a thallus. Nonvascular plants are all placed in the division Bryophyta, including the mosses and liverworts. The vast majority of the plant kingdom is vascular, with tubular, water-conducting cells called xylem tissue. Like a microscopic pipeline system, they are arranged end-to-end from the roots to the leaves. Unlike nonvascular plants, they have true roots, stems and leaves. There are several plant classification systems and we will simply refer to these groups by their informal names, Algae, Bryophytes, Pteridophytes, Gymnosperms and Angiosperms.

2.6.1. Lower Plants

Lower plants usually include Algae and Bryophytes. The word Cryptogams literally means "hidden wedding" and alludes to the fact that the sex life of these plants (Algae, Bryophytes and Pteridophytes) was once not understood. Phanerogams (open wedding) are the seed plants - the gymnosperms and angiosperms. Thallophytes are the plants, whose body is not well differentiated into root/stem/leaves and termed as thallus. Algae fall into this category and fungi did too when they were considered to be plants. Vascular plants are those with vascular tissue (xylem and phloem). Embryophytes, except algae are plants that bear an embryo and are synonymous with land plants.

2.6.2. Higher Plants

The classification of higher plants are given in the following Table 2.1

Table 2.1: Classification of higher plants

CLASS	Angiospermae (Angiosperms)	Plants which produce flowers. It comprises about 90 percent of the Kingdom Plantae. The total number of described species exceeds 230,000, and many tropical species are as yet unnamed.
	Gymnospermae (Gymnosperms)	They do not produce flowers
SUBCLASS	Dicotyledonae (Dicotyledons, Dicots)	Plants with two seed leaves
	Monocotyledonae (Monocotyledons)	Plants with one seed leaf
SUPERORDER	A group of related Plant Families, classified in the order in which they are thought to have developed their differences from a common ancestor. There are six Super orders in the Dicotyledonae (Magnoliidae, Hamamelidae, Caryophyllidae, Dilleniidae, Rosidae, Asteridae), and four in the Monocotyledonae (Alismatidae, Commelinidae, Arecidae, Liliidae). The names of the Super orders end with -idae	

ORDER	Each Super order is further divided into several Orders. The names of the Orders end with -ales
FAMILY	Each Order is divided into Families. These are plants with many botanical features in common, and are the highest classification normally used. The names of the Families end with -aceae
SUBFAMILY	The Family may be further divided into a number of sub-families, which group together plants within the Family that have some significant botanical differences. The names of the Subfamilies end with -oideae
TRIBE	A further division of plants within a Family, based on smaller botanical differences, but still usually comprising many different plants. The names of the Tribes end with -eae
SUBTRIBE	A further division, based on even smaller botanical differences, often only recognizable to botanists. The names of the Subtribes end with -inae
GENUS	This is the part of the plant name that is most familiar, the normal name that we give a plant - Papaver (Poppy), Aquilegia (Columbine), and so on. The plants in a Genus are often easily recognizable as belonging to the same group. The name of the Genus should be written with a capital letter.
SPECIES	This is the level that defines an individual plant. Often, the name will describe some aspect of the plant - the colour of the flowers, size or shape of the leaves, or it may be named after the place where it was found. Together, the Genus and species name refer to only one plant, and they are used to identify that particular plant. The name of the species should be written after the Genus name, in small letters, with no capital letter.
VARIETY	A Variety is a plant that is only slightly different from the species plant, but the differences are not as insignificant as the differences in a form. The name follows the Genus and species name, with var. before the individual variety name.
FORM	A form is a plant within a species that has minor botanical differences, such as the colour of flower or shape of the leaves. The name follows the Genus and species name, with form (or f.) before the individual variety name.
CULTIVAR	A Cultivar is a cultivated variety, a particular plant that has arisen either naturally or through deliberate hybridization, and can be reproduced (vegetatively or by seed) to produce more of the same plant. The name follows the Genus and species name. It is written in the language of the person who described it, and should not be translated. It is either written in single quotation marks or has cv. written in front of the name.

In conclusion, we have seen how life originated on earth and the development of amazing biodiversity. It is our duty to protect this biodiversity for the homeostasis of all forms of life on earth. We can not create it, but can protect it from destruction. The aim of the chapter was not to describe the world of taxonomy or biodiversity but to introduce so that one can understand the cell biology, the basic science of this biodiversity, better. Now let us discuss the chemistry, cellular machineries and their coordinated mechanism of action in coming chapters.

Suggested Readings

- E. Mayer. Elements of Taxonomy.
- E.O. Wilson. Biodiversity, Academic Press, Washington.
- E.O. Wilson. The Diversity of Life (The College Edition), W.W. Northern & Co.
- G.G. Simpson. Principle of Animal Taxonomy. Oxford IBH Pub. Co.
- J.C. Avice. Molecular Markers. Natural History and Evolution, Chapman & Hall, New York.
- M. Kato. The Biology of Biodiversity, Springer.
- Allaby, Michael. The Concise Oxford Dictionary of Zoology. New York: Oxford Press, 1992.
- Canby, Thomas Y. "Bacteria," National Geographic. Aug. 1993, pp. 36-60.
- Goin, Coleman J., and Olive B. Goin. Introduction to Herpetology. London: W. H. Freeman and Co., 1962.
- Margulis, Lynn, and Karlene V. Schwartz. Five Kingdoms. New York: W. H. Freeman and Co., 1988.
- Wilson, E.O. The Diversity of Life. Cambridge, Mass.: Harvard University Press, 1992.
- Whitfield, Philip, Peter D. Moore, and Barry Cox. The Atlas of the Living World. Boston: Houghton Mifflin Co., 1989

CHAPTER 3

Chemical Basis of Life

- Atom: The basic unit of matter
- Isotopes and Ions
- Chemical bonds
- Molecules and Compounds
- Water
- Types of Solution
- Acids and Bases
- The pH Scale
- Buffer solution
- The Chemistry of Life
- Organic Compounds
- Isomerism
- Monomers and Polymers
- Carbohydrates
- Lipid
- Proteins
- Enzymes
- Nucleic Acid
- Chemical Structure of Nucleic acids
- Polymer formation
- Deoxyribonucleic Acid
- Ribonucleic Acid
- Bioenergetics
- Energy
- Gibbs free energy (ΔG) and spontaneity of a chemical reaction
- Oxidation and Reduction Reactions
- NAD^+
- FAD
- Metabolism

"What is the relationship between man, the universe and their creator? This question has always intrigued philosophers and thinkers. One of these was Kanada, who, in about 600 BC at Prabhasa propounded the Vaisesikasutra (Peculiarity Aphorisms). Today, we realize that these sutras are a blend of science, philosophy and religion. Their essence is the atomic theory of matter. If Kanada's sutras are analysed, one would find that his atomic theory was far more advanced than those forwarded later by the Greek philosophers, Leucippus and Democritus. In fact, he gave the name paramanu (atom) to an indivisible entity of matter. According to Kanada, everything is made up of paramanu. When matter is divided, then further divided, till no further division is possible, the remaining indivisible entity is called paramanu. This entity does not exist in a free state, nor can it be sensed through any human organ. It is eternal and indestructible."

3.1 Atom: The Basic Unit of Matter

All matter in the universe is formed by different combinations of 92 naturally occurring substances known as elements. The smallest quantity of an element that still exhibits the characteristics of that element is known as an atom. The idea of the atom was first devised by Democritus in 530 BC. In 1808, John Dalton proposed the modern atomic theory. Atoms composed of even smaller particles called electrons, protons, and neutrons. Each of these particles possesses a different electrical charge. Protons are positively charged, neutrons have no charge and electrons are negatively charged. The protons and neutrons of an atom are located in a central body called a nucleus. Electrons appear around the nucleus within orbital of varying energy (Fig 3.1). Overall, the atom is neutral owing to equal numbers of positively charged protons and negatively charged electrons. The number of protons in their nuclei is the distinguishing feature of an element, known as atomic number.

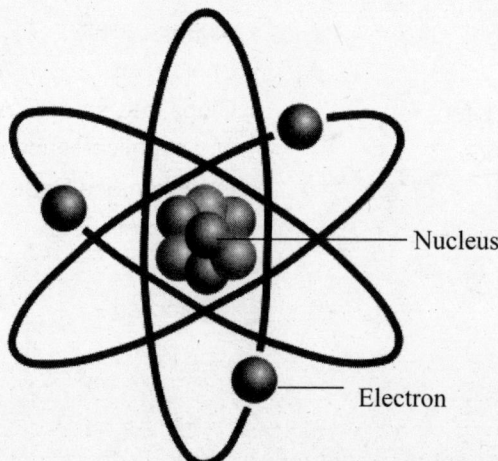

Figure 3.1. Structure of an atom

3.2. Isotopes and Ions

Atoms of the same element having different numbers of neutrons are called isotopes. For example, the most common isotope of hydrogen ($^1H_1$) has no neutrons at all; there is also a hydrogen isotope called deuterium, with one neutron, and another, tritium, with two neutrons. Isotopes can be represented as ^AX_Z. Here X is the chemical symbol for the element, while Z is the atomic number, and A is the number of neutrons and protons combined, called the mass number. For instance, ordinary hydrogen is written $^1H_1$, deuterium is $^2H_1$, and tritium is $^3H_1$. Carbon usually has six protons and six neutrons and can be called carbon-12 because the number of its protons and neutrons add up to 12. Isotopes of carbon are carbon-13 and carbon-14. Isotopes do not have charge, because the numbers of positive and negative particles remain balanced. Even though they have different masses, all isotopes of the same element have similar chemical properties because the number of electrons (not the number of neutrons or protons) determines the way an atom will interact with other atoms.

3.3. Chemical Bonds

Chemical compounds are formed by the joining of two or more atoms. The attractive force which keeps atoms together is known as chemical bond. The bonds present between atoms give the molecules different properties. A stable compound occurs when the total energy of the combination has lower energy than the separated atoms. The more charges a positive ion has, the greater the attraction towards its accompanying negative ion. The greater the attraction, the more energy is released when the ions come together. Energy is needed to remove electrons from atoms. This is called ionization energy. The total ionization energy increases as the electrons are removed. The types of bonds present between the atoms can be:

3.3.1. Ionic bonds: In ionic bonding, electrons are completely transferred from one atom to another. In the process of either losing or gaining negatively charged electrons, the reacting atoms form ions. The oppositely charged ions are attracted to each other by electrostatic forces, which are the basis of the ionic bond. For example, during the reaction of sodium with chlorine: sodium loses its one valence electron to chlorine, resulting in a positively charged sodium ion and a negatively charged chlorine ion. If a sodium atom gives an electron to a chlorine atom, both become more stable.

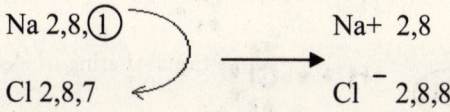

$$Na\ 2,8,\textcircled{1} \longrightarrow Na^+\ 2,8$$
$$Cl\ 2,8,7 \longleftarrow Cl^-\ 2,8,8$$

The sodium has lost an electron, so it no longer has equal number of electrons and protons; it has a charge of +1 since there is one more proton than electron. If electrons are lost from an atom then positive ions are formed, which are called cations.

The chlorine has gained an electron, so it now has one more electron than proton. It therefore has a charge of -1. If electrons are gained by an atom then negative ion is formed, called an anion.

3.3.2. Covalent bonds: A covalent bond is a bond that is formed when two atoms share electrons. A single bond is formed when 1 pair of electrons is shared; a double bond is formed when 2 pairs of electrons are shared; and a triple bond is formed when 3 pairs of electrons are shared. Bonding between non-metals consists of two electrons shared between two atoms. The covalent bond involves an overlap of the electron clouds from each atom. The electrons are concentrated in the region between the two atoms. In covalent bonding, the two electrons shared by the atoms are attracted to the nucleus of both atoms. Neither atom completely loses or gains electrons as in ionic bonding. There are two types of covalent bonding:

(a) Non-polar bonding: It is by equal sharing of electrons. The simplest non-polar covalent molecule is hydrogen. Each hydrogen atom has one electron and needs two to complete its first energy level. Since both hydrogen atoms are identical, neither of the atoms will be able to dominate in the control of the electrons. The electrons are therefore shared equally.

(b) Polar bonding: It is an unequal sharing of electrons. The number of shared electrons depends on the number of electrons needed to complete the octet. Hydrogen chloride forms a polar covalent molecule. The chlorine has 7 and hydrogen has 1 electron in its outer energy shell. Since 8 electrons are needed for an octet, they share the electrons. However, chlorine gets an unequal share of the two electrons, although the electrons are still shared (not transferred as in ionic bonding), it is unequal (Fig. 3.2). The electrons spend more of the time closer to chlorine. As a result, the chlorine acquires a "partial" negative charge. At the same time, since hydrogen loses the electron most but not all of the time, it acquires a "partial" positive charge. The partial charge is denoted with a small Greek symbol for delta.

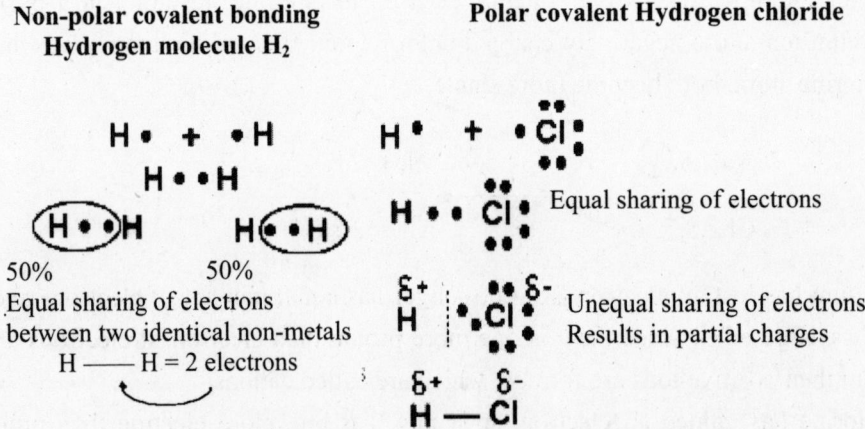

Figure 3.2: Polar and non-polar covalent bonding

3.3.3. Hydrogen bonds: A hydrogen bond is the attractive force between the hydrogen attached to an electronegative atom of one molecule and an electronegative atom of a different molecule. Usually, the electronegative atom is oxygen, nitrogen, or fluorine, which has a partial negative charge. The hydrogen then has the partial positive charge. The hydrogen bond is much weaker than both the ionic bond and the covalent bond. Within macromolecules such as proteins and nucleic acids, it can exist between two parts of the same molecule and figures as an important constraint on such molecules' overall shape.

The most ubiquitous and perhaps simplest example of a hydrogen bond is found among the water molecules (Fig. 3.3). In a discrete water molecule, water has two hydrogen and one oxygen atom. Two molecules of water can form a hydrogen bond between them. The oxygen of one water molecule has two lone pairs of electrons, each of which can form a hydrogen bond with hydrogens on two other water molecules. This can repeat so that every water molecule is H-bonded with four other molecules (two through its two lone pairs and two through its two hydrogen atoms).

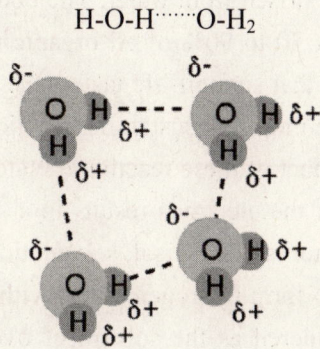

Figure 3.3: Hydrogen boding in water

The high boiling point of water is due to the high number of hydrogen bonds present in it. Water is unique because its oxygen atom has two lone pairs and two hydrogen atoms, meaning that the total number of bonds of a water molecule is four.

Hydrogen bonding also plays an important role in determining the three-dimensional structures adopted by proteins and nucleic acids. In these macromolecules, bonding between parts of the same macromolecule helps to fold into a specific shape, which helps in determining physiological or biochemical role of the molecules. For example the double helical structure of DNA is mainly due to hydrogen bonding between the base pairs, which link one complementary strand to the other and hence enable replication.

3.4. Molecules and Compounds

Atoms combine with each other in chemical reactions to create molecules, which are unique substances with physical and chemical properties distinct from those of their constituent elements. Combining two hydrogen atoms with one oxygen atom creates water, which has very different characteristics than hydrogen or oxygen do alone. Molecules such as water containing more than one type of element can also be called compounds. The molecular formula of water is H_2O. The "H" and "O" stand for the elements, hydrogen and oxygen, and the subscript indicates that water contains two parts hydrogen for every one part oxygen. Similarly, the formula can be created for any compound by writing down the letter symbol of each of its constituent elements and using subscripted numbers to indicate how many atoms of each element are present.

3.5. Water

The Universal Solvent, the existence of life on earth is mainly because of the abundant liquid water. Other planets may have water, but they either have it as a gas (Venus) or ice (Mars). All life on earth is thought to have arisen from water. The bodies of all living organisms are composed largely of water. About 70 to 90% of all organic matter is water. The chemical reactions in all plants and animals that support life take place in a water medium. Water not only provides the medium to make these life sustaining reactions possible, but water itself is often an important reactant or product of these reactions. Water is a polar covalently bonded molecule. This unequal sharing of the electrons results in a slightly positive and a slightly negative side on the molecule. Water is a universal, solvent due to the marked polarity of the water molecule and its tendency to form hydrogen bonds with other molecules. In terrestrial living systems, the water is considered as the solvent of overwhelming biological importance. It provides a fluid in which molecules of nutrients and waste products can be dissolved and transported, helps to regulate the temperature and preserves chemical equilibrium within living cells, and makes up a major fraction of the body weight of every organism.

3.6. Types of Solution

A solution is a homogeneous mixture of two or more substances. The medium in which solutes are dissolved are known as solvent. The substances dissolved in a solvent are called solutes. A solution can exist in a solid, liquid or gas form depending on mixed substances and external conditions such as temperature and pressure. On the basis of solute concentrations the solutions can be:

3.6.1. Saturated solutions have the maximum amount of solute dissolved in them at a given temperature and pressure. No more solute can be made to dissolve.

3.6.2. Unsaturated solutions have less than the maximum amount of solute dissolved in them. This means that more solute could be added to the solution and the additional solute can be still dissolved.

3.6.3. Supersaturated solutions have more than the maximum amount of solute dissolved in them. This is normally not possible. Not all substances can form supersaturated solutions. If a crystal of the solute is added to a supersaturated solution, precipitation of all of the extra solute will occur.

3.7. Acids and Bases

The disassociation of water ($H_2O \rightarrow H^+ + OH^-$) produces equal amounts of hydrogen and hydroxide ions. However, the disassociation of some compounds produces solutions with high proportions of either hydrogen or hydroxide ions. Solutions high in hydrogen ions are known as acids, while solutions high in hydroxide ions are known as bases. Both types of solutions are extremely reactive, likely to form bonds, because they contain so many charged particles. Chemically an acid is a hydrogen ion donor, or a proton donor, as hydrogen ions are consisted of only a single proton. Acids put H^+ ions into solution. The definition of a base is a little more complicated: they are H^+ ion or proton acceptors, which means that they remove H^+ ions from solution. Some bases can directly produce OH^- ions that take H^+ out of solution. NaOH is an example of this type of base ($NaOH \rightarrow Na^+ + OH^-$). A second type of base can directly take H^+ out of an H_2O solution. Ammonia (NH_3) is a common example of this sort of base ($NH_3 + H_2O \rightarrow NH_4^+ + OH^-$).

3.8. The pH Scale

The degree of acidity or alkalinity of a solution is measured in terms of a value known as pH, which is the negative logarithm of the concentration of hydrogen ions:

$$pH = 1/\log[H^+] = -\log[H^+]$$

The pH scale, which ranges from 0 to 14, measures the degree of a solution that is acidic or basic. If the proportion of hydrogen ions in a solution is the same as the proportion of hydroxide ions or equivalent, the solution is considered having a pH of 7, which is neutral. The most acidic solutions (those with a high proportion of H^+) have pH approaching 0, while the most basic solutions (those with a high proportion of OH^- or equivalent) have pH closer to 14. When sodium hydroxide (NaOH) disassociates, it forms only hydroxide ions, making it a base and giving it a pH above 7. Like acids, bases can be strong or weak, depending on how many hydroxide ions they put in solution or how many hydrogen ions they take out of solution. Living things are extremely sensitive to pH and function best (with certain exceptions, such as certain portions of the digestive tract) when solutions are nearly neutral. Most interior living matter (excluding the cell nucleus) has a pH of about 6.8. Blood plasma and other fluids that surround the cells in the body have a pH of 7.2 to 7.3. Numerous special mechanisms aid in stabilizing these fluids so that cells can not be subjected to appreciable fluctuations in pH.

3.9. Buffer Solution

Buffer solution is an aqueous solution consisting of a mixture of a weak acid and its conjugate base or a weak base and its conjugate acid. It has the property that the pH of the solution changes very little when a small amount of acid or base is added to it. Buffers have the capacity to bound ions and remove them from solution(s) whenever their concentration begins to rise. Conversely, buffers can release ions, whenever their concentration begins to fall. Buffers thus help to minimize the fluctuations in pH. This is an important function because many biochemical reactions normally occurring in living organisms either release or use up ions. Buffers resist changes in pH even when acids or bases are added to them. The cell contains many buffers because wide changes in pH can negatively impact the chemical reactions of cell processes.

An acidic buffer solution is simply one which has a pH less than 7. Acidic buffer solutions are commonly made from a weak acid and one of its salts, often a sodium salt. A common example would be a mixture of acetic acid and sodium acetate. An equal molar solution of both the acid and the salt would have a pH of 4.76.

The pH of the buffer solution can be changed by changing the ratio of acid to salt, or by choosing a different acid and one of its salts. An alkaline buffer solution has a pH greater than 7. Alkaline buffer solutions are commonly made from a weak base and one of its salts. A frequently used example is a mixture of ammonia solution and ammonium chloride solution. If these were mixed in equal molar proportions, the solution would have a pH of 9.25.

3.10. The Chemistry of Life

The four elements, carbon (C), oxygen (O), hydrogen (H), and nitrogen (N) constitute more than 98% of all biological matter. Virtually, every important organic compound is made up of these four elements. The carbon atom has six electrons of which four in the outermost energy level. Carbon can form four covalent bonds with other atoms and/or molecules. Carbon atoms can link to other carbon atoms to create long carbon strings that form the backbone of many natural organic molecules. It is the special property of carbon atoms that make them so important. Life is based on the chemistry of carbon, its important role or ability to from four chemical bonds with other elements at the same time. Carbon often attach to other carbon atoms, forming long chains called hydrocarbons. These molecules get their name because the central carbons also bonded to hydrogen. In addition to making a connection to four other atoms, carbon also has the ability to make two or three separate connections with the same single partner (and make its remaining one or two bonds with other substances). These bonds, which are stronger than single bonds, are known as double or triple bonds, respectively.

3.11. Organic Compounds

Organic molecules are the chemicals of life. The compounds are composed of more than one type of element that are found in, and produced by, living organisms. The feature that distinguishes an organic molecule from inorganic molecule is that the organic molecules contain carbon-hydrogen bonds, whereas inorganic molecules do not. Molecules made up of H and C are known as hydrocarbons.

Specific chemical properties of a compound are due to the presence of particular functional groups. Functional groups are clusters of atoms with characteristic structure and functions. Polar molecules (with +/- charges) are attracted to water molecules hence said to be hydrophilic. Non-polar molecules are repelled by water and do not dissolve in water there fore they are hydrophobic in nature. Hydrocarbon is hydrophobic except when it has an attached ionized functional group such as carboxyl (acid) (COOH), and then molecule is considered as hydrophilic. Since cells contain 70–90% water, the degree to which organic molecules interact with water, affects their function. One of the most common groups is the -OH (hydroxyl) group. Its presence enables a molecule to be water soluble.

Carbon has four electrons in outer shell and can bond with up to four other atoms (usually H, O, N, or another C). Since carbon can make covalent bonds with another carbon atom, carbon chains and rings that serve as the backbones of organic molecules are possible. Chemical bonds store energy. The C–C covalent bond has 83.1 Kcal (kilocalories) per mole, while the C=C double covalent bond has 147 kcal/mole. Energy is conserved in two forms: kinetic, or energy in use/motion; and potential, or energy at rest or in storage. Chemical bonds are potential energy, until they are converted into another form of energy, i.e. kinetic energy (according to the two laws of thermodynamics).

3.12. Isomerism

An important property shown by organic molecules is isomerism. The existence of two or more compounds with same molecular formula but different properties (physical, chemical or both) is known as isomerism and the compounds themselves are called isomers. The term isomerism was given by Berzelius. The difference in properties of two isomers is due to the difference in the arrangement of atoms within their molecules. Isomerism may be of two types:

3.12.1. Structural isomerism: When the isomers differ only in the arrangement of atoms or groups within the molecule, without any reference to space, these are known as structural isomers and the phenomenon as structural isomerism. Thus, the structural isomers have the same molecular formula, but possess different structural formulae. Structural isomerism may again be of several types.

(a) Chain, nuclear or skeleton isomerism

This type of isomerism is due to the difference in the nature of the carbon chain (i.e. straight or branched) which forms the nucleus of the molecule, e.g.,

$$CH_3CH_2CH_2CH_3$$

and

$$CH_3\text{-}CH\text{-}CH_3$$
$$|$$
$$CH_3$$

$$CH_3CH_2CH_2\text{-}C\equiv CH$$

and

$$CH_3\text{-}CH\text{-}C\equiv CH$$
$$|$$
$$CH_3$$

(b) Position isomerism

It is due to the difference in the position of the side chain atom or group or an unsaturated linkage in the same carbon chain. Examples are

$$CH_3CH_2\text{-}CH=CH_2$$

and

$$CH_3\text{-}CH=CH\text{-}CH_3$$

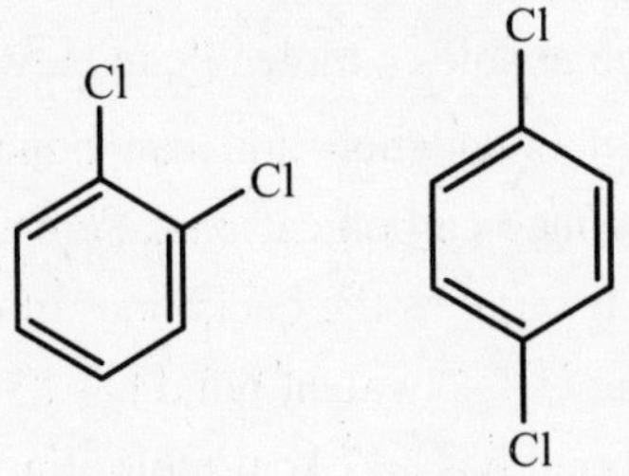

and

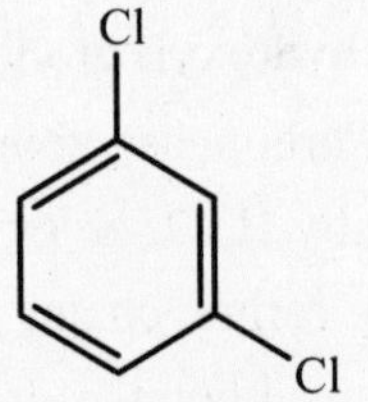

(c) Functional isomerism

This type of isomerism is due to difference in the nature of functional group present in the isomers, e.g.,

C_2H_6O :
- $CH_3\text{-}CH_2OH$ — Ethyl alcohol (alcoholic group)
- $CH_3\text{-}O\text{-}CH_3$ — Dimethyl ether (ether group)

C_3H_6O :
- $CH_3\text{-}CH_2\text{-}CHO$ — Propanal
- $CH_3\text{-}CO\text{-}CH_3$ — Acetone
- $CH_2=CH\text{-}CH_2OH$ — Allyl alcohol

(note the different functional groups in 3 isomers)

(d) Tautomerism

Tautomerism may be defined as the phenomenon in which a single compound exists in two readily inter-convertible structures that differ markedly in the relative position of at least one atomic nucleus, generally hydrogen. The two different structures are known as tautomers of each other. There are several types of tautomerism of which keto-enol tautomerism is the most important. In this type, one form (tautomer) exists as a ketone while the other exists as an enol. The two simplest examples are of acetone and phenol.

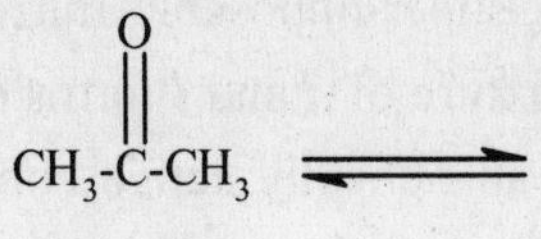

$$CH_3\text{-}\overset{\overset{\displaystyle O}{\|}}{C}\text{-}CH_3 \rightleftharpoons CH_3\text{-}\overset{\overset{\displaystyle OH}{|}}{C}\text{=}CH_2$$

keto form   enol form (negligible amount) 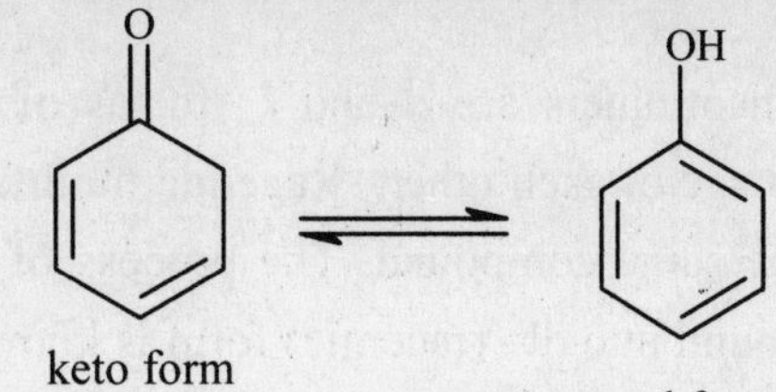   keto form   enol form

3.12.2. Stereo isomerism: When isomers have the same structural formula but differ in relative arrangement of atoms or groups in space within the molecule, these are known as stereoisomers and the phenomenon as stereoisomerism. The spatial arrangement of atoms or groups is also referred to as configuration of the molecule and thus we can say that the stereoisomers have the same structural formula but different configuration. The stereoisomerism is of two types:

(a) Geometrical isomerism

The isomers which possess the same structural formula but differ in the spatial arrangement of the groups around the double bond are known as geometrical isomers and the phenomenon is known as geometrical isomerism. This isomerism is shown by alkenes or their derivatives. In cis-isomer similar groups lie on the same side, while the similar groups when lie on opposite sides, the isomer is known as *trans*.

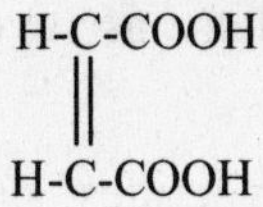

$$\begin{array}{c} H\text{-}C\text{-}COOH \\ \| \\ H\text{-}C\text{-}COOH \end{array} \qquad \begin{array}{c} H\text{-}C\text{-}COOH \\ \| \\ HOOC\text{-}C\text{-}H \end{array} \qquad \begin{array}{c} H\text{-}C\text{-}Cl \\ \| \\ H\text{-}C\text{-}Cl \end{array} \qquad \begin{array}{c} H\text{-}C\text{-}Cl \\ \| \\ Cl\text{-}C\text{-}H \end{array}$$

Maleic acid (cis) 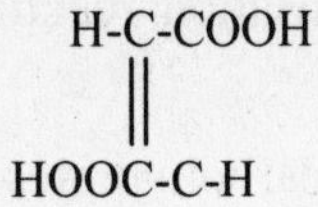   Fumaric acid (trans) 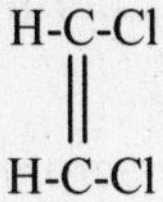   Dichloroethylene 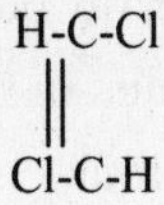   Dichloroethylene

(b) Optical isomerism

This type of isomerism arises from different arrangements of atoms or groups in space, resulting in two isomers which are mirror image of each other. Optical isomers contain an asymmetric (chiral) carbon atom (a carbon atom attached to four different atoms or groups) in their molecules. Optical isomers have similar chemical and physical properties and differ only in their behavior towards plane polarized light. The isomer which rotates the plane polarized light to left is known as laevo (l) while that rotates the plane polarized light to the right is known as dextro (d). For example,

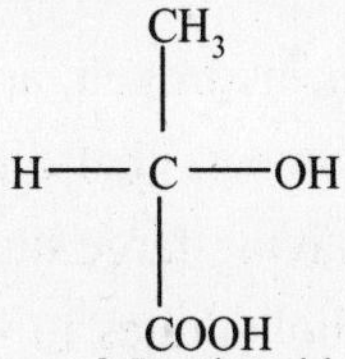

$$\begin{array}{c} CH_3 \\ | \\ H\text{---}C\text{---}OH \\ | \\ COOH \end{array} \qquad \begin{array}{c} CH_3 \\ | \\ HO\text{---}C\text{---}H \\ | \\ COOH \end{array} \qquad \begin{array}{c} CH_3 \\ | \\ H\text{---}C\text{---}NH_2 \\ | \\ COOH \end{array} \qquad \begin{array}{c} CH_3 \\ | \\ H_2N\text{---}C\text{---}H \\ | \\ COOH \end{array}$$

d- Lactic acid 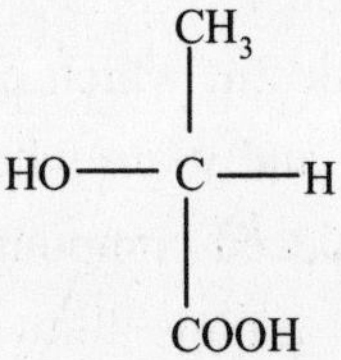   *l*- Lactic acid 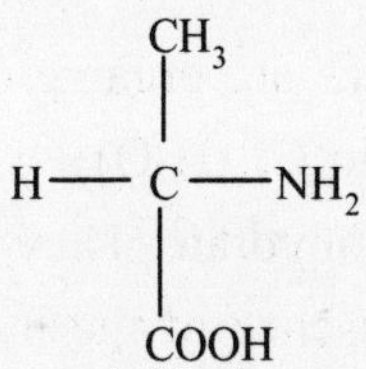   *d*- Alanine 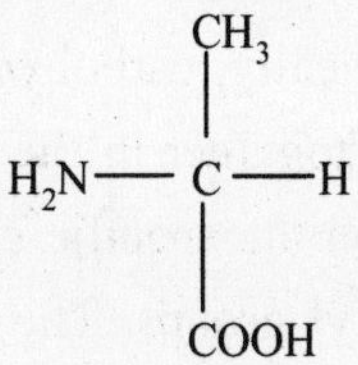   *l*- Alanine

Enantiomers are *d*–and *l* –forms of a compound, which are non–super-imposable mirror image of each other. Racemic modification is an equimolecular mixture of *d* and *l* forms of the same compound. The process of converting *d*– or *l*– form of an optically active compound into dl– (racemic) form is known as racemisation. Since the rotation of *d* is cancelled by equal but opposite rotation of *l*, racemic mixture (*r*) is always optically inactive. Separation of dl–mixture of a compound into *d* and *l* isomers is known as resolution. This can be done by several ways, viz. mechanical, biochemical and chemical method.

3.13. Monomers and Polymers

Organic molecules are the chemicals which are synthesized by living systems. These molecules are often called macromolecules because they may be very large, containing thousands of carbon and hydrogen atoms and they are typically composed of many smaller molecules bonded together. Macromolecules are constructed by covalently bonding monomers (smaller molecules) by condensation reactions (Fig.3.4), where water is removed from functional groups on the monomers. Cellular enzymes carry out condensation (and the reversal of the reaction, known as hydrolysis of polymers). When two monomers join, a hydroxyl (OH) group is removed from one monomer and hydrogen (H) is removed from the other. This produces the water to be given off during a condensation reaction, where as reversal of the mechanism occurs in hydrolysis.

There are four classes of macromolecules (carbohydrates, triglycerides, polypeptides, nucleic acids), which perform a variety of functions in cells.

3.14. Carbohydrates

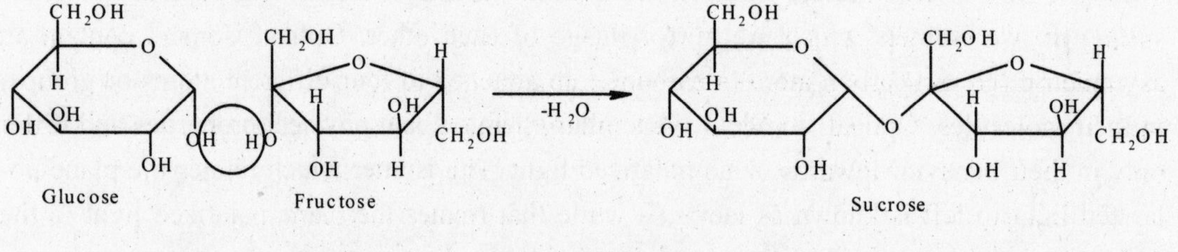

Figure 3.4: Condensation reaction in the formation of macromolecules

Chemically, carbohydrates are organic molecules in which carbon, hydrogen, and oxygen bond together in the ratio $C_x (H_2O)_y$, where x and y are whole numbers that differ depending on the specific carbohydrate. They are reduced compounds having large quantities of hydroxyl groups. The presence of the hydroxyl groups allows carbohydrates to interact with the aqueous environment and to participate in hydrogen bond formation, both within and between chains. The simplest carbohydrates also contain either an aldehyde moiety (termed polyhydroxyaldehydes) or a ketone moiety (polyhydroxyketones). Derivatives of the carbohydrates can contain nitrogen/s, phosphates and sulfur compounds. Carbohydrates can also combine with lipid to form glycolipids or with protein to form glycoproteins.

The aldehyde and ketone moieties of the carbohydrates with five and six carbons will spontaneously react with alcohol groups present in neighboring carbons to produce intramolecular hemiacetals or hemiketals, respectively. This results in the formation of five- or six-membered rings. As the five-membered ring structure resembles the organic molecule furan, the derivatives with this structure are termed as furanoses. Those with six-membered rings, resemble the organic molecule pyran are termed pyranoses and are depicted by either Fischer or Haworth style diagrams. The numbering of the carbons in carbohydrates proceeds from the carbonyl carbon, for aldoses, or the carbon nearest the carbonyl, for ketoses.

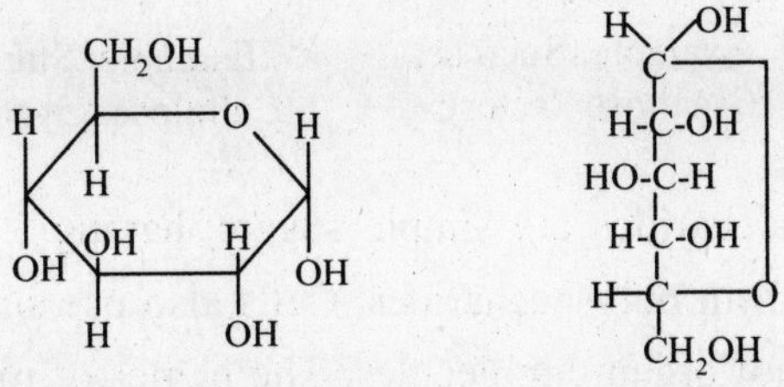

Haworth Projection of
a-D-Glucose

Cyclic Fischer Projection of
a-D-Glucose

The rings can open and re-close, allowing rotation to occur about the carbon bearing the reactive carbonyl, yielding two distinct configurations (α and β) of the hemiacetals and hemiketals. The carbon about which this rotation occurs is the anomeric carbon and these two forms are termed anomers. Carbohydrates can change spontaneously between α and β configurations: a process known as mutarotation. In the Fischer projection, α configuration places the hydroxyl attached to the anomeric carbon to the right, towards the ring, while in the Haworth projection, α configuration places the hydroxyl downward.

Carbohydrates can exist in either of two conformations, as determined by the orientation of the hydroxyl group about the asymmetric carbon farthest from the carbonyl. With a few exceptions, those carbohydrates that are of physiological significance exist in the D-conformation. Carbohydrates are the main energy source for the human body. Animals (including humans) break down carbohydrates during the process of metabolism to release energy. For example, the chemical metabolism of the sugar (glucose) is shown below:

$$C_6H_{12}O_6 + 6 O_2 \rightarrow 6 CO_2 + 6 H_2O + energy$$

Carbohydrates are manufactured by plants during the process of photosynthesis. Plants harvest energy from sunlight and stores in carbohydrate moieties.

$$6\ CO_2 + 6\ H_2O + energy\ (from\ sunlight) \rightarrow C_6H_{12}O_6 + 6\ O_2$$

All carbohydrates can be classified as monosaccharides, oligosaccharides or polysaccharides. Two to ten monosaccharide units, linked by glycosidic bonds, make up an oligosaccharide. Polysaccharides are much larger and contain hundreds of monosaccharide units.

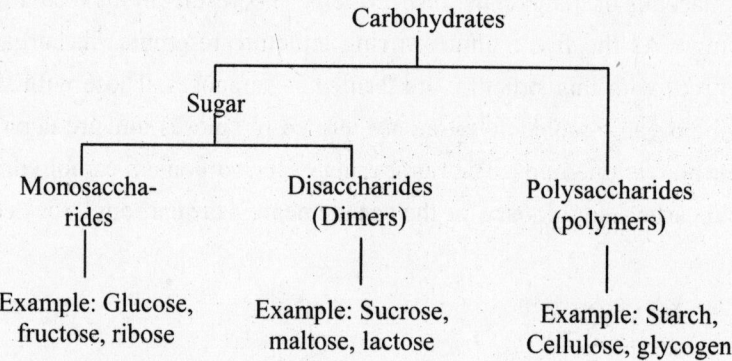

(a) Monosaccharide: Monosaccharides are simple sugars, having 3 to 7 carbon atoms. They can be bonded together to form polysaccharides. Cells also use simple sugars to store energy and construct other kinds of organic molecules. The names of most sugars end with the letters 'ose'. Glucose and other kinds of sugars (fructose, and galactose) may be linear molecules $(C_6H_{12}O_6)$ but in aqueous solution they take ring form.

There are two isomers of the ring form of glucose. They differ in the location of the OH group on the number 1 carbon atom. The number 1 carbon atom of the linear form of glucose is attached to the oxygen on the number 5 carbon atom.

(b) Disaccharides: Disaccharides are composed of 2 monosaccharides joined together by a condensation reaction. There are three common disaccharides:

• **Maltose** (or malt sugar) consists of glucose monomers. Amylase enzyme digests starch molecules to produce maltose.

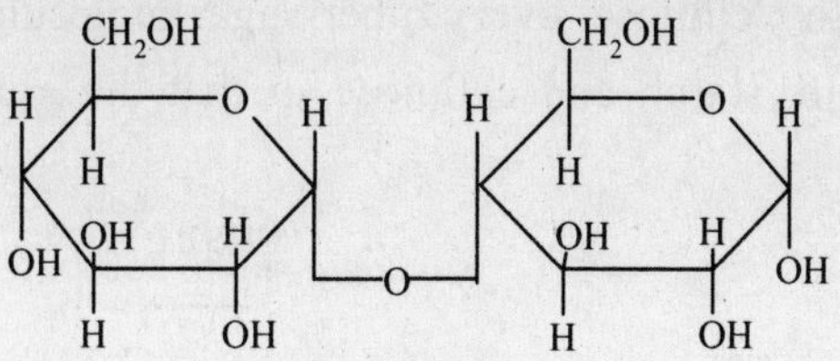

Maltose

- **Sucrose** (or cane sugar) composed of glucose and fructose. Plants synthesize sucrose to transport to non-photosynthetic parts of the plant, because it is less reactive than glucose.
- **Lactose** (or milk sugar) is made up of galactose and glucose. It is found only in mammalian milk

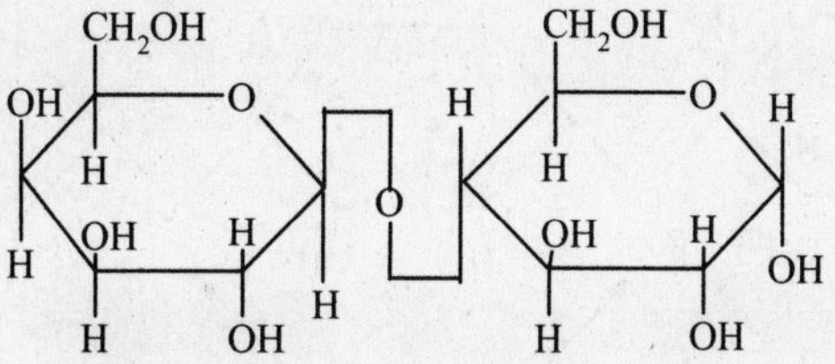

Lactose

(c) Polysaccharides

Monosaccharides may be bonded together to form long chain compounds called polysaccharides. The monomeric building blocks used to generate polysaccharides can be varied; in all cases, however, the predominant monosaccharide found in polysaccharides is D-glucose. Polysaccharides that are composed of a single monosaccharide building block are termed as homopolysaccharides, while polysaccharides composed of more than one type of monosaccharide, they are termed as heteropolysaccharides. For examples, starch and glycogen are composed of glucose monomers bonded together, producing long chains. They serve the function as stored food, starch in plants and glycogen in animal, in the liver and muscles. Glycogen is poly (1-4) glucose with 9% (1-6) branches (Fig. 3.5).

Starch is a long (100s) polymer of glucose molecules, where all the sugars are oriented in the same direction. Unbranched starch is called amylose, while branched starch is known as amylopectin. Amylose is simply poly-(1-4) glucose units in a straight chain. In fact the chain is floppy, and it tends to coil up into a helix. Amylopectin is poly (1-4) glucose with about 4% (1-6) branches. This gives it a more open molecular structure than amylose. As it has more ends, it can be broken more quickly than amylose by amylase enzymes. Amylopectin is a form of starch that is very similar to glycogen except for a much lower degree of branching (about every 20–30 residues). Another example of polysaccharide is cellulose. Cellulose is a long (100's) polymer of glucose molecules. However, the orientation of the sugars is little different. In Cellulose, every other sugar molecule is "upside-down". Glycogen is different from both, starch and cellulose in that the glucose chain is branched or "forked" (Fig. 3.6).

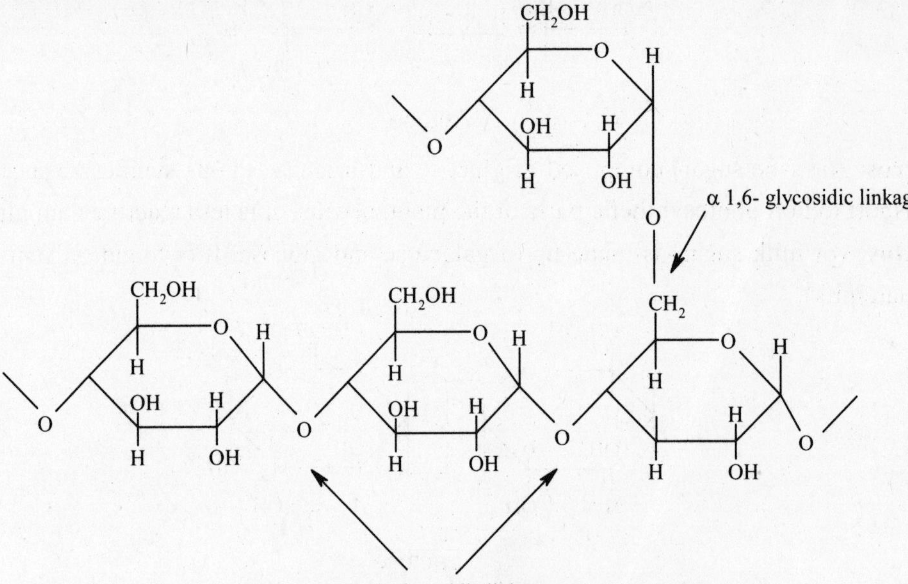

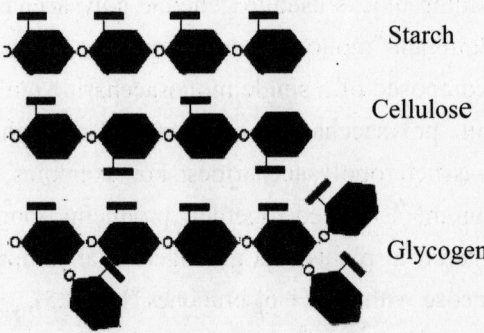

Figure 3.5: Structure of Glycogen

Starch

Cellulose

Glycogen

Figure 3.6: Orientation of monomers in polysaccharides

3.15. Lipids

Lipids are the biomolecules of structural and functional importance. They are the important component of membrane composition and function with a role in long-term energy storage. One gram of fat stores more than twice as much energy as one gram of carbohydrate. Lipids have multiple functions within the body. Phospholipids are important part of cell membranes, which encase each and every cell. The triglycerides are very important for fat metabolism and energy production. There is recent evidence that lipids are also important as signaling molecules within the body, sometimes serving as a marker for programmed cell death. Finally, some lipids take the form of vitamins, which can be important for mitochondria and creating other compounds. Chemically, they are made up of long chain hydrocarbons and are non-polar in nature; hence they are insoluble in water but soluble in non-polar solvents (Fig. 3.7). This group of molecules include fats and oils, waxes, phospholipids, steroids (like cholesterol), and some other related compounds.

3.15.1. Classification of Lipid

Classification of fatty acids is based on the length of the carbon chain (short, medium, or long); the number of double bonds (unsaturated, mono-, or polyunsaturated); and or essentiality in the diet (essential or non-essential). A current designation is based on the position of the end most double bond, counting from the methyl (CH_3) carbon, called the omega end. The most important omega fatty acids are: Omega 6 - linolein and arachidonic acids and Omega 3 - linolenic, icosapentaenoic, and docosahexaenoic acids.

(a) Triglycerides (neutral fats): Triglycerides consist of three long hydrocarbon chains known as fatty acids, attached to each other by a molecule called glycerol, are joined to each other by dehydration synthesis. They are the esters of three molecules of fatty acids plus one molecule of glycerol; the fatty acid may be all different. As they include three fatty acids, fats and oils are also known as triglycerides. They are found in adipose tissue, butterfat, lard, suet, fish oils, olive oil, corn oil, etc. Some fats are saturated, while others are unsaturated.

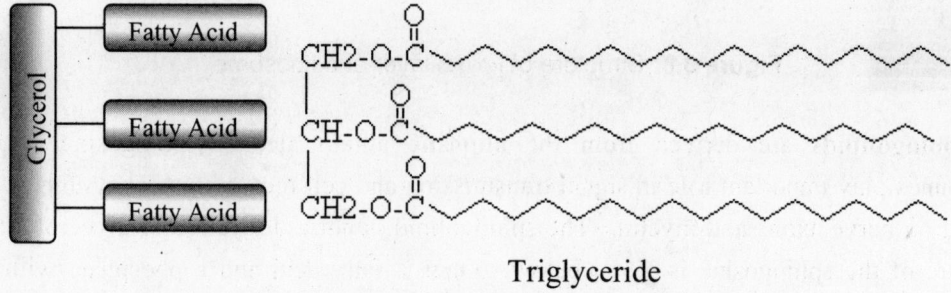

Triglyceride

Figure 3.7: Structure of lipids

These terms refer to the presence or absence of double bonds in the fatty acids of fats. Saturated fats have no double bonds, whereas unsaturated fats contain one or more such bonds. In general, plant fats are unsaturated and animal fats are saturated. Saturated fats are generally solid at room temperature, while unsaturated fats are typically liquid.

(b) Phospholipids (phosphatides): Phospholipids are major components of cell membranes. Like all fats, the hydrocarbon tails of phospholipids do not dissolve in water. However, phosphate groups are polar and soluble in water. The different solubilities of the two ends of phospholipid molecules allow them to form the bilayers that make up the cell membrane (Fig. 3.8). Their structure is similar to that of triglycerides, but they contain only two fatty acids. The third molecule attached to the glycerol is a phosphatidylcholine molecule (choline is one of the vitamin B). Certain phospholipids also contain inositol (another vitamin B) as phosphatidylinositol, as well as phosphatidylethanolamine, another phospholipid that has several functions, such as being a precursor to choline and acetylcholine. Most common phospholipids are lecithin, found in soybeans and egg yolks in highest concentration. It is also found in brain and other organ tissue.

Figure 3.8: Structure of lipid bilayer and liposome

(c) Sphingolipids are derived from the aliphatic amino alcohol sphingosine. These compounds play important role in signal transmission and cell recognition. They impart the coating on nerve axons and myelin. The sphingolipid is not a derivative of glycerol. The structure of the sphingosine is given below. Once a fatty acid and a phosphate with an attached choline are bonded to the sphingosine, forming sphingomyelin (Fig. 3.9).

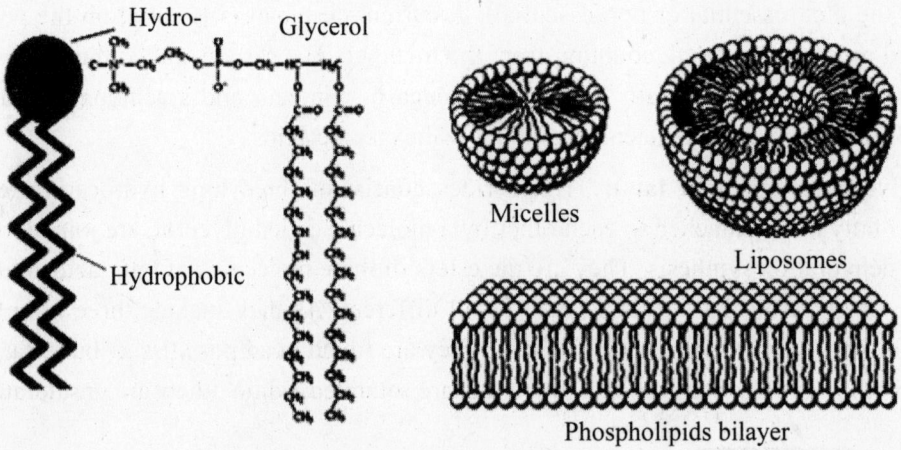

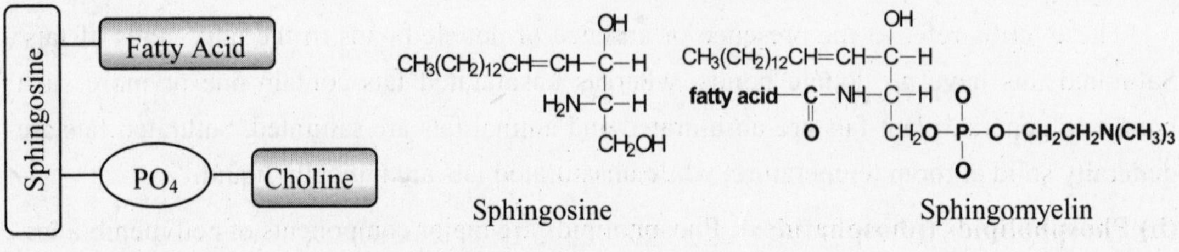

Sphingosine

Sphingomyelin

Figure 3.9: Structure of sphingolipids

(d) Glycolipids: Glycolipids are complex lipids that contain carbohydrates. Cerebrosides are examples which contain the sphingosine backbone attached to a fatty acid and a carbohydrate. The carbohydrates are most often glucose or galactose. Those that contain several carbohydrates are called gangliosides. Glucocerebroside has the specific function in the cell membranes of macrophages (cells that protect the body by destroying foreign microorganisms). Galactocerebroside is found almost exclusively in the membranes of brain cells.

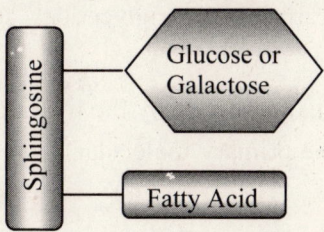

(e) Steroids: Steroids, the primary structure in hormones are substances that play important signaling role in the body. The general structure of cholesterol consists of two six-membered rings side-by-side and sharing one side in common, a third six-membered ring off the top corner of the right ring, and a five-membered ring attached to the right side of that.

Cholesterol is the central steroid from which other steroids such as the sex hormones are synthesized. Cholesterol is only found in animal cells. Examples of steroids include estrogen, progesterone, cortisone, aldosterone, testosterone, and Vitamin D. Steroids differ in the functional groups that are attached to the ring's edges. Cholesterol is the precursor of sex hormones and Vitamin D. Vitamin D is formed by the action of UV radiations in sunlight on cholesterol molecules that have "risen" to near the surface of the skin. Our cell membranes contain a lot of cholesterol, in between the phospholipids, to keep them fluid.

$$HCCH_3(CH_2)CH(CH_3)_2$$

Bile salts which assist in the digestion of lipids and other non-soluble molecules are synthesized in liver from cholesterol. Hormones are another derivative of steroids. Testosterone and estrogen are the hormones which give males and females their unique physical characteristics.

(f) Lipoproteins: These are the complexes of lipids with proteins, which act as a means of carrying lipids, including cholesterol in our blood. LDL or low density lipoprotein is the "bad lipid," being associated with deposition of "cholesterol" on the walls of arteries. HDL or high density lipoprotein is the "good lipid," being associated with carrying "cholesterol" out of the blood system and is more dense/ compact than LDL. The ratio of these two, LDL: HDL is the blood test currently being used to evaluate our risk of cardiovascular disease. The different classes of lipoproteins are:

(i) VLDLs (very-low-density lipoproteins) are made in the intestines and the liver to carry fats throughout the body. VLDLs carry mostly triglycerides, about 5–15% of the cholesterol to the body tissues.

(ii) LDLs (low-density lipoproteins) are made by the liver (and possibly by transformation of VLDLs in the blood) and are the primary molecular complexes that carry cholesterol in the blood to the organs and cells.

(iii) HDLs (high-density lipoproteins) pick up already used or unused cholesterol and cholesterol esters and take them back to the liver as part of a recycling process and the most protective form of lipoprotein in preventing buildup of cholesterol. The site of synthesis of HDL is not certain (probably in the liver). Low HDL levels are indications of risk of cardiovascular diseases. It also appears that HDL may be able to collect cholesterol from artery plaque, thus reversing the atherosclerotic process that leads to heart attacks. HDLs deliver cholesterol to the VLDL, converting them to LDL, which has more density; the liver then removes the LDLs from the blood and converts their cholesterol into bile acids, which are then eliminated.

(g) Waxes: They are composed of esters of long chain fatty acids with alcohol other than glycerol and are of industrial and medicinal importance. Examples are beeswax and lanolin.

3.16. Proteins

Proteins are the molecules of life, which perform wide range of functions inside the body, from structural components to catalysts of much metabolic function as well as chemical reactions and control the immune system. Amino acids are the basic building blocks of proteins (Table 3.1). Fundamentally, amino acids are joined together by peptide bonds to form the basic protein or peptide structures. However, owing to the many 'side groups' that are part of the amino acids other sorts of bonds may additionally form between the amino acid units. These additional bonds twist and turn the protein into convoluted shapes that are unique to the protein and essential to its ability to perform certain functions within the human body. Amino acids are carbon compounds which contain two functional groups: an amino group (NH_2) and a carboxylic acid group (COOH). A side chain (R) attached to the compound gives each amino acid a unique set of characteristics.

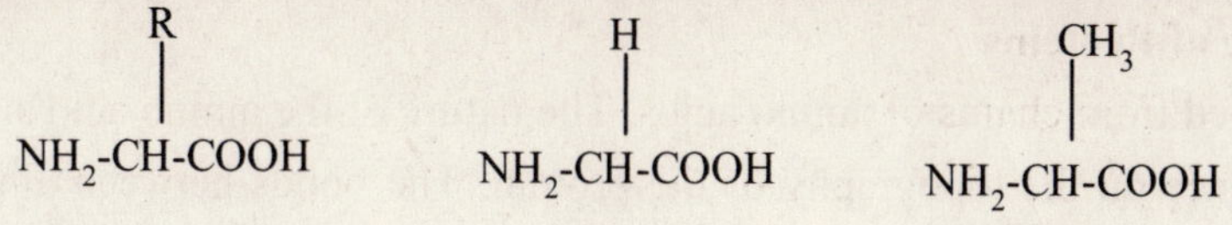

$$R$$
$$|$$
$$NH_2\text{-CH-COOH}$$

$$H$$
$$|$$
$$NH_2\text{-CH-COOH}$$

$$CH_3$$
$$|$$
$$NH_2\text{-CH-COOH}$$

General structure of amino acids   Glycine   Alanine

Though, the amino acids can be classified in different ways; the main two types of classification are given below

Table 3.1: Classification of amino acids on the basis of charge on the amino acid

Classification	Non- polar	Polar	Acidic (Polar)	Basic (Polar)
Amino acids	Glycine, Alanine Valine, Leucine Isoleucine, Proline Methionine, Phenylalanine Tryptophan	Serine Threonine Asparagine Glutamine, Cysteine Tyrosine	Aspartic Acid Glutamic Acid	Lysine Arginine Histidine

3.16.1. Peptides and Polypeptides

Two amino acids can combine together with the elimination of a molecule of water to produce a dipeptide. The formation of peptide bond occurs by the following mechanism.

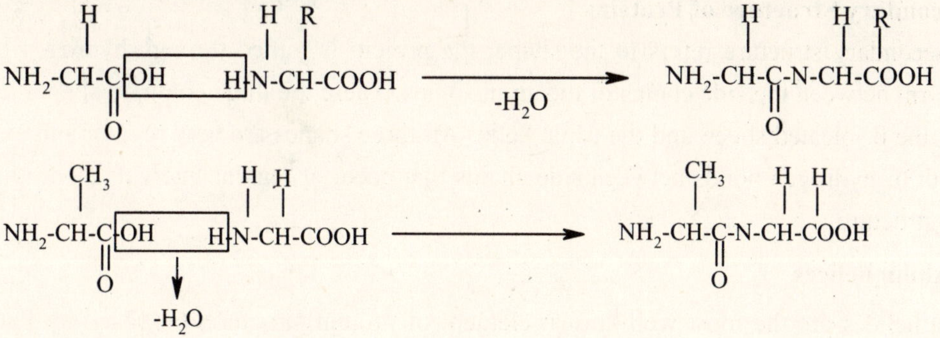

Three amino acids when joined together form a tripeptide, same way the large number of amino acids combine to form a polypeptide. A protein chain may consists of 50 to 2000 amino acid residues. The end of the peptide chain with the -NH₂ group is known as the N-terminal, while the end with the -COOH group is known as C-terminal.

3.16.2. Structure of Proteins

Proteins are formed from chains of amino acids. The nature of the amino acid side chains has significant influence on the topography of the protein. The bonds between amino acid side chains generate a complex protein structure, which is considered in four stages: primary, secondary, tertiary, and quaternary.

i. The primary structure

The primary structure of a protein refers to the sequence of amino acids that makes up the protein. The bonds considered in the primary structure are the peptide bonds between each amino acid. Amino acids when linked to form proteins, the amino group (-NH$_2$) of one amino acid combines with the carboxyl group (-COOH) of the next to form an amide or peptide linkage (-CONH-) which forms -N-C-C-N-C-C-N-C-C-, the backbone structure. The primary structure is read from the NH$_2$- terminal to the -COOH terminal. There are 20 different amino acids in living organisms. Most polypeptides consist of 50- 1000s amino acids. The shape of proteins is critical to their function. The shape is largely a result of the bonds, which form between the side chains of amino acids, making the protein. In short the primary purpose of the side chains in amino acids is to give proteins their shape, which dictates their function.

R-group   Peptide bond

ii. Secondary Structure of Proteins

The secondary structure refers to the shape; the protein is pulled through hydrogen bonds that form between the side chains of the amino acids. There are three common shapes, the α-helix, the β -pleated sheet, and the triple helix. All three shapes are very regular and exist as a result of hydrogen bonds between side chains that occur at regular intervals along the primary structure.

(a) Alpha helices

Alpha helices are the most well known element of protein structure, proposed by Pauling. Alpha-helices have distinctive patterns of hydrogen bonding and phi-psi angles (Fig. 3.10). They are generally between 5 and 20 residues in length, but some proteins are of coiled-coil structures, can be considerably longer. Alpha helices generally have a pitch of about 3.5 residues per turn, but there are forms of helices with tighter (3 residues per turn) and longer

(4 residues per turn). Alpha helices can be coiled about themselves in two coils, three coils and four coils (four helix bundles) conformations. Alpha helices can exist internal in proteins (generally hydrophobic), on the surface of proteins (amphipathic) or in membranes (hydrophobic). Alpha helices can span membranes either singly or in groups.

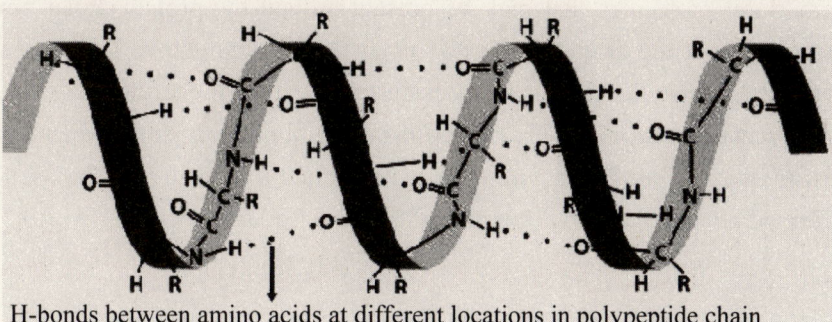

H-bonds between amino acids at different locations in polypeptide chain

Figure 3.10: Alpha helical structure of protein

(b) Beta pleated structure

Beta-strands represent for an extended form in which the side chains alternate on either side of the extended chain. Beta pleated structures are so called because the pleated or folded appearance, when view from the side (Fig. 3.11). Here the polypeptide chain is much more stretched out in comparison to alpha helix. The back bones of beta-strands form hydrogen bond with the backbone of an adjacent beta strand forming a beta-sheet structure. The strands in a beta sheet can be either parallel or anti-parallel and the hydrogen bonding pattern may be different between the two forms.

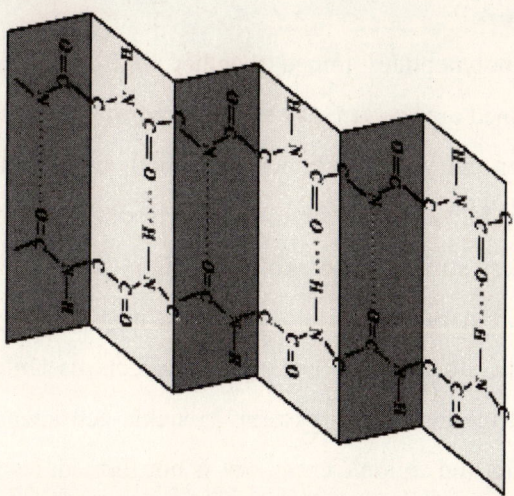

Figure 3.11: Beta pleated structure of protein

(iii) Tertiary Structure

Tertiary structure is the three dimensional conformation of a poly peptide. In other words, they are the folded proteins. Folding occurs during post translational modification. The tertiary structure of proteins is the result of further bonding between side chains within the protein and with water molecules that may be present around the protein. Polar amino acids move to the outside of the shape, while non-polar amino acids move to the inside, when placed in a polar solution. Bonds that are considered as part of the tertiary structure include: Bonds formed between non-polar side chains, disulfide bonds formed between sulfur atoms in cysteine side chains, ionic bonds formed between acidic and basic side chains, and hydrogen bonds formed between carbonyl groups and hydroxyl or amino groups (Fig. 3.12).

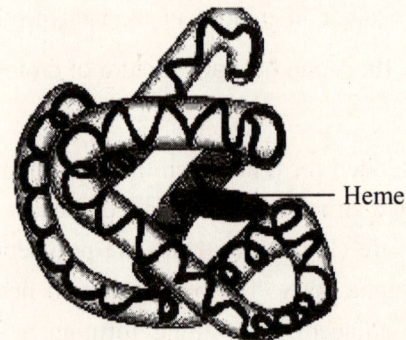

Heme

Figure 3.12: Tertiary structure: β polypeptide of Hemoglobin

(iv) Quaternary Structure

Two or more tertiary polypeptides joined together to form the quaternary structure of proteins. The bonds formed are the same as those found in the tertiary structure of proteins. Hemoglobin, the oxygen carrying component of blood, is an example of a protein in a quaternary structure (Fig.3.13). Hemoglobin is comprised of four polypeptide subunits, two with alpha helix secondary structure and two with beta pleated sheet form. All four components carry a heme group that can bind to oxygen, and all four components must be present to form hemoglobin. The shape of the hemoglobin affects its ability to carry oxygen and travel freely throughout the circulatory system. In sickle-cell anemia a particular glutamic acid is replaced by valine, and an ionic cross-link is not formed, resulting in a severe change of shape of the tertiary structure of the hemoglobin, which is a crescent or sickle in shape that reduces the oxygen carrying capacity of the red blood cells.

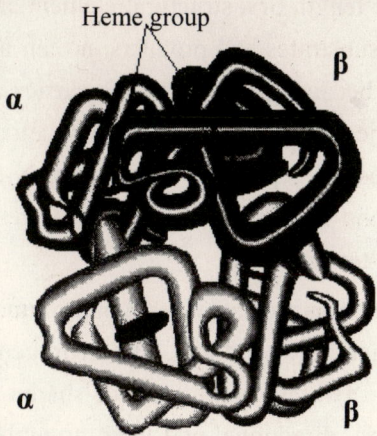

Heme group

α

β

α

β

Figure 3.13: Quaternary structure of hemoglobin

3.16.3. Forces Determining Protein Structure

There are several covalent and non-covalent forces involved which determine protein structure.

(a) Van der Waals interactions: These non-covalent forces result from the attraction of one atom's nucleus for the electrons of another atom in a non-covalent form (no sharing of orbitals). These forces are much weaker than covalent interactions. The interaction distances are much longer than covalent bonds and much shorter than the other non-covalent interactions. Van der Waals interactions occur at distances between 3 and 4 A°. They are very weak beyond 5 A° and electron repulsion prevents atoms from getting much closer than 3 A°. van der Waals interactions are non-directional and very weak. However, significant energy of stabilization can be obtained in the central hydrophobic core of proteins by the additive effect of many such interactions.

(b) Hydrophobic force: The hydrophobic force is really a negative non-covalent force. The presence of hydrophobic side chains in aqueous solution induces the formation of structured water. This reduction in entropy of the water molecules is a very unfavorable resulting in a strong force to keep hydrophobic side chains buried in the interior of the protein. The hydrophobic force is one of the largest determinants of protein structure.

(c) Electrostatic forces: The attraction of oppositely charged side chains can form salt-bridges which stabilize secondary and tertiary structures. The electrostatic force is quite strong, falling off as the square of the distance between the charged atoms. It also depends heavily on the dielectric constant of the medium in which the protein is dissolved.

(d) Dipole moments: Dipole moments are caused by pairs of charges separated by a larger distance than permitting a salt- or ion bridge formation. The dipole moment can give rise to an electric field along the entire length of a structural element and are often used by proteins to attract and position charged substrates and products in their active site. The peptide chain naturally has a dipole moment because the N-terminus carries a partial positive charge and the C-terminus carries partial negative charge. The alpha-helix is known to carry a partial negative charge at its C-terminus and a positive charge at its N-terminus. In order to neutralize this charge distribution, alpha helices often have acidic residues near their N-terminus and a basic residue near their C-terminus.

(e) Hydrogen bonds: Hydrogen bonds occur when a pair of nucleophilic atoms such as oxygen and nitrogen shares hydrogen between them. The hydrogen may be covalently attached to either nucleophilic atom (the H-bond donor) and or shared with the other atom (the H-bond receptor). H-bonds are very directional and their strength deteriorates dramatically as the angle changes. Hydrogen bonding between the carboxyl groups and the amino groups in the peptide backbone gives rise to alpha helix and beta strand conformations.

3.16.4. Covalent Bond Distances and Torsion Angles

The major properties of the covalent bonds that hold proteins together are their bond distances and bond angles. In particular, the bond angles between two adjacent bonds on either side of a single atom, or the dihedral angles between three contiguous bonds and two atoms control the geometry of the protein folding. One of the stabilizing forces in secondary structure of protein is the disulphide linkages. A covalent bridge can be formed by the oxidation of two cysteine residues to a cystine residue. The-S-S-bond is very strong and its presence confers additional stability (Fig. 3.14).

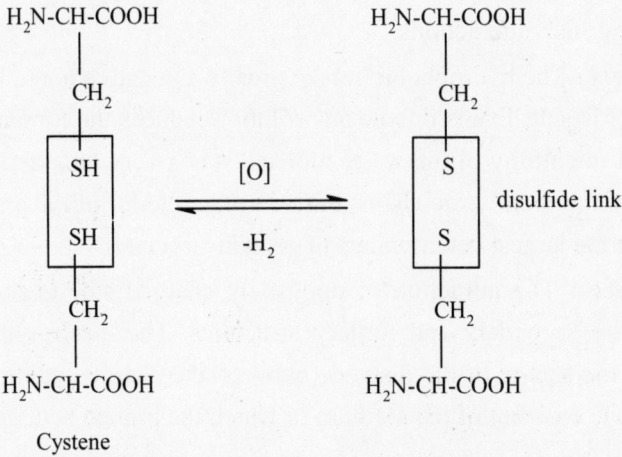

Figure 3.14: Formation of Disulfide Bridge

3.16.5. The Ramachandran Plot

The peptide backbone is constrained by steric hindrance and hydrogen bonding patterns that limit its torsional angles (phi-psi angles) to certain limits. Plots of phi versus psi dihedral angles for amino acid residues are called Ramachandran plots. One can tell if the backbone is following a helical or an extended beta strand structure based on the values of the phi-psi angles over a length of backbone (usually 3-4 residues is sufficient).

In a polypeptide, the main chain N-Cα and Cα-C bonds relatively are free to rotate. These rotations are represented by the torsion angles phi (φ) and psi (ψ) respectively. G. N Ramachandran used computer models of small polypeptides to systematically vary phi and psi with the objective of finding stable conformations. For each conformation, the structure was examined for close contacts between atoms. Atoms were treated as hard spheres with dimensions corresponding to their Van der Waals radii. Therefore, phi and psi angles which cause spheres to collide correspond to sterically disallowed conformations of the polypeptide backbone.

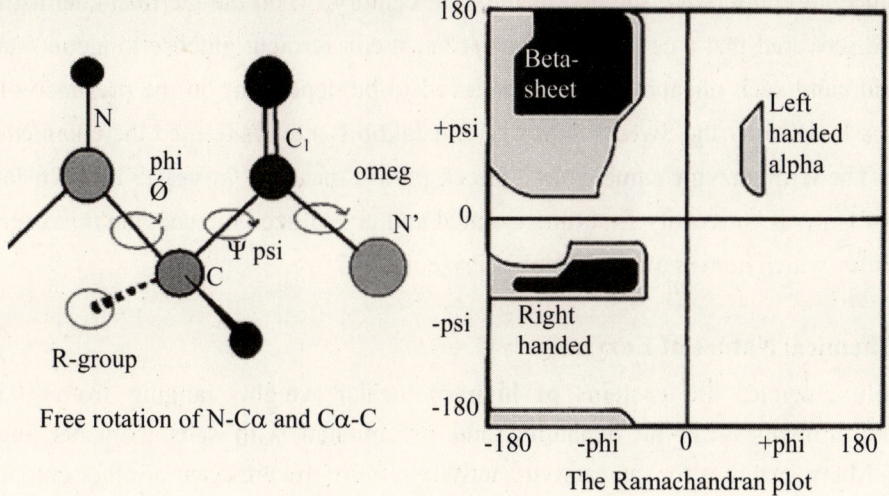

Figure 3.15: Ramachandran plot

In the above diagram (Fig. 3.15), the white areas correspond to conformations where atoms in the polypeptide come closer than the sum of their Van der Waals radii. These regions are sterically disallowed for all amino acids except glycine which is unique in that it lacks a side chain. The dark regions correspond to conformations where there are no steric clashes, i.e., these are the allowed regions namely the alpha-helical and beta-sheet conformations. The light shaded areas show the allowed regions if slightly shorter Vander Waals radii are used in the calculation, i.e., the atoms are allowed to come a little closer together. This brings out an additional region, which corresponds to the left-handed alpha-helix.

Disallowed regions generally involve steric hindrance between the side chain C-β methylene group and main chain atoms. Glycine has no side chain and therefore can adopt phi and psi angles in all four quadrants of the Ramachandran plot. Hence, it frequently occurs in turn regions of proteins where any other residue would be sterically hindered.

3.17. Enzymes

Enzymes are proteins which act as biological catalysts. Catalysis is characterized by the acceleration of a chemical reaction by some substance which itself does not undergo any permanent chemical change. The living cell is the site of tremendous biochemical activity called metabolism. The majority of these biochemical reactions do not take place spontaneously. The catalysts of biochemical reactions are enzymes and are responsible for bringing out almost all of the chemical reactions in living organisms. These reactions without enzymes are exceedingly slow and do not coordinate with the metabolism.

Enzymatic processes such as alcoholic fermentation and the digestion of meat have been known since antiquity. Until the end of the 19th century, when the German chemist Eduard Buchner discovered that a cell-free extract of yeast can ferment glucose to alcohol and carbon dioxide and such phenomena were believed to be dependent on the presence of living organisms. In 1835 by the Swedish chemist Jon Jakob Berzelius termed the chemical action catalytic. The term enzyme came from a Greek phrase meaning 'in yeast'. In 1926 James B. Sumner of Cornell University first time isolated and crystallized the enzyme urease from the jack bean for which he was awarded Nobel Prize in 1947.

3.17.1. Chemical Nature of Enzymes

Chemically enzymes are proteins of high molecular weight (ranging from 10,000 to 2,000,000). Enzymes can be denatured and precipitated with salts, solvents and other reagents. Many enzymes for the catalytic activity require the presence of other compounds - cofactors. This entire active complex is referred to as the holoenzyme; i.e., apo-enzyme (protein portion) and the cofactor (coenzyme, prosthetic group or metal-ion-activator). The cofactors can be a coenzyme, a non-protein organic substance loosely attached to the protein part or a prosthetic group. It can also be a metal-ion-activator, which includes K^+, Fe^{++}, Fe^{+++}, Cu^{++}, Co^{++}, Zn^{++}, Mn^{++}, Mg^{++}, Ca^{++}, and Mo^{+++}. The region on the enzyme molecule in close proximity, where the catalytic event takes place is known as the active site. For example, nicotinamide adenine dinucleotide (NAD) is a coenzyme for a great number of dehydrogenase reactions in which it acts as a hydrogen acceptor. Prosthetic groups necessary for catalysis are usually located in the active site, and it is the place where the substrate (and coenzymes, if any) bind just before the reaction takes place. The substrate can interact with the active site through opposite charges, hydrogen bonding, hydrophobic non-polar interaction, and/or coordinate covalent bonding to the metal ion activator.

3.17.2. Specificity of Enzymes

Enzymatic catalysis begins with the binding of the substrate (or substrates) to the active site on the enzyme. The binding of the substrate to the enzyme causes conformational changes and distribution of electrons in the chemical bonds of the substrate and results in reactions that lead to the formation of products. The products are released from the enzyme surface to regenerate the enzyme for another reaction cycle.

The active site has a unique geometric shape that is complementary to the geometric shape of a substrate molecule, similar to the fit of puzzle pieces. This means that enzymes specifically react with only one or a very few similar compounds, which makes them important diagnostic and research tools. In general, there are four distinct types of enzyme specificities:

(a) Absolute specificity: the enzyme will catalyze only one reaction.

(b) Group specificity: the enzyme will act only on molecules that have specific functional groups, such as amino, phosphate and methyl groups.

(c) Linkage specificity: the enzyme will act on a particular type of chemical bond regardless of the molecular structure.

(d) Stereochemical specificity: the enzyme will act on a particular steric or optical isomer. They have the ability to discriminate between asymmetric molecules of the right-handed and left-handed configurations. An example of a stereospecific enzyme is L -amino acid oxidase. This enzyme catalyzes the oxidation of a variety of amino acids of the type R—CH (NH_2) COOH. The rate of oxidation varies greatly, depending on the nature of the R group.

3.17.3. Lock and Key Theory

Lock and Key theory is first postulated in 1894 by Emil Fischer to explain the specificity of enzymes. In this analogy, the lock is the enzyme while the key is the substrate. Only a correct key (substrate) fits into the key hole (active site) of the lock (enzyme). The enzyme and substrate must fit together like a lock and key. If the fit is not exact then the reaction will not occur. The diagram below shows the lock and key theory (Fig. 3.16).

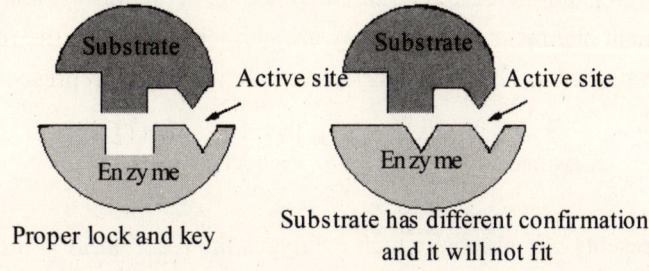

Figure 3.16: Diagrammatic representation of lock and key theory

3.17.4. Induced Fit Theory

The rigid enzyme model assumed by the lock and key theory failed to explain all type enzymatic catalysis hence, a modification called the induced-fit theory has been proposed. The induced-fit theory assumes that the substrate plays a role in determining the final shape of the enzyme and that the enzyme is partially flexible (Fig. 3.17). This explains why certain compounds can bind to the enzyme but do not react because the enzyme has been distorted too much. Other molecules may be too small to induce the proper alignment and therefore cannot react. Only the proper substrate is capable of inducing the proper alignment of the active site.

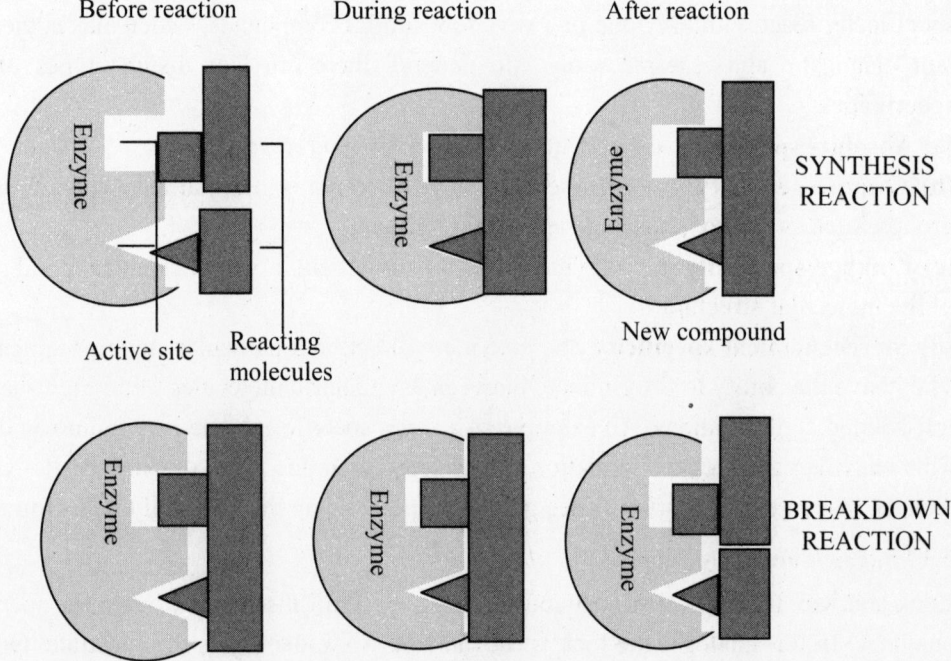

Figure 3.17: Diagrammatic representation of induced fit theory

3.17.5. Enzyme Kinetics

Enzymes are catalysts and increase the rate of a chemical reaction without themselves undergoing any permanent chemical change. They are neither used up in the reaction nor do they appear as reaction products. The basic enzymatic reaction can be represented as follows

$$S + E \longrightarrow P + E \dots\dots(1)$$

Substrate enzyme   Product complex

Where E represents the enzyme which catalyzes the reaction, S is the substrate and P is the product of the reaction. In an enzyme-catalyzed reaction, the substrate first binds to the active site of the enzyme to form an enzyme-substrate (ES) complex, then the substrate is converted into product and finally it is released, thus allowing the enzyme to start all over again (Fig. 3.18). An example is the action of the enzyme sucrase, which hydrolyzes sucrose into glucose and fructose

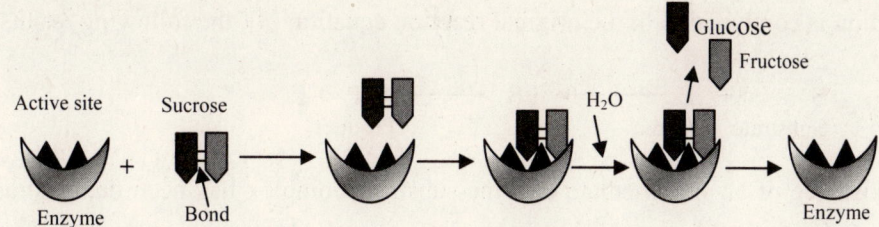

Figure 3.18: Hydrolysis of sucrose into glucose and fructose

3.17.6. Energy Levels

Some amount of energy is needed for a chemical reaction to proceed, before the reactants can change into product, the substrate must overcome an "energy barrier" called the activation energy. The larger the activation energy is, the slower the reaction (Fig. 3.19). This is because only a few substrate molecules will have sufficient energy to overcome the activation energy barrier.

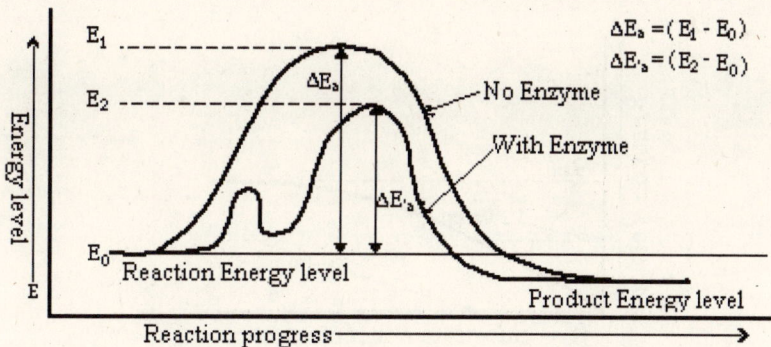

Figure 3.19: Activation energy of enzyme catalyzed reactions

Most biological reactions have large activation energies; hence in the absence of enzymes they proceed too slowly. Enzymes reduce the activation energy of a reaction so that the kinetic energy of most molecules exceeds the activation energy required and hence they can react (Fig.3.19). Swedish chemist Savante Arrhenius in 1888 proposed that the substrate and enzyme form some intermediate substance which is known as the enzyme substrate complex.

The reaction can be represented as:

$$S \quad + \; E \longrightarrow ES \ldots\ldots\ldots\ldots(2)$$

Substrate Enzyme   Substrate Enzyme
complex

If this reaction is combined with the original reaction equation [1], the following results:

$$S \quad + \; E \longrightarrow ES \longrightarrow P + E$$

Substrate Enzyme   Product

The existence of an intermediate enzyme-substrate complex has been demonstrated in the laboratory, for example, catalase and a hydrogen peroxide derivative. In the absence of catalyst, the activation energy for the reaction ($2H_2O_2 \rightarrow 2H_2O + O_2$) is 86kJmol^{-1}. In presence of inorganic catalyst it is 62 kJmol^{-1} while in presence of the enzyme catalase it is just 1 kJmol$^{-1.}$

3.17.7. Factors Affecting the Rate of Enzyme Reactions

(a) Substrate Concentration

The rate of an enzyme-catalyzed reaction is affected by substrate concentration. If the amount of the enzyme is kept constant and the substrate concentration is then gradually increased, the reaction velocity will increase until it reaches a maximum and a further increase in substrate concentration will not increase the velocity (Fig. 3.20).

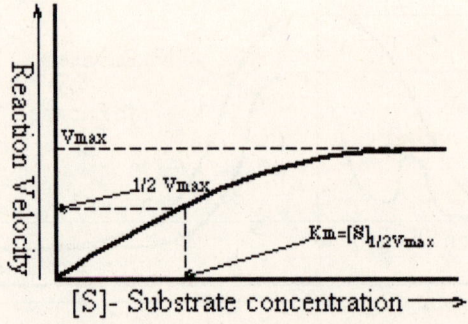

Figure 3.20: Relationship showing velocity and substrate concentration

The increase in rate of the reaction with substrate concentration is because there can be more collision with active sites, so more enzyme-substrate complexes will be formed. At higher concentrations the enzyme molecules become saturated with substrate, and there are few free active sites, therefore further substrate addition will not make much difference.

Michaelis-Menten equation gives the relation between enzyme velocity and substrate concentration, which can be represented as

$$\text{Velocity} = V = \frac{V_{max}\,[S]}{[S] + K_m} \quad \ldots\ldots\ldots(4)$$

Where V_{max} is the maximum rate at infinite substrate concentration that gives a rate of half V_{max}, called K_M. The velocity or the turnover number is defined as the number of molecules of substrate converted to product by one enzyme site per second. These quantities are useful for characterizing an enzyme. A good enzyme has a high V_{max} and a low K_M. It is theorized that when this maximum velocity reaches, the entire available enzyme is converted to ES, the enzyme substrate complex. This point on the graph is designated as V_{max}. K_M is expressed in units of concentration which is usually in molar units.

A simple enzymatic reaction can be represented as

$$E + S \underset{k_{-1}}{\overset{k_1}{\rightleftharpoons}} ES \xrightarrow{k_2} E + P \quad \text{........ (5)}$$

The substrate (S) binds reversibly to the enzyme (E) in the first reaction to form the enzyme substrate complex. In the second step enzyme substrate complex is converted to product and the free enzyme. This reaction is slow; hence it is the rate determining step.

Thus, rate of the reaction = K_2 [ES]............. **(6)**

At equilibrium, the rate of forward reaction will be equal to backward reaction. The rate of product formation thus equals the rate at which ES turns into E+P. In the above equation it is not possible to calculate [ES]. To solve this, let us assume that the concentration of ES is steady during the time intervals used for enzyme kinetic work. It means that the rate of ES formation equals the rate of ES dissociation, i.e. either back to E+S or forward to E+P. It is assumed that the rate of reverse reaction (formation of ES from E+P) is negligible. Therefore, at the steady state, the rate of ES formation = rate of ES dissociation

$$K_1\,[S]\,[E_{free}] = K_{-1}\,[ES] + k_2\,[ES]\ldots\ldots\ldots(7)$$

But, the total concentration of enzyme E_{total} = ES + E.

Now, the equation can be rewritten as

$$K_1\,[S]\,([E_{total}] - [ES]) = K_{-1}\,[ES] + K_2\,[ES]\ldots\ldots\ldots(8)$$

Solving for ES:

$$[ES] = \frac{K_1 [E_{total}] [S]}{K_1 [S] + K_2 + K_{-1}} = \frac{[E_{total}] [S]}{[S] + \dfrac{K_2 + K_1}{K_1}} \quad \cdots\cdots\cdots(9)$$

Therefore the velocity of the enzyme reaction is:

$$Velocity = K_2 [ES] = \frac{K_2 [E_{total}] [S]}{[S] + \dfrac{K_2 + K_1}{K_1}} \quad \cdots\cdots\cdots(10)$$

Now $(k_2 + k_{-1})/k_1 = K_M$, is called as Michaelis-Menten constant. The equation can be further simplified by considering that maximum velocity occurs, when the enzyme is saturated, that is at Vmax $[ES] = E_{total}$. On substituting these values the equation:

$$Velocity = V = \frac{Vmax [S]}{[S] + Km} \quad \cdots\cdots\cdots(11)$$

(b) Enzyme Concentration

As the enzyme concentration increases the rate of the reaction also increases, because there are more enzyme molecules (and so more active sites), available to catalyze the reaction and the reaction will leads to more enzyme-substrate complex formation.

(c) Temperature Effects

The rate of an enzyme-catalyzed reaction increases as the temperature is raised like that of normal chemical reactions. A ten degree centigrade rise in temperature will increase the activity of most of the enzymes by 50 to 100% (Fig. 3.21). Enzymes have an optimum temperature at which they work fast. For mammalian enzymes, the optimum temperature is about 40°C, but there are certain enzymes that work best at very different temperatures, e.g. enzymes from the arctic snow flea work at -10°C, while enzymes from thermophilic bacteria work at 90°C. The rate increases as the enzyme and substrate molecules both have more kinetic energy and hence collide more often and also because more molecules have sufficient energy to overcome the activation energy. Above the optimum temperature the rate decreases as more of the enzyme molecules denature. The thermal energy breaks the hydrogen bonds holding the secondary and tertiary structure of the enzyme together, therefore, the enzyme lose its shape and becomes a random coil - thus the substrate can no longer fit into the active site.

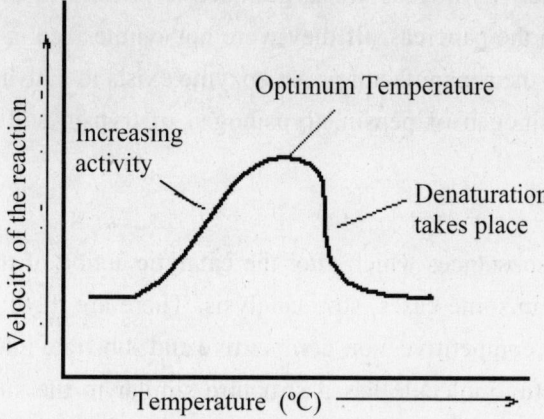

Figure 3.21: Effect of temperature on enzymatic activity

(d) pH

The most favorable pH value or the pH at which the enzyme is most active - is known as the optimum pH. For most enzymes this is about pH 7–8 (normal body pH), but a few enzymes can work at extreme pH, such as gastric protease (pepsin) in our stomach, which has an optimum pH 1. The pH affects the charge of the amino acids at the active site, therefore, the properties of the active site change and the substrate can no longer bind (Fig. 3.22). For example a carboxyl acid R groups will be uncharged at low pH (COOH), but can be charged at high pH (COO⁻).

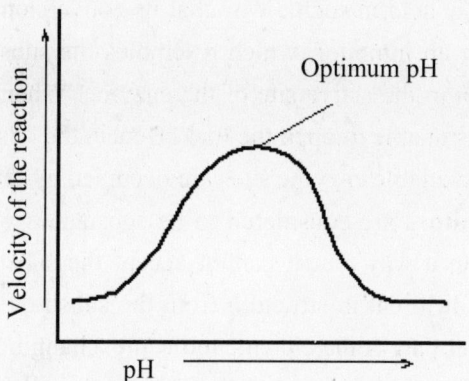

Figure 3.22: Effect of pH on enzyme activity

(e) Covalent modification

An inactive form is converted to an active form by covalent modifications catalyzed by other enzymes. The activity of certain enzymes is controlled by other enzymes, which modify the protein chain by cutting it, or adding a phosphate or methyl group. This modification can turn an inactive enzyme into an active enzyme (or vice versa) and this is used to control many metabolic enzymes. Zymogens are large inactive precursors of proteolytic enzymes. They are synthesized in the pancreas. If they were not synthesized in an inactive form they would digest the site of their manufacture. An enzyme exists to activate each zymogen. The examples include, pepsinogen of pepsin, trypsinogen of trypsin and chymotrypsinogen of chymotrypsin.

(f) Inhibitors

Enzyme inhibitors are substances which alter the catalytic action of the enzyme and consequently slow down, or in some cases, stop catalysis. There are three common types of enzyme inhibition namely competitive, non-competitive and substrate inhibition.

(i) Competitive inhibitor molecule has a structure similar to the substrate molecule, and therefore it can fit into the active site of the enzyme. It competes with the substrate for the active site, hence the reaction is slower. Increasing the concentration of substrate restores the reaction rate and the inhibition is usually temporary and reversible. Competitive inhibitors increase K_M for the enzyme, but have no effect on Vmax, so the rate can approach a normal rate if the substrate concentration is increased considerably.

Most theories concerning inhibition mechanisms are based on the existence of the enzyme-substrate complex (ES). Competitive inhibition occurs when the substrate and a substance resembling the substrate are both added to the enzyme. Competitive inhibition can be well explained by lock and key theory concept, which utilizes the concept of an "active site." The concept holds that one particular portion of the enzyme surface has a strong affinity for the substrate. The substrate is held in such a way that its conversion to the reaction products is more favorable. However an inhibitor, which resembles the substrate, will compete with the substrate for the position in the active site of the enzyme. When the inhibitor prevails, it gains the lock position but is unable to open the lock. Hence, the observed reaction is slowed down because some of the available enzyme sites are occupied by the inhibitor.

(ii) Non-competitive inhibitors are considered to be substances which when added to the enzyme, alter the enzyme in a way that it cannot accept the substrate. A non-competitive inhibitor molecule is quite different in structure from the substrate and does not fit into the active site. It binds to another part of the enzyme molecule, changing the conformation of the whole enzyme, including the active site, so that substrate molecules cannot bind properly. Non-competitive inhibition is equivalent to decreasing the enzyme concentration, so they decrease Vmax, while no effect on K_M. This kind of inhibitor tends to bind tightly and irreversibly – such as cyanide and heavy metal ions.

(iii) Substrate inhibition: Substrate inhibition will sometimes occurs when excessive amounts of substrate are present. Additional amounts of substrate added to the reaction mixture after a level decreases the reaction rate. This is thought to be due to the fact that there are so many substrate molecules competing for the active sites on the enzyme surfaces that they block the sites and prevent any other substrate molecules from occupying them.

(iv) Feedback inhibition (Allosteric effectors): The activity of some enzymes is controlled by certain molecules binding to a specific regulatory (or allosteric) site on the enzyme, distinct from the active site. It is the cellular control mechanism in which an enzyme that catalyzes the production of a particular substance in the cell is inhibited when that substance has accumulated to a certain level, thereby balancing the amount provided with the amount needed or it is suppression of the activity of an enzyme by a product of the sequence of reactions in which the enzyme is participating. When the product accumulates in a cell beyond an optimal amount, it decreases its own production by inhibiting an enzyme involved in its synthesis. After the product has been used or broken down, the inhibition is relaxed and the formation of the product resumes. Enzymes whose ability to catalyze a reaction depends on molecules other than the substances on which they act directly are said to be under allosteric control. Only a few enzymes can do this, and they are often at the start of a long biochemical pathway. They are generally activated by the substrate and inhibited by the product of the pathway, thus only turning the pathway on, when it is needed. This process is known as feedback inhibition.

3.17.8. Classification of Enzymes

Enzymes are classified according to the reactions they catalyze, by the nomenclature committee of the International Union of Biochemistry and Molecular Biology (IUBMB).

(a) Oxidoreductases: These are enzymes which catalyze a variety of oxidation-reduction reactions. Oxidation is the reverse of reduction reactions and that an enzyme has to catalyze the forward and reverse reactions to the same degree, thus the double-barreled name "oxidoreductase." Common examples include dehydrogenase, oxidase, reductase and catalase.

(b) Transferases: These enzymes catalyze the transfer of a group of atoms from one molecule to another. A common example involves transfer of a phosphate between ATP and a sugar molecule. Common names include acetyltransferase, methylase, protein kinase and polymerase.

(c) Hydrolases: As the name suggests, these enzymes catalyze hydrolysis reactions (and their reverse reactions). Common examples are:

Proteases- splits protein molecules

Nucleases- split nucleic acids (DNA and RNA). Based on the substrate type, they are \divided into RNase and DNase.

Phosphatase - catalyzes dephosphorylation, i.e. removal of phosphate groups.

(d) Isomerases: These enzymes catalyze the conversion of a molecule into an isomer that is an atomic rearrangement within a molecule. Examples include epimerase and racemase, like the cis-trans inter-conversion of malate and fumarate.

(e) Lyases: These enzymes catalyze the cleavage of C–C, C–O, C–S and C–N bonds by means other than hydrolysis or oxidation. Common names include decarboxylase and aldolase.

(f) Ligases: These enzymes catalyze reactions which make bonds to join together (ligate) smaller molecules to make larger ones. Examples include peptide synthase, aminoacyl-tRNA synthase, DNA ligase and RNA ligase.

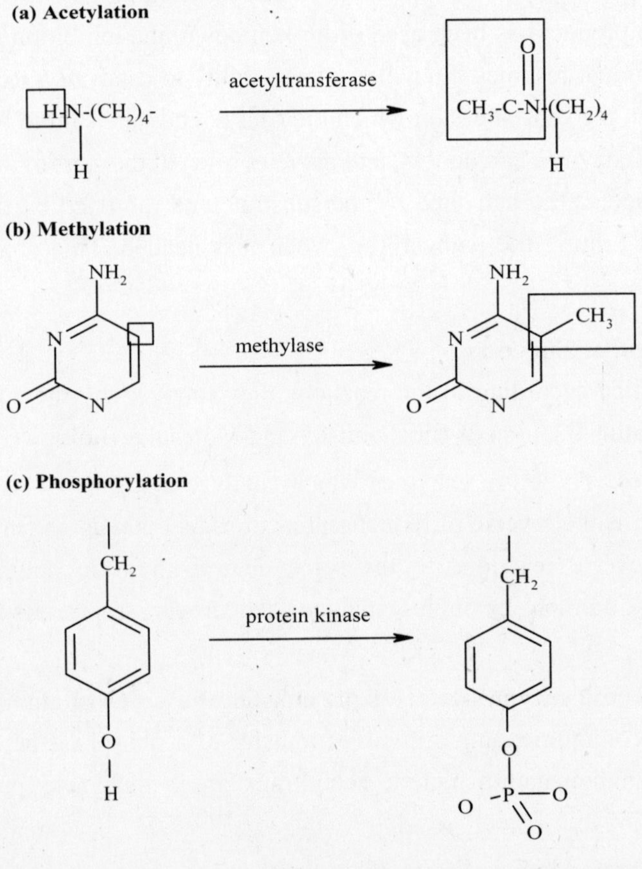

(a) Acetylation

(b) Methylation

(c) Phosphorylation

Each of these classes has more specific subclasses as well. The key to use this classification scheme is to look at the reaction, that the enzyme catalyzes, decide which type of reaction it is, and apply the appropriate name. Each enzyme is assigned an EC (Enzyme Commission) number. For example, the EC number of catalase is EC 1.11.1.6. The first digit indicates that the enzyme belongs to oxidoreductase (class 1) and subsequent digits represent subclasses and sub-subclasses.

Are all enzymes proteins?

As a general definition we learned that all enzymes are proteins. Is it true in all cases? No, there are certain types of naturally-occurring RNA molecules that can behave as enzymes, catalyzing their own assembly, called ribozymes. The RNA catalysts called ribozymes are found in the nucleus, mitochondria, and chloroplasts of eukaryotic organisms. Some viruses, including several bacterial viruses, also have ribozymes. Thomas Cech at the University of Colorado and Sydney Altman at Yale University provided an empirical basis for the concept of the "RNA world", which is explained in the first chapter, by their discovery of ribozymes. Ribozymes have the ability to catalyze the cleavage and formation of covalent bonds in RNA strands at specific sites. Examples include self-splicing rRNA involved in catalyzing RNA processing reactions, i.e., the biochemical reactions that convert a newly synthesized RNA molecule to its matured form.

Ribozymes share many similarities with protein enzymes, as assessed by two parameters that are used to describe a biological catalyst. The Michaelis-Menten constant K_m relates to the affinity that the catalyst has for its substrate, and ribozymes possess K_m values which are comparable to K_m values of protein enzymes. The values of this constant for ribozymes are markedly lower than the values observed for protein enzymes. Nevertheless, ribozymes accelerate the rate of chemical reaction with specific substrates by 10^{11} times compared with the rate observed for the corresponding un-catalyzed, spontaneous reaction. Almost all ribozymes are involved in the processing of RNA.

3.18. Nucleic Acid

Nucleic acids are complex compounds of monomeric nucleotides, composed of phosphoric acid, sugar and nitrogenous base and involved in the preservation, replication, and expression of hereditary information in every living cell. Nucleic acids were so named because they were first found in the nucleus of cells.

Johann Friedrich Miescher in 1870 isolated a weakly acidic substance of unknown function in the nuclei of human white blood cells, and named this material "nuclein", which later came to known as DNA. In the 1920s nucleic acids were found to be major components of chromosomes, small gene-carrying bodies in the nuclei of complex cells. Elemental analysis of nucleic acids showed the presence of phosphorus, in addition to the usual C, H, N and O. It was later found that there were two kinds of nucleic acids, according to the bases that were identified. One type of nucleic acid was obtained from animal glands and later called DNA, while the other type was obtained from yeast cells, and called RNA. It was not until the 1940s that biochemists realized that both DNA and RNA are present in all living cells, whether plant or animal. American chemist Marshall Nirenberg was later credited with translating the code of life and was awarded the Nobel prize in 1968. He demonstrated that RNA could be translated into protein. Initially, it was thought that there was only one kind of RNA, but other types of RNAs with specialized functions were later discovered. On the basis of presence of deoxyribose sugar, chromosomal nucleic acids were called deoxyribonucleic acids, abbreviated as DNA. Analogous nucleic acids, RNA, in which the sugar component is ribose, termed ribonucleic acids. The acidic character of the nucleic acids was attributed to the phosphoric acid moiety.

3.18.1. Chemical Composition of Nucleic Acids

The basic structure of nucleic acids consists of bases, sugar and phosphates. There are three monocyclic bases, cytosine, thymine and uracil, called pyrimidines, and the two bicyclic bases, adenine and guanine, called purines. It can be easily remembered by the notation the longer word (pyrimidine) represents the smaller structure (only one ring), and vice versa. Each has at least one N–H site at which an organic substituent may be attached. Nucleic acids are polynucleotide, formulated as alternating copolymers of phosphoric acid (P) and nucleosides (N). Nucleosides consist of sugar and bases. The base - sugar covalent bond in a nucleoside or nucleotide is an N-glycosidic link because it involves the N of the purine or pyrimidine ring. The sugar that is part of a nucleotide is a 5-carbon atom sugar in its ring form. It will either be ribose in RNA or deoxyribose in DNA. The "de-oxy" simply means that the ribose molecule has lost oxygen from the second carbon, so the more correct name for deoxyribose is 2-deoxyribose. As the last asymmetric carbon atom has an OH to the

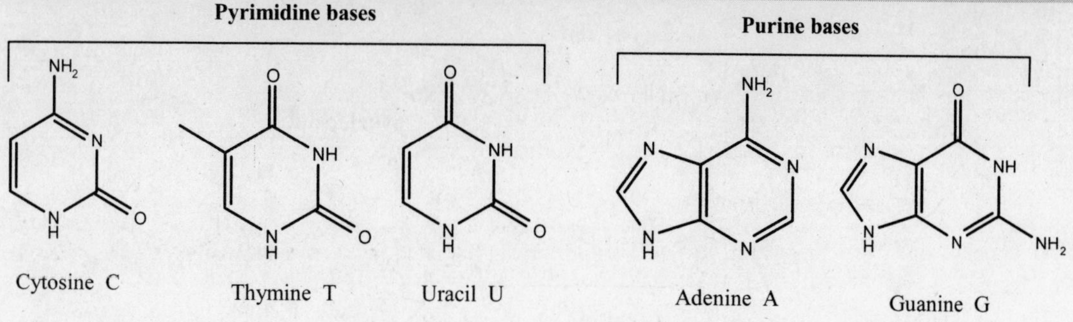

Pyrimidine bases

Purine bases

Cytosine C

Thymine T

Uracil U

Adenine A

Guanine G

right, these molecules are sometimes given the more complete names of D-ribose and also D -2-deoxyribose.

Nucleosides are formed by the N-glycosidic link between sugar and nitrogen base. The phosphate groups are linked to the sugars at the 5′ position. The addition of one to three phosphate groups generates a nucleotide, also known as a nucleoside monophosphate, nucleoside diphosphate, or nucleoside triphosphate (Fig. 3.23).

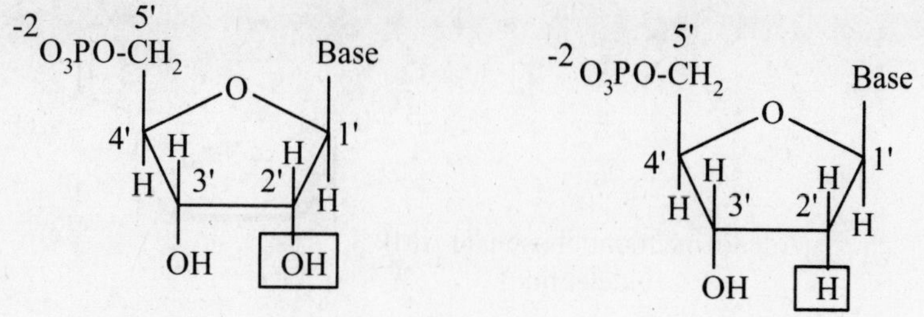

Ribonucleotide

Deoxyribonucleotide

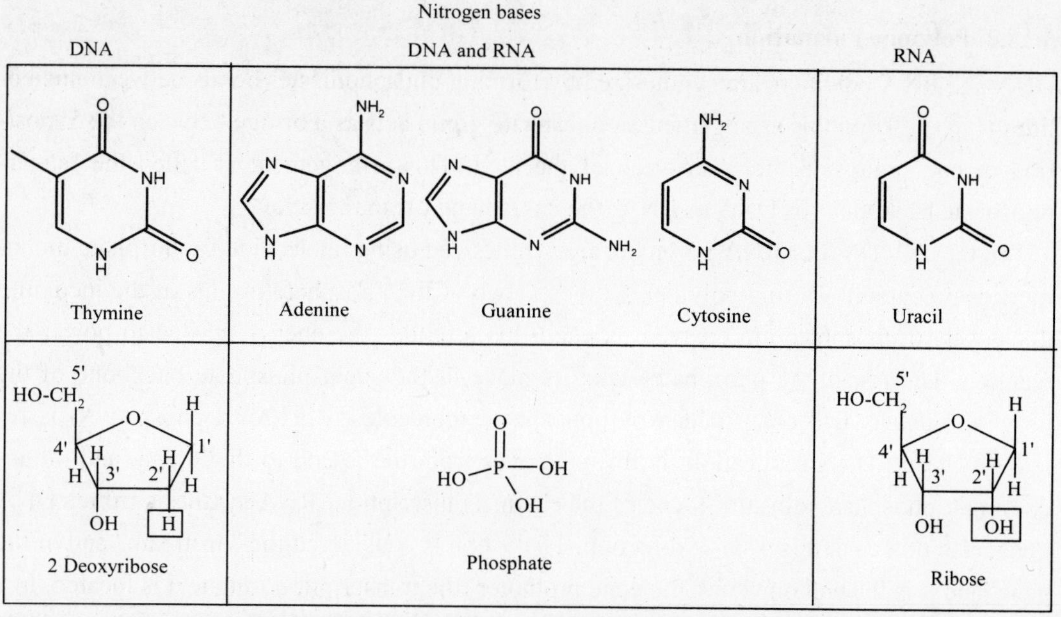

Nitrogen bases

DNA

DNA and RNA

RNA

Thymine

Adenine

Guanine

Cytosine

Uracil

2 Deoxyribose

Phosphate

Ribose

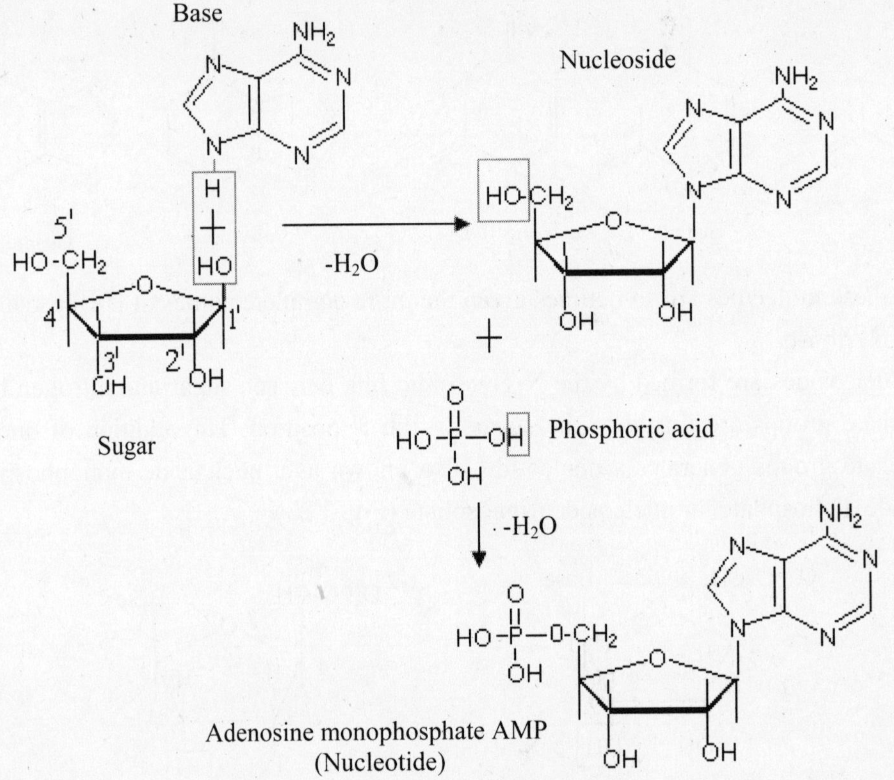

Figure 3.23: Formation of nucleotide

3.18.2. Polymer Formation

DNA and RNA polymers are synthesized by forming phosphodiester bonds between nucleotides (Fig. 3.24). In this arrangement, a phosphate group acts as a bridge between the 5′ position of one sugar and the 3′ position of the next. This arrangement is called the "sugar-phosphate backbone" of DNA or RNA; the bases hang off to the side.

In the cell, DNA or RNA polymers are synthesized using nucleoside triphosphate monomers as precursors. During polymer synthesis, two of the phosphate groups of the incoming nucleoside triphosphate are cleaved off, and this provides the energy needed to power the reaction. The remaining phosphates take its place in the sugar-phosphate backbone of the growing nucleic acid chain and a pyrophosphate molecule (two linked phosphates) is released. During DNA replication, it always moves from the 5′ end to the 3′ end, and the incoming triphosphate joins the 3′ end of the chain. Transcription (RNA synthesis from a DNA gene) also moves in this 5′-to-3′ direction. The 5′ end is considered the "upstream" end of the gene, and it is the end on which the gene promoter (the transcription initiator) is located. In a nucleic acid chain, two nucleotides are linked by a phosphodiester bond, which may be formed by the condensation reaction similar to the formation of the peptide bond. However, the whole nucleic acid chain is usually synthesized by RNA polymerase or DNA polymerase.

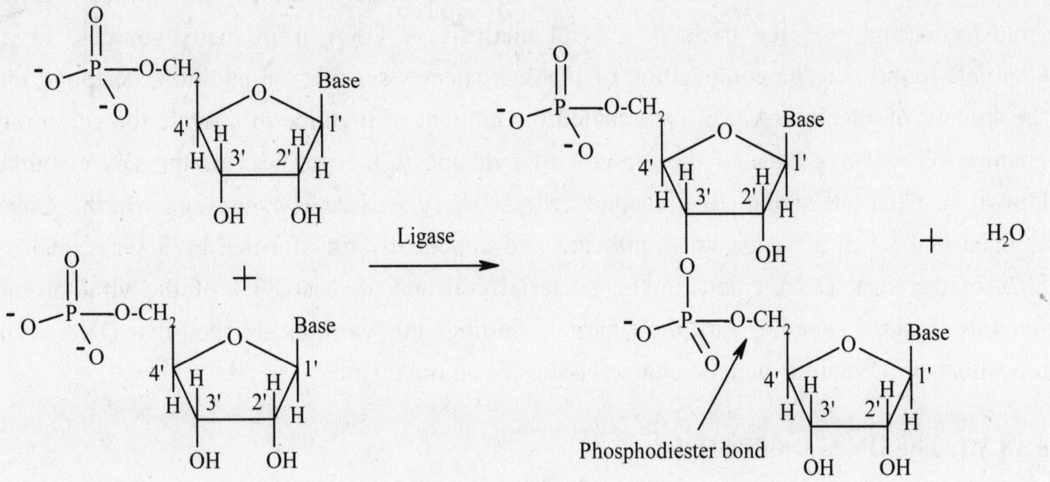

Figure 3.24: Formation of the phosphodiester bond through the condensation reaction

Like peptide chains, a nucleic acid chain has also orientation: its 5' end contains a free phosphate group, while 3' end contains a free hydroxyl group. Synthesis of a nucleic acid chain always proceeds from 5' to 3'. Therefore, unless specified otherwise, the sequence of a nucleic acid chain is written from 5' to 3' (left to right).

In DNA or RNA, a nucleic acid chain is also called a strand. A DNA molecule typically contains two strands, whereas most RNA molecules contain a single strand. The length of a nucleic acid chain is represented by the number of bases. In the case of a double-stranded nucleic acid, bases are paired between two strands. Therefore, its length is given by the number of base pairs (bp). 1 kb = 1000 base pair; 1 Mb = 1 million bases. Oligonucleotides refer to short nucleic acid chains (< 50 bases or bp) while polynucleotides have longer chains.

3.18.3. Deoxyribonucleic Acid

Deoxyribonucleic Acid (DNA) is the genetic material found in the cells of all living organisms. DNA is the fundamental molecule which carries the genetic instructions used in the development and functioning of all known living organisms and some viruses. The main role of DNA molecules is the long-term storage of information. DNA is often compared to a set of blueprints or a recipe, or a code, since it contains the instructions needed to construct other components of cells, such as proteins and RNA molecules. The DNA segments that carry the genetic information are called genes, but other DNA sequences have structural purposes, or are involved in regulating the use of genetic information.

Oswald Avery and colleagues in 1944 demonstrated that bacterial DNA was likely the genetic agent that carried information from one organism to another in a process called "transformation". On the basis of careful analysis of DNA from many sources, Erwin Chargaff found that the composition of DNA is species specific. In addition, he found that the amount of adenine (A) always equaled the amount of thymine (T), while the amount of guanine (G) always equaled the amount of cytosine (C), regardless of the DNA source, known as Chargaff's rule. In a second critical study, Alfred Hershey and Martha Chase showed that when a bacterium is infected and genetically transformed by a virus, at least 80% of the viral DNA enters in the bacterial cell and at least 80% of the viral protein remains outside. Together with the Chargaff findings this work established that DNA is the repository of the unique genetic characteristics of an organism.

3.18.3.1. The DNA- Double Helix

DNA is usually a double-helix and has two strands running in opposite directions. There are some examples of viral DNAs which are single-stranded. Each strand has a backbone made up of (deoxy-ribose) sugar molecules linked together by phosphate groups. All DNA strands are read from the 5' to the 3' end where the 5' end terminates in a phosphate group and the 3' end terminates in a sugar molecule.

In the double-stranded DNA, the A-T base-pair has 2 hydrogen bonds and the G-C base-pair has 3 hydrogen bonds. The G-C interaction is therefore stronger (by about 30%) than A-T. The bases are oriented perpendicular to the helix axis. They are hydrophobic in the direction perpendicular to the plane of the bases (can not form hydrogen bonds with water). The interaction energy between two bases in a double-helical structure is therefore a combination of hydrogen-bonding between complementary bases and hydrophobic interactions between the neighboring stacks of base-pairs (Fig. 3.25).

The backbone of polynucleotides is highly charged (1 unit negative charge for each phosphate group; 2 negative charges per base-pair). If there is no salt in the surrounding medium, there is a strong repulsion between the two strands and they will fall apart. Therefore, counter-ions are essential for the double-helical structure. Counter-ions shield the charges on the sugar-phosphate backbone.

The most common DNA structure in solution is the B-DNA (Fig.3.26). The two strands form a "double helix" structure, was first discovered by James D. Watson and Francis Crick in 1953. In this structure, the B form, the helix makes a turn every 3.4 nm (34A°), and the distance between two neighboring base pairs is 0.34 nm (3.4A°). Hence, there are about 10 pairs per turn. The intertwined strands make two grooves of different widths, referred to as the major groove and the minor groove, which may facilitate binding with specific proteins. The major groove is approximately 50% wider than the minor. Proteins that interact with DNA often make contact with the edges of the base pairs that protrude into the major groove. The chemical groups on the edges of GC and AT base pairs are those available for interaction in the major and minor grooves.

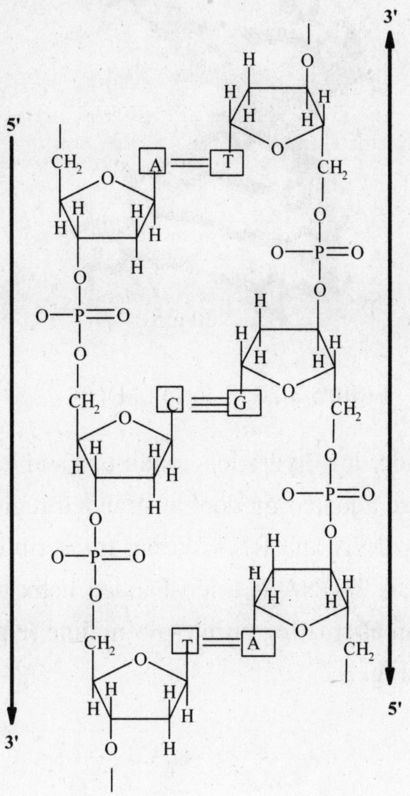

Figure 3.25: Schematic representation of double-stranded DNA

DNA can adopt several other conformations under conditions of applied force or twists, under low hydration conditions (Table 3.2). In a solution with higher salt concentrations or with alcohol added, the DNA structure may change to an 'A' form, which is still right-handed, but every 2.3 nm makes a turn and there are 11 base pairs per turn. Another DNA structure is called the Z form, because its bases seem to as zigzag. Z DNA is left-handed (Fig. 3.27). One turn spans 4.6 nm, comprising of 12 base pairs. The DNA molecule with alternating G-C sequences in alcohol or high salt solution tends to have such structure.

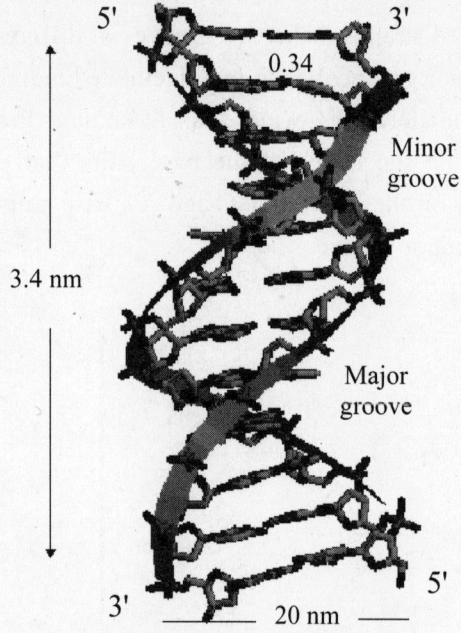

Figure 3.26: B form of DNA

The A-form crystallizes under low hydration conditions and is not normally found in the cell. It is, however, the structure adopted by double-stranded regions in RNA as well as the transient double-helix between DNA and RNA during transcription. Both A- and B-DNA are right-handed helices whereas Z-DNA is a left-handed helix and is commonly found in the regions of DNA that have an alternating purine-pyrimidine (e.g. 5'-CGCGCGCG-3' or 5'-CGCGCATGC-3') sequences (Fig. 3.27).

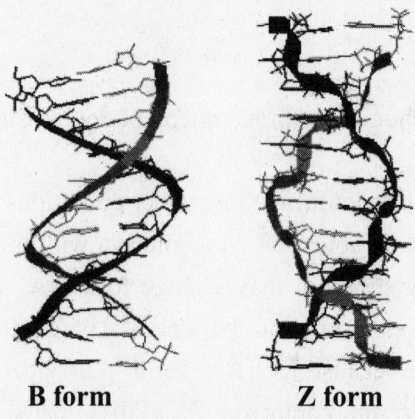

B form   **Z form**

Figure 3.27: Z form of DNA

Table 3.2: Major forms of DNA

Characteristics	A DNA	B DNA	Z DNA
Orientation	Right-handed helix	Right-handed	Left-handed
Shape	Short and broad	Long and thin	Longer and thinner
Helix Diameter	25.5A	23.7A	18.4A
Rise / base-pair	2.3A	3.4A	3.8 A
Base-pair / helical	~11	~10	~12
Helix pitch	25A	34A	47A
Tilt of the bases	20 deg	-1 deg	-9 deg

The coding regions (the genes) in the DNA strand make up represent only a fraction of the total amount of DNA. The stretches that flank the coding regions are called introns, and consist of non-coding DNA. Introns were considered as junk in the early days. Today, biologists and geneticists believe that this non-coding DNA may be essential in order to expose the coding regions and to regulate how the genes are expressed.

3.18.3.2. Chromatin

DNA is found associated with histones and non-histone proteins, to form the chromatin. There are 3×10^9 nucleotide pairs in the human haploid genome, representing about 30,000 genes dispersed over 23 chromosomes for a haploid set.

Histones are the major proteins of chromosomes, containing a high proportion of basic amino acids (arginine and lysine) that facilitate binding to the negatively charged DNA molecule. In addition, chromatin contains an approximately equal mass of a wide variety of nonhistone chromosomal proteins. Histones are not found in eubacteria (e.g., *E. coli*), although the DNA of these bacteria is found associated with other proteins that presumably function like histones to pack the DNA within the bacterial cell. Archaebacteria, however, do contain histones that package their DNAs in structures similar to eukaryotic chromatin. The packaging of DNA into nucleosomes yields a chromatin fiber approximately 10 nm in diameter (Fig. 3.28). The chromatin is further condensed by coiling into a 30-nm fiber, containing about six nucleosomes per turn.

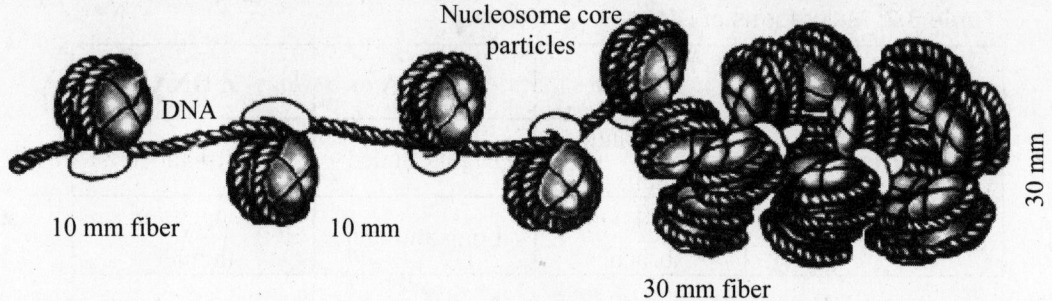

Figure 3.28: Chromatin fibers

Chromatin is found in two varieties: euchromatin and heterochromatin. Originally, the two forms are distinguished cytologically by how intensely they stained - the former is less intense, while the latter stains intensely, indicating their tighter packing. Heterochromatin is usually localized to the periphery of the nucleus.

(a) Heterochromatin

Heterochromatin is a tightly packed form of DNA. Its major characteristic is that the transcription is limited; it is a means to control gene expression, through regulation of the transcription initiation. Heterochromatin is a genetically inactive region of chromomosomes that either lack genes or contain genes that are repressed and replicates in S phase of the cell cycle and is found only in eukaryotes. In some organisms heterochromatin can also be identified by association with small RNA molecules or high levels of DNA methylation. The histone tails can be modified in various ways (including acetylation, methylation, ubiquitination, poly-ADP-ribosylation and phosphorylation), and these modifications are believed to serve as signals as to whether a region will be packed into silent heterochromatin or will remain active as euchromatin. In some organisms heterochromatin can also be identified in association with small RNA molecules or high levels of DNA methylation.

Heterochromatin is believed to serve several functions, from gene regulation to the protection of the integrity of chromosomes; For example, naked double-stranded DNA ends would usually be interpreted by the cell as damaged DNA, triggering cell cycle arrest and DNA repair. However, telomeres, which act as constant triggers of a DNA damage response, are shielded from the DNA damage machinery, as they are packed into heterochromatin.

(b) Euchromatin

Euchromatin comprises the most active portion of the genome within the cell nucleus and found in both eukaryotes and prokaryotes. It is a lightly packed form of chromatin, and is often under active transcription. The lighter staining of euchromatin is due to the less compact structure. It contains structural genes which replicate and transcribe during G1 and S phase of interphase. In particular, it is believed that the presence of methylated lysine on the histone tails acts as a general marker for euchromatin. In prokaryotes, euchromatin is the only form of chromatin present, which indicates that the heterochromatin structure evolved later along with the nucleus.

3.18.4. Ribonucleic Acid (RNA)

Ribonucleic acids are a class of nucleic acids characterized by the presence of the sugar ribose and the organic base uracil instead of thymine as in DNA. Most RNA molecules, including messenger RNA and transfer RNA, act as cellular intermediaries; that is, they convert the genetic information stored in DNA into the proteins. In some viruses, RNA also serves as the hereditary material. It is transcribed from DNA by enzymes called RNA polymerases and further processed by other enzymes. The enzyme progresses along the template strand in the 3' -> 5' direction, synthesizing a complementary RNA molecule with elongation occurring in the 5' -> 3' direction. The DNA sequence also dictates where termination of RNA synthesis will occur. RNA, unlike DNA, is also found in other parts of the cell other than the nucleus. In fact, the majority of the RNA is present in the cytoplasm in various forms. Nuclear RNA is comprised of single-stranded sequences (DNA is double stranded) and has a lower molecular weight than DNA (Fig. 3.29).

The structure of RNA is almost similar to that of DNA but with a slight difference. The structural difference with DNA is that the RNA contains a -OH group both at the 2' and 3' position of the ribose ring, whereas DNA (which stands, in fact, for deoxy-RNA) lacks such a hydroxy group at the 2' position of the ribose. The same bases can be attached to the ribose group in RNA as occur in DNA, with the exception that in RNA thymine does not occur, and is replaced by uracil, which has an H-group instead of a methyl group at the C-5 position of the thymine. Uracil is energetically less expensive to produce than thymine, which may account for its use in RNA. Thus, uracil is appropriate for RNA, where quantity is important but lifespan is not, whereas thymine is appropriate for DNA where maintaining sequence with high fidelity is more critical.

According to the "RNA world" hypothesis, RNA must have come before the first proteins, since without it there would have been no molecule of heredity and therefore no way for other molecules to have been manufactured consistently. RNA alone handled all of the tasks required for a cell to survive, acting both as a genetic material and a catalyst for the various reactions involved in metabolism and for its own assembly. Ribozymes, the catalytic RNA, that can act as their own enzymes, snipping themselves in two and splicing themselves back together. One possibility is that they are used to replicate RNA. Protoribosomes may have taken small strands of RNA from their surroundings and cut and pasted those which matched their template into a new, duplicate strand.

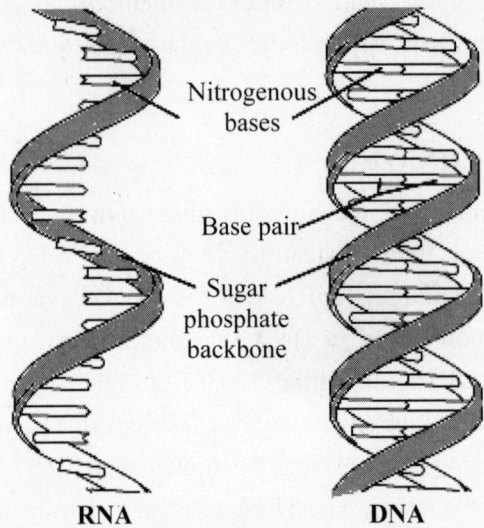

RNA   DNA

Figure 3.29: Structure of RNA

Unlike DNA, whose primary role is to store the genetic information, RNA plays many roles in the cell. RNA is structurally much more flexible than DNA because it is usually a mixture of single-stranded and duplex regions rather than predominantly duplex. The presence of the 2'-hydroxyl chemical group also makes RNA chemically more labile and not generally suitable as a molecule for storage of large amounts of genetic information over long periods of time. RNA is readily cleaved in alkaline conditions and in the presence of divalent metal ions, both of which deprotonate the 2' hydroxyl group, which then attacks the phosphate esterified at the 3' position, resulting in chain scission and a 2',3' cyclic phosphodiester terminal group.

Single-stranded regions of RNA are also very susceptible to attack by ribonucleases in the cell. Many RNAs, especially messenger RNAs, have a life time less than one cell division. This short life time is essential for cells to respond to changing environmental conditions. Other RNAs, such as ribosomal RNAs, tRNAs and small nuclear RNAs have considerable secondary structure and some are protected by complexes with proteins, stabilizing them further.

The three main functionally distinct varieties of RNA molecules are: (1) messenger RNA (mRNA) which is involved in the transmission of DNA information, (2) ribosomal RNA (rRNA) which makes up the physical machinery of the synthetic process, and (3) transfer RNA (tRNA) which also constitutes another functional part of the machinery of protein synthesis.

3.18.4.1. Types of RNA

(a) Messenger RNA (mRNA)

Messenger RNA is RNA that carries information from DNA to the ribosome sites of protein synthesis in the cell. Once mRNA has been transcribed from DNA, it is exported from the nucleus into the cytoplasm (in eukaryotes mRNA is "processed" before being exported), where it is bound to ribosomes and translated into protein and get degraded into its component nucleotides, usually with the assistance of RNases.

As we know the information that mRNA carries is written in genetic code - a sequence of bases. Each code word is called a codon, a sequence of three adjacent nucleotides that specifies one of the twenty amino acids. There are 64 possible codons ($4 \times 4 \times 4$), and each codon codes for an amino acid. More than one codon can code for the same amino acid. For example, GGU, GGC, GGA, and GGG all code for the amino acid glycine. The codon AUG is the start codon and UAA, UAG, and UGA act as the end codon, codons which specify the end of a protein synthesis.

The mRNA in both prokaryotic and eukaryotic cells (Fig. 3.30) has three distinct regions, the 5' Leader, gives physical space to ribosomes so that they can bind to mRNA and move down to the initiation codon, the coding region, is the part of mRNA that actually codes for the protein - the codons and 3′ trailer, which is simply a section that comes after the stop codons. In eukaryotes, mRNA that has just been transcribed from DNA must undergo two post-transcriptional modifications before it can be translated. First is capping, a special methylated version of triphosphate guanine nucleoside is added to the 5' end and addition of a poly-A-tail, a series of 50–150 adenine nucleotides, is added to the 3' end. It helps in the transportation of the mRNA out of the nucleus and determines the number of times mRNA can be translated before it is degraded. Prokaryotic mRNA lacks the methylated cap and the poly-a-tail, and there are no introns so it can be translated right after being transcribed.

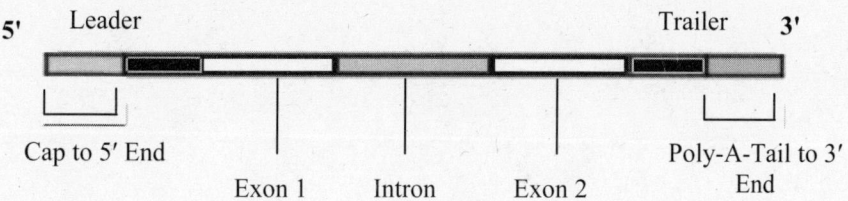

Figure 3.30: Schematic representation of structure of eukaryotic mRNA

Eukaryotic mRNA has regions which do not code for proteins (Fig. 3.30). These regions are called intervening sequences or introns. Regions which do code for something are called exons. After the primary mRNA transcript is produced, introns must be identified and re-moved by splicing with the aid of splicesomes, large RNA-protein complexes that contain many different enzymes and several kinds of RNA so that only exons remain. It is accomplished in the nucleus of a cell splicesomes which contain a short piece of RNA that complements base sequences found at either end of just about every intron.

(b) Transfer RNA (tRNA)

Transfer RNA is a small RNA chain of about 74–93 nucleotides that transfers a specific amino acid to a growing polypeptide chain at the ribosomal site of protein synthesis during translation. It has sites for amino-acid attachment and an anticodon region for codon recognition that binds to a specific sequence on the messenger RNA chain through hydrogen bonding. It is a type of non-coding RNA. The approximate shape of tRNA is known as clover leaf model, since tRNA has 3 loops and one stem (Fig. 3.31).

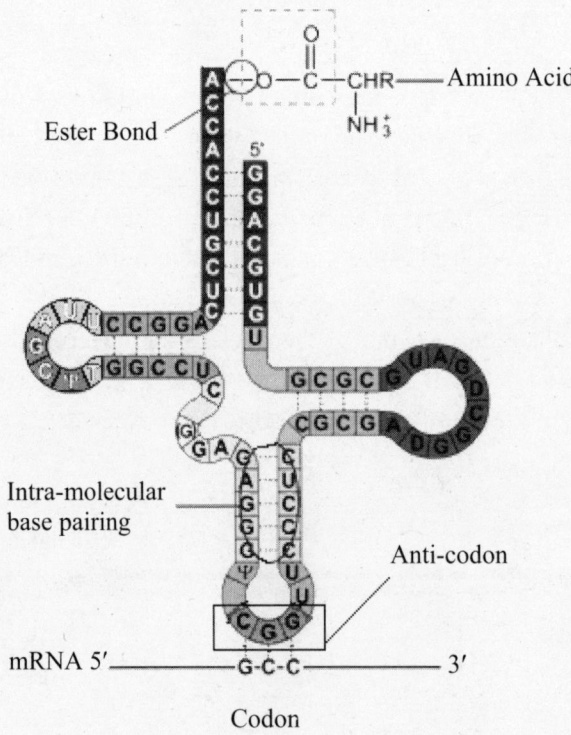

Figure 3.31: Structure of tRNA

One end of the tRNA contains an anticodon loop which pairs with mRNA specifying a certain amino acid. The other end of the tRNA has the amino acid attached to the 3' OH group via an ester linkage. tRNA with an attached amino acid is said to be "charged". The enzyme that attaches the amino acid to the 3'-OH is called an aminoacyl tRNA synthetase. There is a specific tRNA for each amino acid, which are 20 in all.

Only the first 2 nucleotides in the tRNA anticodon loop are strictly required for the decoding of the mRNA codon into an amino acid. The third nucleotide in the anticodon is less stringent in its base-pairing to the codon, and is referred to as the "wobble" base, and the phenomenon is known as wobble hypothesis. Since the genetic code is degenerate, meaning that more than one codon can specify a single amino acid, the anticodon of tRNA can pair with more than one mRNA codon and still be specific for a single amino acid.

(c) Ribosomal RNA (rRNA)

Ribosomal RNA (rRNA) is a component of the ribosomes, the protein synthetic factories in the cell. Eukaryotic ribosomes contain four different rRNA molecules: 18S, 5.8S, 28S, and 5S rRNA, where 'S' is the sedimentation coefficient (Svedberg unit) or density unit that is used in describing the results of ultracentrifugation and reflects the size and shape of a molecule or a particle ($1S = 1 \times 10^{-13}$ cm/sec/dyne). The larger the value of S, the bigger the particle is. Three of the rRNA molecules are synthesized in the nucleolus, and one is synthesized elsewhere. rRNA molecules are extremely abundant. They make up at least 80% of the RNA molecules found in a typical eukaryotic cell. rRNA forms the skeleton of ribosomes. The remainder of the ribosomes is comprised of proteins made in the cytoplasm. They enter the nucleus and then the nucleolus and finally join rRNA. The assembly of ribosomes is completed in the cytoplasm (Fig. 3.32).

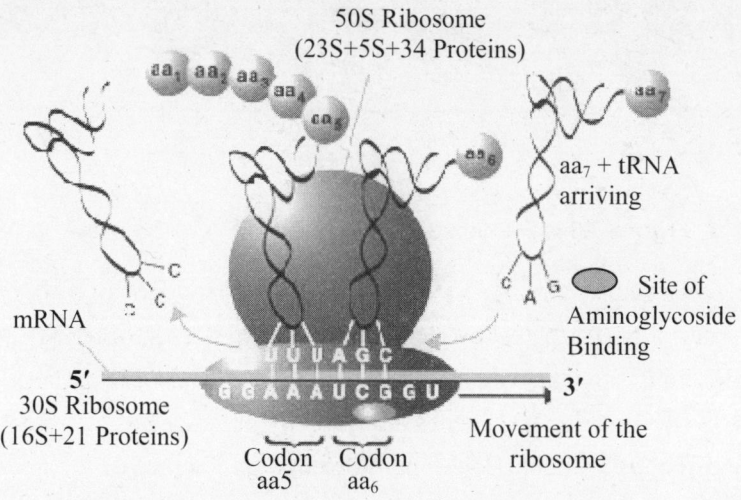

Figure 3.32: Representation of eukaryotic ribosome

Ribosomes have specific attachment sites that allow tRNA molecules and mRNA to be in the proper close contact that they require to synthesize proteins. Two of these sites are tRNA pockets called the P site and the A site. The other sites are mRNA grooves. There is also a site where an enzyme called peptidyl transferase works to form bonds between adjacent amino acids.

In eukaryotic cells ribosomes have two parts (subunit): 60 S and 40 S. The 60 S subunit contains the 28 S rRNA, the 5.8 S rRNA, the 5 S rRNA, and around 45 to 50 different proteins. The 40 S subunit contains the 18 S rRNA and around 30 different proteins. The final total size of the completed ribosome is around 80 S where half of the mass is consisted of proteins.

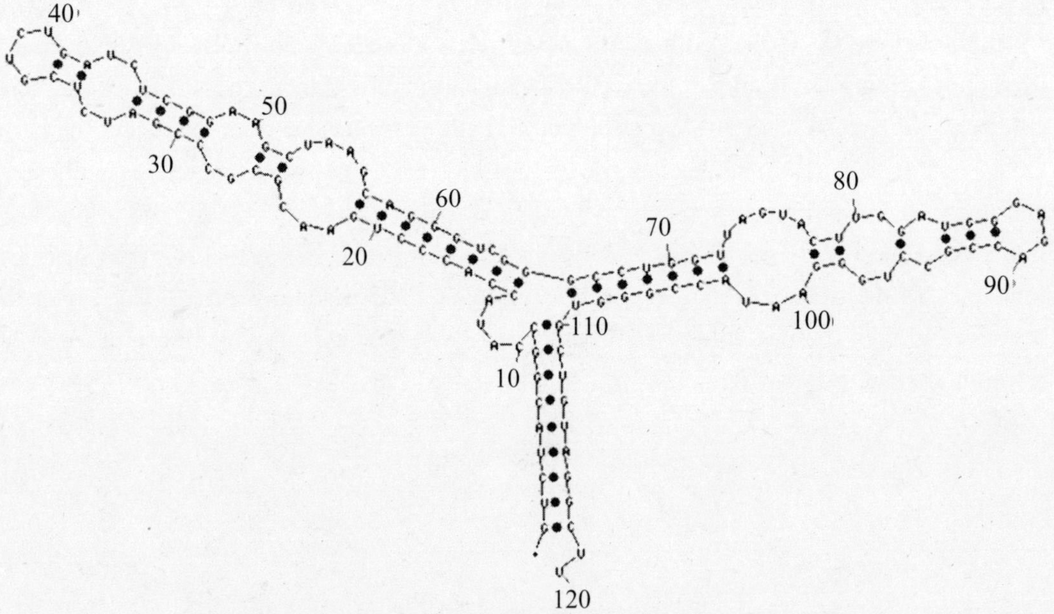

Figure 3.33: Predicted 2° structure for *E. coli* 5S rRNA

In prokaryotes, a small 30S ribosomal subunit contains the 16S rRNA, while the large 50S ribosomal subunit contains two rRNA species (the 5S and 23S rRNAs). The bacterial 16S, 23S, and 5S rRNA (Fig. 3.33) genes are typically organized as a co-transcribed operon. Archaea contains either a single rDNA operon or multiple copies of the operon. The 3' end of the 16S rRNA (in a ribosome) binds to a sequence on the 5' end of mRNA called the Shine-Dalgarno sequence.

(d) Heterogenous Nuclear RNA - hnRNA

Heterogenous nuclear RNA is defined as all nuclear RNA, excluding rRNA having a sedimentation coefficient greater than 8S (Weinberg, 1973). Eukaryote cells synthesize heterogenous nuclear RNA (hnRNA) which has been considered to be the precursor of mRNA. Only some hnRNA, however, serves as precursor of mRNA. Most of the hnRNA synthesized in eukaryote cells is rapidly degraded without becoming mRNA. Ribosomal RNA from mammalian cells has a high G + C content, while the G+C content of hnRNA is considered quite low. About 20–40% of hnRNA molecules are polyadenylated in mammlian cells.

(e) Small nuclear RNA (snRNA)

snRNA consists of short RNA transcripts of 100–300 bp, it associates with proteins to form small nuclear ribonucleoprotein particles (snRNPs) which participate in RNA processing. Small nuclear RNA (snRNA) is the name used to refer to a number of small RNA molecules found in the nucleus. These RNA molecules are important in a number of processes including RNA splicing (removal of the introns from hnRNA) and maintenance of the telomeres, or chromosome ends. They are always found associated with specific proteins and the complexes are referred to as small nuclear ribonucleoproteins (SNRNP) or sometimes as snurps.

(f) Small nucleolar RNA (snoRNA)

As the name suggests, these small (60–300 nts) RNAs are found in the nucleolus where they are responsible for several functions: Some participate in making ribosomes by helping to cut up the large RNA precursor of the 28S, 18S, and 5.8S molecules. Others chemically modify many of the nucleotides in rRNA, tRNA, and snRNA molecules, e.g., by adding methyl groups to ribose. One snoRNA serves as the template for the synthesis of telomeres. In vertebrates, the snoRNAs are made up of introns which are removed during RNA processing.

(g) Micro RNAs (miRNAs)

They are found in all animals (humans have more than 600 miRNA genes) and plants but not in fungi. It contains 19–25 nucleotides. They may be expressed in only certain cell types and at only certain times in the differentiation of a particular cell type. In repression of mRNA translation probably several miRNAs bind simultaneously in the 3'-UTR region.

Architects behind the Discovery of DNA

A primary technique for structural analysis of biological molecule is X-ray crystallography. The wavelength of X-rays is about the same as the space between the atoms in crystalline matter. Deflected X-rays can give an image pattern on a photographic plate, whose angles when analyzed mathematically can lead to the details of each atoms arranged with respect to the other atoms.

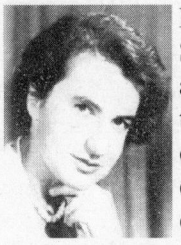

Rosalind Elise Franklin was born in 1920 in London and attended St. Paul's Girls School where she excelled in science, mathematics, and athletics. In 1938, she was awarded a scholarship in physics and chemistry to attend Cambridge University where she undertook studies in X-ray crystallography. After earning her Ph.D. and publishing seminal papers on coal she took a job offer in one of the best labs in Paris. She was a good experimenter, perfected her X-ray techniques, and published, spoke at conferences, and was well liked by her peers. It has been reported that she was a fashion-minded lady of Paris wearing Dior and socializing as a chef for her friends. After 4 years in Paris she decided at 30 years of age to return to London. She was hired by J.T. Randall, Director of King's College biophysics labs, to create an X-ray unit and work on DNA.

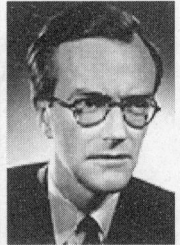

Maurice Wilkins, the assumed overseer of the King's College lab, had in 1951 taken the first X-ray pictures of DNA that led him to suggest the DNA structure might be a helix (similar to just announced Linus Pauling alpha helical structure of proteins). The atmosphere at King's was akin to an old boy's club (the lunch room was from men only) which lead to conflict. In addition, Randall did not clearly delineate a chain of command, and though he had hired Franklin as director of the X-ray lab, Wilkins, who was away when Franklin was hired, believed himself to be in charge.

Rudolf Signer, a Swiss chemist had isolated some quality calf thymus DNA, which he gave in a "jelly jar" to Maurice Wilkins at a scientific meeting sometime in 1951. At the time this was the... " best sample of DNA in the world". Franklin was given Signer's DNA by the King's College biophysics lab director, J.T. Randall.

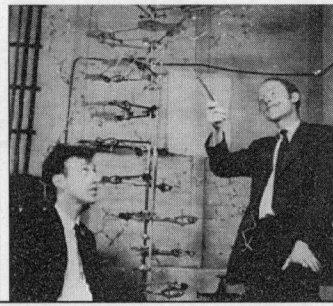

Watson and Crick pursued model building, using balls and sticks. Their first model was a triple helix with the bases pointed outward. However, chemically it wouldn't hold itself together, thus they knew it was incorrect.

At the age of 38 (1958) Rosalind Franklin died of ovarian cancer, probably due to constant exposure to X-rays. In 1962 Francis Crick, James Watson, and Maurice Wilkins shared the Nobel prize.

3.19. Bioenergetics

3.19.1. Energy

Energy is the capacity of a physical system to perform work and it is one of the most fundamental and universal concepts of physical science, but it is remarkably difficult to define in a way that is meaningful to most people. This perhaps reflects the fact that energy is not a "thing" that exists by itself, but is rather an attribute of matter (and also of electromagnetic radiation) that can manifest itself in different ways. It can be observed and measured only indirectly through its effects on matter that acquires, loses, or possesses it.

Basically the energy is of two kinds: kinetic and potential. Kinetic energy is associated with the motion of an object; a body with a mass m and moving at a velocity v possesses the kinetic energy $mv^2/2$. The potential energy is the energy possessed by a body by virtue of its location in a force field— a gravitational, electrical, or magnetic field. For example, when an object of mass m is raised to a height h, its potential energy increases by mgh, where g is a proportionality constant known as the acceleration of gravity.

Energy is measured in terms of its ability to perform work or to transfer heat. Mechanical work is done when a force F displaces an object by a distance d: $w = f \times d$. The basic unit of energy is the Joule. One Joule is the amount of work done when a force of 1 Newton acts over a distance of 1 m; thus 1 J = 1 N-m. The Newton is the amount of force required to accelerate a 1-kg mass by 1 m/sec^2 (1 cal = 4.184 J).

Before dealing with thermodynamics we must be very precise about certain terms. The two most important features of these are system and surroundings. A thermodynamic system is that part of the world, which is under study. Everything that is not a part of the system constitutes the surroundings. The system and surroundings are separated by a boundary. If our system is one mole of a gas in a container, then the boundary is simply the inner wall of the container itself. The boundary need not be a physical barrier. If matter is not able to pass across the boundary, then the system is said to be closed; otherwise, it is open. A closed system may still exchange energy with the surroundings unless the system is an isolated one, in which neither matter nor energy can pass across the boundary. The tea in a closed thermos bottle approximates a closed system over a short time interval.

In dealing with thermodynamics, one must be able to unambiguously define the change in the state of a system when it undergoes some process. This is done by specifying changes in the values of the different state properties using the symbol Δ (delta) as illustrated here for a change in the volume:

$$\Delta V = V_{final} - V_{initial}$$

3.19.2. Gibbs Free Energy (ΔG) and Spontaneity of a Chemical Reaction

Gibbs free energy is the measures of "useful" or process-initiating work obtainable from an isothermal, isobaric thermodynamic system. It is the maximum amount of non-expansion work that can be extracted from a closed system; this maximum can be attained only in a completely reversible process. When a system changes from a well-defined initial state to a well-defined final state, the Gibbs free energy ΔG equals the work exchanged by the system with its surroundings. The free energy change (ΔG) of a reaction determines its spontaneity. A reaction is spontaneous if ΔG is negative (if the free energy of the products is less than the free energy of the reactants).

For a reaction $A + B \leftrightarrow C + D$

$$\Delta G = \Delta G^0 + RT \ln \left(\frac{[C][D]}{[A][B]} \right)$$

Where ΔG= change in free energy, ΔG$^{o'}$ = standard free energy change (with 1 M reactants and products, at pH 7), R = gas constant, T = absolute temperature

At equilibrium, ΔG equals zero. Solving for ΔG$^{o'}$ yields the relationship at left.

K'_{eq}, the ratio [C][D]/[A][B] at equilibrium, is called the equilibrium constant.

$$0 = \Delta G^0 + RT \ln \left(\frac{[C][D]}{[A][B]} \right)$$

$$\Delta G^0 = -RT \ln \left(\frac{[C][D]}{[A][B]} \right) \quad \text{But} \left(\frac{[C][D]}{[A][B]} \right) = K'_{eq}$$

$$\Delta G^0 = -RT \ln K'_{eq}$$

The standard free energy change (ΔG$^{o'}$) of a reaction may be positive and the actual free energy change (ΔG) negative, depending on cellular concentrations of reactants and products. Many reactions for which ΔG$^{o'}$ is positive are spontaneous because other reactions cause depletion of products or maintenance of high substrate concentrations.

An equilibrium constant greater than one, (more products than reactants at equilibrium) indicates a spontaneous reaction (negative ΔG$^{o'}$). Free energy changes of coupled reactions are additive. Examples of different types of coupling:

Type 1: Some enzyme-catalyzed reactions can be expressed in two coupled half-reactions, one spontaneous and the other non-spontaneous. The free energy changes of the half-reactions may be added, to yield the free energy of the coupled reaction. For example, in the reaction catalyzed by the Glycolysis enzyme Hexokinase, the two half-reactions are:

$ATP + H_2O \leftrightarrow ADP + Pi \qquad \Delta G^{o'} = $ -31 kJoules/mol $\rightarrow$ (1)

$P_i + glucose \leftrightarrow glucose\text{-}6\text{-}P + H_2O \qquad \Delta G^{o'} = $ +14 kJoules/mol $\rightarrow$ (2)

Coupled reaction: (1) + (2)

$ATP + glucose \leftrightarrow ADP + glucose\text{-}6\text{-}P \quad \Delta G^{o'} = (\text{-}31 + 14) = $ -17 kJoules/mol

Type 2: Two separate enzyme-catalyzed reactions occurring in the same cellular compartment, one spontaneous and the other non-spontaneous may be coupled by a common intermediate (reactant or product). For example, reactions involving pyrophosphates

$A + ATP \leftrightarrow B + AMP + PP_i \qquad \Delta G^{o'} = $ +15 kJ/mol $\rightarrow$ Enzyme 1

$PP_i + H_2O \leftrightarrow 2\,P_i \quad \Delta G^{o'} = $ –33 kJ/mol $\rightarrow$ Enzyme 2

Overall reaction $\quad A + ATP + H_2O \leftrightarrow B + AMP + 2P_i \qquad \Delta G^{o'} = (+15\text{-}33) = $ –18 kJ/mol

Pyrophosphate (PP_i) is often the product of a reaction that needs a driving force. Its spontaneous hydrolysis, catalyzed by pyrophosphatase enzyme, drives the reaction for which PP_i is a product.

Type 3: Active transport of ions through membrane is coupled to a chemical reaction, e.g., hydrolysis or synthesis of ATP, while the transports of an ion say A^+ creates a potential difference across the membrane. The free energy change (electrochemical potential difference) associated with transport of an ion A^+ across a membrane from side 1 to side 2 is represented as:

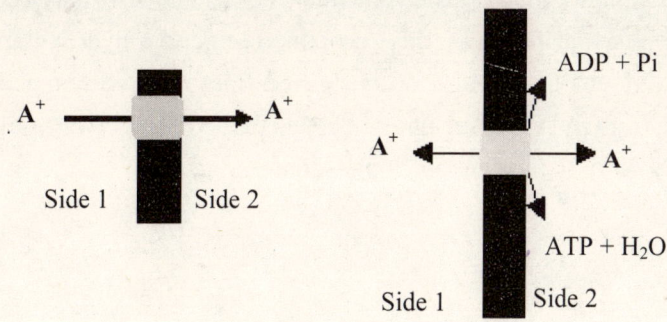

$$\Delta G = RT \ln \left(\frac{[S]_2}{[S]_1} \right) + ZF\Delta\psi$$

Where R = gas constant, T = temperature, Z = charge on the ion, F = Faraday constant, and $\Delta\psi$ = voltage across the membrane.

Each of our cells has an electric potential associated with it. This potential, or voltage, helps to control the migration of ions across the cell membranes. A major example of electrical work is in the operation of the nerves. The nerves when get stimulated, they generate an electrical impulse called an action potential which can communicate information to the brain, or carry a signal from brain to a muscle to initiate its movement.

Since free energy changes are additive, the spontaneous direction for the coupled reaction will depend on the relative magnitudes of ΔG for the ion flux (ΔG varies with the ion gradient and voltage) and ΔG for the chemical reaction ($\Delta G^{o'}$ is negative in the direction of ATP hydrolysis. The magnitude of ΔG also depends on the concentrations of ATP, ADP, and P_i). Two examples of such coupling are:

Active transport: The membrane transport requires energy or ATP. The spontaneous ATP hydrolysis (negative ΔG) is coupled to (drives) ion flux against a gradient (positive ΔG).

ATP synthesis: It takes place in mitochondria, which is also known as the power house of the cell and where the synthesis of ATP occurs. The spontaneous H^+ flux across a membrane (negative ΔG) is coupled to (drives) ATP synthesis (positive ΔG).

3.19.3. How energy is stored in ATP

Phosphoanhydride bonds, link the terminal phosphates (formed by the removal of water between two phosphoric acids or between a carboxylic acid and a phosphoric acid) tend to have a large negative ΔG of hydrolysis and are thus said to be "high energy" bonds.

"High energy" bonds are often represented by the "~" symbol (squiggle), with ~P representing a phosphate group with a high free energy of hydrolysis. Compounds with high energy bonds are said to have high group transfer potential. For example, P_i may be spontaneously removed from ATP for transfer to another compound (e.g., to a hydroxyl group on glucose). Potentially two "high energy" bonds can be cleaved from ATP, as two phosphates are released by hydrolysis from ATP (adenosine triphosphate), yielding ADP (adenosine diphosphate), and ultimately AMP (adenosine monophosphate) (Fig. 3.34).

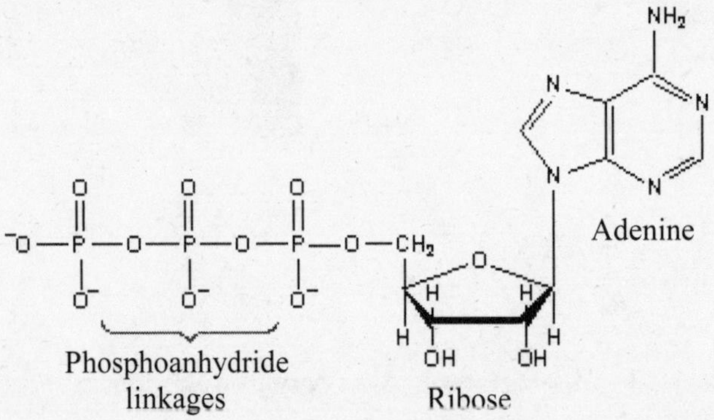

Figure 3.34: Structure of adenosine triphosphate (ATP)

When the third phosphate group of ATP is removed by hydrolysis, a substantial amount of free energy is released. The exact amount depends on the conditions, but generally uses a value of 7.3 kcal per mole. Thus, ATP often serves as an energy source, known as "energy currency of the cell". Another example for molecule containing "high energy" phosphate linkage is phosphocreatine (creatine phosphate), which is used in nerve and muscle cells for storage of ~P bonds. Phosphocreatine is produced when ATP levels are high. When ATP is depleted during exercise in muscle, phosphate is transferred from phosphocreatine to ADP, to replenish ATP.

Phosphocreatine

Creatine kinase catalyzes the chemical change: Phosphocreatine + ADP ☐ ATP + creatine. Phosphoenolpyruvate (PEP), involved in production of ATP in Glycolysis, has a larger negative ΔG of phosphate hydrolysis than ATP.

PEP   enolpyruvate   pyruvate

Removal of phosphate from the ester linkage in PEP is spontaneous because the enroll product spontaneously converts in to a ketone.

The ester linkage in PEP is an exception. Generally, phosphate esters, formed by splitting out water between a phosphoric acid and a hydroxyl group, have a low but negative ΔG of hydrolysis (Fig. 3.35). Thus, generally AMP is not further hydrolyzed in biochemical reactions for energy. The examples of such reactions include the linkage between the first phosphate and the ribose hydroxyl of ATP, the linkage between phosphate and a hydroxyl group in glucose-6-phosphate or glycerol-3-phosphate, the linkage between phosphate and the hydroxyl group of an amino acid residue in a protein (serine, threonine or tyrosine).

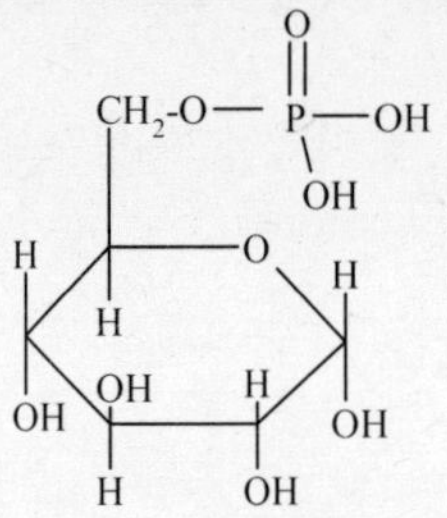

glucose-6-phosphate 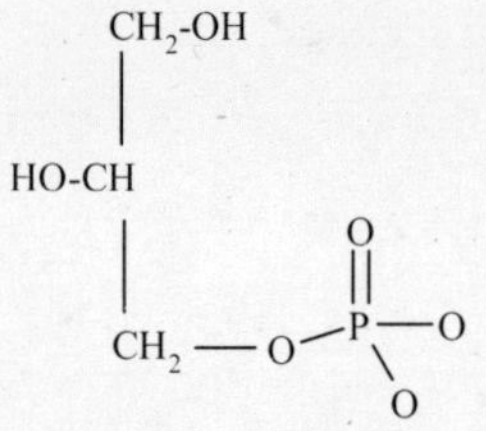   glycerol-3-phosphate

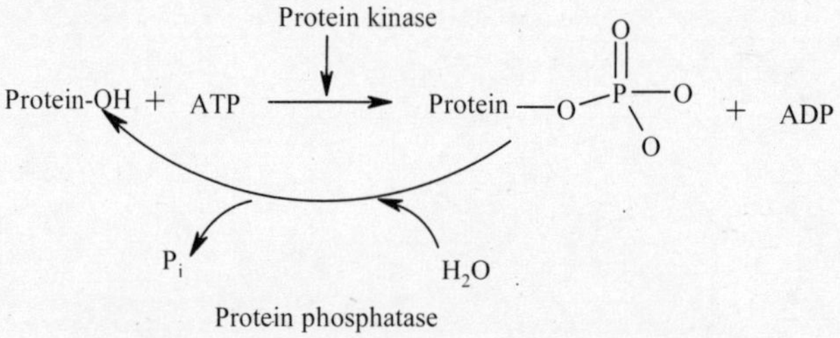

Figure 3.35: Reactions of protein kinases

ATP thus can act as a phosphate donor, and it can be synthesized by transfer of phosphate from other compounds, such as phosphoenolpyruvate (PEP). There are several other examples for molecules containing high energy bond, viz;

Coenzyme A: A thioester bond is formed between a carboxylic acid and a thiol (SH) group, and are of "high energy" linkages e.g., the thiol of coenzyme A (abbreviated CoA-SH). In contrast to phosphate esters, thioesters have a large negative ΔG of hydrolysis.

$$\text{Coenzyme A-SH} + \text{HO-}\overset{\overset{\text{O}}{\|}}{\text{C}}\text{-R} \rightleftharpoons \text{Coenzyme A-S-}\overset{\overset{\text{O}}{\|}}{\text{C}}\text{-R} + \text{H}_2\text{O}$$

The thiol of coenzyme A can react with a carboxyl group of acetic acid (yielding acetyl-CoA) or a fatty acid (yielding fatty acyl-CoA). The spontaneity of thioester cleavage is essential to the role of coenzyme A as an acyl group carrier. Like ATP, acyl-coenzyme A has a high group transfer potential.

$$\text{Coenzyme A-SH} + \text{HO-}\overset{\overset{\text{O}}{\|}}{\text{C}}\text{-CH}_3 \rightleftharpoons \text{Coenzyme A-S-}\overset{\overset{\text{O}}{\|}}{\text{C}}\text{-CH}_3 + \text{H}_2\text{O}$$
$$\text{(acetic acid)} \qquad\qquad\qquad \text{(acetyl CoA)}$$

Coenzyme A includes β-mercaptoethylamine, in amide linkage to the carboxyl group of the B vitamin pantothenate. The –OH group of pantothenate is in ester linkage to a phosphate of ADP-3'-phosphate. cAMP is an another molecule containing high energy bond.

SH
|
CH₂
|
CH₂   β-mercaptoethylamine
|
NH
|
C=O
|
CH₂
|
CH₂   Pantothenate
|
NH
|
C=O
|
HO—C—H
|
H₃C—C—CH₃
|
H₂C—O—P—O—P—O—CH₂

ADP-3`-phosphate

Coenzyme A   **cAMP**

3.19.4. Oxidation and Reduction Reactions

A chemical reaction can be defined as a change in which a substance (or substances) is changed into one or more new substances. In redox reactions both reduction and the oxidation processes go on side-by-side. The oxidation and reduction reactions can be explained in three different ways.

(a) On the basis of oxygen transfer: Oxidation is a gain of oxygen while reduction is loss of oxygen. For example,

$$C_6H_{12}O_6 + 3O_2 \underset{\text{Reduction}}{\overset{\text{Oxidation}}{\rightleftarrows}} 6CO_2 + 6H_2O$$

(b) In terms of hydrogen transfer: Oxidation is loss of hydrogen and reduction is gain of hydrogen

For example, ethanol can be oxidized to ethyl acetate

$$CH_3CH_2OH \xrightarrow{[O]} CH_3CHO + H_2O$$

(c) In terms of electron transfer: Oxidation is loss of electrons and reduction is gain of electrons.

For example

$$NAD^+ + 2\bar{e} + H^+ \xrightarrow{\text{Reduction}} NADH$$

3.19.5. NAD$^+$

Nicotinamide Adenine Dinucleotide functions as an electron acceptor in catabolic pathways. The nicotinamide ring of NAD$^+$, which is derived from the vitamin niacin, accepts 2 e$^-$ and one H$^+$ (a hydride) in going to the reduced state, as NAD$^+$ becomes NADH. NADP$^+$/NADPH is similar, except for an additional phosphate esterified to a hydroxyl group on the adenosine ribose. NADPH functions as an electron donor in synthetic pathways. NAD$^+$ is a coenzyme that reversibly binds to enzymes (Fig. 3.36).

The electron transfer reaction may be summarized as:

$$NAD^+ + 2\acute{e} + H^+ \rightarrow NADH \text{ also be written as } NAD^+ + 2\acute{e} + 2H^+ \rightarrow NADH + H^+$$

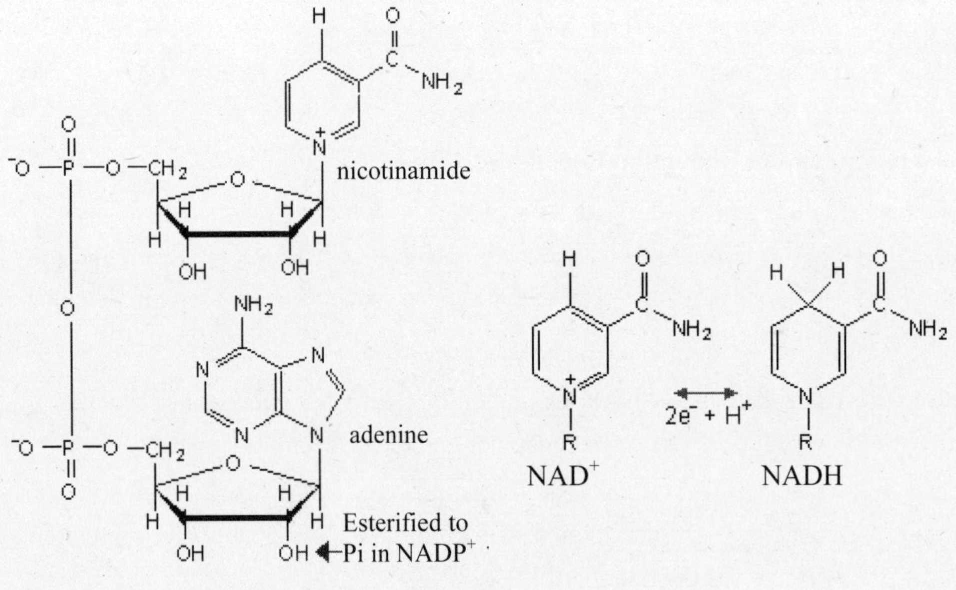

Nicotinamide Adenine Dinucleotide

Figure 3.36: Reactions of NAD

3.19.6. FAD

Flavin Adenine Dinucleotide also functions as an electron acceptor. The portion of FAD that undergoes reduction/oxidation is the dimethylisoalloxazine ring, derived from the vitamin riboflavin. FAD is a prosthetic group that usually remains tightly bound at the active site of an enzyme. FAD normally accepts 2 é and 2 H^+ in going to its reduced state (Fig.3.37):

$$FAD + 2\,é + 2\,H^+ \rightarrow FADH_2$$

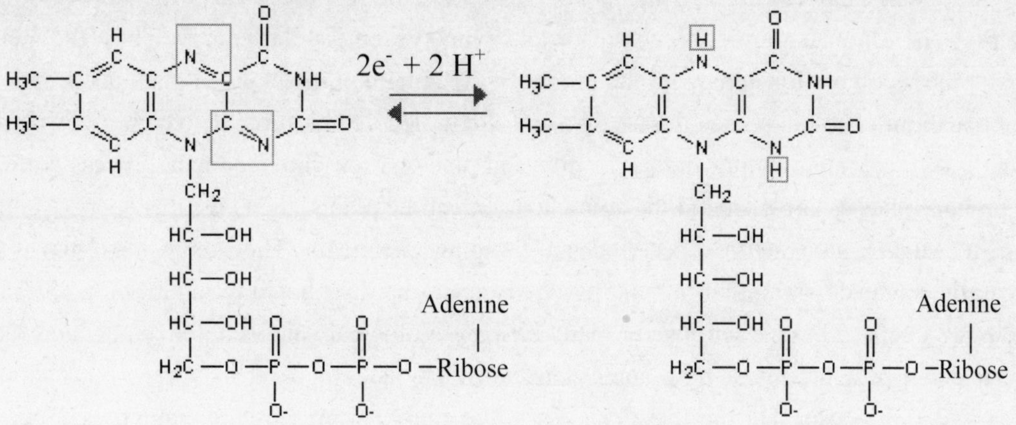

Figure 3.37: Reactions of FAD

3.20. Metabolism

The term metabolism is defined as 'the chemical processes by which nutritive material is built up into living matter, or by which complex molecules are broken down into simpler substances during the performance of special functions'. The various reactions which involve the synthesis of complex molecules are grouped under anabolism, whereas the breakdown of complex molecules is known as catabolism. Both anabolic and catabolic processes include a vast number of different chemical reactions, but there are number of common features. Most of the metabolic processes occur inside the cells of the body, mainly in the cytoplasm, but also inside intracellular organelles such as the mitochondria. Anabolic and catabolic reactions involve the action of enzymes and the utilization of energy.

Metabolism, a vital process for all life forms, is a constant process that begins when an organism being conceived and ends when it dies. In case the metabolism stops, results in death. The process of metabolism is really a balancing act involving two kinds of activities that go on at the same time the building up of body tissues and energy stores (anabolism or constructive metabolism) and the breaking down of energy stores to generate more fuel for body functions (catabolism or destructive metabolism) . Almost all of the chemical reactions in the living body require the expenditure of energy, which is made available mainly by the catabolism of the 'macronutrients' fats and carbohydrates (particularly glucose), and proteins (to a small extent). According to the law of conservation of energy, the total energy of a system remains constant, though energy may transform into another form. In the body's metabolism, the energy released from the oxidation of the macronutrients is used for a series of chemical reactions, instead of being released only as heat.

A fundamental feature of both anabolic and catabolic processes is the utilization of energy. The ultimate source of energy for all living system is solar energy. Thus, the metabolic process on earth begins with the producers, the plants. First, a green plant takes energy from sunlight. The plant uses this energy and the molecule chlorophyll (which gives plants their green color) to build sugars from water and carbon dioxide in a process known as photosynthesis. The men and the animals when eat the plants, they take this energy (in the form of sugar), along with other vital cell-building chemicals. The body's next step is to break the sugar down so that the energy released can be distributed to, and used as fuel by the body's cells. These reactions are made easy by biological catalysts, (enzymes) and they break down proteins into amino acids, fats into fatty acids and carbohydrates into simple sugars (e.g., glucose). During these processes, the energy from these compounds can be released by the body for use or stored in body tissues, especially the liver, muscles, and body fat. During anabolism, small molecules are changed into larger, more complex molecules of carbohydrate, protein and fat. First of all let us consider the synthesis of carbohydrates by plants i.e., the, photosynthesis.

3.20.1. Photosynthesis

Photosynthesis is the physico-chemical process by which producers of nature such as plants, algae and photosynthetic bacteria use light energy to drive the synthesis of organic compounds. This results in the release of molecular oxygen and the removal of carbon dioxide from the atmosphere that is used to synthesize carbohydrates. Photosynthesis provides the energy and reduces carbon required for the survival of virtually all life on our planet, as well as the molecular oxygen necessary for the survival of oxygen consuming organisms. Each year more than 10% of the total atmospheric carbon dioxide is reduced to carbohydrate by photosynthetic organisms.

The energy that drives photosynthesis originates in the center of the sun, where mass is converted to heat by the fusion of hydrogen. A small fraction of the visible light incident on the earth is absorbed by plants. Through a series of energy transducing reactions, photosynthetic organisms are able to transform light energy into chemical free energy in a stable form that can last for hundreds of millions of years (e.g., fossil fuels).

The overall process of photosynthesis is little bit complex, to produce a sugar molecule such as sucrose. The plants require nearly 30 distinct proteins that work within a complicated membrane structure. In plants, these energy factories are called chloroplasts, which collect energy from the sun and use carbon dioxide and water in the process called photosynthesis to produce sugars.

Animals can make use of the sugars provided by the plants in their own cellular energy factories, the mitochondria. The mitochondria produce a versatile energy currency in the form of adenosine triphosphate (ATP), the high-energy molecule. These molecules store enough immediately available energy to allow plants and animals to their necessary work.

Joseph Priestley (1770s) , an English chemist and clergyman showed that plants release oxygen, by his experiment placing a sprig of mint in the chamber and burning a candle in that closed vessel until the flame went out and after several days he showed that the candle could burn again. Later Jan Ingenhousz, a Dutch physician, demonstrated that sunlight was necessary for photosynthesis and that only the green parts of plants could release oxygen. During this period Jean Senebier, a Swiss botanist and naturalist, discovered that CO_2 is required for photosynthesis and Nicolas- de Saussure, a Swiss chemist and plant physiologist, showed that water is essential for photosynthesis. In 1845 Julius Robert von Mayer, a German physician and physicist proposed that photosynthetic organisms convert light energy into chemical free energy (Fig. 3.38).

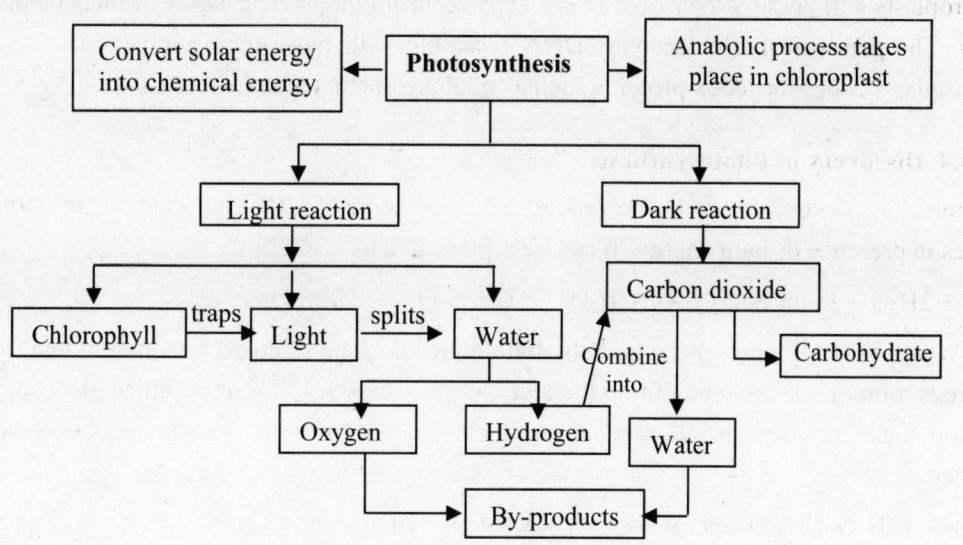

Figure 3.38: Photosynthetic process

3.20.2. Evolution of Photosynthetic Plants

In the beginning, the living systems, thought to had been anoxygenic, used various molecules as electron donors. Green and purple sulfur bacteria are thought to have used hydrogen and sulfur as an electron donor. The use of these molecules is consistent with the geological evidence that the atmosphere was highly reduced at that time or the concentration of oxygen was very low. The main source of oxygen in the atmosphere was oxygenic photosynthesis, and its first appearance is sometimes referred to as the oxygen catastrophe. Geological evidence suggests that oxygenic photosynthesis, such as that in cyanobacteria, became important during the Paleoproterozoic era around 2 billion years ago. Modern photosynthesis in plants and in most photosynthetic prokaryotes is oxygenic. Oxygenic photosynthesis uses water as an electron donor which is oxidized to molecular oxygen (O_2) in the photosynthetic reaction center.

3.20.3. Symbiosis and the Origin of Chloroplasts

Symbiosis is the close and often long-term interactions between different biological species. Chloroplasts have many similarities with photosynthetic bacteria including a circular chromosome, prokaryotic-type ribosomes, and similar proteins in the photosynthetic reaction center. The endosymbiotic theory suggests that photosynthetic bacteria were acquired (by endocytosis) by early eukaryotic cells to form the first plant cells. Therefore, chloroplasts may be photosynthetic bacteria that adapted to life inside plant cells, like mitochondria, chloroplasts still possess their own DNA, separate from the nuclear DNA of their plant host cells. The genes in this chloroplast DNA resemble with those of cyanobacteria. DNA in chloroplasts codes for redox proteins such as photosynthetic reaction centers.

3.20.4. Discovery of Photosynthesis

Chemically, photosynthesis is the process of conversion of CO_2 and water in to carbohydrates in presence of light energy. It can be represented as

$$CO_2 + 2H_2O + \text{Light Energy} \rightarrow [CH_2O] + O_2 + H_2O \quad \ldots\ldots\ldots (1)$$

Where [CH_2O] represents a carbohydrate molecule. The standard free energy needed for the reduction of one mole of CO_2 to the level of glucose is + 478 kJ/mol. Since glucose, a six carbon sugar, is often an intermediate product of photosynthesis. The net equation can be written as,

$$6CO_2 + 12H_2O + \text{Light Energy} \rightarrow C_6H_{12}O_6 + 6O_2 + 6H_2O \ldots\ldots (2)$$

The standard free energy for the synthesis of glucose is + 2,870 kJ/mol.

In 1930s Van Niel, proposed that photosynthesis depends on electron donation and acceptor reactions and that the O_2 released during photosynthesis comes from the oxidation of water and in some photosynthetic bacteria they could use hydrogen sulfide (H_2S) instead of water for photosynthesis and that they release sulfur instead of oxygen. Van Niel's generalized equation is:

$$CO_2 + 2H_2A + \text{Light energy} \rightarrow [CH_2O] + 2A + H_2O \ldots\ldots\ldots (3)$$

In oxygenic photosynthesis, 2A is O_2, whereas in anoxygenic photosynthesis, which occurs in some photosynthetic bacteria, the electron donor can be an inorganic hydrogen donor, such as H_2S (in which case A is elemental sulfur) or an organic hydrogen donor such as succinate (in which case, A is fumarate).

The biochemical conversion of CO_2 to carbohydrate is a reduction reaction that involves the rearrangement of covalent bonds between carbon, hydrogen and oxygen. The energy for the reduction of carbon is provided by energy rich molecules that are produced by the light driven electron transfer reactions. Carbon reduction can occur in the dark and involves a series of biochemical reactions that were elucidated by Melvin Calvin, Andrew Benson and James Bassham in the late 1940s and 1950s. The intermediate steps were traced by using the radioisotope ^{14}C. Calvin was awarded the Nobel prize for Chemistry in 1961 for this work.

In 1954 Daniel Arnon and coworkers discovered that plants and photosynthetic bacteria use light energy to produce ATP, an organic molecule that serves as an energy source for many biochemical reactions. Robert Emerson, Bessel Kok, L.N.M. Duysens, Robert Hill and Horst Witt, proved that plants, algae and cyanobacteria require two reaction centers, photo system II and photo system I, operating in series.

In 1961 Mitchell's proposal that energy is stored as an electrochemical gradient across a vesicular membrane, opened the door for understanding energy transformation by membrane systems. Most of the proteins required for the conversion of light energy and electron transfer reactions of photosynthesis are located in membranes. A key element in photosynthetic energy conversion is electron transfer within and between protein complexes and simple organic molecules. The electron transfer reactions are rapid (as fast as a few picoseconds) and highly specific. Much of our current understanding of the physical principles that guide electron transfer is based on the pioneering work of Rudolph A Marcus, who received the Nobel Prize in Chemistry in 1992 for his contributions to the theory of electron transfer reaction in chemical systems.

3.20.5. Photosynthetic Machinery

In plants, photosynthesis occurs mainly within the leaves. Since photosynthesis requires carbon dioxide, water, and sunlight, all of these substances must be obtained by or transported to the leaves. Carbon dioxide is obtained through tiny pores in plant leaves called stomata. Oxygen is also released through the stomata. Water is obtained by the plant through the roots and delivered to the leaves through vascular plant tissue systems.

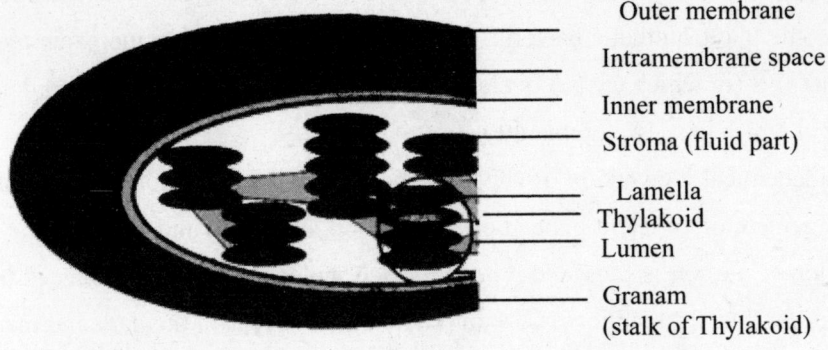

Outer membrane

Intramembrane space

Inner membrane
Stroma (fluid part)

Lamella
Thylakoid
Lumen

Granam
(stalk of Thylakoid)

Figure 3.39: Structure of chloroplast

Chlorophyll, is a green pigment located in structures called chloroplasts, the sites of photo-synthesis. Chloroplasts contain several structures, each having specific functions (Fig. 3.39):

Outer and inner membranes: protective coverings that keep chloroplast structures en-closed.

Stroma: dense fluid within the chloroplast, where the conversion of carbon dioxide to sugar, occurs.

Thylakoid: flattened sac-like membrane structures. It is the site of conversion of light en-ergy to chemical energy.

Grana: dense layered stacks of thylakoid sacs. It is the site of conversion of light energy to chemical energy.

Chlorophyll: a green pigment within the chloroplast (Fig. 3.40). It absorbs light energy.

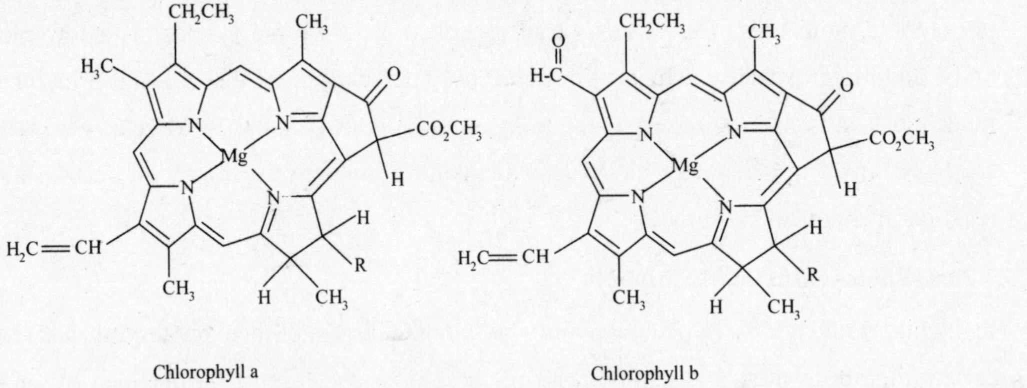

Chlorophyll a

Chlorophyll b

Where R= CH$_2$CH$_2$CO$_2$CH$_2$CH=C(CH$_2$CH$_2$CH$_2$CH)$_3$CH$_3$
CH$_3$ CH$_3$

Figure 3.40: Chemical structure of chlorophyll

Now, it is a question of interest, how these chlorophylls absorb light energy? Chlorophyll traps the light energy, hence called as photoreceptor. It is the green pigment found in plants. The basic structure of a chlorophyll molecule is a porphyrin ring, coordinated to a central atom. This is very similar in structure to the heme group found in hemoglobin, except that in heme the central atom is iron, whereas in chlorophyll it is magnesium. Light absorbed by chlorophyll excites the electrons in the ring. Different wavelengths of light excite the electrons by different amounts. Chlorophylls are very effective photoreceptors because they contain a network of alternating single and double bonds and the orbitals can delocalize the electrons and stabilize the structure. Such delocalized polyenes have very strong absorption bands in the visible regions of the spectrum, allowing the plant to absorb the energy from sunlight.

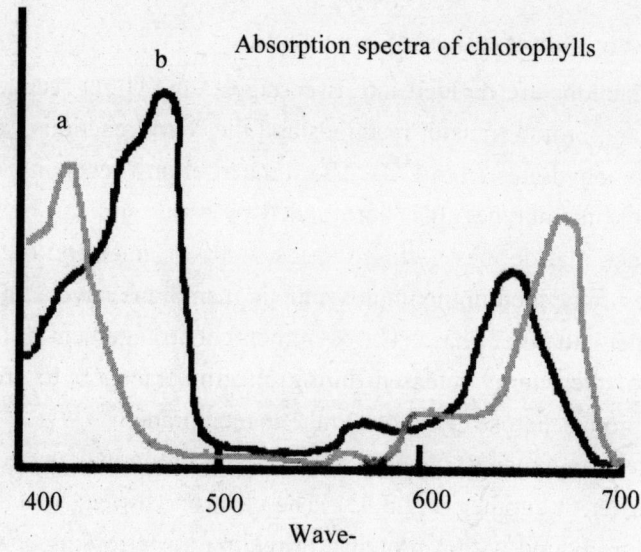

Figure 3.41: Absorption spectra of chlorophyll

There are mainly two types of chlorophyll, named *a* and *b*, which differ in the composition of a side chain (in *a* it is -CH$_3$, while in *b* it is CHO). Chlorophyll a, gives absorption peaks at 430 nm and 662nm, while Chlorophyll b gives peaks at 453 nm and 642 nm. The different side groups in the two chlorophylls 'tune' the absorption spectrum to slightly different wavelengths. Thus, these two kinds of chlorophylls complement each other in absorbing sunlight. For instance, the light which is not significantly absorbed by chlorophyll *a*, at 460 nm, will be strongly absorbed or captured by chlorophyll *b*. The plants can obtain all their energy requirements from the blue and red region of the spectrum, however, there is still a large spectral region, between 500 and 600 nm, where very little light is absorbed

(Fig. 3.41). This light is in the green region of the spectrum, and since it is reflected, this is the reason why plants look green.

The energy in the 'excited electrons' can be passed from one chlorophyll molecule to another, but at the end it will just be lost as fluorescence (i.e. the energy will be re-emitted as light), unless the excited electron itself can be ejected from the chlorophyll molecule. There are two different sorts of reaction centers in plants. In each of these reaction centers, the ejected electron is transferred to an acceptor molecule, which can then pass it on to a different molecule and eventually the electron(s) can be used to fix up carbon dioxide. However, it is not feasible to keep on ejecting electrons from these chlorophyll molecules, electrons must be fed back in to the system to replace those which have been ejected. These electrons come from water, resulting in oxygen being evolved. Thus, this reaction is a non-cyclic electron transport chain.

3.20.6. Steps Involved in Photosynthesis

The photosynthetic reactions are divided into two stages - the "light reactions," which are consisted of electron and proton transfer reactions and the "dark reactions," are consisted of the biosynthesis of carbohydrates from CO_2. The light reactions occur in a complex membrane system (thylakoid membrane). It is surrounded by water and can be thought of as a two-dimensional surface that defines a closed space, with an inner and outer water phase. The protein complexes embedded in the photosynthetic membrane have a unique orientation with respect to the inner and outer phase. The asymmetrical arrangement of the protein complexes allows some of the energy released during electron transport to create an electrochemical gradient of protons across the photosynthetic membrane.

Photosynthetic electron transport consists of a series of individual electron transfer steps from one electron carrier to another (Fig.3.42). The electron carriers, metal ion complexes and aromatic groups are bound within proteins, providing a scaffolding for them. An electron which enters a protein complex at a specific site, is transferred within the protein from one carrier to another, and exits the protein at a different site. Not All electron carriers are bound to the proteins. The reduced forms of plastoquinone or ubiquinone and nicotinamide adenine dinucleotide phosphate (NADPH) or NADH act as mobile electron carriers operating between protein complexes. For electron transfer to occur, these small molecules must bind to special pockets in the proteins known as binding sites. The binding sites are highly specific and are a critical factor in controlling the rate and pathway of electron transfer.

(a) **Light Reaction**

(b) The capture of light energy for photosynthesis is enhanced by networks of pigments in the chloroplasts arranged in aggregates on the thylakoids. These aggregates are called antennae complexes. About 2500 molecules of chlorophyll normally required to produce one molecule of oxygen, and that a minimum of eight photons of light must be absorbed in the process. When a photon reaches the chlorophyll a in the reaction center, that chlorophyll can receive the energy because it absorbs photons of longer wavelengths than the other pigments. Two types of chlorophyll centers have been identified, which are associated with two protein complexes, identified as Photosystem I and Photosystem II.

The light absorption processes associated with photosynthesis take place in large protein complexes known as photosystems. The one known as Photosystem I contain a chlorophyll dimer with an absorption peak at 700 nm known as P700. In addition to the photosystem there are chlorophyll and other pigment containing assemblies, which are called light harvesting complexes. They can funnel additional excitation energy to the photosystem. Photosystem II, which is P-680 reaction center, can absorb light most efficiently at 680 nm.

The light reactions involve several steps. The first step is the conversion of a photon to an excited electronic state of an antenna pigment molecule located in the antenna system. The antenna system consists of hundreds of pigment molecules (mainly chlorophyll and carotenoids) that are anchored to proteins within the photosynthetic membrane and serve a specialized protein complex known as a reaction center. The electronic excited state is transferred over the antenna molecules as an exciton. Some excitons are converted back into photons and emitted as fluorescence; some are converted to heat, while some are trapped by a reaction center protein. Excitons trapped by a reaction center provide the energy for the primary photochemical reaction of photosynthesis - the transfer of an electron from a donor molecule to an acceptor molecule. Both the donor and acceptor molecules are attached to the reaction center protein complex.

In oxygenic photosynthetic organisms, two different reaction centers, photosystem II and photosystem I, work concurrently in series. In the light photosystem II feeds electrons to photosystem I. The electrons are transferred from photosystem II to the photosystem I by intermediate carriers. The net reaction is the transfer of electrons from a water molecule to NADP+, producing the reduced form, NADPH. In addition, the electron transfer reactions concentrate protons inside the membrane vesicle and create an electric field across the photosynthetic membrane. In this process, the electron transfer reactions convert redox free energy into an electrochemical potential of protons. The energy stored in the proton electrochemical potential is used by a membrane bound protein complex (ATP-Synthase) to covalently attach a phosphate group to adenosine diphosphate (ADP), forming adenosine triphosphate (ATP). This phenomenon of conversion of ADP to ATP in presence of light is known as photophosphorylation. The net effect of the light reactions is to convert radiant energy into redox free energy in the form of NADPH and phosphate group-transfer energy in the form of ATP. The NADPH and ATP formed by the light reactions provide the energy for the dark reactions of photosynthesis, known as the Calvin cycle or the photosynthetic carbon reduction cycle.

(b) Dark Reaction

The reduction of atmospheric CO_2 to carbohydrate occurs in the aqueous phase of the chloroplast (stroma) and involves a series of enzymatic reactions. The carbon reduction cycle involves the transfer and rearrangement of chemical bond energy. Carbon dioxide diffuses into the stroma of chloroplasts and combines with a five-carbon sugar, ribulose1, 5-biphosphate (RuBP). This six-carbon unstable intermediate compound immediately breaks down in to two three-carbon molecules (3-phosphoglycerate). This key reaction is catalyzed by Rubisco (D-ribulose 1, 5-bisphosphate carboxylase/oxygenase), a large water soluble protein complex. Later, it goes through the rest of the cycle, regenerating ribulose bisphosphate as well as the three-carbon sugar glyceraldehyde phosphate. It takes three turns of the cycle to produce one glyceraldehyde phosphate, which leaves the cycle to form glucose or other sugars. The fact that this 3-carbon molecule is the first stable product of photosynthesis and form the basis of calling this cycle the C_3 cycle. The energy from ATP and NADPH energy carriers generated by the photosystems is used to attach phosphates to (phosphorylate) the phosphoglycerate (PGA). Eventually, there are 12 molecules of glyceraldehyde phosphate (also known as phosphoglyceraldehyde or PGAL, a 3-C), two of which are removed from the cycle producing a glucose. The remaining PGAL molecules are converted by ATP energy to reform 6 RuBP molecules, thus they start the cycle again. There are about thirteen different enzymes required to complete the Calvin cycle (Fig. 3.42).

Those plants that utilize just the Calvin cycle for carbon fixation are known as C3 plants. In C3 plants the photosynthesis, carbon fixation and Calvin cycle, all occur in a single chloroplast. The energy conversion efficiency of the Calvin cycle is approximately 90%. The reactions do not involve energy transduction, rather than the rearrangement of chemical energy. Each molecule of CO_2 reduced to a sugar $[CH_2O]$ n requires 2 molecules of NADPH and 3 molecules of ATP.

3.20.7. Adaptations for survival in drought /hot condition by plants

The environmental conditions that promote photorespiration are hot, bright, dry days. In these climates, alternate modes of carbon fixation have evolved to minimize photorespiration. The two most important photosynthetic adaptations are exhibited by C_4 and CAM C_4 plants. C_4 plants are so named because they form a four-carbon compound as the first product of the non-light requiring reactions of photosynthesis. Several thousand species in at least 19 families use the C_4 pathway. Agriculturally important C_4 plants are sugarcane and corn, members of the grass family.

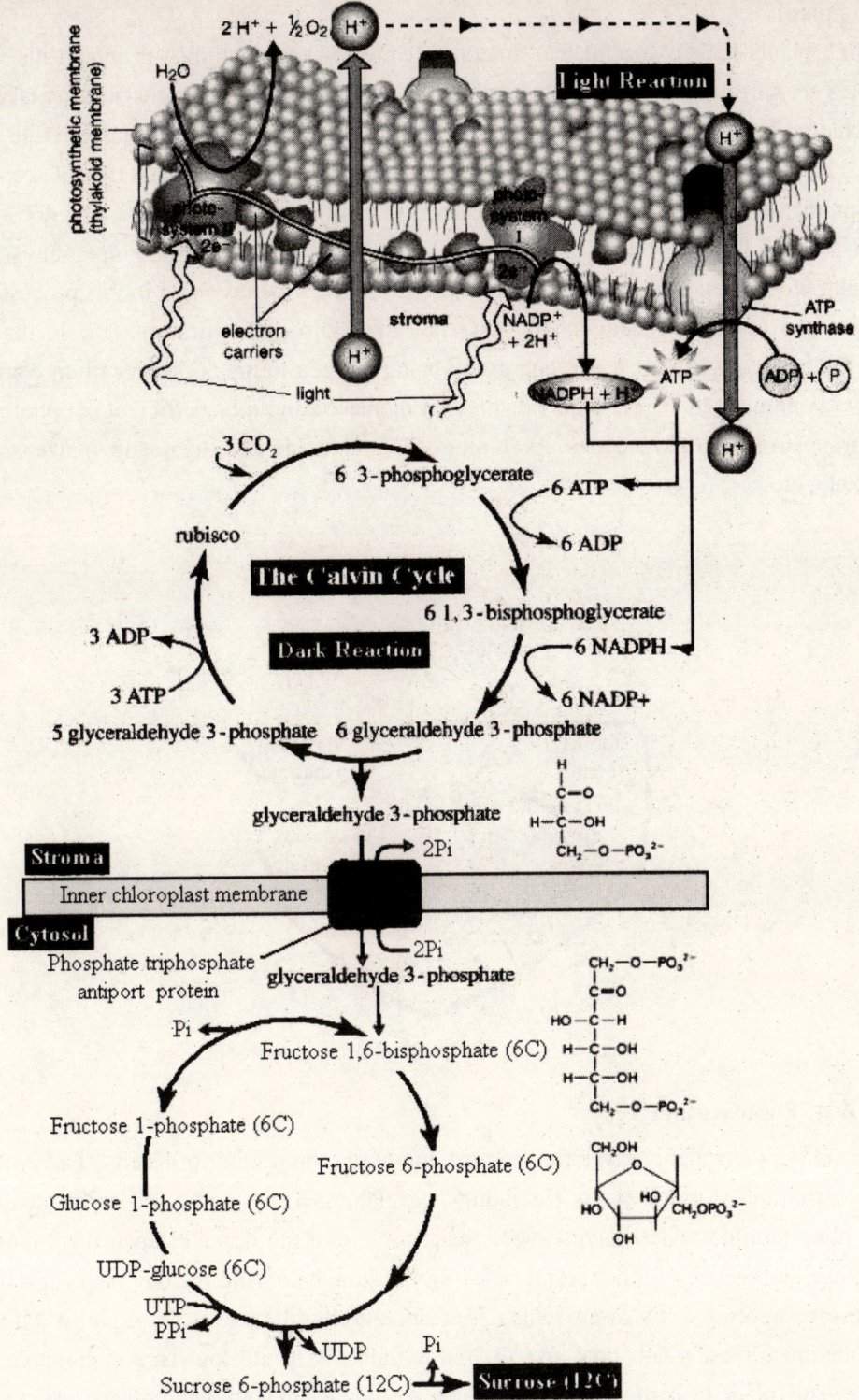

Figure 3.42: Photosynthesis: light and dark reactions

(a) C₄ plants

Most C$_4$ plants have a special leaf anatomy (called Kranz anatomy) in which the vascular bundles are surrounded by bundle sheath cells. In C4 plants, the photosynthesis takes place in a chloroplast of a thin-walled mesophyll cell and a 4-carbon acid is transferred to a thick-walled bundle sheath cell where the Calvin cycle occurs in a chloroplast of that second cell. This protects the Calvin cycle from the effects of photorespiration (Fig. 3.43). A C$_4$ plant is better adapted than a C$_3$ plant in an environment with high day-time temperatures, intense sunlight, drought, or nitrogen or CO$_2$ limitation. The enzyme involved in this process is PEP carboxylase. In this mechanism, the tendency of Rubisco (the first enzyme in the Calvin cycle) to photo-respire, or waste energy by using oxygen to break down carbon compounds to CO$_2$, is minimized. These plants display an increased and more efficient net photosynthesis during strong light intensities. Examples of C$_4$ plants include sugarcane, maize, sorghum, amaranth, etc.

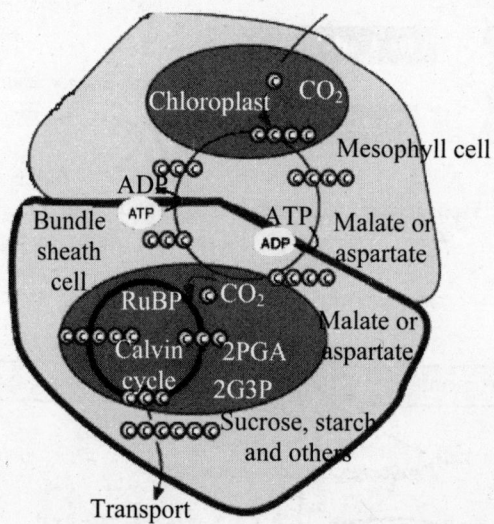

Figure 3.43: C4 cycle of photosynthesis

(b) CAM Photosynthesis

A second photosynthetic adaptation to arid conditions (as found in deserts) has evolved in succulent (water-storing) plants (including ice plants), many cacti, and representatives of other plant families. These plants close their stomata in the day and open them during the night, just the reverse of other plants. Closing the stomata during the day helps desert plants to conserve water, but it also prevents CO$_2$ from entering the leaves. At night, when the stomata are open, these plants take up CO$_2$ and initially fix it into four-carbon compounds like malate. This mode of carbon fixation is called crassulacean acid metabolism, or CAM, after the plant family Crassulaceae, the succulents in which the process was first discovered. The photosynthetic cells of CAM plants store the malate formed in the night in their vacuoles until morning, when the stomata close. In the daytime, when the light reactions can make ATP and $NADPH_2$ for the Calvin cycle, CO_2 is released from the malate made in the night before it is fixed up into sugar in the chloroplasts (Fig. 3.44).

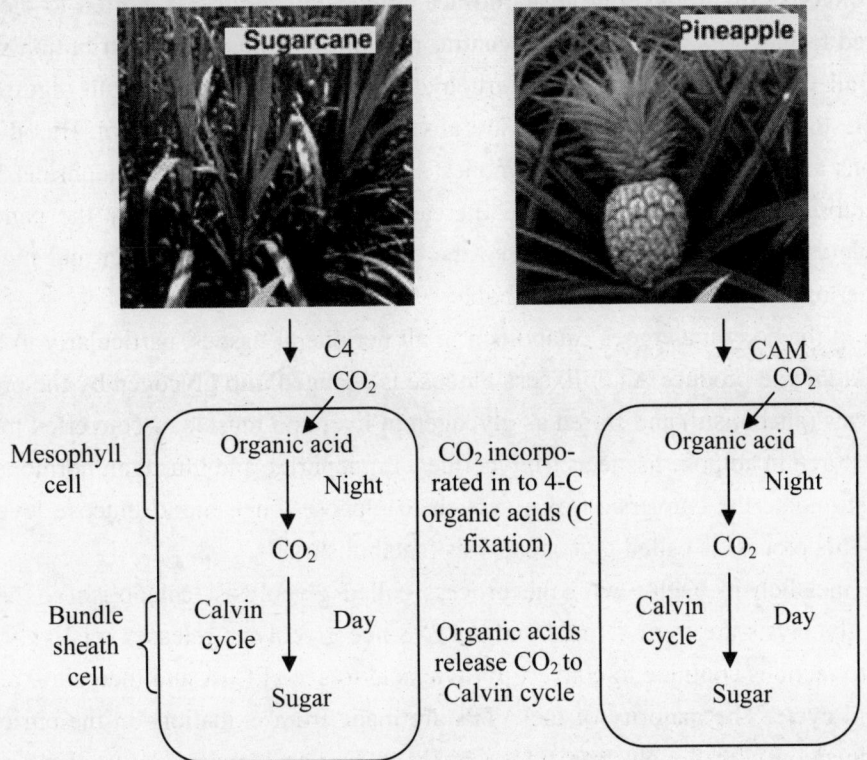

Figure 3.44: CAM plants

Both adaptations are characterized by initial fixation of CO_2 into an organic acid such as malate followed by transfer of the CO_2 to the Calvin cycle. In C_4 plants, such as sugarcane, these two steps are separated spatially; the two steps take place in two cell types. In CAM C_4 plants, such as pineapple, the two steps are separated temporally (time); carbon fixation into malate occurs at night, and the Calvin cycle functions during the day. To prevent water loss, the stomata of these plants are closed by day, to open only at night when temperature decreases and humidity rises. Since the absorption of CO_2 is only possible at night, CO_2 storage and changes in metabolism are necessary to carry out photosynthesis by day. At night CO_2 is stored as malate in the large vacuoles and released for photosynthesis during day. This type of metabolism appeared to occur not only dicot plants, but also in a number of monocots, among others the crop pineapple and the pot plant, *Sanseveria*.

3.21. Carbohydrate Metabolism

In animals, especially in human the major source of dietary carbohydrate is starch from consumed plant material and a small amount of glycogen from animal tissue as well as disaccharides such as sucrose from products containing refined sugar and lactose in milk. Digestion in the gut converts all carbohydrate to monosaccharides which are transported to the liver and converted to glucose. The liver has a central role in the storage and distribution within the body of all fuels, including glucose. Carbohydrate metabolism begins with digestion in the small intestine; here monosaccharides are absorbed into the blood stream. Blood sugar concentrations are controlled by three hormones: insulin, glucagon, and epinephrine. When the concentration of glucose in the blood increases, insulin is secreted by the pancreas, which stimulates the transfer of glucose into the cells, especially in the liver and muscles, although other organs are also able to metabolize glucose.

Glucose in the body undergoes catabolism in all peripheral tissues, particularly in brain, muscle and kidney to produce ATP. Excess glucose is changed into glycogen by the process of glycogenesis (anabolism) and stored as glycogen in liver and muscle or converted to fatty acids and is stored in adipose tissue as triglycerides. Eqinephrine and glucagon hormones are secreted to stimulate the conversion of glycogen to glucose when blood glucose level becomes low. This process is called glycogenolysis (catabolism).

Glucose metabolism begins with the process called glycolysis (catabolism). The end products of glycolysis are pyruvic acid and ATP. Since glycolysis releases relatively little ATP, further reactions continue to convert pyruvic acid to acetyl CoA and then citric acid in the citric acid cycle. The majority of the ATPs are made from oxidations in the citric acid cycle in connection with the electron transport chain. During strenuous muscular activity, pyruvic acid is converted into lactic acid rather than acetyl CoA. During the resting period, the lactic acid is converted back to pyruvic acid. The pyruvic acid in turn is converted back to glucose by the process called gluconeogenesis (anabolism).

3.21.1. Glycolysis

Glycolysis (Embden-Meyerhof pathway) is the initial metabolic pathway of carbohydrate catabolism. It is the most universal process by which cells of all types derive energy from sugars. Glucose is oxidized by all tissues to synthesize ATP. The first pathway which begins the complete oxidation of glucose is called glycolysis. This pathway cleaves the six carbon glucose molecule ($C_6H_{12}O_6$) into two molecules of the three carbon compound pyruvate ($C_3H_3O_3^-$). This oxidation is coupled to the net production of two molecules of ATP per glucose. Glycolysis converts one molecule of glucose into two molecules of pyruvate, along with "reducing equivalents" in the form of the coenzyme NADH. The global reaction of glycolysis is:

$$Glucose + 2\ NAD^+ + 2\ ADP + 2\ P_i \rightarrow 2\ NADH + 2\ pyruvate + 2\ ATP + 2\ H_2O + 4\ H^+$$

In eukaryotes, glycolysis takes place within the cytosol of the cell. Glucose gets into the cell through facilitated diffusion. The first step in glycolysis is phosphorylation of glucose by hexokinase (in liver the most important hexokinase is glucokinase). This reaction consumes 1 ATP molecule. Although the cell membrane is permeable to glucose because of the presence of glucose transport proteins, it is impermeable to glucose 6-phosphate. Glucose 6-phosphate is then rearranged into fructose 6-phosphate by phospho-glucose isomerase. (Fructose can also enter the glycolytic pathway at this point.). Phosphofructokinase-1 then consumes 1 ATP to form fructose 1, 6-bisphosphate. The energy expenditure in this step is justified in 2 ways: the glycolytic process is now irreversible, and the energy supplied to the molecule allows the ring to be split by aldolase into 2 molecules - dihydroxyacetone phosphate and glyceraldehyde 3-phosphate. (Triosephosphate isomerase converts the molecule of di-hydroxy-acetone phosphate into a molecule of glyceraldehyde 3-phosphate.) Each molecule of glyceraldehyde 3-phosphate is then oxidized by a molecule of NAD^+ in the presence of glyceraldehyde 3-phosphate dehydrogenase, forming 1, 3-bisphosphoglycerate. Phosphoglycerate kinase then generates a molecule of ATP while forming 3-phosphoglycerate. At this step, glycolysis has reached the break-even point: 2 molecules of ATP were consumed and 2 new molecules have been synthesized. Phosphoglyceromutase then forms 2-phosphoglycerate; enolase then forms phosphoenolpyruvate and another substrate-level phosphorylation later forms a molecule of pyruvate and a molecule of ATP by means of the enzyme pyruvate kinase (Fig. 3.45).

NAD is used as the electron acceptor in the oxidation reaction. This cofactor is present only in limited amounts and once reduced to NADH, as in this reaction, it must be reoxidised to NAD to permit continuation of the pathway. This re-oxidation occurs by one of two methods:

3.21.2. Anaerobic Glycolysis

In the absence of oxygen, pyruvate is reduced to lactate that is ideally suited to utilization in heavily exercising muscles where oxygen supply is often insufficient to meet the demands of aerobic metabolism. The reduction of pyruvate to lactate is coupled to the oxidation of NADH to NAD.

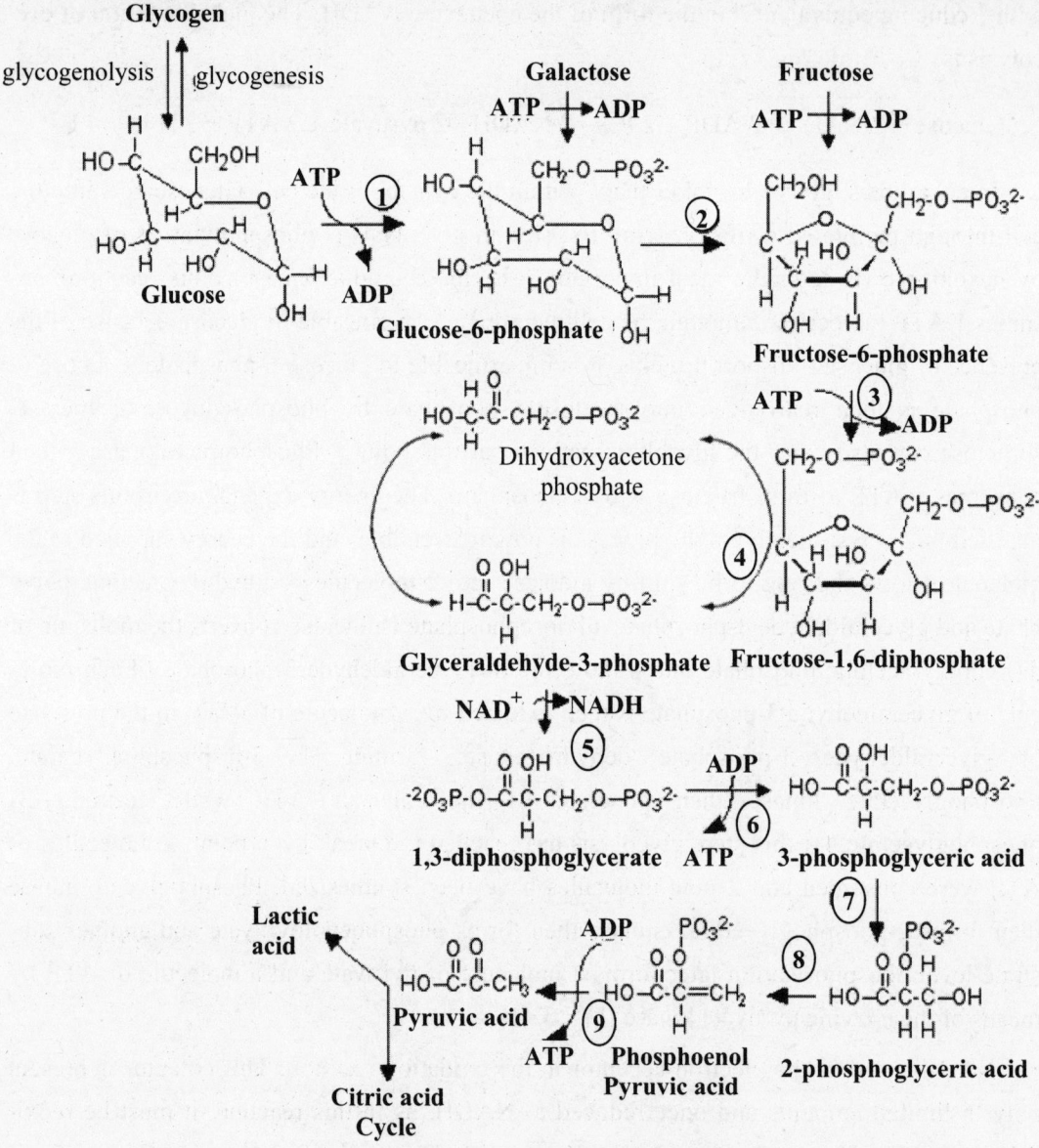

Figure 3.45: Events in glycolytic pathway

3.21.3. Cori Cycle

The lactate formed is transported to other tissues and dealt with by one of the two mechanisms such as converted back to pyruvate or converted back to glucose in the liver. The process of conversion of lactate to glucose is called gluconeogenesis, uses some of the reactions of glycolysis (but in the reverse direction) and some reactions unique to this pathway to re-synthesize glucose. The majority of the enzymes responsible for gluconeogenesis are found in the cytoplasm; the exception is pyruvate carboxylase which is located in the mito-chondria. This pathway requires ATP but has the role of maintaining a circulating glucose concentration in the bloodstream (even in the absence of dietary supply) and also maintaining a glucose supply to fast twitch muscle fibres.

The Cori cycle, named after its discoverers, Carl Cori and Gerty Cori, refers to the metabolic pathway in which lactate produced by anaerobic glycolysis in the muscles moves to the liver and is converted to glucose, which then returns to the muscles and is converted back to lactate (Fig. 3.46). It can be shown by a complex calculation of energy yields that this process of partially oxidizing glucose to lactate in muscle, transporting it to the liver for conversion back to glucose and then re-supplying it to muscle, actually has a much higher energy yield than the 2 ATP/glucose produced by glycolysis alone.

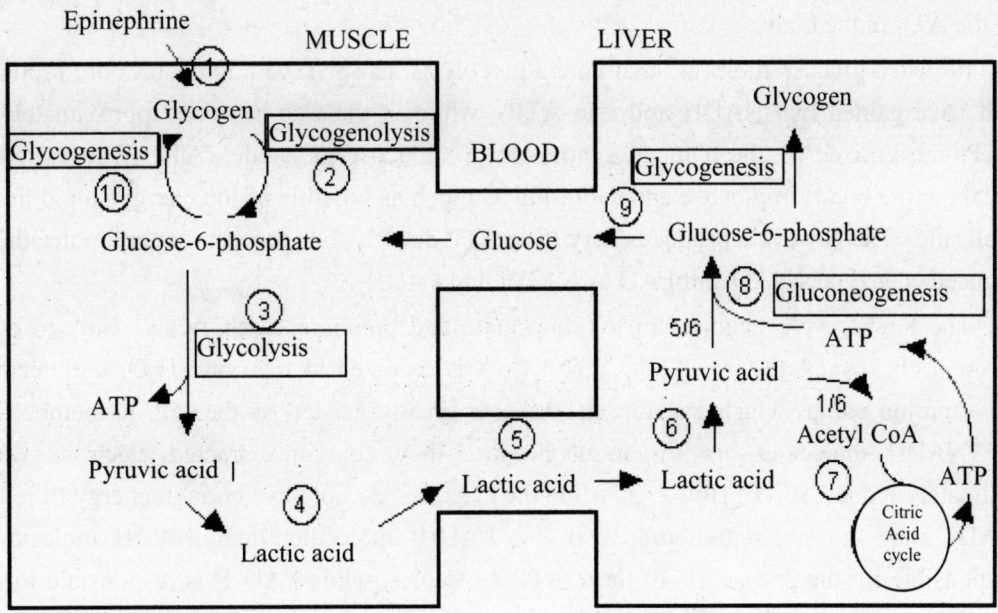

Figure 3.46: Cori cycle

3.21.4. Aerobic Metabolism of Glucose

In aerobic condition pyruvate is transported inside mitochondria and oxidized to acetyl coenzyme A (abbreviated to "acetyl CoA"). This is an oxidation reaction and uses NAD as an electron acceptor. Further, acetyl CoA is oxidized ultimately to CO_2 by citric acid cycle. These reactions are coupled to a process known as the electron transport chain which has the role of harnessing chemical bond energy through a series of oxidation/reduction reactions to the synthesis of ATP and simultaneously re-oxidizing NADH to NAD.

(a) Citric Acid Cycle

The Krebs cycle, also known as the tri-carboxylic acid cycle (TCA), was first recognized in 1937 by the man for whom it is named, German biochemist Hans Adolph Krebs, the winner of Nobel Prize in 1953. In short, the Krebs cycle constitutes the discovery of the major source of energy in all living organisms. The Krebs cycle reactions take place in the matrix of the mitochondria. Some of the final steps of intermediate metabolism take place there, as well. For example, in the matrix as well as the cytoplasm, glutamate (the amino acid glutamic acid) loses its amino group and is oxidized to alpha-ketoglutarate. Under aerobic conditions the end product of glycolysis is pyruvic acid converted to acetyl coenzyme A (acetyl CoA) which is the initiator of the citric acid cycle. In carbohydrate metabolism, acetyl CoA is the link between glycolysis and the citric acid cycle. The citric acid cycle contains the final oxidation reactions, coupled to the electron transport chain, which produce the majority of the ATP in the body.

For each glucose molecule that enters glycolysis, two pyruvate molecules are produced and have gained two NADH and two ATPs, while in the Calvin cycle approximately 54 ATPs are utilized by the plant to synthesize one glucose molecule. ATP is generated by breaking the bonds in glucose and capturing as much as possible of the energy stored in that molecule. The CA cycle produces very little ATP directly, but generates many molecules of reduced coenzymes NAD and FAD as NADH and $FADH_2$.

The Krebs cycle begins with oxalo-acetate and combines with Acetyl CoA to cycle through one complete turn. After Acetyl CoA is oxidized to CO_2 and H_2O, the electrons drive proton pumps which generate ATP that is greatly needed by the cell. Remember that the NADH molecules are important because they contain extracted electrons which ultimately reduce NAD^+. However, when the electrons do not have enough energy to reduce NAD^+, they are stored temporarily in the $FADH_2$ molecule. Each NADH molecule is responsible for the production of three ATP molecules, while $FADH_2$ is responsible for the production of two ATP molecules. In prokaryotic cells, the citric acid cycle occurs in the cytoplasm; in eukaryotic cells the citric acid cycle takes place in the matrix of the mitochondria. The overall reaction for the citric acid cycle is:

$$2 \text{ acetyl groups} + 6 \text{ NAD}^+ + 2 \text{ FAD} + 2 \text{ ADP} + 2 \text{ P}_i \rightarrow 4 \text{ CO}_2 + 6 \text{ NADH} + 6 \text{ H}^+ + 2 \text{ FADH}_2 + 2 \text{ ATP}$$

The citric acid cycle provides a series of intermediate compounds that donate protons and electrons to the electron transport chain by way of the reduced coenzymes NADH and $FADH_2$. The electron transport chain then generates additional ATPs by oxidative phosphorylation. The TCA cycle involves 8 distinct steps, each catalyzed by a unique enzyme.

- The citric acid cycle begins when Coenzyme A transfers its 2-carbon acetyl group to the 4-carbon compound, oxalo-acetate, to form the 6-carbon molecule, citrate.
- The citrate is rearranged to form an isomeric form, isocitrate (Fig. 3.47).
- The 6-carbon isocitrate is oxidized and a molecule of CO_2 is removed producing the 5-carbon molecule α-ketoglutarate. During this oxidation, NAD^+ is reduced to $NADH + H^+$.

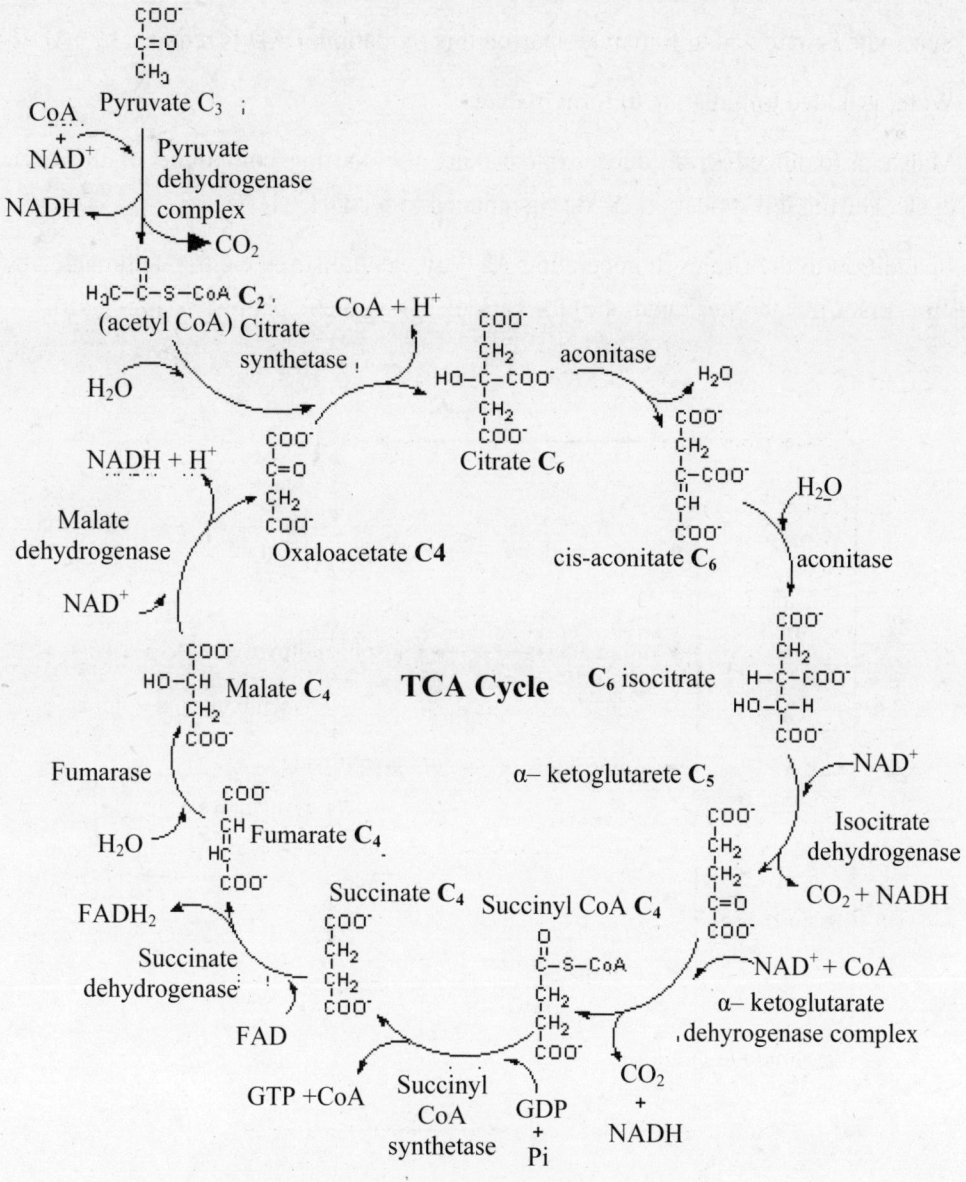

Figure 3.47: Citric acid cycle (TCA)

- Alpha-ketoglutarate is oxidized, carbon dioxide is removed, and coenzyme A is added to form the 4-carbon compound succinyl-CoA. During this oxidation, NAD^+ is reduced to $NADH + H^+$

- CoA is removed from succinyl-CoA to produce succinate. The energy released is used to make guanosine triphosphate (GTP) from guanosine diphosphate (GDP) and P_i by substrate-level phosphorylation. GTP can then be used to make ATP.

- Succinate is oxidized to fumarate. During this oxidation, FAD is reduced to $FADH_2$.

- Water is added to fumarate to form malate.

- Malate is oxidized to produce oxaloacetate, the starting compound of the citric acid cycle. During this oxidation, NAD^+ is reduced to $NADH + H^+$

In addition to their roles in generating ATP by catabolism, the citric acid cycle also supplies precursor metabolites (anabolic) for various biosynthetic pathways (Fig. 3.48).

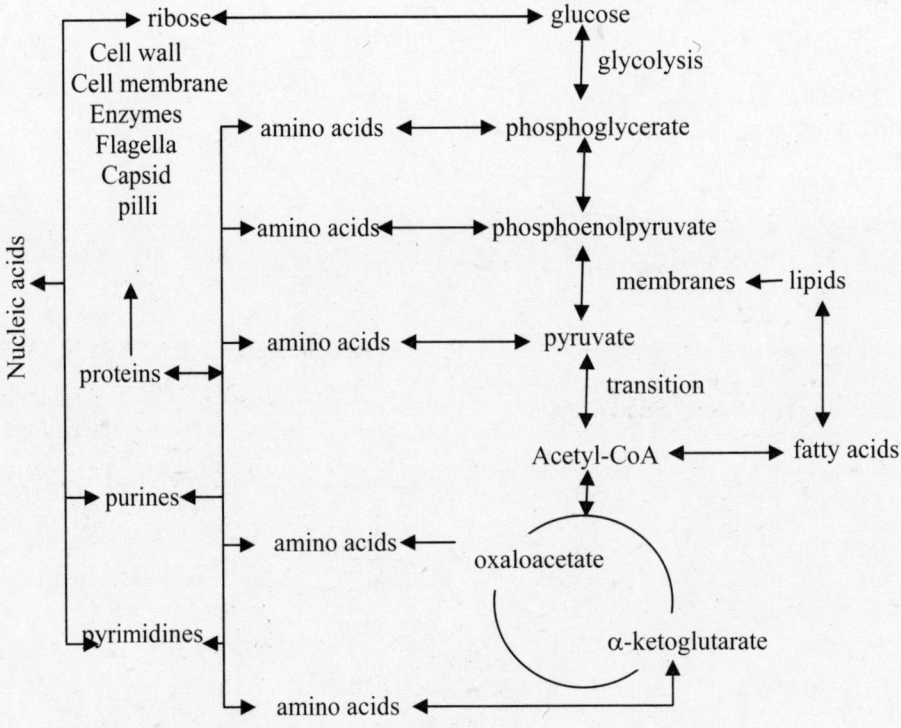

Figure 3.48: Synthesis of precursor metabolites in TCA cycle

Table 3.3: The products of glycolysis, oxidation of pyruvic acid, and Krebs cycle

ATP-Yield in Glycolysis and TCA-Cycle			
Glycolysis		**ATP utilized**	**Net ATP**
Glucose→ Glucose 6- phosphate		-1 ATP	+8 ATP
Fructose 6-phosphate→ Fructose 1, 6-bisphosphate		-1 ATP	
2 mol. [Glyceraldehyde-3-P→ 1, 3-bisphosphoglycerate]	2NADH × 3	+ 6 ATP	
2 mol. [1, 3-bisphosphoglycerate → 3-phosphoglycerate]		+2 ATP	
2 mol. Phosphoenolpyru-vate→ Pyruvate]		+2	
Pyruvate to Acetyl-CoA			
2 mol. [Pyruvate→ Acetyl-CoA]	2NADH × 3	+ 6 ATP	+ 6 ATP
TCA-Cycle (Kreb's Cycle)			
2 mol. [Isocitrate→ α-ketoglutyrate]	2NADH × 3	+ 6 ATP	+ 24 ATP
2 mol. [α- ketoglutyrate→ Succinyl CoA]	2NADH × 3	+ 6 ATP	
2 mol. [Succinyl-CoA→ Succinate]	2GTP	+ 2 ATP	
2 mol. [Succinate→ Fumarate]	2FADH2×2	+4ATP	
2 mol. [L-malate→ Oxaloacetate]	2NADH × 3	+ 6 ATP	

(b) Electron Transport Chain

It is the final part of the phase-II of aerobic respiration. In respiration, oxidation of the substrate occurs by dehydrogenation (i.e., removal) of hydrogen atoms (2H) from the substrate. Most of these hydrogen atoms are accepted by NAD to form reduced co-enzyme NADH. In the aerobic respiration 10 $NADH_2$ are formed (2$NADH_2$ in glycolysis + 8 $NADH_2$ in Krebs cycle) from one molecule of glucose. Also, in Krebs cycle, hydrogen is accepted by FAD to form $FADH_2$ in one step; a total of 2 $FADH_2$ are formed by aerobic respiration of each glucose molecule.

$$\text{NADH}_2 + 1/2\ O_2 \longrightarrow H_2O + NAD$$
$$\text{FADH}_2 + 1/2\ O_2 \longrightarrow H_2O + FAD$$

Terminal oxidation

Each molecule of reduced co-enzyme thus formed in aerobic respiration (glycolysis and Krebs cycle) is finally oxidized by the free molecular oxygen through a process called terminal oxidation (Fig. 3.49).

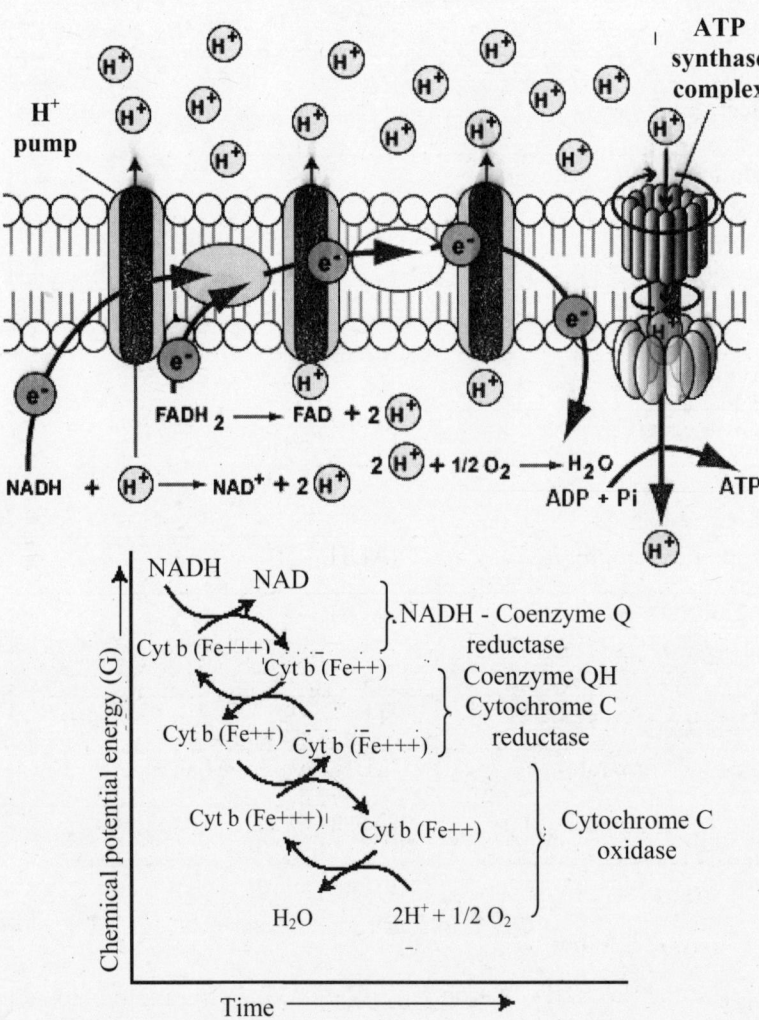

Figure 3.49: Electron transport chain: The energy from the transfer of electrons along the chain transports protons across the membrane and creates an electrochemical gradient. As the accumulating protons follow back across the membrane through an ATP synthase complex, the movement of the protons provides energy for synthesizing ATP from ADP and phosphate. Since oxygen is the final electron acceptor, the process is called aerobic respiration

The respiratory chain (or the ETS) is present in the inner membrane of mitochondrion (i.e., in the cristae membrane). It consists of various enzymes and co-enzymes which act as electron carriers. Embedded in the inner membrane are proteins and complexes of molecules that are involved in the process called electron transport. The electron transport system (ETS), as it is called, accepts energy from carriers in the matrix and stores it to a form that can be used to phosphorylate ADP. Two energy carriers are known to donate energy to the ETS, namely nicotine adenine di-nucleotide (NAD) and flavin adenine di-nucleotide (FAD). NADH binds to complex -I. It binds to a prosthetic group called flavin mononucleotide (FMN), and is immediately re-oxidized to NAD. NAD is recycled, acting as an energy shuttle. FMN receives the hydrogen from the NADH and two electrons. It also picks up a proton from the matrix. In this reduced form, it passes the electrons to iron-sulfur clusters that are part of the complex, and forces two protons into the inter-membrane space. Reduced NAD carries energy to complex I (NADH-Coenzyme Q Reductase) of the electron transport chain. FAD is a bound part of the succinate dehydrogenase complex (complex II).

Electrons cannot pass through complex-I without accomplishing proton translocation. Electron transport carriers are specific, in which each carrier accepts electrons (and associated free energy) from a specific type of preceding carrier. Electrons pass from complex I to a carrier (Coenzyme Q) embedded by itself in the membrane. From Coenzyme Q electrons are passed to a complex -III which is associated with another proton translocation event. Complex-II, the succinate dehydrogenase complex, is a separate starting point, and is not a part of the NADH pathway. From succinate, the sequence is Complex II to Coenzyme Q to Complex III to cytochrome C to Complex IV. Thus, there is a common electron transport pathway beyond the entry point, either Complex I or Complex II. Protons are not translocated at Complex II. There is not sufficient free energy available from the succinate dehydrogenase reaction to reduce NAD or to pump protons at more than two sites. From Complex III the pathway moves to cytochrome C then to a Complex IV (cytochrome oxidase complex). More protons are translocated by Complex IV, and it is at this site that oxygen binds, along with protons, and using the electron pair and remaining free energy, oxygen is reduced to water. Oxygen serves as an electron acceptor, clearing the way for carriers in the sequence to be re-oxidized so that electron transport can continue. The purpose of electron transport is to conserve energy in the form of a chemiosmotic gradient. The gradient, in turn, can be exploited for the phosphorylation of ADP as well as for other purposes. With the cessation of aerobic metabolism cell is damaged immediately and irreversibly.

Summary

Biochemistry aims to explain biological form and function in chemical terms. The major biological phenomena have been revealed by purifying individual chemical component, such as a protein, from a living organism and its structural and chemical characterization.

Proteins are long polymers of amino acids, constitute one of the largest fractions of cells. Some proteins have catalytic activity and function as enzymes; others serve as structural elements, signal receptors, or transporters that carry specific substances into or out of cells. The nucleic acids, DNA and RNA, are polymers of nucleotides. They store and transmit genetic information, and some RNA molecules have structural and catalytic roles in molecular complexes. The polysaccharides are polymers of simple sugars such as glucose. They have two major functions: as energy-yielding fuel stores and as extracellular structural elements with specific binding sites for particular proteins. Shorter polymers of sugars (oligosaccharides) attached to proteins or lipids at the cell surface serve as specific cellular signals. The lipids, greasy or oily hydrocarbon derivatives, serve as structural components of membranes, energy-rich fuel stores, pigments, and intracellular signals. In proteins, nucleotides, polysaccharides, and lipids, the number of monomeric subunits is very large: molecular weights in the range of 5,000 to more than 1 million for proteins, up to several billion for nucleic acids, and in the millions for polysaccharides such as starch.

The covalent bonds and functional groups of a biomolecule are, of course, central to its function, but so also is the arrangement of the constituent atoms of a molecule in three-dimensional space, its stereochemistry. A carbon-containing compound commonly exists as stereoisomers, molecules with the same chemical bonds but different stereochemistry that is, different configuration and the fixed spatial arrangement of atoms. Interactions between biomolecules are invariably stereospecific, requiring specific stereochemistry in the interacting molecules. A nearly universal set of several hundred small molecules is found in living cells; the inter-conversions of these molecules in the central metabolic pathways have been conserved in evolution.

The central issue in bioenergetics (the study of energy transformations in living systems) is the means by which energy from fuel metabolism or light capture is coupled to energy-requiring reactions of the cell. All biological macromolecules are much less thermodynamically stable than their monomeric subunits, yet they are kinetically stable: their uncatalyzed breakdown occurs so slowly that, on a time scale that matters for the organism, these molecules are stable. Virtually every chemical reaction in a cell occurs at a significant rate only because of the presence of enzymes—biocatalysts that, like all other catalysts, greatly enhance the rate of specific chemical reactions without being consumed up in the process. Cellular catalysts are, with a few exceptions, proteins. A further contribution to catalysis occurs when two or more reactants bind to the enzyme's surface close to each other and with stereospecific orientations that favor the reaction. This increases by orders of magnitude the probability of productive collisions between reactants. The thousands of enzyme-catalyzed chemical reactions in cells are functionally organized into many sequences of consecutive reactions, called pathways, in which the product of one reaction becomes the reactant in the next. Some pathways degrade organic nutrients into simple end products in order to extract chemical energy and convert it into a form useful to the cell; together these degradative, free-energy-yielding reactions are designated as catabolism. Other pathways start with small precursor molecules and convert them to progressively larger and more complex molecules, including proteins and nucleic acids. Such synthetic pathways, which invariably require the input of energy, are collectively designated as anabolism. The overall network of enzyme-catalyzed pathways constitutes cellular metabolism. ATP is the major connecting link (the shared intermediate) between the catabolic and anabolic components of this network.

All cells are bounded by a plasma membrane; have a cytosol containing metabolites, coenzymes, inorganic ions and enzymes; and have a set of genes contained within a nucleoid (prokaryotes) or nucleus (eukaryotes). Bacterial cells contain cytosol, a nucleoid and plasmids. Eukaryotic cells have a nucleus and are multicompartmented, segregating certain processes in specific organelles, which can be separated and studied in isolation, details of which are discussed in coming chapters.

Suggested Reading

- Biochemical Methods by Sadasivam & Manickam (1996) New Age International (P) Ltd.
- Biochemistry, 2nd edition, by Laurence A. Moran, K.G. Scrimgeour, H. R. Horton, R.S. Ochs and J. David Rawn (1994), Neil Patterson Publishers Prentice Hall.
- Biochemistry, 2nd edition, by R.H. Garrett and C.M. Grisham (1999). Saunders College Publishing, NY.
- Biochemistry, 4th edition, by L. Stryer (1995). W.H. Freeman & Co.,NY.
- Enzymes: Biochemistry, Biotechnology and Clinical Chemistry by Trevor Palmer (2001) Horwood Publishing.
- Fundamentals of Biochemistry by Donald Voet and Judith G Voet (1999). John Wiley & Sons, NY .
- Fundamentals of Enzymology, 3rd edition, by Nicholas C. Price and Lewis Stevens (1999) Oxford University Press.
- Harper's Biochemistry, 25th edition, by R.K.Murray, P.A.Hayes, D.K.Granner, P.A. Mayes and V.W.Rodwell (2000) Prentice Hall International.
- Introductory Biochemistry by SK.Singla & O.P.Chauhan (1995) Kalyani Publishers, New Delhi.
- Lehninger: Principles of Biochemistry, 3rd edition, by David L. Nelson and M.M. Cox (2000) Maxmillan/ Worth publishers.

- Modern Experimental Biochemistry, 3rd edition, by R. Boyer (2002) Addison-Wesley Longman.
- Outlines of Biochemistry by E.E.Conn, P.K.Stumpf, G. Bruenimg and Ray H.Doi (1987), John Wiley.
- Structure and mechanism in Protein Science, 2nd edition, by Alan Fersht (1999). W.H. Freeman and Co., NY.
- The Chemical Kinetics of Enzyme action by K.J. Laidler and P.S. Bunting, Oxford University Press London.

CHAPTER 4

Cell: The Basic Unit of Life

- Types of cells
  - Prokaryotic cells
  - Eukaryotic cells
  - Viruses
- Ultra structure of the cell
  - Cell Wall
  - Bacterial Cell Surface Structures
  - Plasma membrane
  - Active Transport
  - Transport of large molecules
  - Protoplasm
  - Cytoplasm
- Cellular Organelles
- The Cell Nucleus
- Special types of chromosomes
- Nucleosome model
- Chromosomes in prokaryotes
- The Endoplasmic reticulum
- Ribosomes
- Golgi Apparatus
- Plastids
- Mitochondria
- Lysosome
- Peroxisomes
- Vacuoles
- Cytoskeleton

"I now appreciate how much I learn by being wrong. I can change my mind when confronted with a rational argument, without the need to have the change appear to be purely semantic or to hope it will pass unnoticed. What must it be like to be a priest, general, bureaucrat, lawyer, medicine person, or politician who is never permitted to be wrong? No wonder they learn so slowly. I am grateful to be in a profession where the realization of being wrong is equivalent to an increase in knowledge."

—Melvin Cohn. *Annual Review of Immunology* 12, 2 (1994)

The cell is the basic unit of life. The life of all organisms including man starts from a single cell and the body is a consortium of individual cells of specific functions and features working in a coordinated manner. Each cell is an amazing world of several biochemical activities: it can assimilate nutrients, convert these nutrients into energy, carry out specialized functions, and reproduce as necessary. Even more amazing is that each cell stores its own set of instructions for carrying out each of these activities. The largest known cell is an ostrich egg. There are millions of different types of cells and many organisms such as microscopic amoeba and bacteria are single celled. In the present chapter we are going to discuss about the structure and function of cellular machineries.

Microscopes opened up new doors in the field of biology by allowing scientists to gaze into the cellular world. Credit for the first compound microscope is usually given to Zacharias Jansen, of Middleburg, Holland, around the year 1595. English scientist Robert Hooke, in 1665 first observed cells and coined the term "cell" in the slices of cork through a microscope. Actually, Hooke only observed cell walls because cork cells are dead and without cytoplasmic contents. The term came from the Latin word *cella* which means "store room" or "small container". At the same time, Anton van Leeuwenhoek (1632–1723) pioneered the invention of one of the best microscopes. Leeuwenhoek was the first to observe, draw, and describe a variety of living organisms, including bacteria gliding in saliva, one-celled organisms cavorting in pond water, and sperm swimming in semen.

Modern ideas about cells appeared in the 1800s, when improved light microscopes enabled scientists to observe more details of cells. The cell theory, or cell doctrine, states that all organisms are composed of similar units of organization, cells. The concept was formally articulated in 1839 by Schleiden and Schwann and has remained as the foundation of modern biology. It wasn't until 1838 that Matthias Schleiden stated that all plant material was made up of cells. The following year, Theodor Schwann came to the same conclusion about animals. Their findings are now known as the cell theory. German pathologist Rudolf Virchow (1821–1902) altered the thought of cellular biology with his powerful dictum, *"Omnis cellulae e cellula"*... "All cells only arise from pre-existing cells." This was new information to most scientists and had not been understood before even for Schwann, who thought that new cells arose from particles in the fluid surrounding the cells. The idea predates other great paradigms of biology including Darwin's theory of evolution (1859), Mendel's laws of inheritance (1865), and the establishment of comparative biochemistry (1940).

In the following years, experiments conducted by Louis Pasteur provided the proof for Virchow's proposal. Pasteur carried out experiments to determine how substances like milk and wine became curdled or fermented. Through carefully controlled environments, he proved that exposure to airborne particles caused the change. In other words, he proved that organisms did not arise spontaneously, but had to be provided by some means, in this case in the air. Now the basic concepts of cell theory can be summarized in the three following statements.

- The cell is the basic unit of life.
- All living organisms are composed of cells. They may be unicellular or multi- cellular.
- Cells arise from pre-existing cells.
- Over time and with the development of the electron microscope, the theory has continued to evolve. As more and more living material was observed at higher and higher magnifications, much more was learned about cells and the cell theory, leading to the

modern cell theory. The modern cell theory includes the two basic components of the classic cell theory and it includes the following postulates.

- The cell is structural and functional unit of all living things. When cells divide, the hereditary information they contain, as DNA, is passed from cell to cell.
- Energy flow (metabolism) occurs within cells.
- All cells have basically the same chemical composition.
- The activity of the organism is determined by the activity of the independent cells.

Table 4.1: Landmarks of cell biology

Year	Events
1595	Jansen credited with 1st compound microscope
1626	Redi postulated that living things do not arise from spontaneous generation.
1655	Hooke described 'cells' in cork.
1674	Leeuwenhoek discovered protozoa. He saw bacteria some 9 years later.
1833	Brown described the cell nucleus in cells of the orchid.
1838	Schleiden and Schwann proposed cell theory.
1840	Albrecht von Roelliker realized that sperm cells and egg cells are also cells.
1856	N. Pringsheim observed how a sperm cell penetrated an egg cell.
1857	Kolliker described mitochondria.
1858	Rudolf Virchow expounds his famous conclusion: *omnis cellula e cellula* that is cells develop only from existing cells
1869	Miescher isolated DNA for the first time.
1879	Flemming described chromosome behavior during mitosis.
1883	Germ cells are haploid, chromosome theory of heredity.
1898	Golgi described the golgi apparatus.
1926	Svedberg developed the first analytical ultracentrifuge.
1938	Behrens used differential centrifugation to separate nuclei from cytoplasm.
1939	Siemens produced the first commercial transmission electron microscope.
1941	Coons used fluorescent labeled antibodies to detect cellular antigens.
1952	Gey and co-workers established a continuous human cell line.
1953	Crick, Wilkins and Watson proposed structure of DNA double-helix.
1955	Eagle systematically defined the nutritional needs of animal cells in culture.
1957	Meselson, Stahl and Vinograd developed density gradient centrifugation in cesium chloride solutions for separating nucleic acids.

1965   Cambridge Instruments produced the first commercial scanning electron micro-scope.

1976   Sato and colleagues published papers showing that different cell lines require different mixtures of hormones and growth factors in serum-free media.

1981   Transgenic mice and fruit flies are produced. Mouse embryonic stem cell line established.

1987   First knockout mouse created.

1998   Mice are cloned from somatic cells.

2000   Human genome DNA sequence draft.

The development of electron microscope, which uses high-energy electrons instead of light waves to view specimens, made a drastic revolution in the field of cytology and molecular biology. New generations of electron microscopes have provided resolution, or the differentiation of separate objects, with the resolution being thousands of times more powerful than that available in light microscopes. This powerful resolution revealed cell organelles such as the endoplasmic reticulum, lysosomes, the Golgi apparatus, and the cytoskeleton.

The discovery of the structure of DNA in 1953 by American biochemist James D. Watson and British biophysicist Francis Crick ushered in the era of molecular biology. Today, investigation inside the world of cells of genes and proteins at the molecular level constitutes one of the largest and fastest moving areas in the science. One particularly active field in recent years has been the investigation of cell signaling, the process by which molecular messages find their way into the cell via a series of complex protein pathways operate within the cell. Another major research area, cell biology, concerns programmed cell death, or apoptosis and cancer treatments. Millions of times per second in the human body, cells commit suicide as an essential part of the normal cycle of cellular replacement and maintenance.

4.1. Types of Cells

On the basis of cell theory, it is clear that all living things are constructed of cells; at least one (unicellular) or many (multi-cellular). In multi-cellular organisms, a group of cells that work together to perform a particular function is called a tissue. In the next higher level of organization, various tissues that perform coordinated functions form organs. Finally, organs that work together to perform general processes form body systems. Multi-cellular organisms contain a vast array of highly specialized cells. Plants contain root cells, leaf cells, and stem cells. Humans have skin cells, nerve cells, and sex cells. Each kind of cell is structured to perform a highly specialized function. For example, microvilli, present in small intestine promote the absorption of foods. Nerve cells consist of a cell body and long attachments, called axons that conduct nerve impulses. Dendrites are shorter attachments that receive nerve impulses. Other types of cells, sensory cells, detect information from the outside environment and transmit that information to the brain. Sensory cells often have unusual shapes and structures that contribute to their function. The rod-shaped cells in the retina of the eye, enables human to detect light, have a light-sensitive region that contains numerous disks. Within each disk is embedded a special light-sensitive pigment that captures light. When the pigment receives light from the outside environment, nerve cells in the eye are triggered to send a nerve impulse in the brain.

However, there are certain organisms called protists such as *Paramecium* and *Chlamydomonas* exist as single-celled, in which all the metabolic functions are performed by a single cell itself. On the basis of cellular organization cells are classified in to two major groups: prokaryotes and eukaryotes. Let us consider each type separately.

4.1.1. Prokaryotic Cells

Prokaryotes are cells that have no membrane-bound nucleus and instead of having chromosomal DNA, their genetic information is in a circular loop called a plasmid. Bacterial cells are very small, roughly the size of an animal mitochondrion (about 0.5–1µm in diameter and 10 µm long). Small size of microorganisms is that the surface area/volume ratio of bacteria is exceedingly high compared to the same ratio for larger organisms of similar shape. The shape of a bacterium is governed by its rigid cell wall. Typical bacterial cells are spherical (cocci; singular, coccus); straight rods (bacilli; singular, bacillus); or spiral that are helically curved (spirilla; singular, spirillum). Although most bacterial species have cells that are of a fairly constant and characteristics shape, some have cells that are pleomorphic, i.e., that can exhibit a variety of shapes.

A spherically shaped bacterium is known as a coccus, a term derived from the Greek kokkos, meaning, 'berry'. Cocci tend to be quite small, being only 0.5–1µm in diameter. They are usually round, may be oval, elongated or indented on one side. Those cocci that remain in pairs after reproducing are called diplococci. Cocci that remain in chains are called streptococci (*Streptococcus pyogenes*). Another arrangement of cocci is the tetrad, consisting of four cocci forming a squire. A cube- like packet of eight cocci is called a sarcinia, *Micrococcus luteus*, a common inhabitant of the skin, is one example. Other cocci may divide randomly and form an irregular grape like cluster of cells called a staphylococcus, such as *Staphylococcus aureus*, cause of food poisoning and numerous skin infections.

Bacillus are rod-shaped bacteria and the cylindrical cell may be as long as 20 µm or as short as 0.5 µm. Certain bacilli are slender, such as those of *Salmonella typhi* that cause typhoid fever; the agent of anthrax (*Bacillus anthracis*), are rectangular with squired ends; others such as the diphtheria bacilli (*Corynebacterium diphtheriae*), are club shaped. Most rods occur singly, but some are arranged in to long chains called *streptobacilli* (strepto = chains).

The third major shape of bacteria is the spiral, which can take one of three forms. Certain spiral bacteria called *vibrios* are curved rods that resemble commas. Other spiral bacteria called spirilla (sing., spirillum) have a helical shape with a thick, rigid cell wall and flagella that assist movement. Those spiral- shaped bacteria known as spirochetes have a thin, flexible cell wall but no flagella in the traditional sence.

In addition to the bacillus, coccus and spiral shapes, other variations also exist. In the genus *Caulobacter*, there are appendaged bacteria; members of the genous *Nocardia* consist of branching filaments; and some Archaea have squire and cluster shapes.

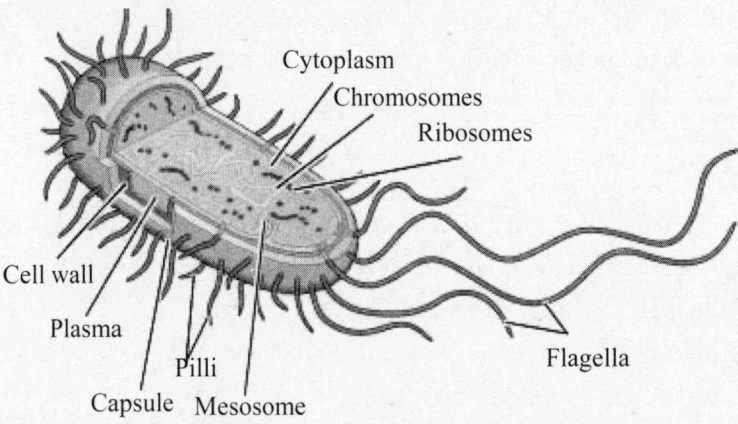

Figure 4.1: A typical bacterial cell

Bacterial cells have a cell wall made up of peptidoglycan. Some bacteria have whip like locomotory structures attached to the cell wall called flagella. Some others also have pilli, short, finger like projections that help the bacteria to attach to tissues, one of the main features necessary for pathogenesis. Bacteria that cause pneumonia, for instance, attach to the tissues of the lung (Fig. 4.1).

Bacteria perform many important functions on earth. They serve as decomposers, agents of fermentation, and play an important role in our digestive system. Also, bacteria are involved in many nutrient cycles such as the nitrogen cycle, which restores nitrate into the soil for plants. Unlike eukaryotic cells that depend on oxygen for their metabolism, prokaryotic cells enjoy a diverse array of metabolic functions. For example, some bacteria use sulphur instead of oxygen in their metabolism. Even there are several anaerobic microbes which can survive in the absence of oxygen.

4.1.2. Eukaryotic Cells

Eukaryotic cells (Eu = "true", karyon = "nucleus") comprise all life forms except kingdom Monera. Eukaryotes have a distinct membrane bound nucleus and organelles. An organelle is a small structure that performs a specific set of functions within the eukaryotic cell while in prokaryotes they lack distinct nucleus or organelles.

The basic structure of all cells is the same. All cells have an outer covering called a plasma membrane. The plasma membrane holds the cell together and permits the passage of substances into and out of the cell. With a few minor exceptions, plasma membranes are basically the same in prokaryotes and eukaryotes. The interior of both kinds of cells is called the cytoplasm. Within the cytoplasm of eukaryotes are embedded the cellular organelles. Both types of cells contain small structures, called ribosomes, the site of synthesis of proteins. Ribosomes are not bounded by membranes and are not considered as organelles. Now on the basis of presence of certain specialized organelles having specific functions like chloroplast, eukaryotic cells are of two types: plant cell and animal cell (Fig. 4.2).

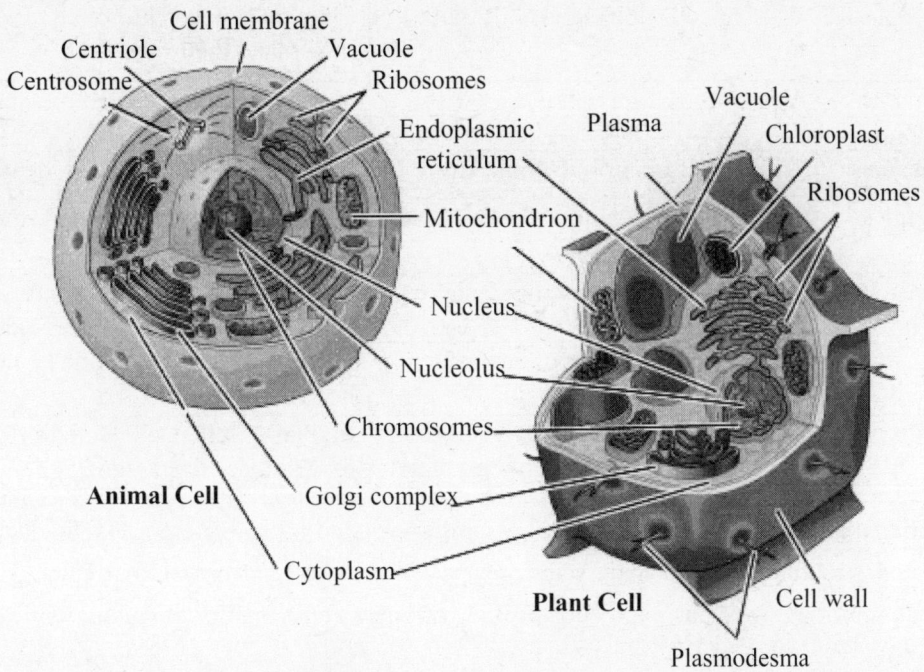

Figure 4.2: Structure of plant and animal cell

Table 4.2: Comparison between plant and animal cell

Characters	Animal cell	Plant cell
Shape	Round (irregular shape)	Rectangular (fixed shape)
size	Animal cell is smaller than plant cell	Plant cell is larger than Animal cell
Cell wall	Animal cell is covered by a thin cell membrane. It is made up of Lipo-protein	Plant cell is covered by a thick cell wall. Cell wall is made up of cellulose and hemicellulose.
Vacuole	In animal cell, Vacuole is small, temporary and not so prominent	In plant cell, Vacuole is big, prominent and permanent
Plastid	Plastid is absent in animal cell	Plastids are present only in plant cell.
Centrosome	Centrosome is present is animal cell. It helps in the process of cell division	Centrosome is absent in plant cell
Mitochondria	The number of Mitochondria is approximately more in animal cell.	The number of Mitochondria is less in plant cell than animal cell.
Cilia	Present	It is very rare
Chloroplast	Animal cells don't have chloroplasts	Plant cells have chloroplasts because they make their own food
Plasma Membrane	Yes; only cell membrane	Yes; cell wall and a cell membrane
Lysosomes	Lysosomes occur in cytoplasm	Lysosomes usually not evident
Centrioles	Present in all animal cells which help in mitosis	Only present in lower plant forms
Glyoxysomes	Animal cells do not have glyoxysomes	Plant cells have glyoxysomes
Amino acids	Animal cell can synthesize only some kinds of Amino acids	In Plant Cell all the Amino acids can be synthesized
Cell division	In Animal Cell, Cell Division occurs by furrow in place of cell plate	In Plant Cell, Cell Division occurs by cell plate formation.

Animal and plant cells have some key similarities and noted differences. Understanding basic cell structure helps to understand how plant cells differ from animal cells. They do differ in important ways, as plant cells provide different functions for the plant, while animal cells provide for the body (Table 4.2).

One of the primary differences between animal and plant cells is that, the plant cells have a cellulose cell wall. This protects the plant cell wall from osmotic shocks. A plant cell has to be able to accept large amounts of liquid through osmosis, without being destroyed. Animal cells do not have rigid cell wall (Fig.4.2). This allows animal cells to form and adopt various shapes. A type of animal cell called the phagocytic cell can even absorb other structures. This ability is not inherent in plant cells. Further, unlike animal cells, plant cells have chloroplasts containing chlorophyll by using them they perform the function of photosynthesis which is absent in animal cells.

Plant cells also contain a larger central vacuole (enclosed by a membrane) as compared to animal cells. Also, while animal cells depend on an analogous system of gap-junctions that allows communication between cells, the plant cells use linking pores in their cell wall to connect to each other and pass information. Plant cells are of three different types. The parenchyma cells help in storage, photosynthesis-support and other functions and collenchyma cells are only present during the time of maturity and have only a primary wall. The sclerenchyma cells help in mechanical support. There are about 210 distinct types of cells present in the human body.

4.1.3. Viruses

Viruses (meaning toxin or poison) are extremely small infectious agents that invade cells of all types. A virus is a tiny bundle of genetic material - either DNA or RNA - carried in a shell called a viral coat, or capsid, which is made up of protein. Some viruses have an additional layer around this coat called an envelope. When a virus particle enters a cell and begins to reproduce itself, this is called a viral infection. The virus is usually very, very small compared to the size of a living cell. The information carried in the viruses DNA allows it to take over the operation of the cell, using it as a factory makes more copies of its own.

Viruses are generally considered as a connecting bridge between living and non-living cells. One of the fundamental hallmarks of life is the ability to reproduce. Viruses can only reproduces inside a host cell thus some argue that they are not alive. However, similar to viruses, there are a few prokaryotes that are obligate parasites and cannot reproduce without a host. But these prokaryotes show another hallmark of life that viruses otherwise lack growth. Once assembled, a virus does not change in size or chemical composition. They lack the machinery for producing energy to drive such biological processes. Viruses do, however, show some characteristics of living things. They are made up of proteins and glycoproteins like cells. They contain genetic information needed to produce more viruses in the form of DNA or RNA. They evolve to adapt to their hosts.

All living things are susceptible to viral infections, plants, animals or bacteria can all be infected by a virus specific for that type of organism. Moreover, within an individual species there may be a hundred or more different viruses which can infect that species alone. There are viruses which infect only humans such as smallpox and influenza, some viruses which infect only a certain kind of plant that is the tobacco mosaic virus and some viruses which infect only a particular species of bacteria (the bacteriophage, which infects *E. coli*).

One of the amazing truth is antibiotics do not harm a virus; for this reason, many treatments for the common cold virus just help ease the symptoms; they don't kill the virus. In your body, the immune system can react to the surface of virus particles, and produce neutralizing antibodies. Vaccines can be made from virus particles and injected into your body; the small infection that results won't make you sick, but it allows your body's immune system to learn to recognize the virus, so that if you are infected later with the real one, your body can fight it. However, mutations within viral DNA cause their surfaces to continually change composition and shape, so that the antibodies may not continue to be effective. This is particularly true with the common cold virus, which is constantly changing, so a vaccine won't be of much use.

Architecture of virus

Virus particle are generally either polyhedral (many planer surface) or helical structure, or they are sometimes rather complex combinations of these two shapes. Polyhedral viruses often appear almost spherical, but closer examination shows that their capsid are actually composed of identical subunits arranged in patterns of icosahedral symmetry (that is 20 sided polyhedrons in which each side is an equilateral triangle).

The symmetry of viruses is a property of the protein capsids that enclose and protect the viral nucleic acid (genome). Each capsid is composed of subunits called capsomeres. Each capsomere is turn is made up of a number of protein molecules. Although a capsid may comprise hundreds of capsomeres, the simplest possible icosahedral virion contains only 60 identical protein molecules arranged in 5 identical capsomears. Helical viruses, such as the tobacco mosaic virus consists of nucleic acid within a cylindrical capsid composed of many identical capsomeres in a spiral arrangement. Many virions have a much more complicated morphology. The nucleic acid of some animal viruses, i.e., the enveloped viruses, is contained within a helical or polyhedral protein capsid, which in turn is surrounded by a membranous outer envelope. This envelope can be complex and consist of several layers of lipid and proteins.

Some of the bacterial viruses are also structurally complex. For example, T-even phage (T2, T4 and T6), a group of phages that infact *Escherichia coli,* are composed of a polyhedral head attached to a helical, hollow tail. The nucleic acid of this phage is a single molecule of double-stranded DNA packed tightly with in the head. Both the efficiency of packaging and the incredible amount of DNA contained within the tiny virion.

Viruses differ considerably in size. The smallest viruses are similar in size to large protein molecules or ribosomes, and their nucleic acid contains only a few genes. The more complex virions may be larger than some of the minute bacteria.

4.1.3.1. Structure of Virus Particles

As most viruses are extremely well adapted to their host organism, virus structure varies greatly. However, there are some general structural characteristics that all viruses share. Viruses are very small in size. Some are not as large as a cell ribosome. Their size is so small that individual virus particles can not be visualized with the light microscope. The range of particle size is from about 20 nanometers for a small virus (e.g. poliovirus) to about 0.3 micrometers for a very large virus [e.g. smallpox (variola) virus].

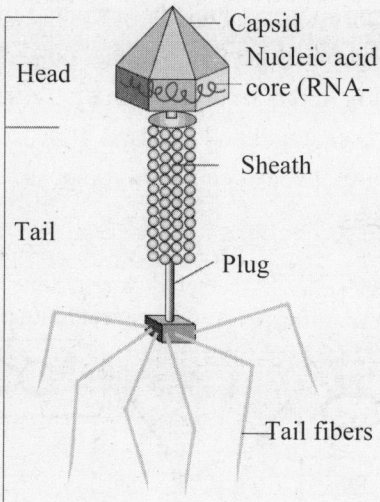

Figure 4.3: Structure of virus particle

Generally, all viruses have a capsid or head region, made up of proteins and glycoproteins, in which the genetic material is present, that can be either DNA or RNA. The construction of capsid varies greatly among viruses, with most being host specific (Fig. 4.3.). Most of the viruses that infect animals have a membranous envelope surrounding their capsid. This allows viruses to penetrate host cells through membrane fusion. In addition to the head region, some viruses, mostly those that infect bacteria, have a tail region. The tail is an often elaborated protein structure. It aids in binding to the surface of the host cell and in the introduction of virus genetic material in to the host cell.

4.1.3.2. Viral Infection

Viruses cannot exist without a host cell. They have to enter in to a host cell for replication, which is known as viral infection. With the possible exception of bacteriophages, the viruses which can kill bacteria, all viruses are considered to be harmful, because their reproduction causes the death of the host cells. If a virus contains DNA, it inserts its genetic material into the host cell's DNA. If the virus contains RNA, it must first turn its RNA into DNA using the host cell's machinery, before inserting it into the host DNA. Once, it has taken over the cell, the viral genes are then copied thousands of times using the machinery of the host cell. Then, the host cell is forced to encapsulate this viral DNA into new protein shells; the new viruses created are then released, destroying the cell.

In general there are six basic steps in their replication cycles. These are: 1) attachment; 2) penetration; 3) un-coating; 4) replication; 5) assembly; 6) release. Viruses are attached to the host cell through special glycoprotein on the exterior of the capsid, envelope or tail. Next, penetration occurs, either of the whole virus or just the contents of the capsid. If the entire capsid enters, the genetic material must be uncoated to make it available to the cell's replication machinery. Replication of genetic material takes place as well as the production of capsid and tail proteins (Fig.4.4). Once all of the necessary parts have been replicated, individual virus particles are assembled and released. Release often takes place in a destructive manner, bursting and killing the host cell, the lytic phase of the viral life cycle.

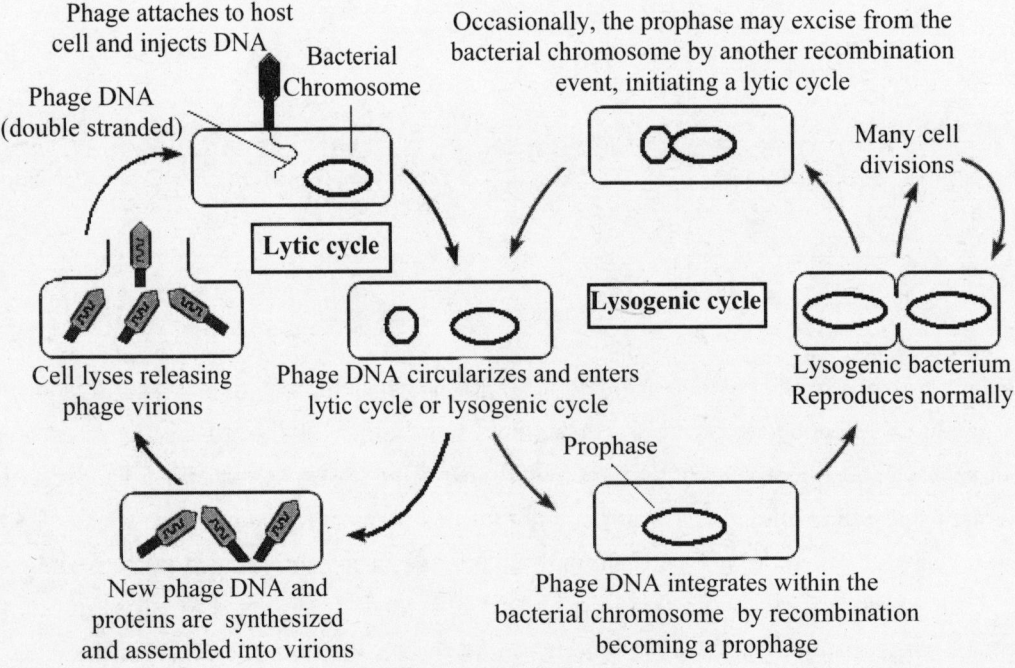

Figure 4.4: Life cycle of Viruses

Some viruses have a slightly more complicated replication cycle involving lytic and lysogenic phases. In the lysogenic phase, however, viral genetic material that has entered the host cell becomes incorporated in the cell and lies dormant. It is passed on to the progeny of the infected cells. Eventually, the lytic phase starts again, and cells that were never infected themselves, but carry the viral genetic material begin to produce new virus particles.

> **Why HIV virus is so dangerous?**
>
> The HIV virus is particularly dangerous because it attacks the cells of the immune system (T-cells), the system that helps to fight diseases. Although, HIV does not itself directly cause the condition known as AIDS, the eventual death of the immune cells in the body due to infection with HIV allows other infections to harm a person.

Table 4.3: Difference between bacteria and viruses

Characters	Viruses	Bacteria
Definition	A virus is an ultramicroscopic, infectious agent that replicates only within the cells of living hosts, mainly bacteria, plants, and animals	Bacteria are one celled organisms that are either spherical, spiral, or rod shaped.
Nature	Viruses must have a living host to multiply	Most bacteria can grow on non-living surfaces
Multiplication	Viruses invade their host's cells and turn the cell's genetic material from its normal function to producing the virus itself	Bacteria carry all the machinery needed for their growth and multiplication
Outermost structure	Protein coat or viral envelope	Peptidoglycan cell wall or capsule/slime layer in some
Nucleic acid	DNA or RNA. can be double-stranded or single-stranded, circular or linear	DNA and RNA. Exist as double-stranded and circular in shape.
Living attributes	Considered living and non-living	Living organism
Enzymes	Yes, in some	Yes
Size	Smaller (20–400 nm)	Larger (1000 nm)
Beneficial?:	Viruses are not beneficial. However, a particular virus may be able to destroy brain tumors (see references). Viruses can be useful in genetic engineering.	Some beneficial bacteria (e.g. certain bacteria required in the gut)

4.2. Ultra structure of the cell

4.2.1. Cell wall

A cell wall is the outer most rigid layer of the cell, located external to the cell membrane, which provides the cell, structural support, protection, and acts as a filtering mechanism. In multi-cellular organisms, it permits the organism to build and to hold its shape (morphogenesis). The cell wall also limits the entry of large molecules that may be toxic to the cell. It further permits the creation of a stable osmotic environment by preventing osmotic lysis and help to retain water. It is found in plants, bacteria, archaea, fungi, and algae, while it is absent in animal and most protists.

The structural component of the cell wall varies according to the type of cells. In plants, the cell wall is made up of carbohydrate polymer, cellulose and in bacteria it is of peptidoglycan, while in fungi, the cell wall is made up of chitin.

[A] Plant cell wall

The cell wall of plant is one of the most important distinguishing features. In addition to the protection of the intracellular contents, it gives rigidity to the plant, provides a porous medium for the circulation and distribution of water, minerals, and other nutrients, and houses a number of specialized molecules that regulate growth and protect the plant from diseases. The thickness, as well as the composition and organization of the cell wall can vary significantly. The cell wall has three major regions:

- **Middle lamella:** It is pectin layer which cements the cell wall of two adjoining cells together. Plants need this lamella to give them stability so that they can form plasmodesmata between the cells. It is the first layer which is deposited at the time of cytokinesis. The Middle lamella is mainly made up of calcium and magnesium pectate.

- **Primary wall:** It is deposited by cells before and during active growth. The actual content of the wall components varies from species to species with the age. All plant cells have a middle lamella and primary wall.

- **Secondary wall:** Some cells deposit additional layers inside the primary wall. This occurs especially after the growth stops or when the cell begins to differentiate. This wall is mainly for support and is comprised primarily of cellulose and lignin. It has distinct layers S1, S2 and S3, which differ in the orientation, or direction of the cellulose microfibrils.

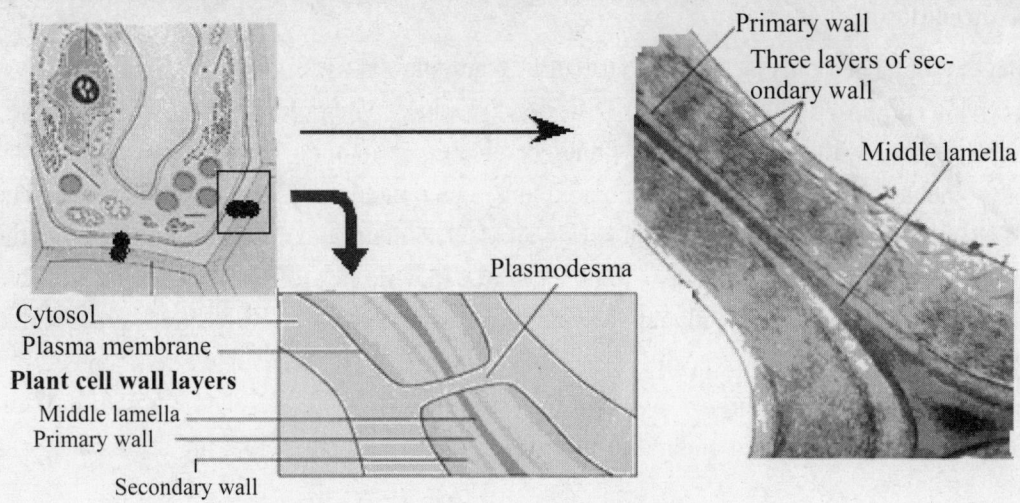

Figure 4.5: Cell wall structure of higher plants

Chemical composition of plant cell wall

Cellulose: Cellulose is the major component of plant cell walls. It is an un-branched polymer with about ten thousand glucose units per chain. Hydroxyl groups (-OH) project out from each chain, forming hydrogen bonds with neighboring chains which creates a rigid cross-linking between the chains, making cellulose as the strong support material. Despite the combined strength of cellulose, it is fully permeable to water and solutes which makes it ideal for allowing water and solutes into and out of the cell. It is the most abundant organic substance found in the living world and has been estimated to be more than half of the total organic carbon available on the planet (Fig. 4.5).

Cellulose readily forms hydrogen bonds with itself (intra-molecular H-bonds) and with other cellulose chains (inter-molecular H-bonds). A cellulose chain forms hydrogen bonds with about 36 other chains in order to yield a micro-fibril. This is somewhat analogous to the formation of a thick rope from thin fibers. Micro-fibrils are 5-12 nm wide and offer the wall strength (Fig. 4.6). They have a tensile strength equivalent to steel. Some regions of the micro-fibrils are highly crystalline while others are more "amorphous".

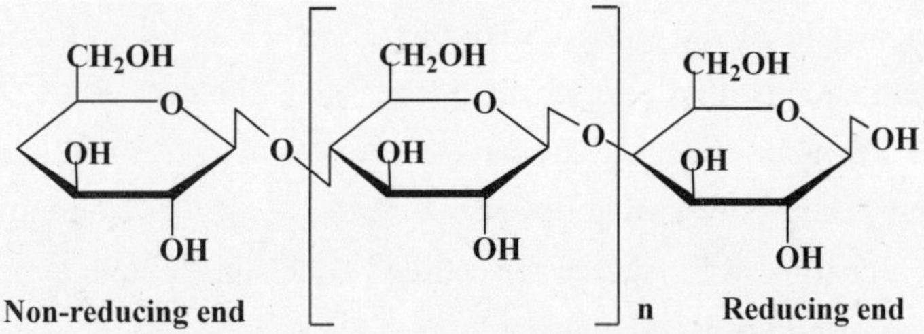

Figure 4.6: Chemical structure of the cellulose

Hemicelluloses

They are branched polysaccharides structurally homolgous to cellulose because they have a backbone composed of 1, 4-linked β-D-hexosyl residues. The predominant hemi-cellulose in many primary walls is xyloglucan. Other hemicelluloses found in primary and secondary walls include glucuronoxylan, arabinoxylan, glucomannan, and galactomannan. They are characterized by being soluble in strong alkali. The main feature of this group is that they do not aggregate with themselves - in other words, they do not form micro-fibrils. However, they form hydrogen bonds with cellulose and hence the reason they are called "cross-linking glycans". Hemi-cellulose molecules are often branched. Like the pectic compounds, hemi-cellulose molecules are highly hydrophilic. They become exclusively hydrated and form gels. Hemi-cellulose is abundant in primary walls and also found in secondary walls (Fig. 4.7).

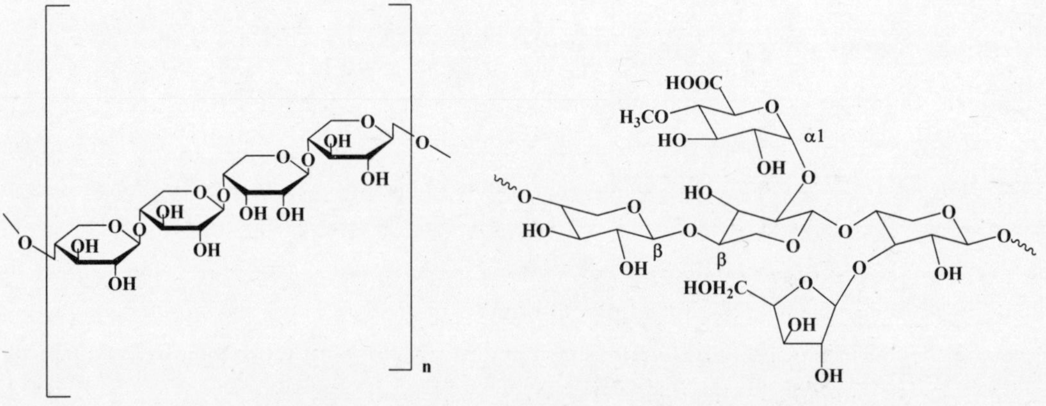

Figure 4.7: Chemical structure of hemi-cellulose

Pectin:

It is a family of complex polysaccharides that contain 1, 4-linked α-D-galacturonic acid. There are three represent classes of pectic polysaccharides. They are comparatively less hydrated than pectic acid but soluble in hot water. It is another major component of middle lamella but also found in primary walls (Fig. 4.8). This is made up of a modified sugar, galacturonic acid and in the plant the carboxyl groups are esterified with methyl (CH_3) groups. Divalent cations, like calcium, also form cross-linkages amongst adjacent polymers creating a gel. Pectic polysaccharides can also be cross-linked by dihydrocinnamic or diferulic acids. The pectic polysaccharides serve a variety of functions including determining wall porosity, a charged wall surface for cell-cell adhesion (middle lamella), cell-cell recognition, pathogen recognition and others.

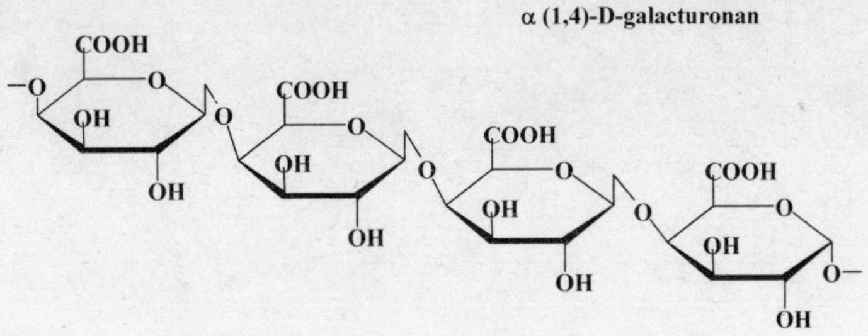

α (1,4)-D-galacturonan

Figure 4.8: Chemical structure of pectin

Proteins:

Wall proteins are typically glycol-proteins (polypeptide backbone with carbohydrate side chains). The proteins are particularly rich in the amino acids hydroxyl-proline (hydroxyproline-rich glycoprotein, HPRG), and glycine (glycine-rich protein, GRP). These proteins form rods (HRGP, PRP) or beta-pleated sheets (GRP). HRGP (Extensin)is induced by wounding and pathogen attack. Protein appears to be cross-linked to pectic substances and may have sites for lignifications. The proteins may serve as the scaffolding used to construct the other wall components.

Lignin:

Lignin is a complex polymer of phenyl-propane units, which are cross-linked to each other with a variety of different chemical bonds. This complexity has thus far proven as resistant to microbial degradation. Nonetheless, some organisms, particularly fungi, have been identified with the necessary enzymes that break up lignin apart.

Lignin is a major chemical compound present in the cell walls of tracheids, xylary fibres and sclereids of plants. Lignin polymers are mostly made up of phenyl-propanoid units linked to each other through different kinds of bonds. Lignin polymers are probably network structures with molecular weights on the order of 10,000 amu. Lignin is the most abundant organic material on earth after cellulose. It is believed that lignin gives wood its stiffness and improves water transport (Fig. 4.9). Lignin is thought to act as a kind of glue in the plant cell walls and give plants very effective protection against parasite attack. Lignin makes up about one-quarter to one-third of the mass of dry wood. In the chemical pulping process, lignin is removed from wood pulp before it is turned into paper, and the extracted lignin is used as a binder in particle board, adhesive for linoleum, and raw material for processing into chemicals (such as DMSO and vanillin). The type of lignin (such as lingo-sulfonates and kraft lignins) used in industry depends upon the method that was used to extract it.

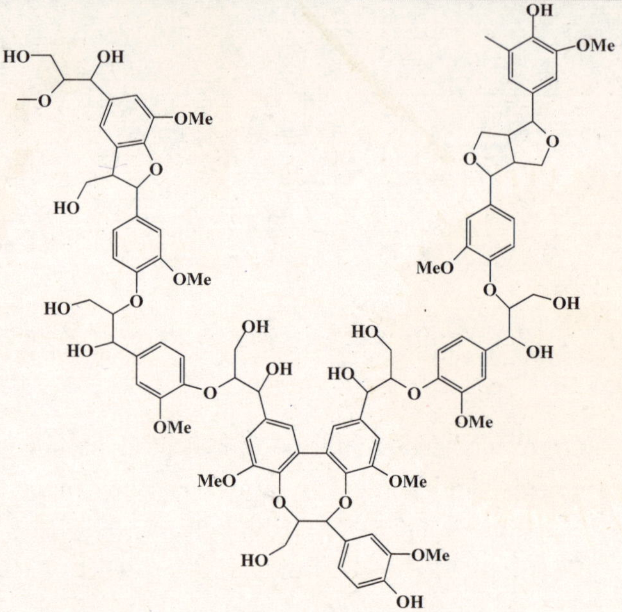

Figure 4.9: Chemical structure of lignin

Suberin and Cutin:

Suberin is fairly hydrophobic and its main function is to prevent water from penetrating the tissue. A variety of lipids are associated with the wall for strength and water-proofing. Cutin is a waxy polymer that is the main components of the plant cuticle which covers all aerial surfaces of plants.

Water: The cell wall is largely hydrated and comprised of between 75—80% water. This is responsible for some of the wall properties. For example, hydrated walls exhibit greater flexibility and extensibility than non-hydrated walls.

[B] Algal cell wall

Algae are a large and diverse class of simple, typically autotrophic organisms. The cell wall composition and structure of algae differs significantly from that of higher plants. Neither in composition nor in biosynthesis do they have any common features with the cell walls of plants.

In many classes of algae cellulose is the main structural element of the wall, though re-markable variations of the fibrillary structure may exist. In some classes of algae there are only dispersed textures, while in others (especially many Chlorophyta-species) a higher de-gree of organization (layers of parallel micro-fibrils) is present. No clear difference between primary and secondary cell wall exists in most algae.

Manosyl: Manosyl constitutes the main structural elements in a number of marine green algae (*Codium, Dasycladus, Acetabularia*, etc.) as well as in the walls of some red algae (*Porphyra, Bangia*). They are linear and the mannosyl residues are (1–4) glycosidically linked.

Xylanes: They are the polymers where the β-D-xylosyl residues are linked through (1–3) and (1-4) glycosidic bonds. In contrast to other polymers, xylans are partially ramified. In species with xylan-containing walls there exists a layered structure and an orientation of the microfilaments. They contain mostly linear polymers.

Alginic Acid: The cell walls of Phaeophyta (brown algae) mainly consist of alginic acid and its salts, the alginates, consist exclusively of uronic acids: mannuronic acid and beta-L-glucuronic acid in varying ratios along with small amounts of β-D-glucuronic acid. It is a linear copolymer consisting mainly of residues of β (1, 4)-linked D-mannuronic acid and α -1,-4-linked L-glucuronic acid. These monomers are often arranged in homo-polymeric blocks separated by regions approximating an alternating sequence of the two acid monomers (Fig.4.10).

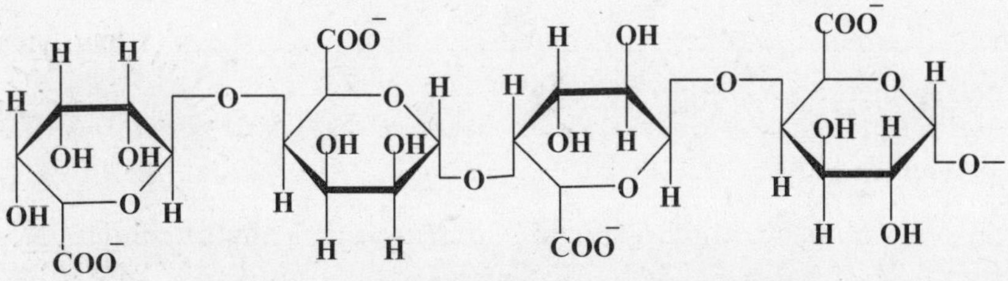

Figure 4.10: Chemical structure of alginic acid

The alginates of brown algae exist both within the cell wall and in the intercellular substance. Their part in the cell wall may be as high as 40 per cent of the dry matter. They have a high affinity for divalent cations (calcium, strontium, barium, magnesium) and a tendency to gel.

Sulfonated Polysaccharides: They occur partially in the cell wall itself and partially in the intercellular substance. Sulfonated galactanes are typical for many red algae, depending on their origin they are called agarose, carrageenan, porphyran, furcelleran and funoran. Chemically they are polysaccharides whose monomers are esterified to sulfuric acid residues and moreover they are partially methylated.

Carrageenan and furcelleran contain exclusively D-compounds. Agar, whose basic unit is agarose, is obtained mainly from *Gelidium* and *Gracillaria*, both genera of red algae. The extraordinary binding types of agarose and carrageenan lead to specific tertiary structures.

Chemically, agarose is a polysaccharide, whose monomeric unit is a disaccharide of D-galactose and 3, 6-anhydro-L-galactopyranose (fig. 4.11).

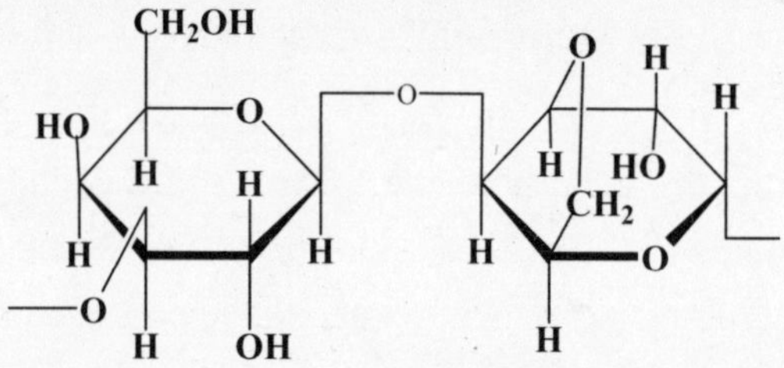

Figure 4.11: Chemical structure of agarose

Silicon: It is one of the main components of the diatom shell. It also occurs in the cell walls of other groups of algae. Silicon is a cell wall component in some brown algae and in the green algae *Hydrodictyon*. Diatoms take up silicon as silicate.

Calcium: Calcium seems to be common in species of tropical and marine waters. Some species participate in reef formation. Calcium is always deposited as calcium carbonate and occurs in two different crystalline states: calcite and aragonite. Calcite is produced in the walls of some groups of red algae and in Charophyceae, while aragonite is produced by some green (*Acetabularia*, etc.), brown and red algae. Both states do not occur simultaneously in one species.

[C] Fungal cell wall

The fungal cell wall is a complex structure composed typically of chitin (fig. 4.12), 1,3- β- and 1,6-β-glucan, mannan and proteins, although the wall composition frequently varies markedly between species of fungi, there is evidence of extensive cross-linking between these components. Fungi have chitin cell walls, which make them more like animals than plants. Conversely, the water molds have cellulose cell walls that make them more plant-like, so they have been separated from the fungi in modern classification.

Approximately 80% of the wall consists of polysaccharides. Most fungi have a fibrillar structure build up of chitin chitosan (Zygomycota only), and ß-glucans, and a variety of hetero-polysaccharides (Fig. 4.13). The fibres are contained in a complex gel-like matrix. Proteins constitute a small fraction of wall material, rarely more than 20%, and often as glycoprotein. Not all proteins have a structural role to play. Hydrophobins are expressed constitutively and become bound in the wall, when the hyphae emerge in air. Lipids are found in walls, usually in very small concentrations. Along with hydrophobins, lipids and waxes appear to function in the process of control over movement of water, especially the prevention of desiccation of cells. Walls also contain a range of other minor components, including pigments and salts. The pigments, melanin is particularly intriguing. Melanin, important for protecting the hyphae and spores from UV stress, is essential for pathogenesis and attachment to surfaces of emerging hyphae from spores.

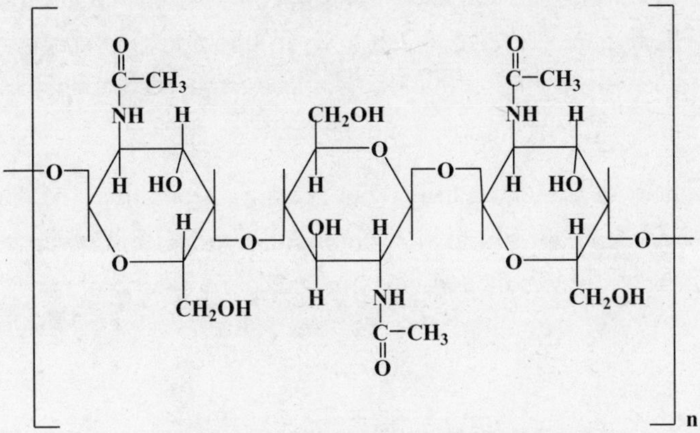

Figure 4.12: Molecular structure Chitin

The constituents of cell walls are synthesized in the cytoplasm, linked in the walls at the hyphal tip, polymerized and cross-linked in the wall matrix. Chitin and the glucans are synthesized at the plasma membrane by the enzymes embedded in the membrane itself. Nucleotide sugar precursors are accepted from the cytoplasm, linked and passed to the wall. The wall glycol-proteins are synthesized in the endoplasmic reticulum carried through the Golgi to the plasma membrane, where vesicles release the glycoprotein to the wall. Enzymes cross-linking fibrils in the wall are released through the plasma membrane.

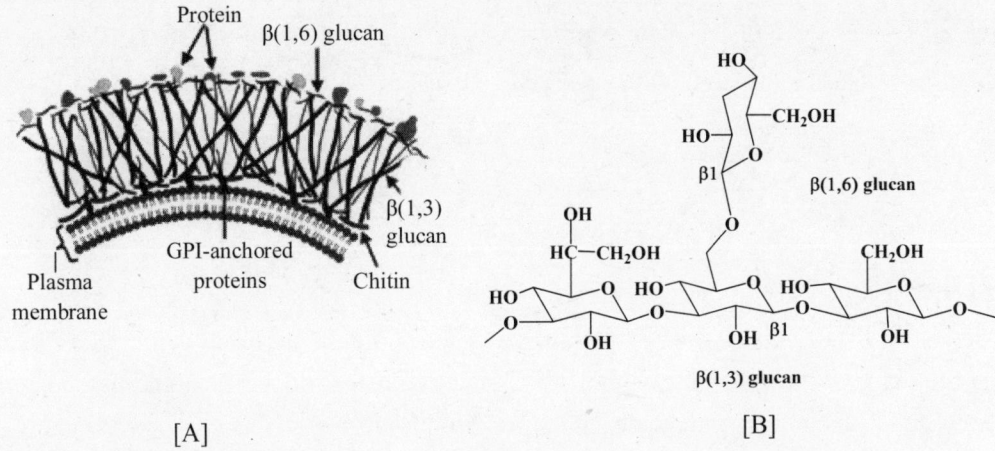

[A]

[B]

Figure 4.13: (A) Fungal cell wall (B) Glycophosphatidylinositol (GPI)

Hydrophobins: Hydrophobins constitute up to 10% of total wall protein. The amphipathic structure (having hydrophobic and hydrophilic domains) provides the molecules with an extraordinary potential array of functions. This construction reduces movement of water through the wall of the hyphae providing some protection from desiccation. It may also increase the strength of the wall. The exposed hydrophobic domain enables attachment to hydrophobic surfaces. The hyphae can also attach to hydrophobic (e.g. waxy) plant surfaces, enabling attachment of spores prior to formation of appressoria. The attachment properties make hydrophobins extremely important in morphogenic development.

Glomalin: Some members of the Glomeromycota produce a putative glycoprotein in the walls. This compound has been called glomalin. Glomalin is important because of its possible correlation with aggregation of soil particles and the purported resilience of the molecule.

[D] Protists cell wall

Protists are all eukaryotes (cell with nuclei). All protists live in moist surrounding, unicellular, while some are multi-cellular. Some are heterotrophs (can not make their own food; have to eat something) some are autotrophs (make their own food) some can not move (sessile), while others can move. These are divided into three categories, i.e., animal-like, plant-like and fungus-like protists. The cells of many protists are surrounded by a filamentous layer of oligosaccharides. This forms the cell coat. It is in fact a part of the cell membrane. In many cases the cell coat becomes deposited with salts of calcium and silica (Fig.4.14). The cell coat mainly provides protection to the cell from infection by pathogens. It also helps in the recognition of similar cells.

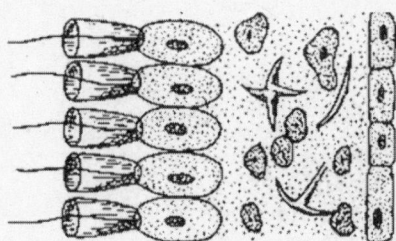

Figure 4.14: Protest cell wall

[E] Bacterial cell wall

The cell wall lies outside the cell membrane. The rigid peptidoglycan is important in defining the shape of the cell and giving the cell a mechanical strength. Bacteria may be conveniently divided into two groups, depending upon their ability to retain a crystal violet-iodine dye complex when cells are treated with acetone or alcohol (Gram reaction, named after

Christian Gram). This reaction, however, reveals fundamental differences in the structure of bacteria. Cells with many layers of peptidoglycan can retain a crystal violet-iodine complex when treated with acetone. These are called Gram-positive bacteria and appear blue-black or purple when stained using Gram's method (Fig. 4.15). Gram-negative bacteria have only one or two layers of peptidoglycan and cannot retain the crystal violet-iodine complex. They require counterstaining with another dye (safranin) to be seen using Gram's method.

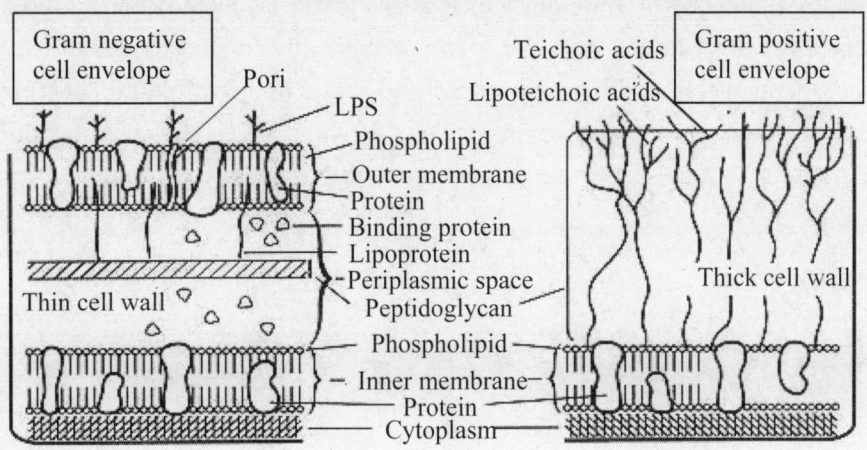

Figure 4.15: Cell wall of Gram positive and Gram negative bacteria

Gram negative bacteria have a much thinner cell wall. The wall is high in lipid content and low in peptidoglycan. The crystal-violate escapes from cell when the decolorizer is added because of the lack of peptidoglycan. The outer membrane of gram negative bacteria is composed of a high concentration of lipids, polysaccharides and proteins. Most Gram-positive bacteria have a relatively thick (about 20 to 80 nm), continuous cell wall, which is composed largely of peptidoglycan (also known as mucopeptide or murein). In thick cell walls, other cell wall polymers such as the teichoic acids, polysaccharides, and peptidogly-colipids are covalently attached to the peptidoglycan. In contrast, the peptidoglycan layer in Gram-negative bacteria is thin (about 5 to 10 nm thick); in *E coli*, the peptidoglycan is probably only a monolayer thick. Outside the peptidoglycan layer in the Gram-negative envelope, there is an outer membrane structure (about 7.5 to 10 nm thick). In most Gram-negative bacteria, this membrane structure is anchored non-covalently to lipoprotein molecules, which in turn, are covalently linked to the peptidoglycan. The lipo-polysaccharides of the Gram-negative cell envelope form outer part of the outer membrane structure.

(a) **Peptidoglycans:**

(b) Both Gram-positive and Gram-negative bacteria possess cell wall peptidoglycans, which confer the characteristic cell shape and provide the cell with mechanical protection.

Peptidoglycans are unique to prokaryotic organisms and consist of a glycan backbone of muramic acid and glucosamine (both N-acetylated; N- acetyl muramic acid (NAM) and N- acetyl glucosamine (NAG)), and peptide chains highly cross-linked with bridges in Gram-positive bacteria (*Staphylococcus aureus*) or partially cross-linked in Gram-negative bacteria (*E. coli*). The main function of peptidoglycan is to preserve cell integrity by withstanding the turgor pressure inside the cell. Inhibition of peptidoglycan biosynthesis by mutations or antibiotics such as penicillin or degradation by lysozyme in growing cells results in cell lysis (Fig. 4.16). Peptidoglycan contributes to the maintenance of a defined cell shape (rod or sphere) and serves as a scaffold for anchoring other cell envelope components such as proteins and teichoic acids. However, peptidoglycan is found absent in some bacteria (*Mycoplasma* sp., *Planctomyces*, *Rickettsia* and *Chlamidiae*).

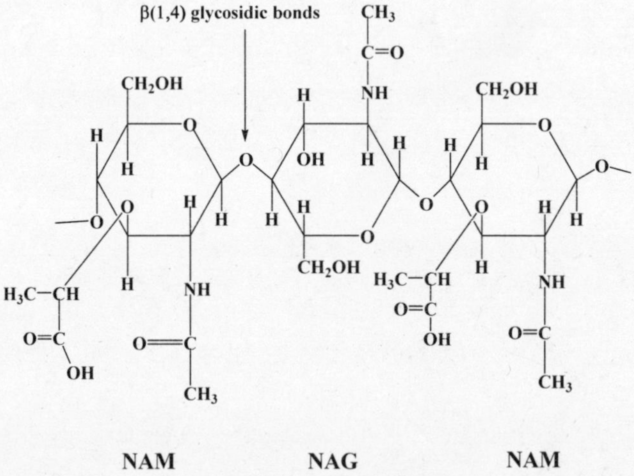

Figure 4.16: Chemical structure of peptidoglycan

(b) Teichoic Acids:

Membrane associated teichoic acids (lipoteichoic acids) are polymers of amphiphilic glycophosphates with the lipophilic glycolipid and anchored in the cytoplasmic membrane. They are antigenic, cytotoxic and adhesions (*Streptococcus pyogenes*). Teichoic acids are polyol phosphate polymers, with either ribitol or glycerol linked by phosphordiester bonds bearing a strong negative charge. They are covalently linked to the peptidoglycan in some Gram-positive bacteria. They are strongly antigenic, but are generally absent in Gram-negative bacteria. Teichoic acids are covalently linked to the peptidoglycan.(Fig. 4.17). These highly negatively charged polymers of the bacterial wall can serve as a cation-sequestering mechanism.

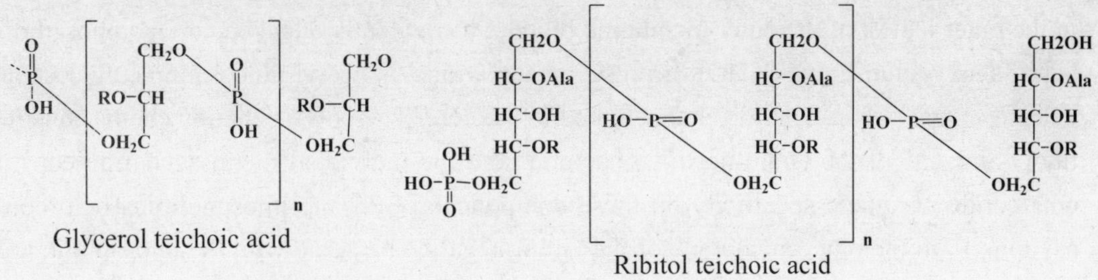

Glycerol teichoic acid

Ribitol teichoic acid

Figure 4.17: Structures of cell wall teichoic acids

(c) Lipo-polysaccharides (LPS):

One of the major components of the outer membrane of Gram-negative bacteria is lipo-polysaccharide (endo-toxin), a complex molecule consisting of a lipid anchor, a polysaccharide core, and chains of carbohydrates. Sugars in the polysaccharide chains confer serologic specificity. So far, only one Gram-positive organism, *Listeria monocytogenes*, has been found to contain an authentic LPS. Endo-toxins possess an array of powerful biologic activities and play an important role in the pathogenesis of many Gram-negative bacterial infections. In addition to causing endo-toxic shock, LPS is pyrogenic, can activate macrophages and complement, mitogenic for B lymphocytes, induces interferon production, causes tissue necrosis and tumor regression and has adjuvant properties.

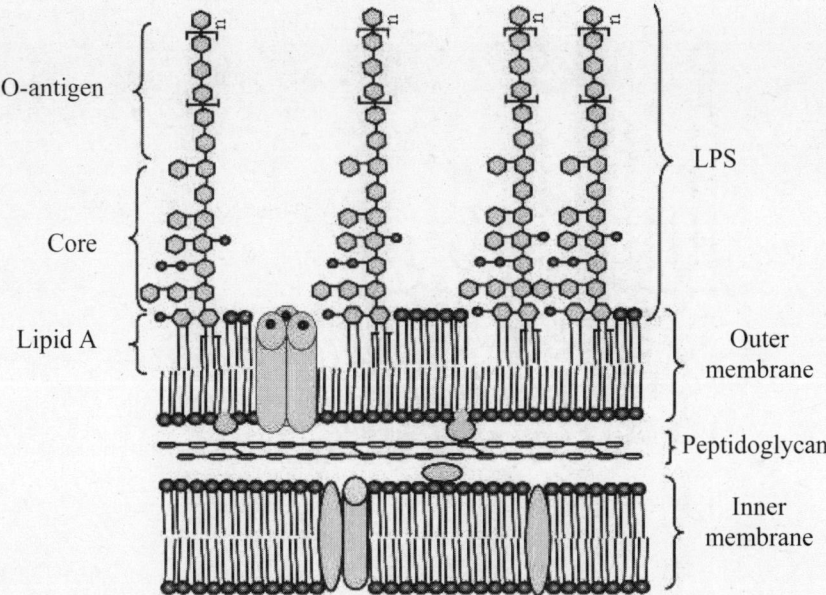

Figure 4.18: Organization of LPS

Usually, the LPS molecules have three regions: the lipid structure required for insertion in the outer leaflet of the outer membrane bilayer; a covalently attached core composed of 2-keto-3deoxyoctonic acid (KDO), heptose, ethanolamine, N-acetyl-glucosamine, glucose, and galactose; and polysaccharide chains linked to the core. The polysaccharide chains constitute the O-antigens of the Gram-negative bacteria, and the individual monosaccharide constituents confer serologic specificity on these components. LPS and phospholipids help confer asymmetry to the outer membrane of the Gram-negative bacteria, with the hydrophilic polysaccharide chains outermost. Each LPS is held in the outer membrane by relatively weak cohesive forces (ionic and hydrophobic interactions) and can be dissociated from the cell surface by action of surface-active agents (Fig. 4.18).

[F] Wall-less forms

Two groups of bacteria devoid of cell wall peptidoglycans are the Mycoplasma species, which possess a surface membrane structure, and the L-forms that arise from either Gram-positive or Gram-negative bacterial cells that have lost their ability to produce the peptidoglycan structures.

[G] Cell wall of acid fast bacteria

Acid-fast bacteria are gram-positive. Acid fast bacterial cell wall is composed of a thin, inner layer of peptidoglycan and large amount of glycolipids, such as mycolic acid, arabinogalactan-lipid complex, and lipoarabinomannan. It is approximately 60 percent lipid and contains much less peptidoglycan (Fig. 4.19).

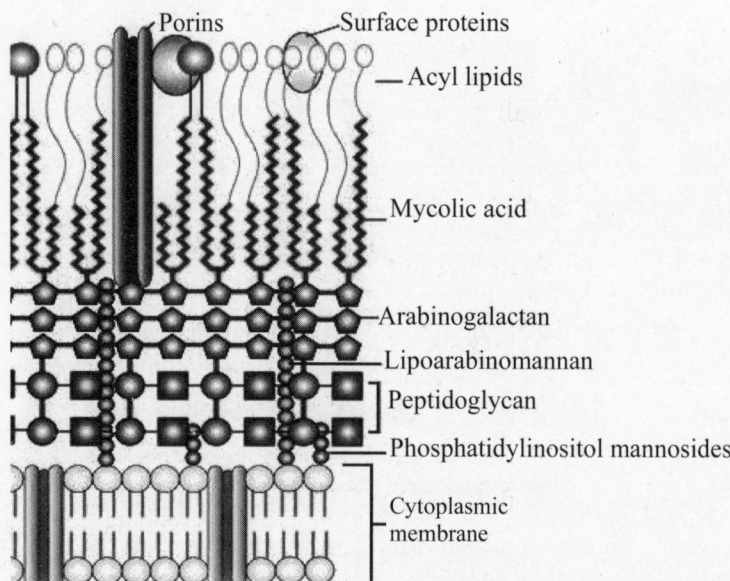

Figure 4.19: Cell wall organization of Acid fast bacterial cell wall

The lipids make acid-fast organisms impermeable to most other stains and protect them from acids and alkalis. During the acid-fast staining procedure, the acid-fast cell wall enables the bacterium to resist de-colorization with acid alcohol and retain the original stain carbol fuchsin. Like the outer membrane of the gram-negative cell wall, porins are required to transport small hydrophilic molecules through the outer membrane of the acid-fast cell wall. There are far fewer porins in the acid-fast cell wall compared to the gram-negative cell wall and the pores are much longer. The peptidoglycan prevents osmotic lysis and the mycolic acids and other glycol-lipids impede the entry of chemicals which cause the organisms to grow slowly and be more resistant to chemical agents and lysosomal components of phago-cytes than most bacteria. This is thought to contribute significantly to the lower permeability of acid-fast bacteria.

[H] Archaea bacterial cell wall

Archaeal cell walls lack peptidoglycan, except one group of methanogens. In this, the pepti-doglycan is a modified form, different from that found in bacteria. There are four types of cell wall currently known among the Archaea.

- Pseudo-peptidoglycan (also called pseudomurein) is the main structural component of cell wall of some methanogens (*Methanobacterium* and *Methanothermus)*. Pseudo-peptidoglycan consists of polymer chains of glycan cross-linked with short peptides. However, unlike peptidoglycan, the sugar N-acetylmuramic acid is replaced by N-acetyltalosaminuronic acid, and the two sugars are bonded with a $\beta,1$-3 glycosidic link-age instead of $\beta,1$-4, also cross-linking peptides are L-amino acids rather than D-amino acids as in bacteria.

- The second type of cell wall is composed entirely of a thick layer of polysaccharides, which may be sulfated in case of *Methanosarcina* and *Halococcus*.

- Third type of Archaeal cell wall consists of glycoprotein, which occurs in the hyperther-mophiles, *Halobacterium*, and some methanogens. In *Halobacterium*, the proteins in the wall have a high content of acidic amino acids, giving the wall an overall negative charge and thrive only under conditions with high salinity since structure is stabilized by the presence of large quantities of positive sodium ions that neutralize the charge.

- In the fourth type, the wall is composed of only of surface-layer proteins, known as an S-layer. S-layers are monomolecular crystalline arrays of proteinaceous subunits and are common in bacteria, where they serve as either the sole cell-wall component or an outer layer in conjunction with peptidoglycan and murein. Most Archaea are Gram-negative, though at least one Gram-positive member is known. *Methanomicrobium* and *Desulfu-rococcus* are belonging to this category.

4.2.2. Bacterial Cell Surface Structures

Two types of surface appendages can be recognized on certain bacterial species: the flagella, which are organs of locomotion, and pili, which are also known as fimbriae. They are found on many species of bacilli but rarely on cocci. Pilli occur almost exclusively on Gram-negative bacteria and are found on only a few Gram-positive organisms (*Corynebacterium renale*). Some bacteria have both flagella and pilli.

Flagella

The flagella of motile bacteria differ in structure from eukaryotic flagella. A basal body anchored in the plasma membrane and cell wall gives rise to a cylindrical protein filament. The flagellum moves by whirling about its long axis. The number and arrangement of flagella on the cell are diagnostically useful. Flagella are embedded in the cell membrane, extend through the cell envelope and project as a long strand. Flagella consist of a number of proteins including flagellin. They move the cell by rotating with a propeller like action.

Pili (Fimbriae)

Pili are slender, hair-like, proteinaceous appendages found on the surface of many (particularly Gram-negative) bacteria. They are important in adhesion to host surfaces. Pili are tubules that are used to transfer DNA from one cell to another cell.

Endospores

Endospores are heat-resistant, dehydrated resting cells that are formed intra-cellular by and contain a genome and all essential metabolic machinery. The endospore is enclosed in a complex protective spore coat. Endospores contain calcium dipicolinate (dipicolinic acid) which is involved in the heat resistance of the spores. Spores are commonly found in the genera *Bacillus* and *Clostridium*. The outer proteinaceous coat surrounding the spore provides much of the chemical and enzymatic resistance. Beneath the coat resides a very thick layer of specialized peptidoglycan called the cortex. Proper cortex formation is needed for dehydration of the spore core, which offers resistance to high temperature.

Capsules and slime layers

These are structures surrounding the outside of the cell envelope. They usually consist of high molecular-weight viscous polysaccharide; however, in certain bacilli they are composed of a polypeptide (poly-glutamic acid). They are not essential to cell viability and some strains within a species are known to produce a capsule, whilst others do not. Capsules of pathogenic bacteria inhibit their ingestion and killing by phagocytes. The capsule of *Bacillus anthracis* (the causal agent of anthrax) is unusual in that it is composed of glutamyl polypeptide.

4.2.3. Plasma Membrane

The cell membrane (also called the plasma membrane in eukaryotic cells) is the boundary layer between the cell cytoplasm and the cells external environment. It is made up of Lipids and Proteins held together mainly by non-covalent interaction. Plasma membrane encloses the cell, defines its boundaries and maintains the essential differences between the cell and extracellular environment and also between the cellular organelles and cytosol. To perform also certain specialized functions, this membrane makes some compartments inside the cytoplasm as in mitochondria, chloroplasts, golgi apparatus, lysosomes and other membrane bound organelles in all the eukaryotic cells.

Cell membranes are dynamic, fluid structures and most of their molecules are able to move about in the plane of the membrane. The fundamental structure of the membrane is the phospholipid bilayer, which forms a stable barrier between two aqueous compartments. These compartments are the inside and the outside of the cell. Proteins embedded within the phospholipid bilayer carry out some specific functions of the plasma membrane, including selective transport of molecules, cell-cell recognition and in anchoring some cytoskeletal fibres to give the cell its shape. Membrane bound enzymes perform certain specific reactions which are needed for certain cellular activities. Ion gradients across membranes, established by the activities of specialized membrane proteins, can be used to synthesize ATP, to drive the transmembrane movement of selected solutes, or, in nerve and muscle cells, to produce and transmit electrical signals.

The chemical composition of the membrane is not constant for all cell types. There is considerable variation in the amount of proteins and lipids present in the membrane structure of different organisms. The ratio of protein to lipid varies from 80:20 in bacteria to 20:80 in some nerve cells. In most of the membranes, however the ratio is about 50:50. The lipid components of the membrane are phospholipids, glycolipids or steroids. Due to this diversity in membrane-composition, different ideas or models have been proposed to know the structure and organization of membrane.

On the basis of it's lipid permeability character, Overton, 1895 regarded it as a lipoidal membrane. Gorter and Grandel, 1925 regarded it as a lipid bimolecular layer. Thereafter several important models were proposed which are discussed here.

Butter-Sandwich Model

Davson and Danielli in1935 proposed that the plasma membrane is made up of two monomolecular protein layers sandwiching a bimolecular lipid layer. The membrane proteins may be globular or α-helical or in a folded β-chain form on both sides. There may be β-chain on one side and globular on the other side. The membrane has protein lined pores of 7 Å diameters. The lipid molecules of the membrane are arranged in a tail facing orientation.

Unit Membrane Concept

Robertson, 1953 suggested that the plasma membrane is made up of two monomolecular protein layers sandwiching a bimolecular lipid layer. However, the two protein layers differ in their constitution. The outer layer has mucoproteins whereas the inner side has non-mucoid proteins. The lipid molecules are arranged in tail facing manner. In plasma membrane, the total protein layer having heads of lipids embedded in 25 Å thick but the clear protein layer is 20 Å thick. The clear lipid layer is 25 Å thick but the total lipid layer is 35 Å thick. The total thickness of plasma membrane is about 75 Å.

Benson's Model

Benson in 1966 proposed that the plasma membrane lipids and proteins show a hydrophobic association. There is a folded protein chain in which the tails of lipids molecules are inserted. The charged heads of lipid molecules lie on the surface of the membrane.

There are many other models available which explain the structure of the membrane. According to Frey-Wyssling and Muhlethaler, 1965, there is a bimolecular layer of globular lipoprotein molecules. Later, Muhlethaler et al., (1966) regarded that the membrane is a lipid bilayers having globular protein molecules of 40 Å size partly embedded in it. While Lenard and Singer, 1966 considered the membrane to be a lipid-protein-lipid structure. Lucy (1968), regarded that the membrane has lipid globules and bilayers embedded in a proteinaceous matrix.

Fluid-Mosaic Model

The current model of membrane structure, proposed by Jonathan Singer and Garth Nicolson in 1972, views membrane as a fluid mosaic in which proteins are inserted in to lipid bilayer. While phospholipid provides the basic structural organization of membranes, membrane proteins carry out the specific functions of the different membranes of the cell. These proteins are divided in to two general classes, based on the nature of their association with the membrane. Integral membrane proteins are embedded directly within the lipid bilayer. Peripheral membranes proteins are not inserted in to the lipid bilayer but are associated with the membrane indirectly, generally by interactions with integral membrane proteins (Fig.4.20).

Most integral membrane proteins (called transmembrane proteins) span the lipid bilayer, with portions exposed to both the sides of the membrane. The membrane- spanning portions of these proteins are usually α-helical regions of 20 to 25 non polar amino acids. The hydrophobic side chains of these amino acids interact with the fatty acid chains of membrane lipids, and the formation of an α helical neutralizes the polar character of the peptide bonds. The only other proteins structure known to span lipid bilayers is the β-barrel, formed by the folding of β sheets in to a barrel like structure, which is found in some transmembrane proteins of bacteria, chloroplasts and mitochondria. Like phospholipids, transmembrane proteins are amphipathic molecules, with their hydrophilic portions exposed to the aqueous environment on the both sides of the membrane. Most transmembrane proteins of eukaryotic plasma membranes have been modified by the addition of carbohydrates, which are exposed on the surface of the cell and may participate in cell-cell interactions.

Proteins can also be anchored in membranes by lipids that are covalently attached to the polypeptide chain. Distinct lipid modifications anchor proteins to the cytosolic and extracellular face of the membrane either by the addition of 14-carbon fatty acids (myristic acid) to their amino terminus or by the addition of either a 16 carbon fatty acid (palmitic acid) or 15 or 20 carbon prenyl groups to the side chains of cysteine residues. Alternatively, proteins are anchored to the extracellular face of the plasma membrane by the addition of glycolipids to their carboxy terminus.

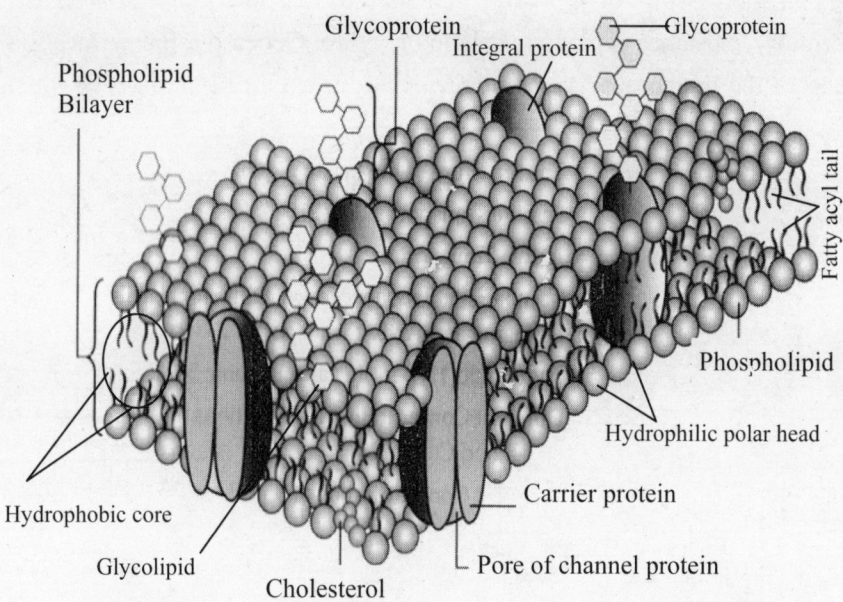

Figure 4.20: Three dimensional structure of Plasma membrane

According to their position in the plasma membrane, the proteins fall into two main types : Integral or intrinsic proteins and peripheral or extrinsic proteins, both of which may be either ectoproteins, lying exposed to external or extra cytoplasmic surface of the plasma membrane or endoproteins, lying or sticking out to the inner or cytoplasmic surface of the plasma membrane. The intrinsic proteins tend to associate firmly with the membrane, while the extrinsic proteins have a weaker association and are bound to lipids of membrane by electrostatic interaction.

On the basis of their functions, proteins of plasma membrane can also be classified into three main types: structural proteins, enzymes and transport proteins. Structural proteins are extremely lipophilic and form the back bone of the plasma membrane. Enzymes of plasma membrane are either ectoenzymes or endoenzymes. Transport proteins transport specific substances across the plasma membrane and other cellular membranes. There are two major classes of membrane transport proteins: Carrier proteins (also called carriers, permeases, or transporters) bind to specific solute to be transported and undergo a series of conformational changes in order to transfer the bound solute across the membrane. Channel proteins, on the other hand, need not bind the solute. Instead, they form hydrophilic pores that extend across the lipid bilayer; when these pores are open, they allow specific solutes (usually inorganic ions of appropriate size and charge) to pass through them and thereby cross the membrane. Transport through channel proteins occurs at a very much faster rate than carrier proteins.

4.2.3.1. Membrane Transport

Compartmentalization is one of the main functions of cell membrane, transport nutrients, ions, and excretory substances from one side to the other. Generally, the permeation of small molecules across the membrane is quite different from engulfing molecules which are too large to penetrate the membrane (Fig. 4.21).

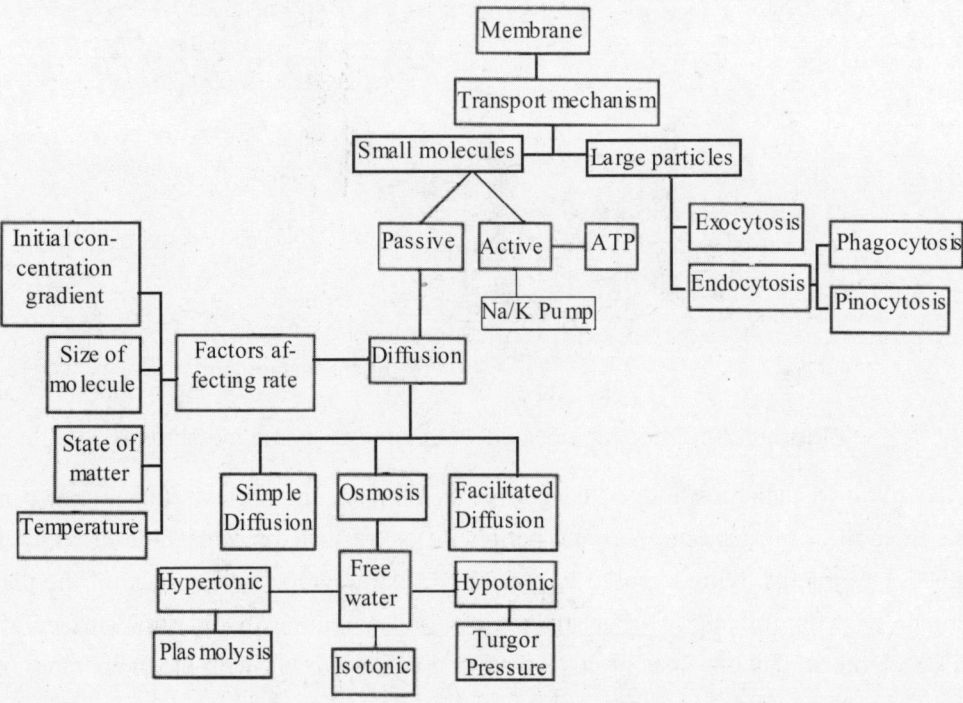

Figure 4.21: Scheme of membrane transport

4.2.3.2. Transport of small molecules

Based on the expenditure of energy membrane, transports are divided in to two: active and passive transports.

(a) Passive transport: Passive transport does not require an expenditure of metabolic energy, and materials flow down the concentration gradient. Examples of passive transport are diffusion, osmosis, and facilitated diffusion (Fig. 4.22).

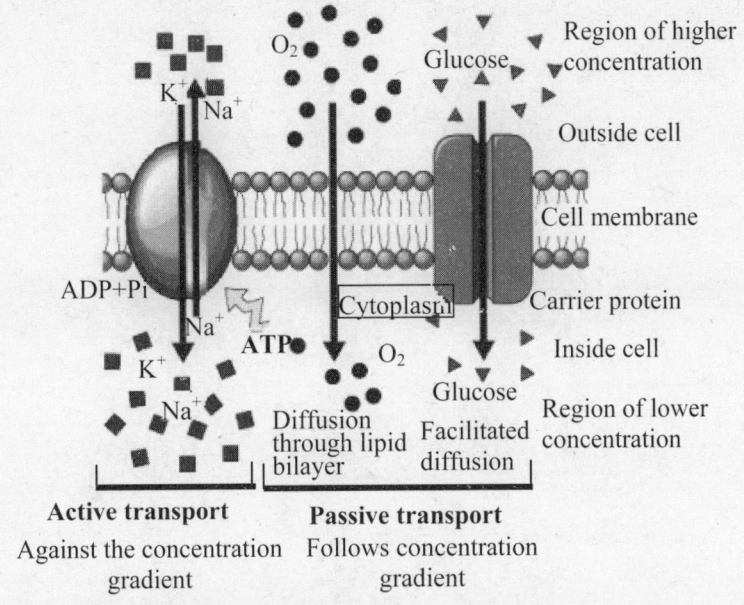

Figure 4.22: Passive and active membrane transport

(i) Simple diffusion: Diffusion is the movement of substances with the concentration gradient. As it does not need any helper molecules or energy, hence it is passive.

(ii) Osmosis: Lipid membranes are semi-permeable; some substances pass through freely (water), while some do not (ions). Diffusion of water down its concentration gradient is called osmosis. Water moves from an area of higher solute concentration to an area of lower solute concentration, that is, toward the area where there is more solute, and thus less water. The area of less solute is called the hypotonic solution, while the area of more solute is called the hypertonic solution. If a semi-permeable membrane separates the hypotonic solution from the hypertonic solution, water will move across the membrane from the hypotonic to the hypertonic solution. No metabolic energy is involved (Fig. 4.23).

Consider two water solutions, one rich in ions (hyper tonic) and the other not (hypotonic), which are separated by a semi-permeable membrane. Water can move across the membrane in both directions, but because ions attract water and impede its random diffusion, water is retarded on the ion-rich side; therefore the rate from the ion-rich side is less than the rate of ions permeating the membrane from the other side.

The net movement of water toward the ion-rich solution builds up hydrostatic pressure, called osmotic pressure, which at some point will counteract the attraction of ions. The two sides will then be at equilibrium. Whenever two solutions are separated by a semi permeable membrane, net movement of water will be towards the solution more concentrated in substances that do not permeate the membrane.

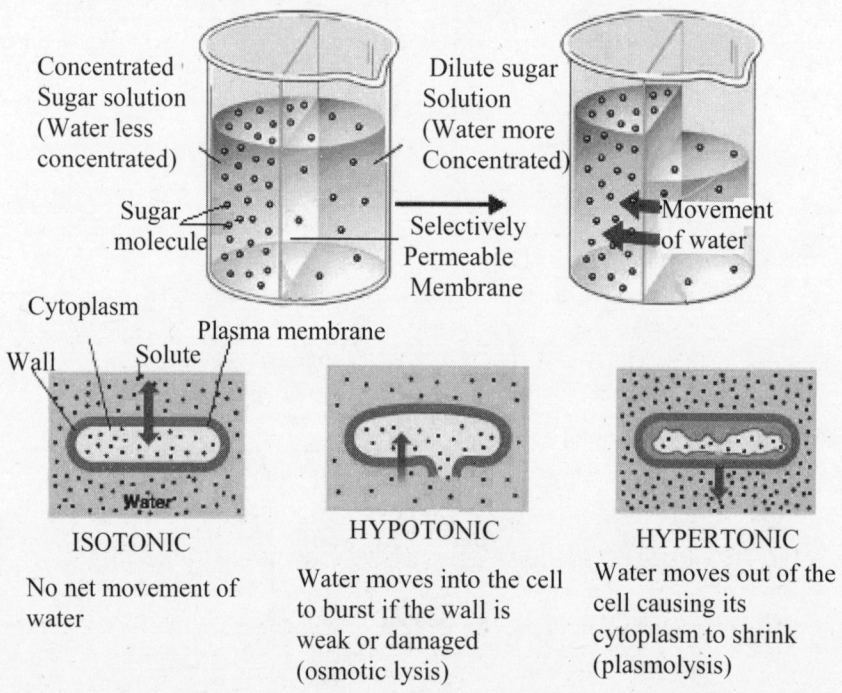

Figure 4.23: Diagrammatic representation of osmosis

(iii) Facilitated diffusion

Facilitated diffusion is the diffusion of a substance across a membrane, enhanced by transport protein in the membrane (Fig.4.24). The involvement of the transport protein makes facilitated diffusion a type of carrier-mediated transport, although it is passive. The transport membrane is specific to the substance being transported, that is, it only transports a particular substance. For example glucose, which is needed in large amounts by cells for energy, is one substance commonly transported into cells by facilitated diffusion.

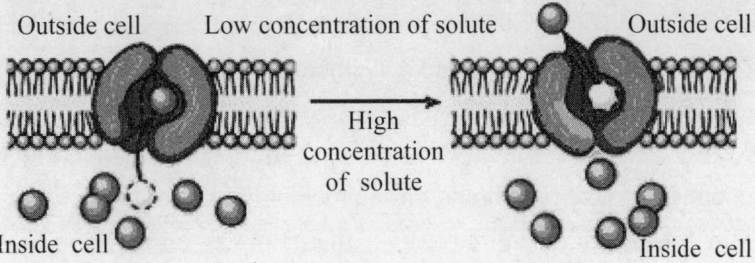

Figure 4.24: Facilitated diffusion of glucose

The kinetics of facilitated (with a helper) transport is different from those of simple diffusion. In the latter, the rate of diffusion is proportional to the concentration of the diffusing molecules; the more of them, the more will diffuse across the membrane per unit time. In facilitated diffusion, however, the rate is limited by the availability of the helper molecules. Once all the helpers are saturated, the increasing concentration of diffusing molecules will only increase a waiting line for the helper and will not increase the rate of transport (Fig. 4.25).

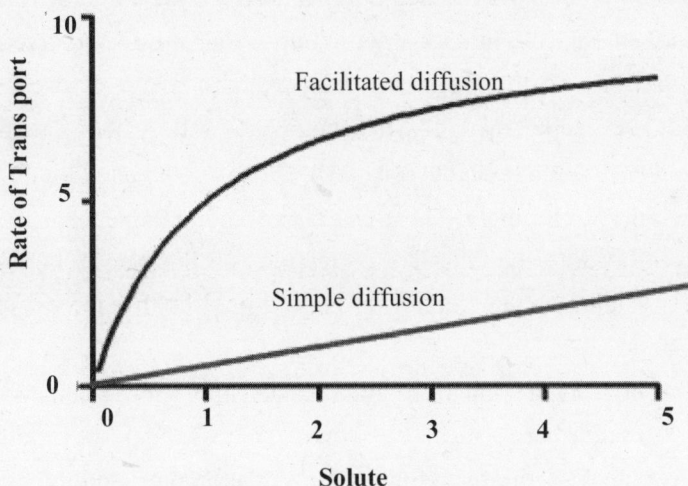

Fig. 4.25: Graphical representation of rate of diffusion

4.2.3.3. Transport of uncharged Molecules and Ions

Gases like O_2, N_2, diffuse easily through membrane because they have no charge (partial or complete) to interact with water. Hydrophobic molecules (oils) have also no trouble permeating membrane. Ions do not penetrate because of charge and the solvation layer that would have to diffuse with them. Thus when considering transport of ions we must take into account their concentration gradient as well as the electrical gradient, the combined potential is called electrochemical potential. In most cells there is an unequal distribution of ions: Na^+ 10 mM inside; 150 mM outside; K^+ 150 mM inside; 5 mM outside. Electrochemical potential in the cell means that the Na and K ions experience different forces. The concentration gradient favors influx of Na and efflux of K, but a membrane potential of -70 mV potential favors influx of cations of any kind.

Ionophores are structures which work as transporters and dissipate ion gradients. Some form pores (channels) in the membrane through which ions can diffuse in or out of the cell, e.g., Gramicidin A is a peptide antibiotic with alternating D- and L-amino acids that forms a channel large enough for protons, Na^+ and K^+ ions to pass through, but is blocked by Ca^{2+}. The trans-membrane channels that permit facilitated diffusion can be opened or closed. They are said to be "gated". Some gated ion channels are:

(a) Ligand-gated ion channels: Many ion channels open or close in response to binding a small signaling molecule or "ligand". Some ion channels are gated by extracellular ligands; some by intracellular ligands. In both cases, the ligand is not the substance that is transported when the channel opens.

External ligands bind to a site on the extra-cellular side of the channel. For example, Acetylcholine (ACh) the binding of the neurotransmitter acetylcholine at certain synapses opens channels that admit Na^+ and initiate a nerve impulse or muscle contraction, while internal ligands bind to a site on the channel protein exposed to the cytosol. For example, "Second messengers", like cyclic AMP (cAMP) and cyclic GMP (cGMP), regulate channels involved in the initiation of impulses in neurons responding to odors and light respectively.

(b) Mechanically-gated ion channels: These channels respond to mechanical impulses. For example, sound waves bending the cilia-like projections on the hair cells of the inner ear open up ion channels leading to the creation of nerve impulses that the brain interprets as sound.

(c) Voltage-gated ion channels: In neurons and muscle cells, some channels open or close in response to changes in the charge (measured in volts) across the plasma membrane. As an impulse passes down a neuron, the reduction in the voltage opens sodium channels in the adjacent portion of the membrane. This allows the influx of Na^+ into the neuron and thus the continuation of the nerve impulse. Some 7000 sodium ions pass through each channel during the short period (about 1 millisecond) that it remains open.

4.2.3.4. Carriers: Permeases

Proteins that act as carriers are too large to move across the membrane. They are trans-membrane proteins with fixed topology. An example is the GLUT1 glucose carrier, in plasma membranes of various cells, including erythrocytes. GLUT1 is a large integral protein, predicted via hydro-pathy plots to include 12 trans-membrane α-helices.

Carrier proteins such as Glucose permease in erythrocytes are more complex than channels (Fig.4.26). The transported molecule (glucose) moves down its concentration gradient. Once inside the cell, the molecule is transformed into another, impermeant species, thus lowering the inside concentration and maintaining the concentration gradient.

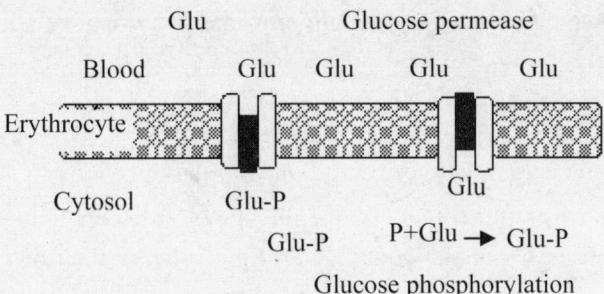

Figure 4.26: Glucose permease

4.2.4. Active Transport

There are numerous situations in living organisms when molecules move across cell membranes from an area of lower concentration toward an area of higher concentration. In order to accomplish this, membranes have evolved elaborate schemes to pump the substance from the area of smaller concentration to a compartment with higher concentration. All these schemes cost the cell energy and thus are called active transport. If a molecule is to be transported from an area of low concentration to an area of high concentration, work must be done to overcome the influences of diffusion and osmosis. Since, in the normal state of a cell, large concentration differences in K^+, Na^+ and Ca^{2+} are maintained, it is evident that active transport mechanisms are at work (Fig. 4.27).

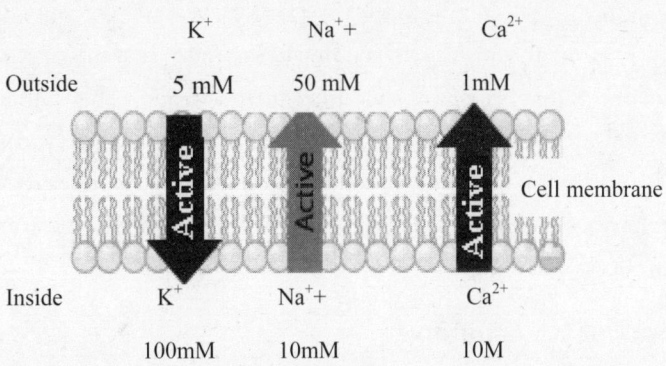

Figure 4.27: Active transport of ions: the sodium-potassium pump moves toward an equilibrium state with the relative concentrations of Na^+ and K^+

Many crucial processes in the life of cells depend upon active transport. Active transport mechanisms may draw their energy from the hydrolysis of ATP, the absorbance of light, the transport of electrons, or coupling with other processes that are moving particles down their concentration gradients. A vital active transport process that occurs in the electron transport process in the membranes of both mitochondria and chloroplasts is the transport of protons to produce a proton gradient. This proton gradient powers the phosphorylation of ATP associated with ATP synthase.

(a) Direct Active Transport

The cytosol of animal cells contains a concentration of potassium ions (K^+) as much as 20 times higher than that in the extra-cellular fluid. Conversely, the extracellular fluid contains a concentration of sodium ions (Na^+) as much as 10 times greater than that within the cell. These concentration gradients are established by the active transport of both ions and in fact, the same transporter, called the Na^+/K^+ ATPase, does both jobs. It uses the energy from the hydrolysis of ATP to actively transport 3 Na^+ ions out of the cell and for each 2 K^+ ions pumped into the cell

(b) Na/K ATPase (pump)

The process of moving sodium and potassium ions across the cell membrane is an active transport process involving the hydrolysis of ATP to provide the necessary energy. It involves an enzyme referred to as Na^+/K^+-ATPase. The function of Na/K ATPase is to set up the electrochemical gradient of the membrane. It does so by pumping Na out of the cell and pumping K into the cell (Fig. 4.28). The net effect is to create a chemical potential consisting of two concentration gradients (for Na and for K), as well as electrical potential because three positive charges are pumped out while two positive charges are pumped in. A negative potential inside the cell is thus created.

This process is responsible for maintaining the large excess of Na^+ outside the cell and the large excess of K^+ ions on the inside. It accomplishes the transport of three Na^+ to the outside of the cell and the transport of two K^+ ions to the inside. This unbalanced charge transfer contributes to the separation of charge across the membrane. The sodium-potassium pump is an important contributor to action potential produced by nerve cells. This pump is called a P-type ion pump because the ATP interactions phosphorylate the transport protein and causes a change in its conformation.

Biological significance of Na/K pump

The crucial roles of the Na^+/K^+ ATPase are reflected in the fact that almost one-third of all the energy generated by the mitochondria in animal cells is used just to run this pump. It helps in establishing a net charge across the plasma membrane with the interior of the cell being negatively charged with respect to the exterior. This resting potential prepares nerve and muscle cells for the propagation of action potentials leading to nerve impulses and muscle contraction. The accumulation of sodium ions outside of the cell draws water out of the cell and thus enables it to maintain osmotic balance (otherwise it would swell and burst from the inward diffusion of water). The gradient of sodium ions is harnessed to provide the energy to run several types of indirect pumps. H^+ ATPase is another pump mechanism present in the body. The parietal cells of stomach use this pump to secrete gastric juice. These cells transport protons (H^+) from a concentration of about 4×10^{-8} M within the cell to a concentration of about 0.15 M in the gastric juice (giving it a pH close to 1). Both of these pumps can be made to run backward. That is, if the pumped ions are allowed to diffuse back through1 the membrane complex, ATP can be synthesized from ADP and inorganic phosphate.

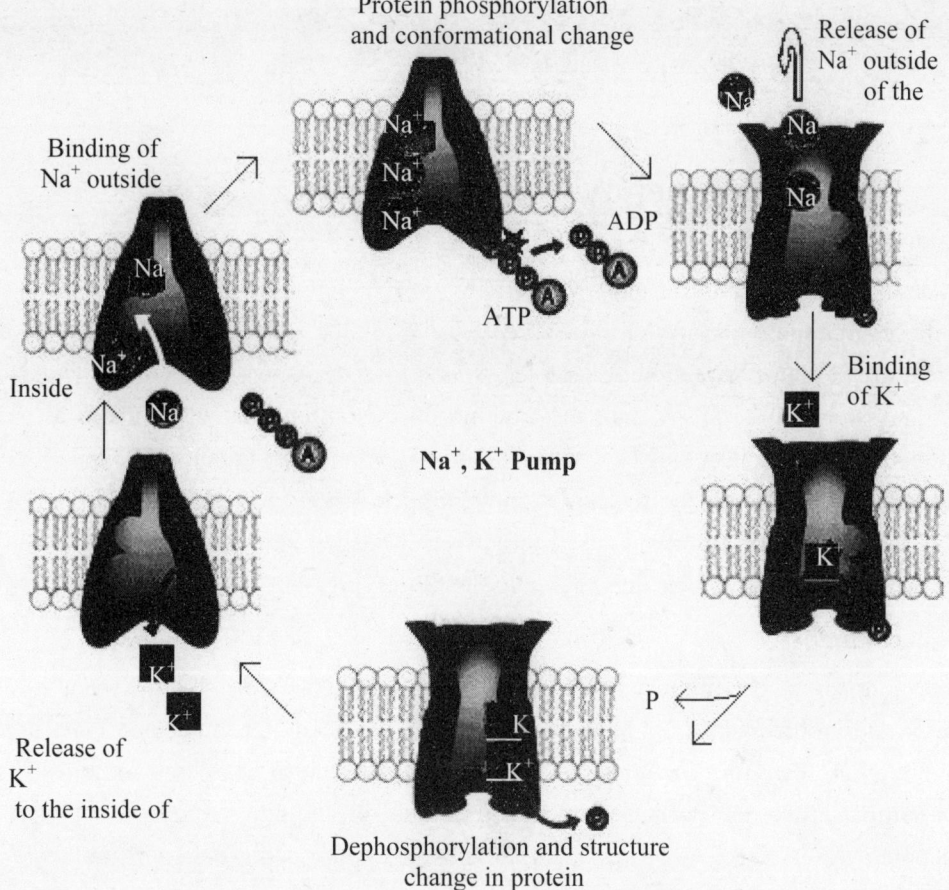

Figure 4.28: Events occurs in sodium-potassium pump

4.2.4.1. Indirect Active Transport

Indirect active transport uses the downhill flow of an ion to pump some other molecule or ion against its gradient. The driving ion is usually sodium (Na^+) with its gradient established by the Na^+/K^+ ATPase. ATP is not directly involved, but it sets up the electrochemical gradient used to propel the driver. It can be of three types, uniport, symport or antiport (Fig. 4.29). In uniport single solute moves from one side of the membrane to the other.

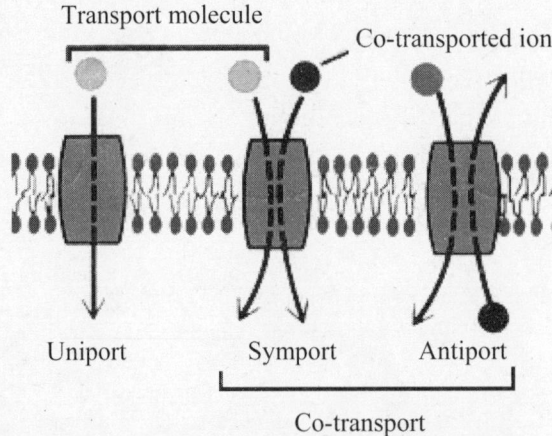

Figure 4.29: Indirect active transport

(a) Symport

In this type of indirect active transport, the driving ion (Na^+) and the pumped molecule pass through the membrane pump in the same direction, i.e., is the passenger and the driver are transported in the same direction. Examples of symport transporters include; The $Na^+/$ glucose transporter: This trans-membrane protein allows sodium ions and glucose to enter the cell together. The sodium ions flow down their concentration gradient, while the glucose molecules are pumped. Later the sodium is pumped back out of the cell by the Na^+/K^+ AT-Pase. The $Na^+/$glucose transporter is used to actively transport glucose out of the intestine and also out of the kidney tubules and back into the blood (Fig. 4.30).

(b) Anti-port pumps

In anti-port pumps, the driving ion (again, usually sodium) diffuses through the pump in one direction providing the energy for the active transport of some other molecule or ion in the opposite direction. Examples include Mg^{2+} ions are pumped out of cells by a sodium-driven anti-port pump; Ca-Na anti-port takes place in cardiac muscle and sucrose-H anti-port in plant vacuoles. The Na^+/K^+ ATPase is also an anti-port pump using the energy of ATP to pump Na^+ out of the cell, while K^+ in. This sodium/proton anti-port pump enables the plant to sequester sodium ions in its vacuole. Transgenic tomato plants that over express this sodium/proton anti-port pump are able to thrive in saline soils, too salty for conventional tomatoes.

Some inherited ion-channel diseases

A growing number of human diseases have been discovered to be caused by inherited mutations in genes encoding channels.

(a) Chloride-channel diseases: e.g.: Cystic fibrosis: inherited tendency to kidney stones (caused by a different kind of chloride channel than the one involved in cystic fibrosis)

(b) Potassium-channel diseases: e.g.: some inherited life-threatening defects in the heartbeat and a rare inherited tendency to epileptic seizures in the newborn.

(c) Sodium-channel diseases: e.g.: inherited tendency to certain types of muscle spasms, Liddle's syndrome: Inadequate sodium transport out of the kidneys, because of a mutant sodium channel, leads to elevated osmotic pressure of the blood and resulting hypertension (high blood pressure).

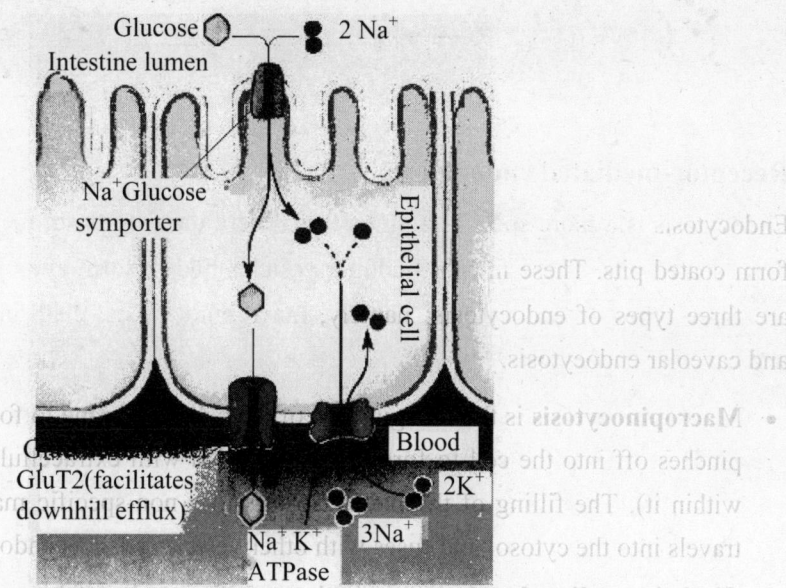

Figure 4.30: The Na$^+$/glucose transporter in intestinal lumen

4.2.5. Transport of large molecules

Membranes transport molecules too big to permeate the membrane by engulfing the substance and forming internal vesicles. Uptake of substances by such a mechanism is called endocytosis and the secretion is called exocytosis.

(a) Exocytosis: In exocytosis, the transport vesicle fuses with the plasma membrane, making the inside of the vesicle as continuous with the outside of the cell. Exocytosis is used in secretion of protein hormones (insulin), serum proteins and extracellular matrix (collagen).

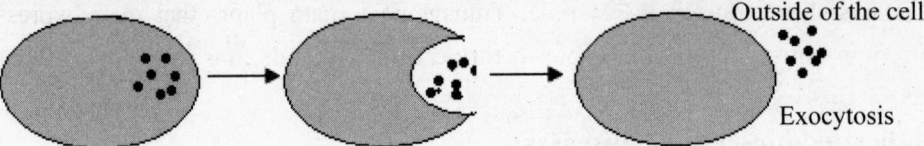

Outside of the cell

Exocytosis

(b) Endocytosis: It is a process whereby cells absorb material (molecules such as proteins) from the outside by engulfing it with their cell membrane. It is used by all cells of the body because most substances important to them are large polar molecules, and thus cannot pass through the hydrophobic plasma membrane. The function of endocytosis is the opposite of exocytosis. The absorption of material from the outside environment of the cell is commonly divided into two processes: phagocytosis and pinocytosis.

Outside of the cell

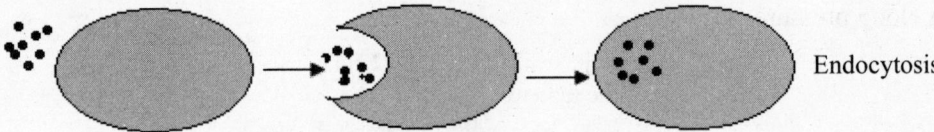

Endocytosis

Receptor-mediated endocytosis

Endocytosis is a more specific active event where the cytoplasm membrane folds inward to form coated pits. These inward budding vesicles bud to form cytoplasmic vesicles. There are three types of endocytosis: namely, macropinocytosis, clathrin-mediated endocytosis, and caveolar endocytosis.

- **Macropinocytosis** is the invagination of the cell membrane to form a pocket which then pinches off into the cell to form a vesicle filled with extracellular fluid (and molecules within it). The filling of the pocket occurs in a non-specific manner. The vesicle then travels into the cytosol and fuses with other vesicles such as endosomes and lysosomes.

- **Clathrin-mediated** endocytosis is the specific uptake of large extracellular molecules such as proteins, membrane localized receptors and ion-channels. These receptors are associated with the cytosolic protein clathrin which initiates the formation of a vesicle by forming a crystalline coat on the inner surface of the cell's membrane (Fig. 4.31).

- **Caveolae** consist of the protein caveolin-1 with a bi-layer enriched in cholesterol and glycolsphingolipids. Caveolae are flask shaped pits in the membrane that resemble the shape of a cave (hence the name caveolae). Uptake of extra-cellular molecules is also believed to be specifically mediated via receptors in caveolae.

(c) Phagocytosis (literally, cell-eating) is the process by which cells ingest large objects, such as cells which have undergone apoptosis, bacteria, or viruses. The membrane folds around the object, and the object is sealed off into a large vacuole known as a phagosome. Removal of foreign materials or dead cells by immune cells is a form of endocytosis. For example, phagocytes are macrophages that line blood channels of liver (spleen) and eat up aging RBCs; monocytes penetrate inflamed tissue and remove the invading bacteria. Amoebas also use this process.

(d) Pinocytosis (literally, cell-drinking) is the process of taking up liquid from the surrounding environment. It is a non-specific uptake of extra-cellular solution tiny pockets are formed along the membrane, filled with liquid, and then pinched off. This process is concerned with the uptake of solutes and single molecules such as proteins.

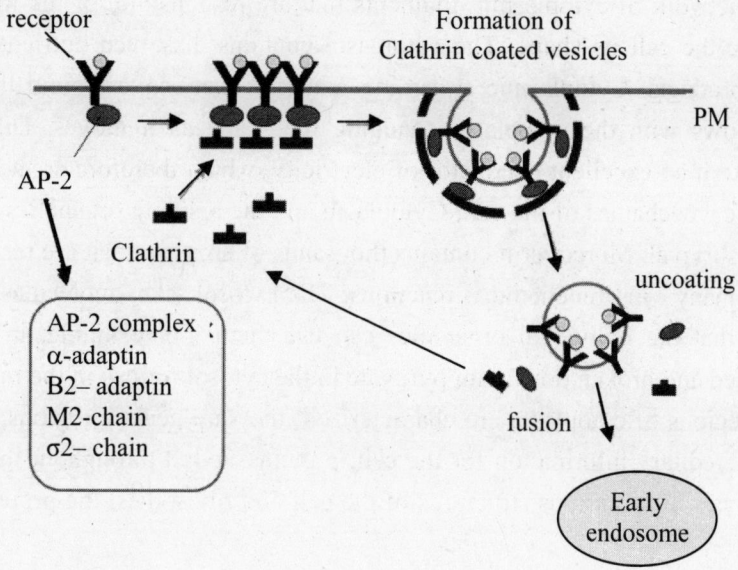

Figure 4.31: Mechanism of clathrin-dependent endocytosis. Clathrin and cargo molecules are assembled into clathrin-coated pits on the plasma membrane together with an adaptor complex called AP-2 that links clathrin with transmembrane receptors, concluding in the formation of mature clathrin-coated vesicles (CCVs). CCVs are then actively uncoated and transported to early/sorting endosomes.

4.2.6. Protoplasm

The term protoplasm includes both the substance within the cell and associated with the cell membrane. It is the "living part" of the cell. It can be differentiated into cytoplasm and the nucleus. J.E. Purkinje, in 1840, used the term protoplasm to describe the juicy, slimy gelatinous contents of the cell. The chemical properties of protoplasm can be divided into inorganic and organic substances. Inorganic substances are water, which make up 90% of the protoplasm, mineral salts, such as NaCl-salt, and gases like oxygen and carbon dioxide. Organic substances include proteins, carbohydrates, lipids, nucleic acids and enzymes.

4.2.7. Cytoplasm

Cytoplasm is homogeneous, clear jelly-like materials that fill the cells. The cytoplasm consists of cytosol and the cellular organelles, except the nucleus. The cytosol is made up of water, salts and organic molecules and many enzymes that catalyze reactions. It plays an important role in a cell, in which the organelles are suspended and held together by plasma membrane. It comprises 54% of the cells total volume.

The cytoplasm plays a mechanical role, i.e. to maintain the shape, the consistency of the cell and to provide suspension to the organelles. In other words cytoplasm is the home of the cytoskeleton, a network of cytoplasmic filaments that are responsible for the movement of the cell and give the cell its shape. The cytoplasm contains dissolved nutrients and helps dissolve waste products. Cytoplasmic streaming materials can move around the cell. The nucleus often flows with the cytoplasm changing the shape as it moves. Different salts present in it make it an excellent conductor of electricity, which therefore creates a medium for the vesicles, or mechanics of the cell. Cytoplasm and the residing organelles play a critical role in cell's survival. Moreover it contains thousands of enzymes that are responsible for the catalysis of many vital biochemical reactions. The cytosol takes molecules and breaks them down, so that the individual organelles can use them. For example, in respiration, glucose is ingested and broken down into pyruvate in the cytosol for use in the mitochondria. Three specific regions of cytoplasm are characterized; they are genetic regions, the regions containing the hereditary information for the cell; proteins, found throughout the cell either as reaction catalysts or in various structures of the cell and ribosomes, the protein synthesis machinery.

4.3. Cellular Organelles

4.3.1. The Cell Nucleus

The nucleus is a highly specialized organelle that serves as the information processing and administrative center of the cell. This organelle has two major functions: it stores the cell's hereditary material, or DNA, and it coordinates the cell's activities, which include growth, intermediary metabolism, protein synthesis, and reproduction (cell division).

Robert Brown (1833), first described the nucleus from the cells of *Tradescantia* (belongs to family *Commelinaceae*) and recognized as a constant feature of all animal and plant cells. Generally a cell contains just one nucleus (uninucleate), however, there may be several nuclei in a cell (multinucleate). Usually the nucleus, the largest organelle in the cell is round and located in the centre of the cell. But its position may change from time to time according to the metabolic status of the cell. In certain cells such as the glandular cells the nucleus remains located in the basal portion of the cell. On the basis of presence or absences of this membrane-enclosed organelle, cells are classified as eukaryotic and prokaryotic. The prokaryotic cells of bacteria do not have true nucleus, there the single, circular DNA molecules remains in contact with cytoplasm but in case of eukaryotes they have a well organised nucleus as found in other groups. However, certain eukaryotic cells such as sieve tubes of higher plants and mammalian erythrocytes contain no nucleus.

Nucleus containing eukaryotic cell is supposed to be evolved by symbiotic relationship between the archaea and bacteria. The archaeal origin of the nucleus is supported by observations that archaea and eukarya have similar genes for certain proteins, including histones. Another model viral eukaryogenesis explains that the membrane-bound nucleus, along with other eukaryotic features, originated from the infection of a prokaryote by a virus. This suggestion is based on similarities between eukaryotes and viruses, such as linear DNA strands, mRNA capping, and tight binding to proteins (analogizing histones to viral envelopes). Recent model, the exo-membrane hypothesis suggests that the nucleus instead of originated from a single ancestral cell that evolved a second exterior cell membrane; the interior membrane enclosing the original cell then became the nuclear membrane and evolved increasingly elaborate pore structures for passage of internally synthesized cellular components such as ribosomal subunits.

Morphology

Usually the cells contain single nucleus but the number of nucleus may vary from cell to cell. On the basis of number of nuclei present, cells are classified as mononucleate, binucleate and poly nucleated cells. Most plant and animal cells contain single nucleous, such cells are known as mononucleate cells. The cells which contain two nuclei are known as binucleate cells. Such cells occur in certain protozoans such as *Paramecium* and cells of cartilage and liver. Poly-nucleated cells may contain 3–100 nuclei. The poly-nucleted cells are known as syncytial cells (eg: osteoblast cells and striated muscle fibers which contains 100 nuclei per cell) or coenocytes (e.g. siphonal algae *Vaucheria*). Coenocytes are found in fungi and some protists, such as algae and slime mold. Some plant structures, such as endosperm, are coenocytic as well.

The shape of the nucleus normally related to the shape of the cell, but certain nuclei are almost irregular in shape. The spheroid, cuboid or polyhedral cells contain spheroid nuclei. The nuclei of the cylindrical, prismatic or fusiform cells are ellipsoid in shape. The size of the nucleus of a cell depends on the volume of the cell, amount of DNA and proteins and metabolic phase of the cell.

4.3.2. Ultra Structure of the Nucleus

The nucleus is composed of four main parts, the nuclear envelope, nuclear sap or nucleoplasm, the nucleolus and the chromatin fibers (Fig. 4.32).

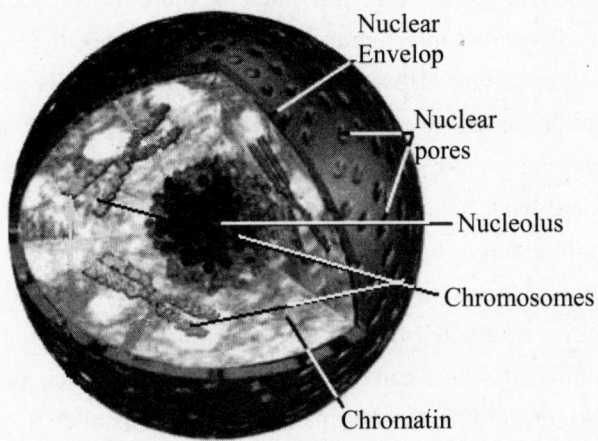

Figure 4.32: Structure of the nucleus

(a) The Nuclear Envelope: The nuclear envelope is a double-layered membrane that encloses the contents of the nucleus during most of the cell's life-cycle. The nuclear membrane in higher plants and animals disappears in late prophase during cell division and reforms around the daughter chromosomes during telophase. Based on the electron microscopic images the dimensions of each membrane are about 75 to 90 A° thick and lipoprotenatious in nature. The space between the layers is called the peri-nuclear space (100–170 A°) and appears to connect with the rough endoplasmic reticulum. The envelope is perforated with tiny holes called nuclear pores. These pores regulate the passage of molecules between the nucleus and the cytoplasm. It is attached to a network of tubules, called the endoplasmic reticulum, where protein synthesis occurs. The inner surface has a protein lining called the nuclear lamina, which binds to chromatin and other nuclear components. During mitosis, or cell division, the nuclear envelope disintegrates, but reforms as the two cells complete their formation and the chromatin begins to unravel and disperse (Fig. 4.33).

(b) Nuclear Pores: The nuclear pores appear circular in surface view and have a diameter between 10 nm to 100 nm. Recent electron microscopic studies have found that a nuclear pore has far more complex structure, so it is called nuclear pore complex. Each pore complex has an estimated molecular weight of 50 to 100 million daltons. These pores regulate the passage of molecules such as building blocks of DNA and RNA as well as molecules that provide the energy for constructing genetic material. The nuclear pore complex is generally permeable for molecules of 5 to 500 Daltons size. The NPCs provide peripheral channels of about 9 nm in diameter (Fig. 4.34). The structure of the NPC has been extensively investigated by electron microscopy and a consensus model of its central framework has emerged. Accordingly, the vertebrate NPC exhibits an 8-fold symmetric (i.e., perpendicular to the plane of the NE) tripartite architecture with a total mass of ~125 MDa. Its ~55 MDa central framework is a ring-like assembly built of eight multi-domain spokes consisting of two roughly identical halves each so that its asymmetric unit (i.e., one half-spoke) represents one 16th of its mass or roughly the size of a ribosome. This central framework is sandwiched between a ~32 MDa cytoplasmic and a ~21 MDa nuclear ring. From the cytoplasmic ring eight short, kinky fibrils emerges out, whereas the nuclear ring anchors a basket (or fish-trap), assembled from eight thin, ~50 nm long filaments joined distally by a 30 to 50 nm-diameter ring. The ring-like, ~822-symmetric central framework embraces the central pore of the NPC which acts as a gated channel.

Thus nucleotides, ions and many other molecules have easy access into the nucleus. But proteins of more than 50 KD (size of ~5nm) cannot diffuse passively; they are transported through ATP dependent (active process) pathways. The central channel is exclusively used for the transport of larger cargo by expansion and contraction mode. One hundred histones are imported per minute per pore complex, non-histones 200, and riboproteins 150 per minute and export ~5 ribosomes per minute per pore complex as well as mRNAs one per minute. The approximate import of different proteins from cytoplasm into the nucleus is around 6000 to 10000. The pore complex transports the ribosomes of 120 × 200 Å sizes. The traffic through the nuclear envelope is mediated by a protein family which can be divided into exportins and importins. Binding of a molecule (a "cargo") to exportins facilitates its export to the cytoplasm, while importins facilitate import into the nucleus.

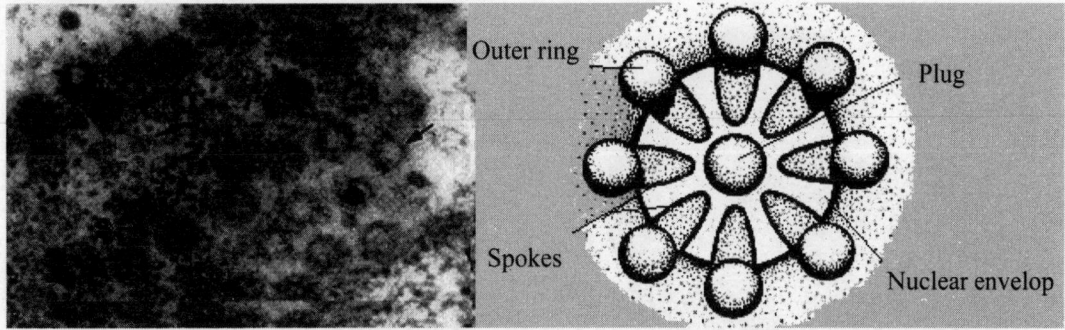

Figure 4.33: Electron micrograph: showing the nuclear envelope in a "face on" view. From this angle the NPCs are seen as round circles. On right view from the top of the pore

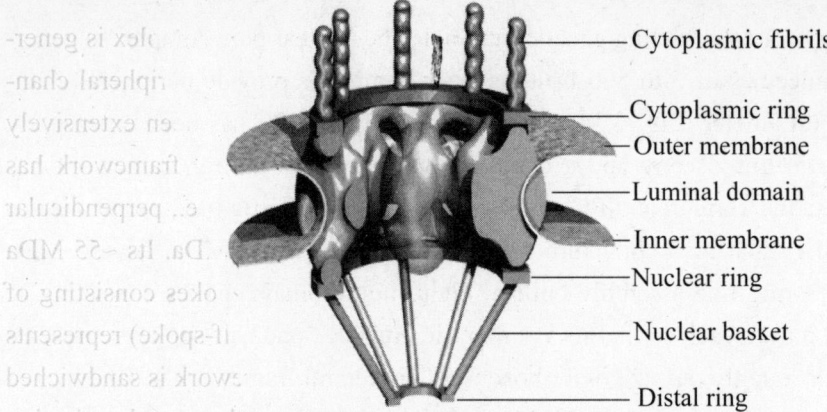

Cytoplasmic fibrils
Cytoplasmic ring
Outer membrane
Luminal domain
Inner membrane
Nuclear ring
Nuclear basket
Distal ring

Figure 4.34: Nuclear pore complex (NPC)

(c) Nucleoplasm: Nuclear sap is colorless, transparent, granular, and highly viscous, semi fluid matrix found inside the nucleus is called nucleoplasm. Within the nucleoplasm, most of the nuclear material consists of chromatin, the less condensed form of the cell's DNA that organizes to form chromosomes during mitosis or cell division. It consists of mainly the nucleoproteins and other organic and inorganic substances like nucleic acids, proteins, enzymes and minerals. The nuclear proteins are simple and basic in nature. They are nucleoprotamines and nucleohistones. Nucleoprotamines have low molecular weight (about 4000 Dalton) and the most abundant amino acid in these proteins is arginine (pH 10 to 11). It usually remains bounded with the DNA molecules with salt linkage.

(d) The Nucleolus: The nucleolus is a membrane-less organelle within the nucleus that manufactures ribosomes, the cell's protein-producing structures. Through the microscope, the nucleolus looks like a large dark spot within the nucleus (Fig. 4.35). A nucleus may contain up to four nucleoli, but within each species the number of nucleoli is fixed. The number of nucleoli in the nucleus depends on the species and the number of chromosomes. After a cell divides, a nucleolus is formed when chromosomes are brought together into nucleolar organizing regions.

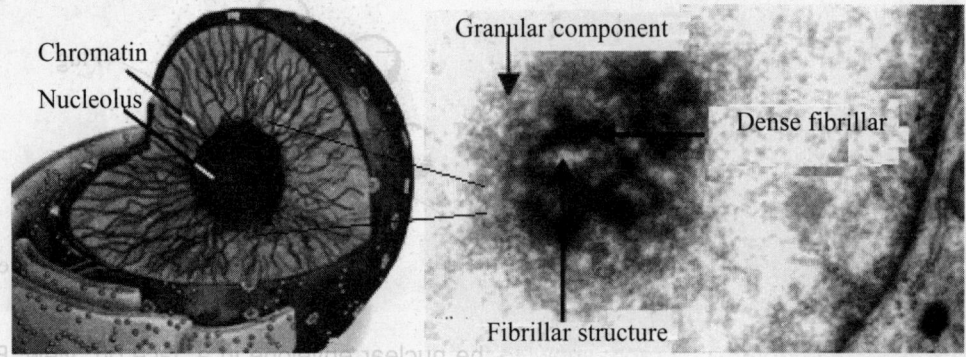

Chromatin
Nucleolus
Granular component
Dense fibrillar
Fibrillar structure

Figure 4.35: Ultra structure of nucleolus; electron micrograph of nucleolus (right)

The size of the nucleolus is found to be related with the synthetic activity of the cell. Cells like sperm which have little or no synthetic activity found to contain smaller or no nucleoli. The position of the nucleoli is eccentric. Chemically nucleolus contains DNA of nucleolar organizer, four types of rRNAs, 70 types of ribosomal proteins and RNA splicing nucleoproteins. It also contains phospholipids, orthophosholipids and calcium ions and these calcium ions supposed to maintain its intact organization.

Nucleoli are typically composed of three morphologically distinct regions which can be visualized by electron microscopy (EM):

1. **Fibrillar Centers** (FC): It is the lightly stained inner most region of nucleolus composed of 'fibrils' that occupies 1-2% of the total volume. The RNA genes of nucleolar organizer of chromosomes are located in this region.

2. **2. Dense Fibrillar Centers** (DFC): It surrounds the FC's, composed of 'densely packed fibrils' and occupies a large fraction of the nucleolus (about 17%). The biogenesis of RNA takes place in this region.

3. Granular region (GR): It is the largest and outer most fraction of the total nucleolus volume (about 75%). At this region the processing and maturation of pre-ribosomal particles occurs.

(e) Chromatin and chromosomes: They are thread-like structures located inside the nucleus of animal and plant cells. The term chromosome comes from the Greek words for color (chroma) and body (soma). Each chromosome is made up of protein and a single molecule of deoxyribonucleic acid (DNA). Packed inside the nucleus of every human cell is nearly 6 feet of DNA, which is divided into 46 individual molecules, one for each chromosome and each about 1.5 inches long. Packing all this material into a microscopic cell nucleus is an extraordinary feat of packaging. Inside the nucleus it is combined with proteins and organized into a precise, compact structure, a dense string-like fiber called chromatin (Fig. 4.36).

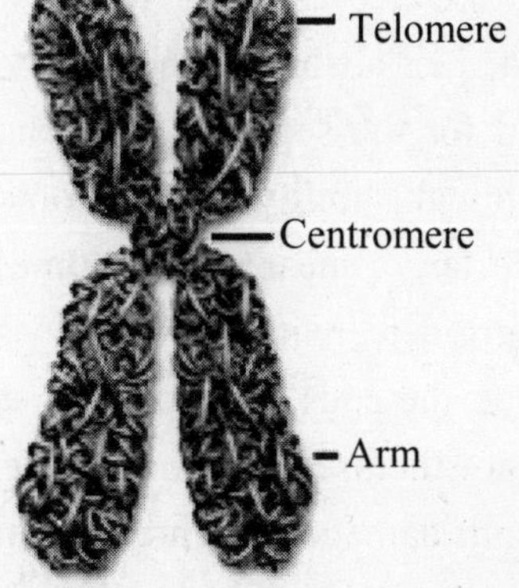

Figure 4.36: Chromosome structure

The chromosome number varies with species. In humans there are 46 chromosomes or 23 pairs (diploid), in every cell except the mature egg and sperm which have a set of 23 chromosomes (haploid). If the chromosomes in a single cell were stretched out and laid end to end, the DNA would be two meters long.

The region where two sister chromatids of a chromosome appear to be joined or "held together" during mitotic metaphase is called centromere. It is the dark-stained region when chromosomes are stained. Based on the position of centromere it can be of different type; In general, if the centromere is near the middle, the chromosome is metacentric, if it is towards one end, the chromosome is acrocentric or sub-metacentric, if it is very near the end, the chromosome is telocentric (Fig. 4.37). All house mouse chromosomes are telocentric, while human chromosomes include both metacentric and acrocentric, but no telocentric. Within the centromere region, most species have several locations where spindle fibers attach, and these sites consist of DNA as well as protein. The actual location where the attachment occurs is called the kineto-chore and is composed of both DNA and protein.

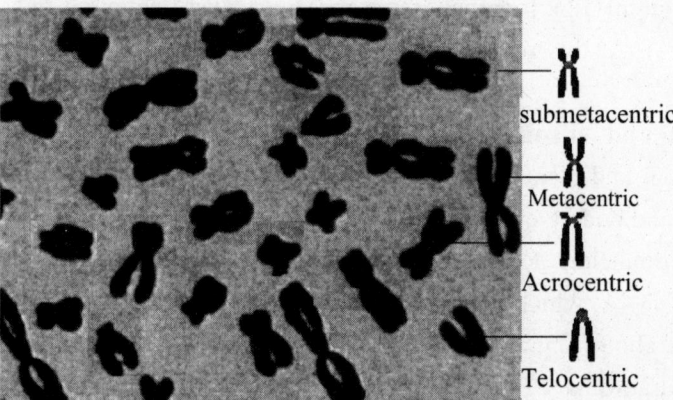

Figure 4.37: Different type of chromosomes on the basis of location of centromere

Centromeres and telomeres are two essential features of all eukaryotic chromosomes. Each provide a unique function, i.e., absolutely necessary for the stability of the chromosome. Centromeres are required for the segregation of the centromere during meiosis and mitosis. Teleomeres provide terminal stability to the chromosome and ensure its survival.

Eukaryotes possess multiple large linear chromosomes contained in the cell's nucleus. Each chromosome has one centromere, with one or two arms projecting from the centromere. Telomeres are sequences at the ends of chromosomes. They do not contain the codes for proteins. So telomeres are not themselves genes, these are repetitive sequences protect the ends of the chromosome from damage, and prevent the chromosomes from fusing into rings, or binding haphazardly to other DNA in the cell nucleus. In the nuclear chromosomes, the uncondensed DNA exists in wrapped around histones (structural proteins), forming a composite material called chromatin. Chromatin is found in two varieties: euchromatin and heterochromatin. Originally, the two forms were distinguished cytologically by how intensely they stained - the former is brightly stained while the latter darkly stained intensely, indicating tighter packing. Heterochromatin is usually localized to the periphery of the nucleus. Detailed chemistry of chromatins is already explained in chapter 3.

4.3.3. Nucleosome Model of Chromatin Assembly

The nucleosome hypothesis proposed by Roger Kornberg in 1974 was a paradigm shift for understanding eukaryotic gene expression. The assembly of DNA into chromatin involves a range of events, beginning with the formation of the basic unit, the nucleosome, and ultimately giving rise to a complex organization of specific domains within the nucleus. The first step is the assembly of the DNA with a newly synthesized tetramer (H3-H4), are specifically modified (e.g. H4 is acetylated at Lys5 and Lys12 (H3-H4)), to form a subnucleosomal particle, which is followed by the addition of two H2A-H2B dimers. This produces a nucleosomal core particle consisting of 146 base pairs of DNA bind around the histone octamer. This core particle and the linker DNA together form the nucleosome (Figs 4.38 and 4.39).

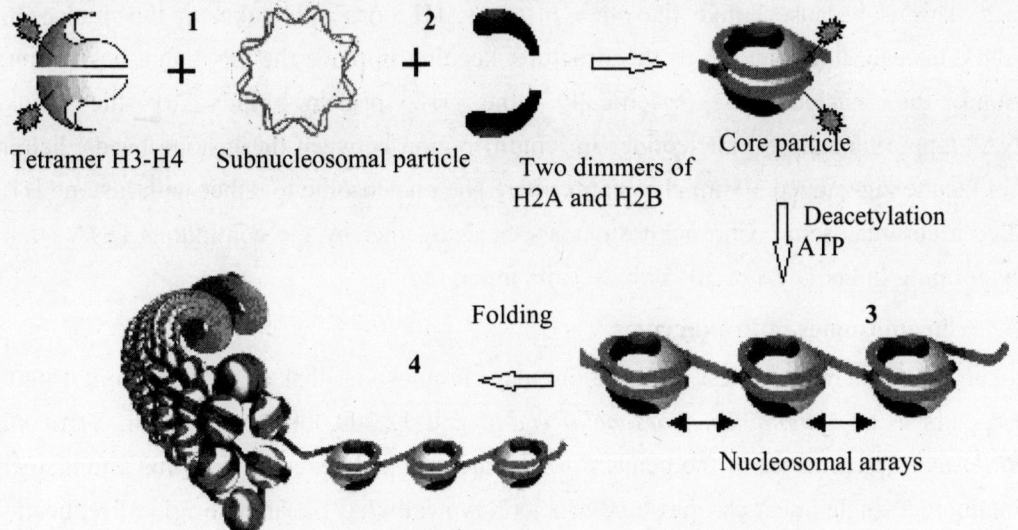

Figure 4.38: The assembly of DNA into chromatin

The next step is the maturation step that requires ATP to establish regular spacing of the nucleosome cores to form the nucleo-filament. During this step the newly incorporated histones are de-acetylated. Next the incorporation of linker histones is accompanied by folding of the nucleo-filament into the 30 nm fibre, the structure of which remains to be elucidated. Two principal models exist: the solenoid model and the zig-zag. Finally, further successive folding events lead to a high level of organization and specific domains in the nucleus.

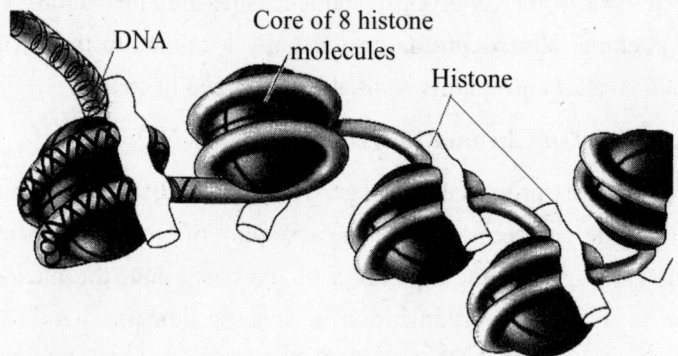

Figure 4.39: Nucleosome model of chromatin assembly

Two molecules of each of the four core histone proteins form the histone octamer via formation of one tetramer of H3 and H4 and two dimers of H2A and H2B. Each of these entities is held together by a so called hand-shake motif of protein structure, forms a "beads on a string" like structure. H1 is involved with the packing of the "beads on a string" sub-structures into a high order structure. H1 is present in half the amount of the other four histones. This is because unlike the other histones, H1 does not make up the nucleosome "bead". Instead, it sits on top of the structure, keeping in place the DNA that has wrapped around the nucleosome. Specifically, the H1 protein binds to the "linker DNA" (approximately 80 nucleotides in length) region between the histone beads, helping stabilize the zig-zagged 30 nm chromatin fiber. The nucleosome together with histone H1 is called a chromatosome. Chromatosomes are held together by the continuous DNA strand, thus forming linker DNA of 30–50 base pairs in length.

4.3.4. Chromosomes in Prokaryotes

Prokaryotes generally possess a single circular chromosome that can range about 160,000 base pairs as in *Candidatus, Carsonella ruddii* and 12,200,000 base pairs in *Sorangium cellulosum*. Spirochaetes of the genus *Borrelia* are a notable exception to this arrangement, containing a single linear chromosome. Bacteria typically have a single origin of replication, whereas some archaea contain multiple replication origins. The genes in prokaryotes are often organized in operons, and do not usually contain introns, unlike eukaryotes. DNA of prokaryotes is organized into a structure called the nucleoid. This structure is, however, dynamic and is maintained and remodeled by the actions of a range of histone-like proteins, which associate with the bacterial chromosome. In archaea, the DNA in chromosomes is even more organized, with the DNA packaged within structures similar to eukaryotic nucleosomes.

4.3.5. Special Types of Chromosomes

The eukaryotes contain some unusual and special types of chromosomes in some body cells or at some particular stage of their life cycle. The special eukaryotic chromosomes are following types:

(a) Giant chromosomes

(b) It is found in certain tissues e.g., salivary glands of larvae, gut epithelium, Malphigian tubules and some fat bodies of some Diptera (*Drosophila, Sciara, Rhyncosciara*). These chromosomes are very long and thick (up to 200 times their size during mitotic metaphase in the case of *Drosophila*). Hence they are known as Giant chromosomes.

(b) Polytene chromosomes

They are first discovered by Balbiani in 1881 and named by Koller in dipteran's salivary glands and thus also known as salivary gland chromosomes. But their significance was realized only after the extensive studies by painter during 1930's (Fig. 4.40).

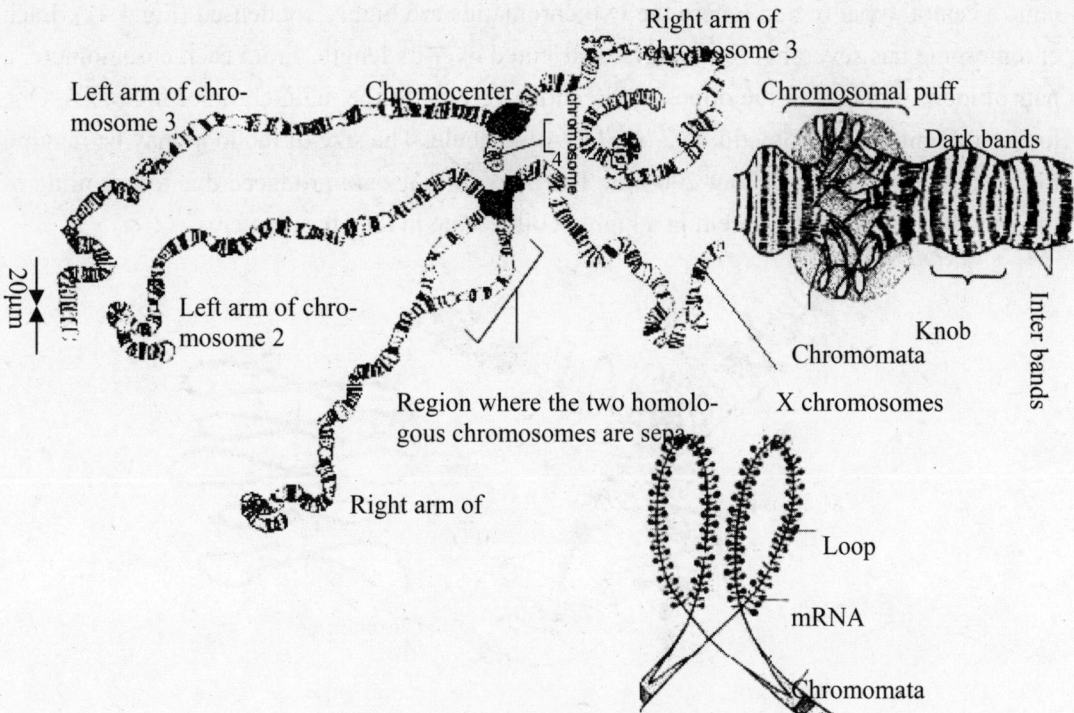

Figure 4.40: Polytene chromosomes

Giant chromosomes have also been discovered in suspensors of young embryos of many plants, but these do not show the bands so typical of salivary gland chromosomes. It is 1000 times larger than somatic chromosomes. The larger size of the chromosomes is due to the presence of many longitudinal strands called chromonemata. Hence, they are also called Polytene chromosomes (many standard). The many strands of the giant chromosomes are due to repeated division of the chromosome without the cytoplasmic division. This type of division is called endomitosis. The bands of Polytene chromosomes become enlarged at certain times to form swellings called puffs or Balbiani rings. The formation of puffs is called puffing. In the regions of puffs the chromonemata uncoil and open out from many loops. Thus puffing is caused by the uncoiling of individual chromomeres in a band. The puffs indicate the site active genes when mRNA synthesis takes place.

(c) Lamp brush chromosomes

Lamp brush chromosomes were first observed by Flemming in 1882. The name lampbrush was given by Ruckert in 1892, because of its similarity in appearance to the brushes used to clean lamp chimneys in centuries past. These are found in oocytic nuclei of vertebrates (sharks, amphibians, reptiles and birds) as well as in invertebrates (*Sagitta, Sepia, Ehinaster* and several species of insects). Lampbrush chromosomes are up to 800 μm long; thus they provide very favorable material for cytological studies. Each lamp-brush chromosome contains a central axial region where the two chromatids are highly condensed (Fig.4.41). Each chromosome has several chromomeres distributed over its length. From each chromomere, a pair of loops emerges in the opposite directions vertical to the main chromosomal axis. One loop represents one chromatid, i.e., one DNA molecule. The size of the loop may be ranging the average of 9.5 μm to about 200 μm. The pairs of loops are produced due to uncoiling of the two chromatin fibers present in a highly coiled state in the chromomeres.

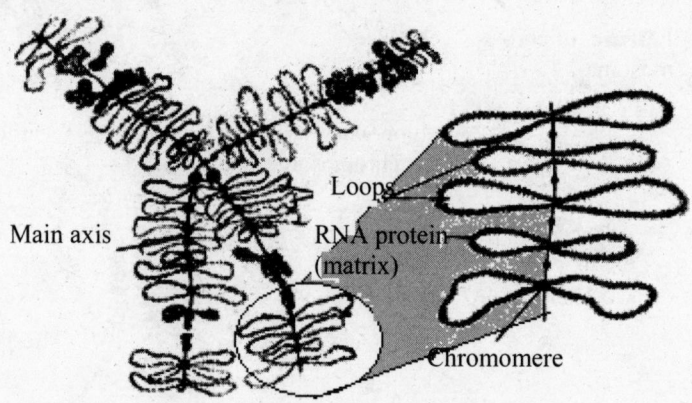

Figure 4.41: Lamb Brush Chromosomes

(d) Barr Bodies

In 1940 two Canadian scientists noticed a dark staining mass in the nuclei of cat brain cells. These dark staining spots are found in female but not in males. This held for cats and humans. They thought the spot was a tightly condensed X chromosome. A woman with the chromosome constitution 47, XXX should have 2 Barr bodies in each cell. XXY individuals are male, but have a Barr body. XO individuals are female but have no Barr bodies.

4.4. The Endoplasmic Reticulum

The endoplasmic reticulum (ER) is a network of disk-like tubules, sacks and vesicles found in eukaryotic cells. Its main function is to operate as a transport system. It consists of lipid bi-layers, which contain embedded proteins. This internal system of membrane is continuous with the double membrane that surrounds the cell's nucleus. Therefore, the encoded instructions that the nucleus sends out for the synthesis of proteins flow directly into the endoplasmic reticulum. Within the cell, the endoplasmic reticulum synthesizes lipids and proteins. The endoplasmic reticulum is responsible for the production of the protein and lipid components of most of the cell's organelles. The ER is additionally responsible for moving proteins and other carbohydrates to the Golgi apparatus, to the plasma membrane, to the lysosomes, or wherever else needed. The ER is made up of three types of structures: cisternae (diameter 400–500 Å), tubules (500-1000 Å) and vesicles (250-5000 Å).

All the three structures are bound by a single unit membrane of about 50 Å thicknesses. In most cells the endoplasmic reticulum is thought to consist of only one continuous membrane enclosing only a single space. However, in protozoa, some unicellular algae, and possibly some fungi, the endoplasmic reticulum occurs as separate, multiple vesicles. Several morphologically and functionally distinct domains of this continuous membrane system can be distinguished. The outer nuclear membrane in turn is continuous with the rough endoplasmic reticulum, which contains specialized regions, termed transitional elements, and is continuous with the smooth endoplasmic reticulum. Endoplasmic reticulum is chiefly made up of a phospholipid membrane. The rough and smooth endoplasmic reticula and the transitional element enclose a space called the intra-cisternal space, or lumen. Both intra-cisternal and peri-nuclear spaces form a single compartment. The amount of smooth and rough endoplasmic reticulum varies greatly among different cell types. The ER is folded and stacked layer upon layer within the cell and is connected to the cell's nuclear membrane. Under a microscope, the endoplasmic reticulum is seen as a highly folded structure surrounding the cell nucleus. The endoplasmic reticulum often makes up more than 10 percent of a cell's total volume. The endoplasmic reticulum is generally divided into two major sections: the rough endoplasmic reticulum and the smooth endoplasmic reticulum.

4.4.1. Rough Endoplasmic Reticulum

The term rough endoplasmic reticulum is based on the morphologic appearance of attached ribosomes, which are absent in smooth endoplasmic reticulum. Another morphologic distinction is the organization of the rough endoplasmic reticulum in interconnected flattened sacs (called cisternae), whereas the smooth endoplasmic reticulum forms a tubular network (Fig. 4.42). Rough endoplasmic reticulum branches out and expands as protein synthesis increases, providing more surface area for ribosome to spread out and create more proteins.

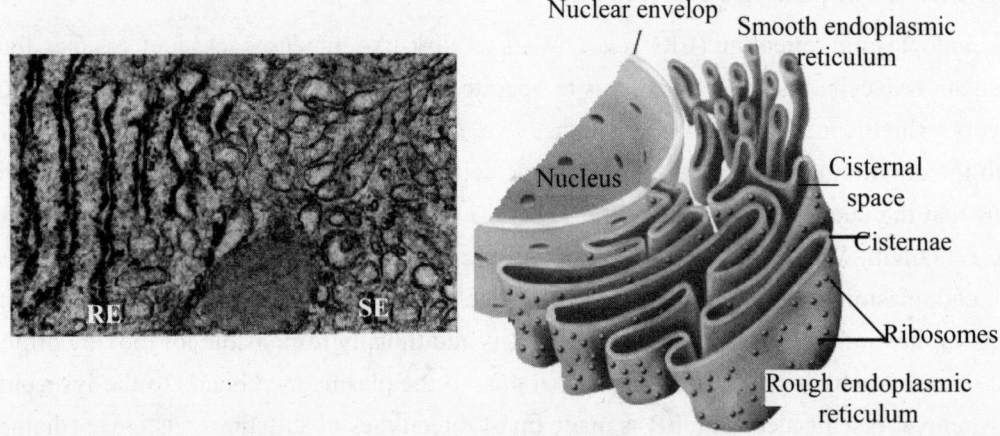

Figure 4.42: Electron micrograph of Endoplasmic reticulum (left); Structure of Endoplasmic reticulum (Right)

During protein synthesis, the ribosomes on the rough ER create new proteins and the ER then folds them properly and sorts them according to function and destination. The rough ER carries out its protein folding activity deep within the cisternal space. There, newly made proteins are twisted and folded into the configurations necessary for them to carry out their function in the cell. For sorting, the rough ER works in conjunction with the Golgi apparatus, to target the newly synthesized proteins to their proper locations. Most proteins produced by ribosomes of the rough endoplasmic reticulum are destined for secretion out of the cell.

The rough endoplasmic reticulum is the site of translocation of secretory and lysosomal proteins from the cytosol to the intra-cisternal space, and of integration into the membrane of integral membrane proteins. Except for integral membrane proteins of chloroplast, mitochondria, and per-oxisomes, essentially all other integral membrane proteins are integrated into the endoplasmic reticulum and either remain there or are subsequently distributed to other cellular membranes. Once a protein is synthesized on a ribosome, it is enclosed within a vesicle, a small, membrane-bound "bubble." The vesicle travels to the Golgi body. Within the Golgi body, the proteins within the vesicle are further modified before they are exported from the cell. Cells that specialize in protein secretion contain large amounts of rough endoplasmic reticulum. For instance, cells of the pancreas that produce the protein insulin have abundant rough endoplasmic reticulum.

Blobel and Sabatini (1971) had formulated the signal hypothesis to explain how proteins are targeted to and then translocated across or integrated into the endoplasmic reticulum membrane. In case of membrane proteins, the existence of an additional topogenic sequence, the so-called stop-transfer sequence, was postulated. This sequence is thought to trigger opening of the channel to the lipid bi-layer to abort translocation and thus integrate the protein into the lipid bi-layer.

4.4.2. Smooth Endoplasmic Reticulum

Smooth ER has a few different functions in the cell, and its functions can vary with cell type. Smooth endoplasmic reticulum does not have ribosomes and is the site of lipid metabolism. Here, macromolecules containing lipids are broken down into their constituent parts. In addition, it functions in the synthesis of lipid-containing macromolecules. It is not as common in cells as rough endoplasmic reticulum. They provide surface area for the action of enzymes and storage space. These enzymes are used in the synthesis of carbohydrates and lipids. In liver cells the smooth ER produces enzymes that help to detoxify certain compounds. For instance, liver cells remove alcohol and drugs from the bloodstream. In muscles the smooth ER assists in the contraction of muscle cells. Similarly, cells of the ovaries and testes, which produce the lipid-containing hormones estrogen and testosterone, contain large amounts of smooth endoplasmic reticulum.

Another function of smooth endoplasmic reticulum is to control the movement of newly synthesized proteins to their proper location in the cell or to the membrane to be sent outside the cell. This is done by a process called budding, where small vesicles of smooth ER are pinched off to carry the proteins to their new location. Various functions of endoplasmic reticulum makes it an important organelle for maintaining normal cell functioning.

4.5. Ribosome

Ribosomes are cytoplasmic granules composed of RNA and protein. It is a protein biosynthetic factory that translates the DNA genetic information into an amino acid sequence (the primary structure of proteins). They were first observed by Palade (1955) in the electron microscope as dense particles or granules. In 1958, Richard and Roberts gave the organalles its name 'Ribosome'. The ribosomes are the smallest cell organelle measuring 170- 230Å in diameter. Unlike other cell organelles, they are not bound by any unit membrane. The main components of ribosomes are proteins and RNA (rRNA). Fabrication of protein is the primary task of ribosomes. A ribosome may be located in many places within the cell. They occur either freely in the matrix of mitochondria, chloroplast and cytoplasm (i.e., cytoplasmic matrix) or others is bound to cellular membranes. Membrane-bound ribosomes are responsible for the characteristic roughness of the endoplasmic reticulum when seen under a microscope. The proportion of membrane-bound ribosomes varies considerably. In a liver cell, 75% ribosomes are membrane bound and 25% lie freely in the cytoplasmic matrix. However, in the He La cells only 15% ribosomes are membrane bound.

Protein synthesis requires the assistance of two other RNA molecules in addition to the ribosomal RNA. Messenger RNA (mRNA) provides instructions from the cellular DNA for building a specific protein. Transfer RNA (tRNA) brings the protein building blocks, amino acids, to the ribosome. Once the protein backbone amino acids are polymerized, the ribosome releases the protein and it is transported to the Golgi apparatus. There, the proteins are completed and released inside or outside the cell.

4.5.1. Biogenesis

Eukaryote ribosomes are produced and assembled in the nucleolus. Three of the four strands are produced there, but one is produced outside the nucleolus and transported inside to complete the ribosome assembly. Ribosomal proteins enter the nucleolus and combine with the four strands to create the two subunits, which forms the completed ribosome. The ribosome units leave the nucleus through the nuclear pores and unite once in the cytoplasm. Some ribosomes will remain free-floating in the cytoplasm, creating proteins for the cell's use. Others will attach to the endoplasmic reticulum and produce the proteins that will be "exported" from the cell.

The scheme for the biosynthesis of ribosomes is as follows: The RNA cistron of nucleolar DNA transcribes 45S precursor RNA in the presence of the enzyme RNA polymerase. The ribose sugar of certain regions of 45S RNA undergoes methylation (addition of methyl groups). In the methylated regions which gives rise to 28S and 18S RNA of the ribosomes. The non-methylated regions have a higher content of guanine and cytosine than the methylated regions. Cleavage at site removes the transcribed spacer sequence from the 5'P end of 45S RNA. Cleavage at site 2 separates 18S rRNA. Cleavage at site 3 results in a large segment containing 28S RNA and 5.8S RNA along with spacer segments. Cleavage 4 results in the final trimming of this segment. 5S RNA is synthesized outside the nucleolus. Ribosomal proteins are synthesized in the cytoplasm and translocated to the nucleus where they become associated with RNA.

Structural core proteins first associate with 45S RNA to form 80S ribo-nucleoprotein particles. Other proteins are probably bound later. The series of degradations by which 45 S RNA forms 18S, 5.8S and 28S RNA occurs within the ribo-nucleoprotein particles. Ultimately the 40S and 60S subunits of the ribosome are formed, containing 18S and 28S+5.8S

RNA, respectively. 5S RNA, which is synthesized outside the nucleolus, also becomes associated with the large 60S subunit. The two types of subunits pass through pores in the nuclear membrane to the cytoplasm. The 40S subunit binds to mRNA in the cytoplasm to form a 40S-mRNA complex. The 60S subunit now becomes associated with the 40S-mRNA complex to form the 80S ribosome with bound mRNA. In prokaryote cells the subunit RNA precursors are trimmed to form 16 S and 23S RNA. These become associated with protein to form the 30S and 50S subunits, respectively, of the 70S ribosome.

4.5.2. Structure of Ribosome

Composition of ribosomes can be divided into two parts – 2/3 part of r-RNA (ribosomal RNA) and 1/3 part RNP (Ribosomal protein or Ribonucleo protein). RNA performs all activities of ribosome that are catalyst based and the protein that resides over the surface stabilizes the organelle. Polypeptide chain is fabricated by translating mRNA (messenger RNA) with the aid amino acids that tRNA (transfer RNA) delivers. Since ribosomes have their active part composed of sub-structures of RNA, they are also termed ribozymes. Structure of ribosome and its sub units are almost similar for both Eukaryotes and Prokaryotes.

Ribosomes in prokaryotes are 70S, where each ribosome comprises of 30S (small) and 50S (large) subunits. 50S further comprises of 5S subunit of RNA (comprising of almost 120 nucleotides) along with subunits of 23S RNA (almost 2900 nucleotides) and 34 protein subunits. 30S subunit of RNA comprises 1540 nucleotide that is bounded through 21 units of protein.

Ribosomes in eukaryotes are 80S, where each ribosome comprises of 40S (small) and 60S (large) subunits. 60S comprises of 5S subunit of RNA (almost 120 nucleotides) along with units of 28S RNA (almost 4700 nucleotides), subunit of 5.8S (close to 160 nucleotides) and ~49 units of protein. 40S has 18S RNA (approximately 1900 nucleotide) and ~33 units of protein.

Ribosomes found in mitochondria and chloroplasts of eukaryotes are closer to prokaryote ribosome rather than the 80S eukaryote ribosome, that supports the endo-symbiotic theory. Vertebrate mitochondria for example, contain 55S ribosome, each with a large 40S subunit and a small 30S unit. The sedimentation coefficients 80S, 70S and 55D are rounded off values (Fig. 4.43). Actual S values in different organisms may be slightly higher or lower. Mitochondrial ribosomes have been called mitoribosomes to distinguish them from cytoplasmic ribosomes or cytoribosomes. Mitoribosomes occur in a wide variety of forms, the predominant form in multicellular organisms being the 55S ribosome. Under certain conditions mitoribosomes have been obtained in aggregates of 2-7 ribosomes, forming poly-ribosomes.

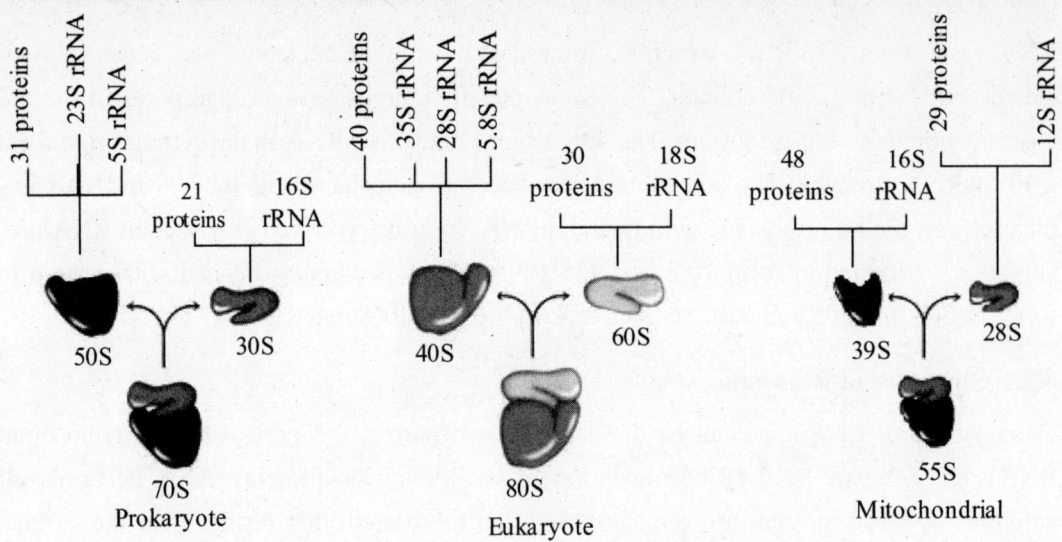

Figure 4.43: Comparative structure of different ribosomes

The unit "S" means Svedberg units, a measure of the rate of sedimentation of a particle in a centrifuge, where the sedimentation rate is associated with the size of the particle. It is important to note that Svedberg units are not additive - two subunits together can have Svedberg values that do not add up to that of the entire ribosome. This is resulting from the loss of surface area when the two subunits are bound. In addition, the ungainly shape of the fully assembled ribosome has different aqua-dynamic properties from the two unbound subunits.

Dissimilarities in eukaryotic and prokaryotic ribosomes are useful in antibiotic treatments against bacterial infections without causing any harmful effect on the neighboring cells. 70S ribosomes, that of bacterial descendants is susceptible to these antibiotics. Mitochondria have risobomes that are similar in nature to 70S of bacteria. However, their double impermeable membrane bounded structure does not permit antibiotics to affect the organelle. Among the antibiotics that interfere with protein synthesis are chloramphenicol, erythromyocin, streptomycin, and the tetracycline. For instance, the chloramphenicol reacts with the 50S structure of the 70S prokaryote ribosome, by inhibiting the formation of the peptide bonds in the growing polypetide chain. The tetracycline interferes with the attachment of the tRNA, which carries the amino acids, to the ribosome, thus preventing the addition of amino acids to the growing polypeptide chain.

4.5.3. Different Type of Ribosomes

(a) 70S Ribosomes: The 70S *E. coli* ribosomes contain 63% RNA and 37% proteins (almost 2:1). Bacterial ribosomes may constitute up to 40% of the dry weight of the cell and 90% of its RNA. Metal ions, chiefly magnesium ions, play an important role in holding the two sub-units together, and also in maintaining the structure of the two subunits. Below a certain level of Mg^{2+} the two subunits of the ribosome separate. The dissociation of the subunits is reversible and the two subunits can re-associate on raising the Mg^{2+} level. A stabilizing role is also attributed to Ca^{2+}, Mn^{2+} and Co^{2+}.

The 30S and 50S subunits of the ribosome have different binding properties. In *E. coli* the 30S subunit binds mRNA to form a 30S -mRNA complex before being attached to the 50S subunit. The 50S subunit, however, cannot bind mRNA if the 30S subunit is not present. The segment of mRNA binding to the 30S subunit is about 27 nucleotides in length. Each 70S ribosome has two binding sites for tRNA, the amino acyl (A site) or acceptor site and the peptidyl (P site) or donor site. The A site receives the tRNA-amino acid complex and the P site binds the growing poly-peptidyl--tRNA. The A site is in the middle of the protected mRNA fragment. The mRNA passes through a tunnel between the two subunits (Fig. 4.44). Between the two subunits is a groove or channel through which the newly formed polypep-tide chain comes out.

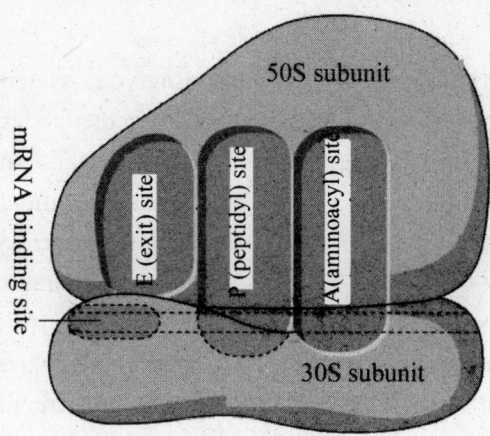

Figure 4.44: The ribosome

(b) 55S Ribosomes: Mitochondria and chloroplasts which have independent protein synthe-sis machinery also contain ribosomes. These ribosomes were formerly thought to be of the 70S prokaryote type. The sedimentation coefficient of mitochondrial ribosomes has, how-ever, been shown to be about 55S, with a large subunit of 40S and a small subunit of 30S. The large subunit contains 16-17S and 5S RNA and the small subunit 12-13S RNA.

(c) 80S Ribosomes: Eukaryotic ribosomes are called '80S ribosomes', although actual S val-ues may be lower or higher than 80S. The sedimentation coefficient is 79S-80S in fungi and 80S in mammals. The small subunit is 40S and the large subunit 60S. The sedimentation coefficient of the large (60S) subunit is 56.3S. It contains one molecule each of 5S, 5.8S and 28S RNA and 49 proteins. RNA constitutes 59.4% of the subunit. The RNA- protein ratio is 1: 1.

The ribosome is responsible for manufacturing the proteins. In each living cell, the information contained in the DNA is "transferred" to a messenger RNA (mRNA). The structure of a ribosome is complex, and it is responsible for making the millions of proteins that are needed by cells.

The mRNA leaves the nucleus and travels to the endoplasmic reticulum (or the cytosol) where the two ribosome subunits assemble around it and start synthesizing proteins. This is done by a process called "translation," which is basically translating the mRNA information into an amino acid sequence. Cell that requires numerous protein for its proper functioning, require comparatively more ribosomes. To function actively in protein synthesis, they must be bound into complete ribosomes. A number of ribosomes may be attached to the same messenger, each manufacturing its own chain of polypeptides, called a polysome. Prokaryotic and eukaryotic ribosomes do not differ in any fundamental way; both perform the same functions by the same set of chemical reactions.

4.6. Golgi Apparatus

In 1897, Camillo Golgi, who was investigating the nervous system by using a new self-developed staining technique, observed a cellular structure that he termed the internal reticular apparatus under his light microscope, which is later universally known as the Golgi apparatus. The Golgi apparatus found universally in both plant and animal cells, is typically comprised of a series of five to eight cup-shaped, membrane-covered sacs called cisternae that look something like a stack of deflated balloons. The Golgi apparatus is often considered the distribution and shipping department for the cell's or more or less the "postal office" of the cell. It process all incoming lipids, proteins, etc., and controls their export as well. These strangely shaped organelles act as a molecular sorting station, directing many of the proteins and carbohydrates used by the body to their correct locations after tagging them with structural modifications and destination information.

4.6.1. Origin

There are views that Golgi complex has originated from the plasma membrane or from nuclear envelope or from the annulated lamella. However, most of the workers believe in its origin from the ER, particularly from the rough ER by the loss of ribosome.

4.6.2. Morphology

The golgi apparatus is morphologically very similar in both plants and animal cells but the number of golgi complex in a cell is variable. The size of the golgi varies with the metabolic state of cell and hence it is called as pleomorphic. It hypertrophies during hyperfunction but reduces considerably during hypofunction. The golgi complex generally lies between the nucleus and periphery usually showing specific orientation.

4.6.3. Chemistry

The Golgi complex is a lipoproteinaceous structure. It also has very low levels of nucleic acid and polysaccharides. Morphologically, the Golgi stands between ER and plasma membrane. The main enzymes of Golgi are thiamine pyrophosphatase (TPPase) and glycosyl transferase, the latter being most characteristic. The Golgi membrane has a single electron transport chain containing cytochrome b_5, the enzyme acyl transferase and choline phosphotransferase are absent in Golgi membrane thus differing from ER.

4.6.4. Structure

Dalton and Felix (1954) elucidated the structure of Golgi complex, which consist of three membranous components: A Golgi cisternae, Golgi vesicles and Golgi vacuoles. All the three structures are bound by a single unit membrane of 70Å thickness. The Golgi apparatus consists, like the ER of membranous structures. It is made up of a stack of flatterned cisternae and similar vesicles. The Golgi cisternae or saccules or lamillar units are flattened membrane bound structures placed one over the other. The number of cisternae in a complex generally varies from 3-8 but rarely there may be as many as 30 cisternae (Fig. 4.46). The distance between two unit membranes in a cisternae is about 150 Å. Its *cis* face is the side facing the ER, while the *trans* face is directed towards the plasma membrane. The *cis* and *trans* faces have different membranous compositions (Fig. 4.45).

In between Golgi cysternae, is found dense inter-cisternal material. The inter-cisternal material may be elongated measuring 60-80 Å in diameter or granular. Perhaps it is a cementing material which holds the cisternae together. Golgi vesicles pinched off from cisternae have a dimension of 400-800 Å diameter.

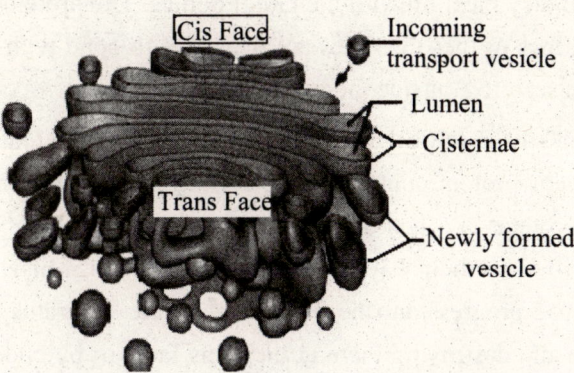

Figure 4.45: Structure of Golgi apparatus

A Golgi complex shows polarity having a proximal or forming face and a distal or maturing face. While the forming face shows convexity, the maturing face exhibits concavity. The forming face is generally closer to nuclear envelope or ER. The forming face is characterized by presence of certain transition vesicles or tubules converging upon the Golgi cisternae. Thus, in a surface view the Golgi cisternae appear reticulate or fenestrated. These transition vesicles are thought to give rise to the ER associated with the maturing face is a region consisting of smooth ER and developing lysosome.

4.6.5. Functions

Golgi apparatus is responsible for handling the macromolecules that are required for proper cell functioning. It processes and packages these macromolecules for use within the cell or for secretion. Primarily, the Golgi apparatus modifies proteins that it receives from the rough endoplasmic reticulum; however, it also transports lipids to vital parts of the cell and creates lysosomes. Some of the modifications made inside the Golgi complex include: attaching polysaccharides to proteins to form glycol-proteins, cutting proteins into smaller active fragments, incorporating phosphates onto protein molecules and addition of a sulfate group to molecules.

Other functions of the Golgi apparatus include the production of glycosaminoglycans, which go on to form parts of connective tissues. The Golgi will use a xylose link to polymerize the glycosaminoglycans onto proteins to form proteoglycan. It then performs sulfation onto the proteoglycans in order to aid in signaling abilities and giving the molecule a negative charge. The Bcl-2 genes that are located within the Golgi apparatus also play a significant role in preventing apoptosis, or the destruction of the cell. The Golgi complex in plant cells produces pectins and other polysaccharides specifically needed by for plant structure and metabolism.

In the endoplasmic reticulum, proteins synthesized by ribosomes are sent through the canals of the ER, where they meet up with the Golgi bodies. The proteins are then packaged in vesicles. The membranes of these vesicles are then able to bond with the cell membrane, where their contents are secreted outside the cell.

The transport vesicles from the ER fuse with the cis face of the Golgi apparatus (to the cisternae) and empty their protein content into the Golgi lumen (the internal space of the Golgi apparatus). The proteins are then transported through the Golgi apparatus towards the trans face and are modified on their way. The transport mechanism itself is not yet clear; it could happen by cisternae progression (the movement of the apparatus itself, building new cisternae at the cis face and destroying them at the trans face) or by budding (small vesicles transport the proteins from one cisterna to the next, while the cisternae remain unchanged).

Once the proteins reach the trans face, they are embedded into transport vesicles and brought to their final destinations. For example in the formation of glycol-proteins used in cell membranes proteins in vesicles from the ER will be directed to Golgi apparatus. In the Golgi apparatus carbohydrates are attached to them creating glycol-proteins. After they have been secreted in to the cell, the vesicles fuse to the cell membrane and release their contents (Fig. 4.46).

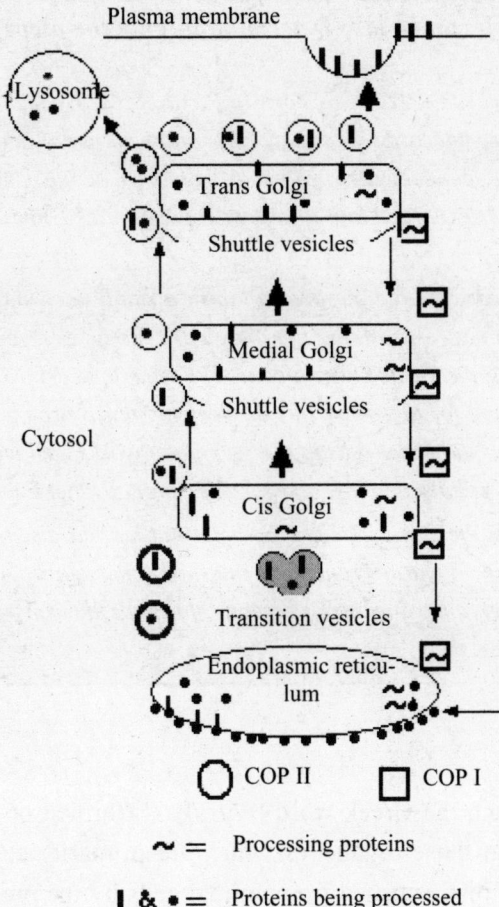

Figure 4.46: Processing and transportation of proteins

The cisternal maturation model states that the vesicles fuse to each other at the cis face of the Golgi apparatus and are essentially pushed along as new vesicles fuse together behind them. Newly synthesized proteins traverse the Golgi stack until they reach the trans-most Golgi compartment, which is termed the trans-Golgi network. The trans-Golgi network sorts the proteins into several types of vesicles. Using a variety of signals, the Golgi separates the products from the processing enzymes that made them and returns the enzymes back to the endoplasmic reticulum. Clathrin-coated vesicles carry certain proteins to lysosomes. Other proteins are packaged into secretory vesicles for immediate delivery to the cell surface. Still other proteins are packaged into secretory granules, which undergo regulated secretion in response to specific signals. This sorting function of the Golgi apparatus allows the various organelles to grow while maintaining their distinct identities.

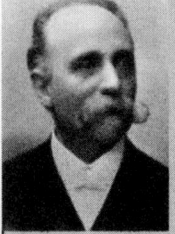

Even a kitchen can be lab: Determination not the place of work

Camillo Golgi (1843–1926) was born in Pavia, Italy. He graduated from the University of Pavia Medical School at age 22, and went on to adopt a high interest in neurology. Golgi conducted neurological research at the University of Pavia till financial difficulties forced him to accept a position as Chief Medical Officer in a mental hospital.

Determined to continue research, Golgi created a lab in a small kitchen. There, he developed his famous black reaction, a technique of staining neurological cells by encasing them in potassium dichromate and then impregnating them with silver nitrate. The technique deposited black outlines on cells in a random fashion, allowing for discovery of cell elements that were previously obscured by other staining techniques. Though the exact reason the technique works remains a mystery, it is so effective that the black reaction is still used today, and earned Golgi a Nobel Prize in Medicine.

In 1898 Golgi announced to the Pavia Medical Society that he had discovered a delicate network inside cells which he termed "apparato reticolare interno" (internal reticular apparatus). The network was soon named the Golgi apparatus and is essential for both the transmission and reception of information between cells.

4.7. Plastids

The term plastid is derived from the Greek word '*plastikas*' (formed or moulded) and was applied by Schimper (1885) to those organelles which are primarily concerned with food storage. Plant cells are readily distinguished from animal cells by the presence of two types of membrane bounded compartments – vacuoles and plastids. Plastids are present in all living plant cells and in *Euglena* (a protozoan). They are small bodies found free in the cytoplasm. Plastids are often more or less spherical or disc-shaped (1 μm to 1 mm in diameter), but may be elongated or lobed or show amoeboid characteristics. All plastids in a particular plant species contain multiple copies of same relatively small genome (DNA) and 70S- type ribosomes. They are self-replicating organelles containing a protein – synthesizing capacity comparable to that of mitochondria. They perform most important biological activities as the synthesis of food and storage of carbohydrates, lipids and proteins. Plastids are absent in the cells of fungi, bacteria, animals and male sperm cells of certain higher plants.

Chloroplasts were described in seventeenth century by Nehemiah Grew and Antonie van Leeuwenhoek. The term plastid was applied by Schimper in 1885; he also classified the plastids of plants. A. Mayer in 1883, F. Schmitz in 1884 and A.F.W. Schimper in 1885 made detailed cytological studies of these cell orgenells and showed that chloroplasts always arise from pre-existing chloroplast. In 1981, Wilstatter and Stoll isolated and characterized the green pigments- chlorophylls *a* and *b*. K. Porter and S. Granick (1947) described the ultra-structure of grana of chloroplasts. Dutrochet (1837) recognized that chlorophyll was essential to oxygen evolution by plants. Liebig, in 1845 indicated that carbon dioxide was the source of all organic compounds synthesized by green plants. In 1845, von Mayer recognized that green plants convert the solar energy into the chemical energy of organic matter. In 1862, Sachs was first to point out that the seat of photosynthesis is chloroplast. Hill, 1937 was first to provide evidence that photochemical reaction in a plant cell occurs inside the chloroplast. Arnon, 1954 suggested that light reaction occurs in the granum, while dark reaction in stroma. This was later, confirmed by Park and Pon in 1963. By using ^{18}O, Ruben, Hassid and Kamen, in 1941 confirmed that oxygen evolved in photosynthesis comes from water and not from CO_2.

4.7.1. Biogenesis

Origin of plastids can be explained by endo-symbiotic theory. Plastids are generally inherited through maternal side as in the case of mitochondria. During the development of plant structures, pro-plastids multiply and they are evenly or unevenly distributed among daughter cells. Every cell in the plant body possesses plastids. The pattern of inheritance itself indicates that plastids are derived from pre existing plastids. When pro-plastids are exposed to light they gradually turn green and enlarge in size. This is accompanied with the development of granal structures. During these stages, the inner chloroplast membrane produces a number of finger shaped invaginations. They in turn pinch off a number of membranous vesicles, which accumulate in the centre. The vesicles start fusing with one another and finally organize into clusters of thylakoid membranes, called Grana. Once the development of chloroplast is completed the invaginations of inner membranes disappear.

4.7.2. Classification

On the basis of structure, presence or absence of pigments and the functions, plastids have been classified into Leucoplasts, Chromoplasts and Chloroplasts.

(a)Leucoplasts

Leucoplasts (comes from Greek word *leuco* meaning white and *plast* = living) are the colourless plastids which are found in embryonic and germ cells. They are also found in meristematic cells and in those regions of the plant which are not exposed to light, such as roots and seeds and are found in storage parenchyma and other colourless tissues. They are colourless due the absence of pigments. Based on the kind of substance they store, they are further classified into following types

Amyloplasts. The amyloplasts (L.,amyl = starch; Gr., plast= living) are those leucoplasts which synthesize and store the starch. The outer membrane of the amyloplast encloses the stroma and contains one to eight starch granules. Starch granules of amyloplasts are typically composed of concentric layers of starch. If amyloplasts are exposed to sunlight they will be transformed into colored plastids, which suggest that these plastids have retained all the genetic potentiality to develop and perform photosynthesis. Leucoplasts do also occur within colourless leaves (variegated leaves) or plant parts.

Elaioplasts. The elaioplasts store the lipids (oils) and occure in seeds of monocotyledons and dicotyledons. They also include sterol- rich sterinochloroplast.

Proteinoplasts. The proteinoplasts are the protein storing plastids which mostly occur in seeds and contain few thylakoids.

(b) Chromoplasts

Chromoplasts (Gr., chroma = colour; plast = living) contain different colored plastids containing carotenoids and other pigments. Depending upon the dominant pigments present in plastids, they are further classified into Rhodoplasts rich in red pigment, i.e. phycoerythrin. Phaeoplasts and Xanthoplasts contain yellow pigments, i.e. xanthophylls and carotinoids. The plastids of the red and brown algae are traditionally counted among the chromoplasts although they contain chlorophyll. The green colour is concealed by the red phyco-erythrin (Rhodophyceae) or the brown fucoxanthin (Phaeophyta).

(c) Chloroplasts

The Chloroplasts (Gr., chloro= green; plast= living) is most widely occurring chromoplast of the plants. It occurs mostly in the green algae and higher plants. The chloroplasts contains the pigment chlorophyll a and chlorophyll b and DNA and RNA.

4.7.3. Photosynthetic Pigments

Plant pigments are basically simple lipids containing many isoprenoid units. Among the plant pigments present in plastids, chlorophylls and carotinoids are found in 3:1 proportions. The composition of pigments varies significantly among different groups of plant kingdom. Chl a, Chl b, β-carotene and xanthophylls are found in most of the green plants. But lower plants contain diverse pigments composition. Chl- a acts as a primary pigment and all others including phycoerythrin and phycocyanin are considered as accessory pigments.

Chlorophyll molecules are made up of hydrophilic head and a hydrophobic tail. The head consists of four pyrole rings joined to each other by a single master ring of CH bridges to from a porphyrin ring. The inorganic Mg^{2+} ion is found in the centre of the ring (Fig. 4.48). Chlorophyll also contains an additional long chain of saturated hydrocarbons called phytol chain. Chl- a is distinguished from Chl- b in having CH_3 group in II ring, while Chl-b possesses CHO.

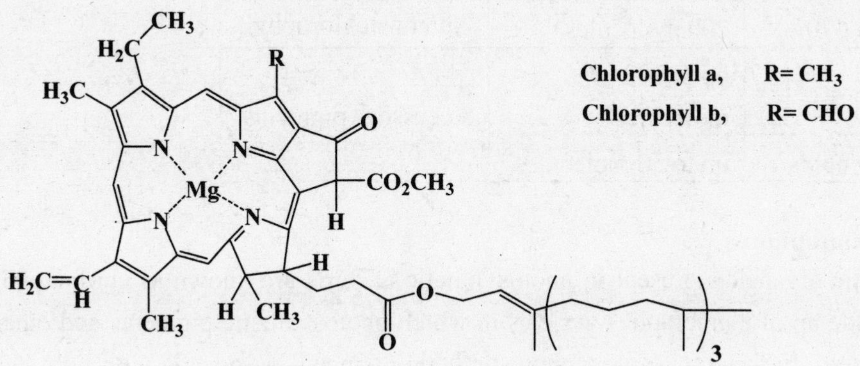

Figure 4.48: Chemical structure of chlorophyll

The most common photosynthetic pigments present in higher plants and green algae are:

(i) Chlorophyll-a (blue-green) = $C_{55}H_{72}O_5N_4Mg$

(ii) Chlorophyll-b (yellow-green) = $C_{55}H_{70}O_6N_4Mg$

(iii) Carotenoids - Carotenes (orange-red) = $C_{40}H_{56}$

(iv) Xanthophylls (yellow) = $C_{40}H_{56}O_2$

For photosynthesis, these pigments can absorb and use light belonging to the visible spectrum only. Both chlorophyll-a and chlorophyll-b show maximum light absorption in the blue-violet and in the red regions of the visible range of wavelengths of light. Carotenoids absorb light in the blue and blue-green regions. They also protect the chlorophyll from undergoing photo-oxidation when exposed to very high intensity light.

4.7.4. Light Trapping Systems

During the photochemical phase, light is trapped by the photosynthetic pigments present in the quantasomes of the grana thylakoids. These pigments are organized into two pigment systems called pigment system I (PS I) and pigment system II (PS II).

(I) PS I is composed of the following pigment molecules:

Chl-a 700 (P700)- one molecule - Reaction center
Chl-a 683 - 200 molecules - Antenna chlorophyll
Carotenoids - 50 molecules - Accessory pigments

(II) PS II is composed of the following pigment molecules:

Chl- a 680	one molecule	Reaction center
Chl- a 670	200 molecules	Antenna chlorophyll
Chl- b	up to 200 molecules	Accessory pigments
Carotenoids	up to 50 molecules	

4.7.5. Chromatophores

Photosynthetic organelles present in photosynthetic bacteria are known as chromatophores. They are made up of membranous vesicles in which photosynthetic pigments and other factors are located. In these structures, photosynthetic pigments, associated with light harvesting proteins and other required enzymes are aggregated into photosynthetic units.

4.7.6. Chloroplasts

Chloroplasts are green coloured plastids for they contain greater amounts of chlorophyll pigments. They are ubiquitously present in green plants and they are mainly responsible for providing food for themselves and to other animals in the world. These structures are mostly restricted to photosynthetic parts of the plants.

4.7.6.1. Distribution

In higher land plants, the number of chloroplasts varies from cell to cell and from organ to organ, i.e. 30-200 per cell and most of them are nearly spherical or ovoidal in shape. Size of eukaryotic chloroplasts is 4-5 nm but it may vary from plant to plant. Plants growing in shade contain large chloroplasts in their cells than that of growing in intense light. In certain algae like *Caulerpa* and *Vaucheria,* chloroplasts are generally clustered in the region of the cell where it is exposed to sunlight. Even in higher plants such as tropical grasses etc, chloroplasts found in bundle sheath cells and those found in the surrounding mesophyll cells are crowded towards each other.

In meristematic cells proplastids are constantly dividing and keep pace with cell division. Once proplastids develop into chloroplasts, they rarely divide in higher plants. But in *Spirogyra* and many algae fully developed plastids, divide at the time of cell division and they are equally distributed among the daughter cells. For example, in *Chlamydomonas,* chloroplasts divide into two, four or more at the time of reproduction just like bacterial division.

In lower plants, plastids got a characteristic shape, specific number and contain pyrenoids; *Chlamydomonas* possesses only one cup shaped chloroplast while *Chlorella* cells contain a single plate shaped chloroplast. Chloroplasts in *Spirogyra* are ribbon shaped spirally coiled. While *Zygnema* cells contain two star shapes chloroplasts.

4.7.6.2. Structure

The chloroplasts are disc-shaped structures bounded by double unit membranes where each membrane is 50 Å thick. The two membranes are separated by 100-300 Å wide periplastidial space. Chloroplast membranes are made up of lipid protein composition. Internally, the chloroplasts are distinguishable into grana and stroma. A chloroplast usually contains some 10-100 grana. A granum looks like a stack of coins placed one above the other (Fig. 4.49). The grana are interconnected by tubular membranes called the lamellae. The distance between two superimposed grana lamellae has been estimated to be between 25–75 Å. Each chloroplast may contain 10–30 such granal clusters; a single granum consists of 20-60 thylakoids. The thylakoids contain the photosynthetic pigments - green chlorophyll a and b and the yellow to red carotenoids. The granal membranes including both thylakoid and intergranal membranes, posses 20-30% of the lipids and the rest of it is all proteins. The most common lipids found in these membranes are ethanolamine, sulfolipids, phytosterols, glycolipids and pigments. The thylakoid lamellae are composed of alternating layers of lipids and aqueous proteins (Fig. 4.50). The chlorophyll molecules are arranged in such a way that their hydrophilic heads extends into the aqueous protein layer while the lipophilic tails are embedded in the lipid layer. The pigments are organized into numerous photosynthetic units called quantasomes. Each quantasome contains about 230 to 300 chlorophyll molecules. Quantasomes are capable of trapping light energy and converting it into chemical energy (ATP) during the photochemical reactions (light reaction) of photosynthesis. The grana also contain various co-enzymes and electron acceptors necessary for the process. Hence, grana are the site of the light reactions (phase-I) in photosynthesis. Granal membrane contains more than 200 polypeptides; most of them are structural proteins, light harvesting antenna proteins and electron transporting proteins. Light harvesting proteins (LHP) are a group of proteins that are associated with various pigments and they are responsible for harvesting and transferring solar energy. Most of the proteins exhibit hydrophilic as well as intrinsic hydrophobic properties. The organization of quantosomes found in chloroplasts of bundle sheaths of C4 is quite different from that of other normal chloroplasts. These chloroplasts contain only stromal lamellae. Photosynthetic units like PS I and PS II have different chemical composition.

Still each of these units are made up of 250-300 Chl molecules complexes with LHP antenna proteins and other cofactors required for specific photochemical reactions. The role of PS I ad PS II present in thylakoid membranes is to perform NADP reduction, non-cyclic photo-phosphorylation and oxygen liberation. On the contrary, the intergranal lamellae containing just PS I systems perform just cyclic photo-phosphorylation (Fig. 4.49).

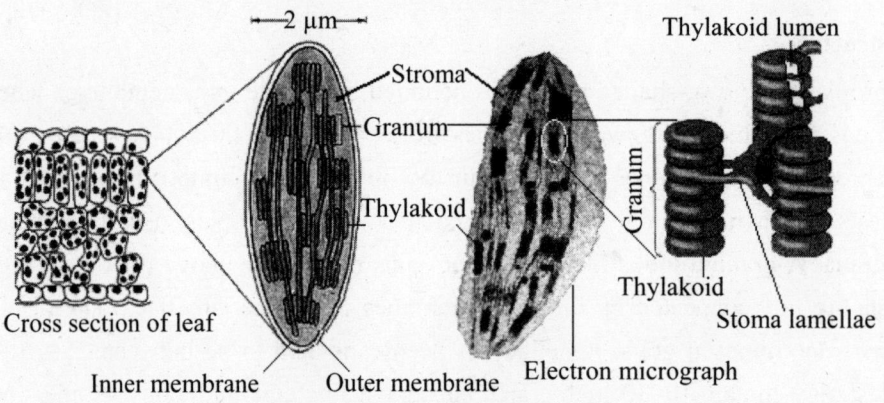

Figure 4.49: Chloroplast structure

Though, this is the general structure for most of the chloroplasts, certain plants belonging to tropical grass members like sugarcane, zea mays, sorghum, crab grass and even some dicots like *Amaranthus* contain chloroplasts of two types. Chloroplasts found in mesophyll cells have the same granal organization as described above, but lack in thylakoids. In its place only stromal lamellae are found. Such dimorphic chloroplasts though found in the same leaf exhibit different functions (see description of C4 plants in chapter 3).

Chloroplast is filled with a liquid called stroma, is the semi viscous, amorphous fluid present within the chloroplast. Besides grana, the stromatic fluid contains a host of enzymes, plastid DNA, RNAs and 70S ribosomes. These enzymes are responsible for carbon fixation, amino acid synthesis, pigment synthesis etc. Hence, stroma is the site of the dark reactions (phase-II) of photosynthesis. The "dark reactions" do not directly require light, but they do require energy produced from light during the light reactions. Some of the biosynthetic pathways in the stroma are under the control of various factors like light, phytochromes, temperature and photoperiods (Fig. 4.50).

In case of C4 plants, the stromatic fluid of chloroplasts found in mesophyll cells contain enzymes for Hatch and Slack pathway. Such enzymes are totally absent in the stroma of C3 chloroplasts. On the other hand, C4 chloroplasts found in bundle sheath cells possess enzymes for C3 pathway and also contain malate dehydrogenase. It has also enzymes for the synthesis of gibberellic acid and abscisic acid.

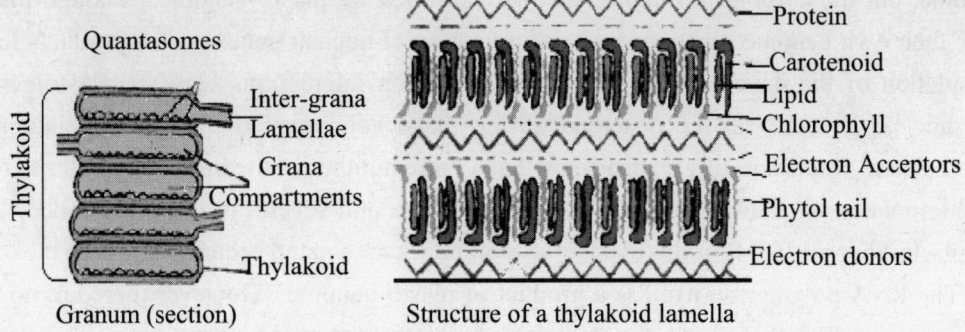

Figure 4.50: Thylakoid lamellae

4.7.6.3. Chloroplast Genome

Chloroplasts contain their own genetic system, like mitochondria, which supports the endo-symbiotic theory. Chloroplast genomes are larger and more complex than those of mitochondria, ranging from 120 to 160 kb and containing approximately 120 genes. Plastid DNAs are circular duplex molecules with a total length of 45 mm, however in some cases DNA of 15 mm have been isolated. Each plastid consists of 6-30 copies of circular DNAs and most of them are in super coiled state.

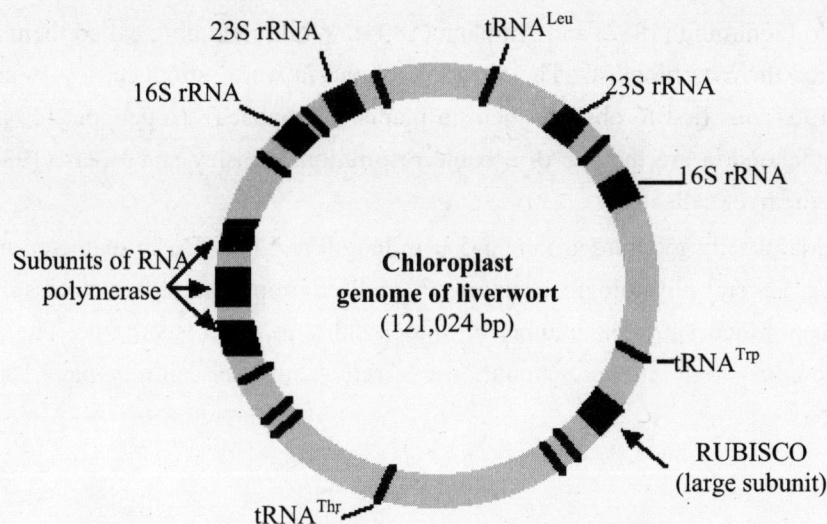

Figure 4.51: Chloroplast Genome

Plastids by virtue of having its own genetic material and ribosomal translating machinery exhibits semi autonomous state within the cells. Inheritance of chloroplasts is maternal and non-Mendelian cytoplasmic type. The Mendelian pattern is controlled by nuclear genome, but the cytoplasmic inheritance is controlled by plasto-genome. Though plastids have their own genome, they need the co-ordination of nuclear genes and its products for the completion of the development of chloroplasts. Such interactions between plasto-genome and nuclear genome can be observed during the development of pro-plastids into green chloroplasts. Studies in this regard show that a large number of the protein complexes found in chloroplasts are found to be nuclear gene products and several proteins are coded for by the plasto-genome like ferrodoxin and plastoquinones associated proteins (Fig.4.51).

The RNA polymerase itself is a product of plasto-genome. However there are no clear cut reports to show that plasto-genome products control the nuclear gene expression required for plastid development.

4.8. Mitochondria

The mitochondria are filamentous or granular cytoplasmic organelles found in all eukaryotic cells, but absent in bacterial cells. The number of mitochondria varies from one to 10, 000 per cell. The average number is generally 200. The mitochondria have lipoprotein framework which contains many enzymes and co- enzymes required for energy metabolism and called power house of the cell.

Mitochondria, small cellular organelle are found in the cytoplasm of eukaryotic cells. They were first observed by Kolliker (1880) in striated muscles, but the credit of discovery is generally given to Flemming (1882) and Altmann (1894). While flemming called them as filia, Altmann named them as bioplast. The term mitochondria were introduced by Benda (1897). Meeves, 1904 was first to observe them in plants (Nymphaea). Hogeboom (1948) discovered that mitochondria are the site of aerobic respiration. Bensley and Hoerr (1934) isolated them from the liver cells.

The mitochondria usually measure around 3-5 μ in length and 0.5- 2 μ in diameter and may be 8-10 μ long. Several physiological factors (P^H, cell environment, osmotic pressure) have some influence on their size. The number of mitochondria in a cell is variable. The algae, *Microsterias,* contains only one mitochondrion in a cell. A rat liver cell may have 1000 – 2500 mitochondria.

Biogenesis

Mitochondria possess genetic material and ribosomes. Mitochondrial DNA is circular and employs characteristic variants of the standard eukaryotic genetic code. Mitochondria divide independently of the cell through binary fission, the method of cell division typical of pro-karyotes. These evidences support the endo-symbiotic theory of mitochondrial origin. Essentially this widely accepted hypothesis postulates that the ancestors of modern mitochondria were independent bacteria that colonized the interior of the ancient precursor of all eukaryotic life. The cytoplasm of nearly all eukaryotic cells contains mitochondria, although there is at least one exception, the protest, *Pelomyxa carolinensis*. They are especially abundant in cells and parts of cells that are associated with active processes. For example, in flagellated protozoa or in mammalian sperm, mitochondria are concentrated around the base of the flagellum or flagella. In cardiac muscle, mitochondria surround the contractile elements. Hummingbird flight muscle is one of the richest sources of mitochondria.

Mitochondria contain the biochemical machinery involved in cellular respiration which take energy from breakdown of glucose and produce energy-rich ATP molecule which is used as a source of energy in the metabolic reactions in the rest of the cell. Hence, mitochondria are described as the 'power houses' of cells. They contain the enzymes required for the citric-acid cycle, ATP synthesis, and the oxidation of fatty acids

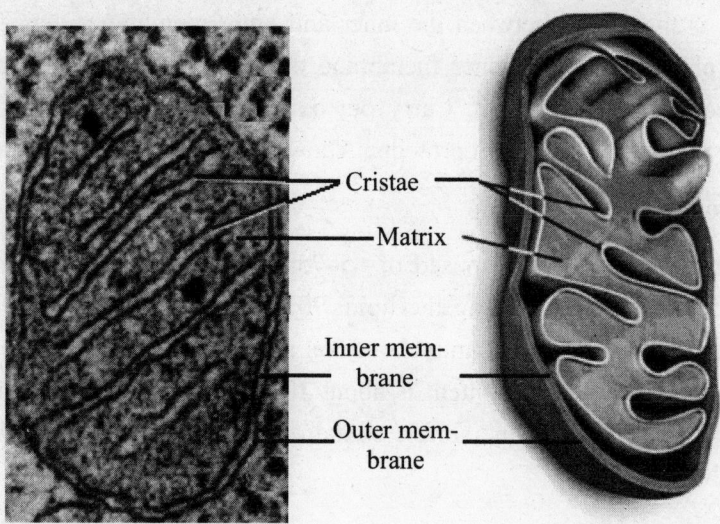

Figure 4.52: Structure of mitochondria: electron micrograph (left)

4.8.1. Structure

The mitochondria are specialized, oval-shaped cellular compartments having a double membrane (Fig. 4.52). Mitochondria can vary greatly in both size (0.5 micrometers - 10 micrometers) and number (1 - ~1000) per cell. However, regardless of their size, number per cell, plant or animal origin, they have varied similar structures. The mitochondria are bound by double unit membrane where each membrane is 60Å thick. The two membranes are separated by 40-70 Å wide perimitochondrial space or outer chamber. The outer membrane is smooth, relatively simple phospho-lipid bilayer, containing protein structures called porins which allows the passage of molecules up to 10 kilo-daltons. Ions, nutrient molecules, ATP,

ADP, etc. can pass through the outer membrane. The matrix contains the enzymes that are responsible for the citric acid cycle reactions. They freely permeable only to oxygen, carbon dioxide, and water. Its structure is highly complex, including all of the complexes of the electron transport system, the ATP synthetase complex, and transport proteins. The inner membrane has numerous folded to form the cristae. The cristae greatly increase the total surface area of the inner membrane. The inner surface of the cristae membrane (i.e. the surface towards the matrix) is covered with numerous (infinite) stalked particles. These are called F_1 particles, elementary particles or sub units. These particles project into the matrix. Each F_1 particle has three parts, viz., the head piece, the stalk and the base piece. The respiratory chain is situated in the cristae membrane where the F_1 particles are present. The chain consists of enzymes and co-enzymes which form the electron transport system (ETS) in the mitochondrion. These enzymes and co-enzymes of the ETS act as the electron acceptors in the aerobic respiration reactions and oxidative phosphorylation (Fig. 4.53). The inter-membrane space, as implied, is the region between the inner and outer membranes, has an important role in oxidative phosphorylation. Inner membrane contains proteins with three types of functions: (1) Electron-transport chain: Carry out oxidation reactions; (2) ATP synthase: Makes ATP in the matrix; (3) Transport proteins: Allow the passage of metabolites.

Chemical composition

Chemically the mitochondria are composed of 65–75% proteins (30% structural and 40% enzymatic) and 25–30 % lipids. Among the lipid, 90% are phospholipid and 10% carotenoids, cholesterol, vitamin E etc. The mitochondrion also contains traces of S, Fe, Cu, Ca, Mg and some vitamins. The DNA content is about 1%. The lipid composition of the two membranes is variable. The outer membrane contains 40% lipid whereas the inner membrane has only 20%.

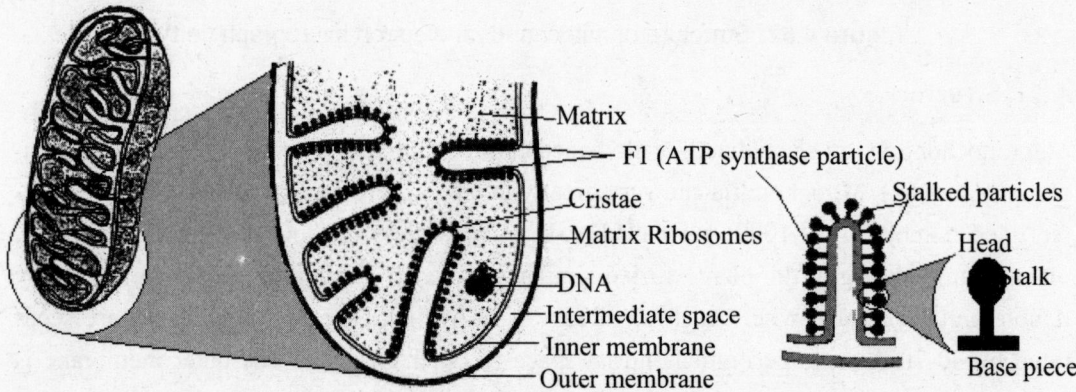

Figure 4.53: Ultra structure of mitochondria

4.8.2. ATP synthase

Boyer and Walker received the Nobel Prize in 1997 for elucidating the mechanism of ATP synthase. This is all-important reactions in which the proton-motive force, produced by proton translocation, is coupled to the synthesis of ATP from ADP and phosphate. ATP synthase is a complex structure consisting of two domains F_O and F_1. F_1 is a spherical structure, sticks out into the matrix and is anchored to the membrane, consists of three α- and three β-subunits, all of which can bind nucleotides, but only the β-subunits can take part in the reactions (Fig. 4.54). F_O is a cylindrical structure capable of rotation when driven by translocated protons and is linked to a central stalk that can revolve inside F_1.

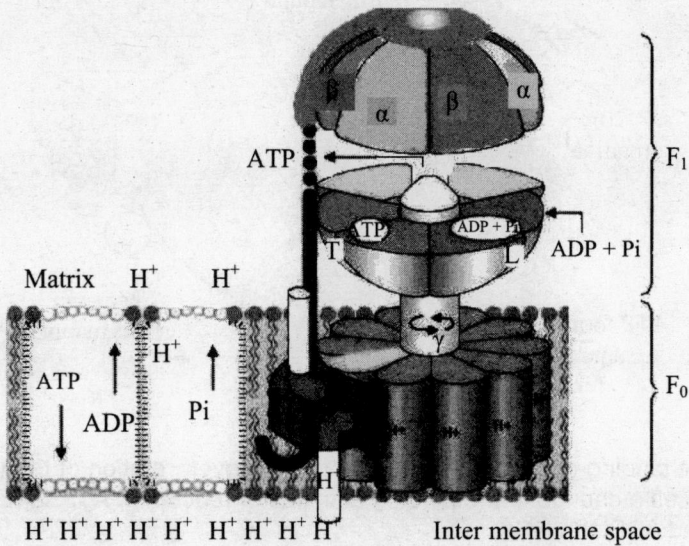

Figure 4.54: structure of ATP synthase (F_1 particle is the catalytic subunit; The F_O particle attaches to F_1 and is embedded in the inner membrane

In F_1F_O ATP synthase, the F_O portion is within the membrane and the F_1 portion is above the membrane. The F_1 fraction derives its name from the term "Fraction 1" and F_O (written as a subscript "O", not "zero") derives its name from being the oligomycin binding fraction. The antibiotic oligomycin inhibits the F_O unit of ATP synthase. A soluble portion, the F_1 ATP-ase, contains 5 subunits, in a stoichiometry of $3\alpha{:}3\beta{:}1\gamma{:}1\delta{:}1\varepsilon$. Three substrate binding sites are in the β-subunits (Fig. 4.55). Additional adenine nucleotide binding sites in α-subunits are regulatory.

According to the current model of ATP synthesis (known as the alternating catalytic model), the proton-motive force across the inner mitochondrial membrane, generated by the electron transport chain, drives the passage of protons through the membrane via the F_O

region of ATP synthase. A portion of the F_O (the ring of C-subunits) rotates as the protons pass through the membrane. The c-ring is tightly attached to the asymmetric central stalk (consisting primarily of the gamma subunit) which rotates within the $\alpha_3 \beta_3$ of F_1 causing the 3 catalytic nucleotide binding sites to go through a series of conformational changes that leads to ATP synthesis.

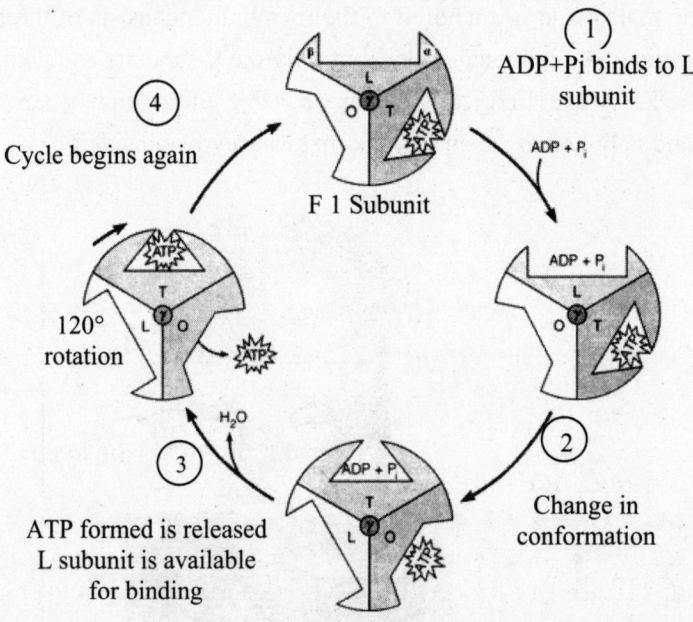

Figure 4.55: The binding-change mechanism of Paul Boyer, rotation of the γ-subunit relative to α, β-ring induces a change in the binding affinities of reactants. ATP forms spontaneously from tightly bound ADP and Pi

The mechanism that drives ATP synthesis seems to depend upon a binding charge conception in which catalytic sites on the β-subunits have different affinities for nucleotides and are designated loose (L), tight (T), and open (O). The loose (L) sites bind the substrates (ADP and phosphate) reversibly. The T sites then bind the reactants so tightly that ATP is formed. The O sites, which have a low affinity for substrates, then release the ATP already formed in the T state. The central stalk is driven by the retro-location of protons through F_O (counter-clockwise as seen from above), and rotates in 120° stages. At each stage, each of the β-subunits in turn changes conformation: L changes to T (after binding ADP and phosphate), T to O, and O to L (after releasing ATP). The new L site then binds new ADP and phosphate and begins a new reaction sequence. One complete revolution of F_O, therefore, results in the formation of 3 ATP, one from each of the β-subunits (~3.3 H^+ needed for the formation of one ATP from ADP and Pi).

4.8.3. Mitochondrial DNA

Mitochondrial DNA is a double stranded circular molecule, which is inherited from the mother in all multi-cellular organisms, though some recent evidence suggests that in rare instances mitochondria may also be inherited via a paternal route. Typically, a sperm carries mitochondria in its tail as an energy source for its long journey to the egg. When the sperm attaches to the egg during fertilization, the tail falls off. Consequently, the only mitochondria the new organism usually gets are from the egg its mother provided. There are about 2 to 10 transcripts of the mt-DNA in each mitochondrion. Compared to chromosomes, it is relatively smaller, and contains the genes in a limited number.

The size of mitochondrial genomes varies greatly among different organisms, with the largest found among plants, including that of the plant *Arabidopsis,* with a genome of 200 kbp in size and 57 protein-encoding genes. The smallest mtDNA genomes include that of the protist *Plasmodium falciparum*, which has a genome of only 6 kbp and just 2 protein-encoding genomes. Humans and other animals have a mitochondrial genome size of 17 kbp and 13 protein genes.

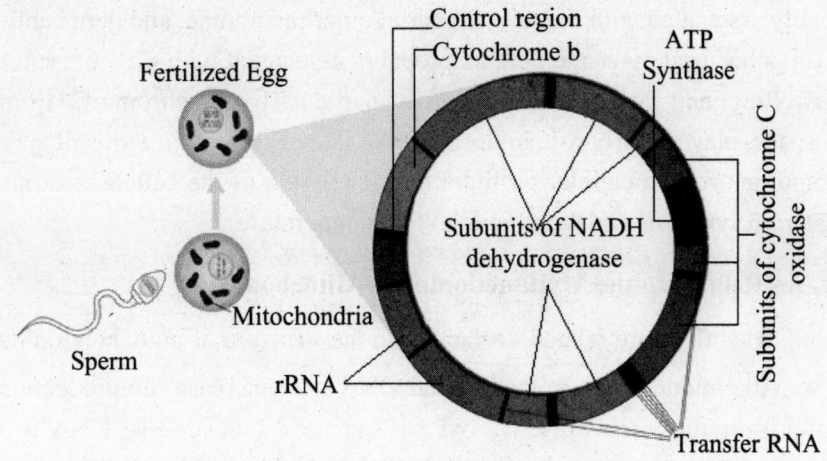

Figure 4.56: Mitochondrial DNA

Mitochondrial DNA consists of 5-10 rings of DNA and appears to carry 16,569 base pairs with 37 genes (13 proteins, 22 t-RNAs and two r-RNA) which are concerned with the production of proteins involved in respiration. Out of the 37 genes, 13 are responsible for making enzymes, involved in oxidative phosphorylation, a process that uses oxygen and sugar to produce adenosine tri-phosphate (Fig. 4.56). The other 14 genes are responsible for making molecules, called transfer RNA (t-RNA) and ribosomal RNA (r-RNA). In some metazoans, there are about 100 - 10,000 separate copies of mt-DNA present in each cell.

Unlike nuclear DNA, mitochondrial DNA doesn't get shuffled every generation, so it is presumed to change at a slower rate, which is useful for the study of human evolution. Mitochondrial DNA is also used in forensic science as a tool for identifying corpses or body parts and has been implicated in a number of genetic diseases, such as Alzheimer's disease and diabetes. Changes in mt-DNA can cause maternally inherited diseases, which leads to faster aging process and genetic disorders.

Mitochondria convert the potential energy of food molecules into ATP by the Krebs cycle, electron transport and oxidative phosphorylation in presence of oxygen. The energy from food molecules (e.g., glucose) is used to produce NADH and $FADH_2$ molecules, via glycolysis and the Krebs cycle. The protein complexes in the inner membrane (NADH dehydrogenase, cytochrome c reductase, cytochrome c oxidase) use the released energy to pump protons (H^+) against a gradient.

Mitochondria have several important functions besides the production of ATP. Some mitochondrial functions are performed only in specific types of cells. For example, mitochondria in liver cells contain enzymes that allow them to detoxify ammonia, a waste product of protein metabolism. Mitochondria also play a role in apoptosis, the mechanism by which the body gets rid of damaged cells. Proteins that control the survival or death of cells are specifically associated with the mitochondrial outer membrane, and permeability changes across the mitochondrial inner membrane, probably associated with Ca^{2+} transport and mitochondrial swelling, and the release of proteins, particularly cytochrome C, from the intermembrane space, play an early role in deciding the fate of the cell in terms of survival. Also, it has an important role in cellular proliferation, regulation of the cellular redox state, heme synthesis, steroid synthesis and maintaining body temperature.

4.8.4. Diseases Related to the Malfunctioning of Mitochondria

The following conditions are related to changes in the structure of mitochondrial DNA.

Cancers: Somatic mutations in mitochondrial DNA may increase the production of potentially harmful molecules called reactive oxygen species. Mitochondrial DNA is particularly vulnerable to the effects of these molecules and has a limited ability to repair itself. As a result, reactive oxygen species easily damage mitochondrial DNA, causing a build-up of additional somatic mutations. Somatic mutations in mitochondrial DNA have been reported in some forms of cancer, including breast, colon, stomach, liver, and kidney tumors. These mutations also have been associated with cancer of blood-forming tissue (leukemia) and cancer of immune system cells (lymphoma).

Ataxia, Neuropathy and Retinitis pigmentosa: The MT-ATP6 gene provides instructions for making a protein that is essential for normal mitochondrial function like the sub unit of ATP synthase, which is responsible for the last step of oxidative phosphorylation, in the formation of ATP. Neuropathy, ataxia, and retinitis pigmentosa are supposed to be due to the mutations in mitochondrial gene, MT-ATP6 since it alters the structure or function of ATP synthase.

Other changes: Inherited changes in mitochondrial DNA can cause problems with growth, development, and function of the body's systems. These mutations disrupt the mitochondria's ability to efficiently generate energy for the cell. Conditions caused by mutations in mitochondrial DNA often involve multiple organ systems. The effects of these conditions are most pronounced in organs and tissues with high energy requirements (such as the heart, brain, and muscles). Although the health consequences of inherited mitochondrial DNA mutations vary widely, some frequently observed features include muscle weakness and wasting, problems with movement, diabetes, kidney failure, heart disease, loss of intellectual functions (dementia), hearing loss, and abnormalities involving the eyes and vision. There are also several diseases conditions which are related to mitochondria like cyclic vomiting syndrome, Leber hereditary optic neuropathy, which affects the nerve that relays visual information from the eye to the brain.

4.9. Lysosome

The electron microscope revealed the presence of some particles intermediate between mitochondria and ribosomes. De Duve (1955) had given the name as lysosomes. It is a membrane-bound organelle, found in the cytoplasm of eukaryotic cells, which contains digestive enzymes. Lysosomes are found in all eukaryotic cells, but are numerous in disease-fighting cells, such as leukocytes (white blood cells). It helps in the disposal of unwanted materials of the cell by breaking down cell components that are no longer needed as well as molecules or even bacteria that are ingested by the cell. The interior of a lysosome is strongly acidic, and its enzymes are active at an acidic P^H. They were earlier identified as pericanalicular bodies. Matile (1964) was first to demonstrate their presence in plants, particularly in the fungus *Neurospora*. Since they contain digestive enzymes they are also called as suicidal bags or lytic bags. About 15–20 lysosomes are found in a cell.

4.9.1. Biogenesis

Lysosomes are often budded from the membrane of the Golgi apparatus, but in some cases they develop gradually from late endosomes, which are vesicles that carry materials brought into the cell by a process known as endocytosis. Lysosomal enzymes are synthesized on the rough endoplasmic reticulum (RER) and packaged into pre-lysosomal vesicles by the Golgi bodies (Fig. 4.57). The enzymes are glycosylated in the rough endoplasmic reticulum and a mannose group is phosphorylated in the Golgi to target them to lysosomal vesicles. In lysosomal biogenesis, pre-lysosomal vesicles that bud directly from the Golgi fuse to form mature, primary lysosomes.

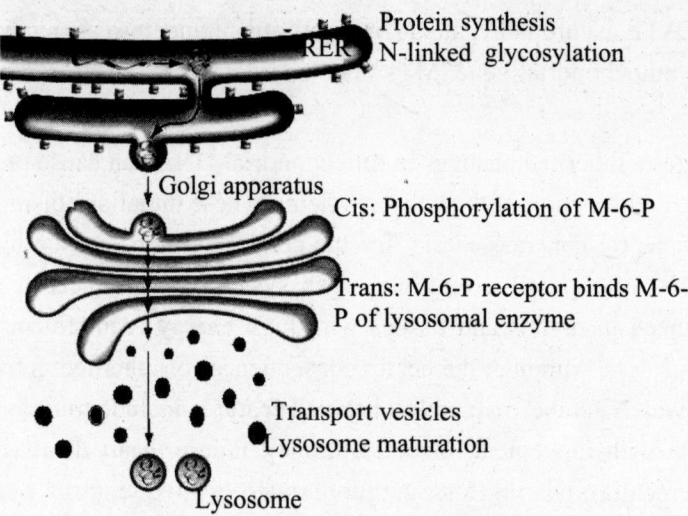

Protein synthesis
N-linked glycosylation

Golgi apparatus

Cis: Phosphorylation of M-6-P

Trans: M-6-P receptor binds M-6-P of lysosomal enzyme

Transport vesicles
Lysosome maturation

Lysosome

Figure 4.57: The formation of lysosomes

4.9.2. Occurrence

It is mostly occurs in most animal and few plant cells but not found in bacteria and mature mammalian erythrocytes. Few lysosomes occur in muscle cells or cells of pancreas. They are also numerous in epithelial cells of absorptive, secretory and excretory organs (i.e., intestine, liver and kidney) but it is mostly concentrated in leucocytes, especially granulocytes.

4.9.3. Structure

The lysosomes are round vacuolar structures which remain filled with dense material and are bounded by single unit membrane. The lysosome has no characteristic shape. They measure 0.2 to 0.8μ in size. Since, size and shape of lysosomes vary from cell to cell and time to time i.e., they are polymorphic. They are bound by a single unit membrane of 70Å thickness. This membrane shows controlled permeability, i.e. it is impermeable to substrates whose lytic enzymes present inside it. De Duve and Wattiux classified the lysosomes into four major types:

1. Primary lysosome or Proto-lysosomes: They are also called as storage granules and first to be differentiated probably from the ER or indirectly from Golgi. They contain specific enzymes.

2. Secondary lysosomes or Telo-lysosomes.

3. Pre-lysosomes or Phagosomes.

4. Post-lysosomes or residual bodies.

However, the lysosomes are generally divided into two categories – primary and secondary lysosomes and the latter is further divided into three types: hetero-phagosomes, residual bodies and auto-phagosome.

(a) Heterophagosomes: Also called as secondary lysosome. They contain acid hydrolases. A digestive vacuole called phagosome is formed as a result of pinocytosis (cell drinking) or phagocytosis (cell eating). The phagosome fuses with the primary lysosme so as to form the secondary lysosome or heterophagosome. They show positive phophatase reaction. The phenomenon of digesting extra cellular material by lysosome is called as heterophagy.

(b) Residual bodies: They contain indigestible material. They are formed when the digestion is incomplete, perhaps due to the absence of some enzymes.

(c) Autophagosomes: Also called as autophagic vacuoles or cytolysosomes. They contain some part of the cell in the process of digestion such as ER, mitochondria etc. Digestion of these intracellular components is described as cellular autophagy.

4.9.4. Enzymes

The lysosomes contain lytic or destructive enzymes. These enzymes work under acidic medium and hence they are collectively called as acid hydrolases. It is due to accumulation of H^+ maintained by a proton pump inside the organelle. A lysosome may contain one or more of these enzymes:

- **Nucleases**: They are meant for the digestion of nucleic acid
- **Phosphatase:** They are meant for the digestion of phosphate polymers.
    - Acid phosphatase: For the digestion of phosphate monoesters.
    - Acid phosphodiesterase: For the digestion of phosphodiesterase.
- **Lipases:** They are meant for the digesting lipids.
    - Esterases: For digesting fatty acid esters.
    - Phospholiases: For digesting phospholipids.
- **Proteases:** They are meant for destroying proteins e.g., cathepsins, collagenases, peptidases etc.
- **Glycosidases:** They are meant for the digestion of carbohydrates e.g., β-galactosidases, α-mannosidase, α-glucosidase etc.
- **Sulphatases:** They are meant for the digestion of sulphate esters e.g., acrylsulphatse A and B. The release of lysosomal enzymes occurs under extremes of pH and critical levels of Ag^{++} and Cu^{++}.

Like other micro-bodies, lysosomes are spherical organelles contained by a single layer membrane. This membrane protects the rest of the cell from the digestive enzymes contained in the lysosomes, which would otherwise cause significant damage. The cell is further safeguarded from exposure to the biochemical catalysts present in lysosomes by their dependency on an acidic environment. With an average pH of about 4.8, the lysosomal matrix is favourable for enzymatic activity, but the neutral environment of the cytosol renders most of the digestive enzymes inoperative, so even if a lysosome is ruptured, the cell as a whole may remain uninjured. The acidity of the lysosome is maintained with the help of hydrogen ion pumps, and the organelle avoids self-digestion by glucosylation of inner membrane proteins to prevent their degradation (Fig. 4.58).

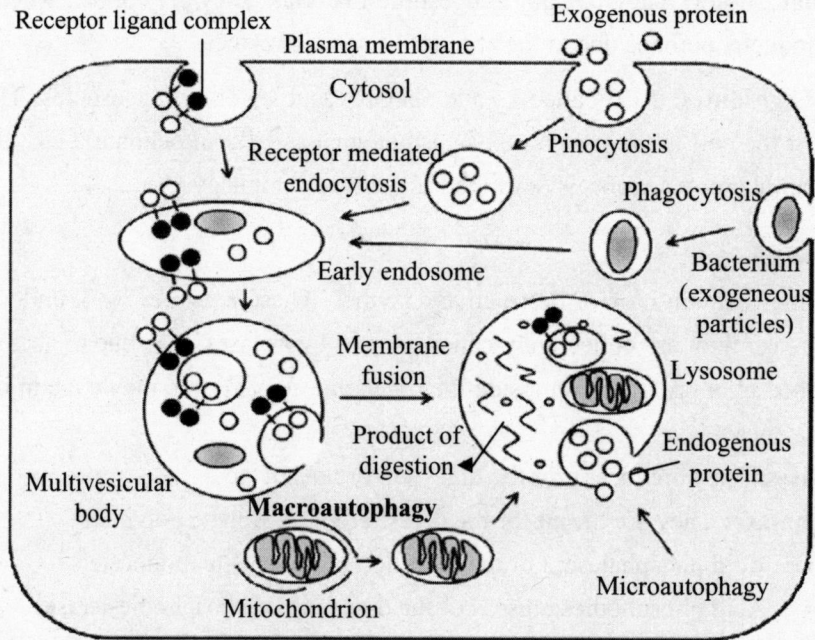

Figure 4.58: The digestive processes that are mediated by the lysosome: specific receptor-mediated endocytosis; pinocytosis (the nonspecific engulfment of extracellular fluid); phagocytosis (the engulfment of extracellular particles); and autophagy (the engulfment of intracellular proteins (microautophagy) and organelles (macroautophagy)).

4.9.3. Function

The main functions of lysosomes are;

- **Digestion of Ingested Materials:** Cells ingest materials by various endo-cytotic means including the classic phagocytosis ("cell eating") and pinocytosis ("cell drinking"). Inside the cell, the material that is taken up is enclosed in an endosome (phagosome or pinosome, respectively). The endosome then fuses with a primary lysosome to form a digestive vacuole. In the digestive vacuole the hydrolases of the lysosome will act on the ingested material to break down. After digestion is completed, the vacuole is called a residual vacuole because it is full of residual, indigestible components. The contents of the residual vacuole are released outside the cell by exocytosis.

- **Cell Death:** Lysosomes mediate events in the controlled or programmed death of cells called apoptosis. They also come into play during necrosis, the pathologic death of cells and tissues.

- **Autophagy:** The survival of cells requires that cellular constituents are constantly turning over. New molecules and structures are made while old unnecessary components are removed. During starvation, cells use auto-phagy to break down cellular components to provide energy for their survival. In the case of organelles, the mitochondrion, for example, is separated from other cellular constituents by an isolation membrane to become an auto-phagosome. The auto-phagosome fuses with primary lysosomes to form an auto-phagic vacuole within which the mitochondrion is digested. The resulting residual vacuole is exo-cytosed.

- **Receptor-Mediated Endocytosis:** Lysosomes play an important role in the uptake and modification of critical molecules such as cholesterol. They also mediate events of receptor recycling and the shutting down of events of cell communication. This sequence of events involves a receptor binding to its ligand followed by their uptake into coated vesicles.

Some human diseases are caused by lysosome enzyme disorders. Tay-Sachs disease, for example, is caused by a genetic defect that prevents the formation of an essential enzyme and breaks down ganglioside lipids. An accumulation of undigested ganglioside damages the nervous system, causing mental retardation and death in early childhood.

4.10. Peroxisomes

Peroxisomes are small membrane-bound, self-replicating organelle found in nearly all eukaryotic cells. They contain oxidative enzymes, such as D-amino acid oxidase, ureate oxidase, and catalase. They are a major site of oxygen utilization and prevent the body from toxic substances like hydrogen peroxide, or other metabolites. They resemble lysosome; however, they are not formed in the Golgi complex. Peroxisomes are distinguished by a crystalline structure inside a sac which also contains amorphous gray material. They enlarge and bud to produce new per-oxisomes.

Peroxisomes were first described by Mollenhauer, Moore and Kelly in 1966. Peroxisomes were first observed as small, single-membrane bound organelles (micro-bodies) in kidney cells of the mouse. After centrifugation of cell homogenate peroxisomes were found in the crude organellar pellet, together with mitochondria and lysosomes. But, they could be separated out from other organelles by subsequent equilibrium density centrifugation, due to their remarkable high density. Characterization of this fraction showed the presence of H_2O_2 producing oxidases (among which enzymes to degrade fatty acids) and catalase to decompose H_2O_2 (hence the name peroxisomes). Since they are rich in enzymes like per-oxidase, oxidizer and catalases, they are called as peroxisomes. Those peroxisomes contain the enzymes of glyoxylate cycle (i.e., glycolate metabolism), are called as glyoxysomes. They have been isolated from algae, yeasts, leaves and seeds of higher plants, protozoans, amphibians, birds and mammals.

4.10.1. Origin

In all probability the peroxisomes arise from the E.R. The E.R. membrane dialates and finally the peroxisomes are pinched off. The peroxisomal enzymes are synthesized on ribosomes on rough E.R. membrane.

4.10.2. Morphology

They are oblate or spheroidal in shape measuring 0.2–1.2 µm in diameter. The average diameter of peroxisome occurring in rat liver cells ranges between 0.6–0.7µm. They are bound by a single lipoproteinaceous unit membrane of about 60Å thickness. They contain granular contents condensing in the centre. Their membrane is permeable to amino acids, uric acids, hydroxyl acids etc., but shows controlled permeability to pyridine nucleotides.

4.10.3. Structure

Peroxisomes have a single limiting unit membrane of lipid and protein molecules, which encloses their granular matrix. In some cases the matrix contains numerous threads or fibrils, while in others they are observed to contain either an amorphous nucleoid or a dence inner core which in many species shows a regular crystalloid structure. Peroxisomes are similar in appearance to lysosomes, but the two have very different origins. Lysosomes are generally formed in the Golgi complex, whereas peroxisomes self-replicate. Unlike self-replicating mitochondria, however, peroxisomes do not have their own internal DNA molecules. Consequently, the organelles must import the proteins they need to make copies of themselves from the surrounding cytosol.

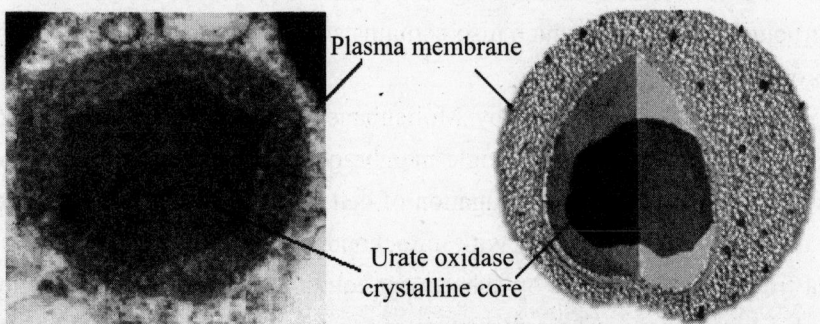

Figure 4.59: Transmission electron micrograph of a peroxisome

The enzymes and other proteins destined for peroxisomes are synthesized in the cytosol. Each contains a peroxisomal targeting signal (PTS) that binds to a receptor molecule that takes the protein into the peroxisome. Two peroxisomal targeting signals have been identified: a 9-amino acid sequence at the N-terminal of the protein and a tri-peptide at the C-terminal (Fig. 4.59).

4.10.4. Functions

Peroxisomes contain a variety of enzymes, which primarily function together to remove toxic substances, and in particular, hydrogen peroxide (a common by-product of cellular metabolism) from the cell. These organelles contain enzymes that convert the hydrogen peroxide to water, rendering the potentially toxic substance safe for release back into the cell. Some types of peroxisomes, such as those in liver cells, detoxify alcohol and other harmful compounds by transferring hydrogen from the poisons to molecules of oxygen (a process termed oxidation). They are also known to be essential in many vital pathways, including: metabolism of free oxygen radicals, synthesis of cholesterol and ether lipids, bile acid formation, catabolism of long chain fatty acids, catabolism of purines, prostaglandins, leucotriens, and alcohol detoxification in liver and metabolism of estradiol. Peroxisomes are also present in plant cells where they participate in symbiotic nitrogen fixation and photorespiration The glyoxysomes show glyoxylate cycle. The phenomenon of photorespiration can be seen in C3 - plants. It is the chief site of photo respiration. Three organelles are found associated with the phenomenon of photorespiration, namely peroxisomes, chloroplasts and mitochondria. The peroxisomes also participate in β- oxidation.

4.10.5. Peroxisomal Disorders

Two major categories of metabolic disorders have been discovered to be caused by molecular defects in peroxisomes. The first category consists of disorders of per-oxisome biogenesis in which the organelle fails to develop normally, causing defects in numerous peroxisomal proteins. The second category involves defects of single per-oxisomal enzymes. The most serious of these disorders is Zellweger syndrome, which is characterized by an absence or reduced number of peroxisomes in the cells. This disorder results from the inheritance of two mutant genes for one of the receptors (PXR1) needed to import proteins into the peroxisome.

4.11. Vacuoles

Vacuoles (means "empty space") are cavities in the cytoplasm (especially in plant cells) surrounded by a cytoplasmic membrane, the tonoplast, and filled with a watery fluid called the cell sap containing water and various substances in solution or suspended state. Plants cells have very large distinct vacuoles while in animals, vacuoles are smaller in size. The Plant vacuoles tend to be so large that they push all other organelles against the cell wall. In plant cells vacuoles may occupy 80% or more of the volume of the cell. A cell may have one or two, small or large vacuoles. The presence of the vacuole is a very conspicuous feature of mature plant cells. They occur in cytoplasmic matrix of the cell starting off as a few small vacuoles in young plant cells. These vacuoles grow and merge as the cell matures (Fig. 4.60).

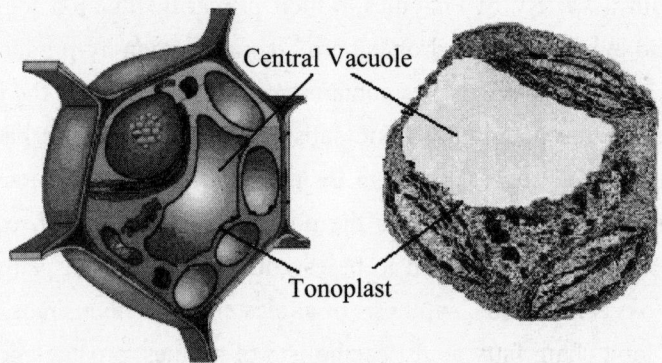

Central Vacuole

Tonoplast

Figure 4.60: Structural representation of vacuoles; electron micrograph (right)

4.11.1. Structure and Function

Vacuole is membrane-bound organelle with little or no internal structure but they serve several functions. Plant cells use their vacuoles for transport and storing nutrients, metabolites, and waste products. The membrane surrounding the plant cell vacuole, tonoplast, is a very active and dynamic membrane. As a membrane, it mainly involved in regulating the movements of ions around the cell, and isolating materials that might be harmful or a threat to the cell. Transport of protons from the cytosol to the vacuole stabilizes cytoplasmic pH, while making the vacuolar interior more acidic creating a proton motive force which the cell can use to transport nutrients into or out of the vacuole. Proteins found in the tonoplast (aquaporins) control the flow of water into and out of the vacuole through active transport, pumping potassium (K^+) ions into and out of the vacuolar interior.

The salts present in vacuoles add to the osmotic activity of the vacuole therefore contributing to the turgor pressure. Turgor pressure exerted by vacuoles is required for cellular elongation: as the cell wall is partially degraded by the action of expansions, the less rigid wall is expanded by the pressure coming from within the vacuole. It is also essential in supporting plants in an upright position. Another function of a central vacuole is that it pushes all contents of the cell's cytoplasm against the cellular membrane and thus keeps the chloroplasts closer to light so that the light absorbing efficiency is improved.

Vacuoles store organic acids, carbohydrates, proteins, and minerals. Some of these compounds are important for human nutrition like simple sugars such as sucrose found in many fruits, the stems of sugarcane, and the roots of sugar beets. In the leaves and stems of forage grasses, vacuoles store complex polysaccharides that are the principal energy source for herbivores. The other compounds found to accumulate in vacuoles include anthocyanin pigments, alkaloids, enzyme inhibitors, and toxins. Waste products and xenobiotics, including herbicides, are often shuttled into vacuoles by specialized membrane transporters. Once in the vacuole, these compounds are digested or detoxified. They also aid in destruction of invading bacteria or of mis-folded proteins.

Vacuoles of certain specialized cells can store products such as rubber and opium. The contractile vacuoles found in animal cells play an important role in the excretion of water and salts. Fresh water protozoans exhibit the presence of one or two contractile vacuoles that take part in osmo-regulation.

4.12. Cytoskeleton

The existence of cytoskeleton in the structure of the protoplasm was proposed by Koltzoff in 1928. They are complex network of protein filaments extend throughout the cytoplasm and mesh of different proteins in cells. As its name implies it helps to maintain cell shape and is important in cell motility. It is a dynamic three-dimensional structure that fills the cytoplasm. This structure acts as both muscle and skeleton, for movement and stability. The internal movement of cell organelles, locomotion and muscle fiber contraction cannot take place without the cytoskeleton. It is believed that cytoskeleton is the characteristic feature of eukaryotic cells but recent research proved that prokaryotic cells have proteins that form a cytoskeleton. In the course of the human genome project more than 800 probably cytoskeleton related genes are found. On the basis of three types of protein filaments, cytoskeletons are of three types such as microtubules, intermediate filaments and microfilaments.

4.12.1. Microfilaments

Microfilaments are fine, thread-like protein fibers, 5–7 nm in diameter, represent the active or motile part of the cytoskeleton (Fig. 4.62). They appear to play a major role in cyclosis and amoeboid motion. They are composed predominantly of a contractile protein called actin, which is the most abundant cellular protein. These filaments are cross-linked into networks or bundles. The semi flexible microfilaments make cells mobile, to divide in mitosis (cytokinesis) and are responsible for muscular contraction. The flexible intermediate filaments strengthen the cell additionally.

In most cases a shell of microfilaments supports the plasma membrane. Microfilaments are a polymer of actin protein subunits plus attached proteins like cross-linkers. Most multi-cellular organisms have several actin iso-forms. Humans have six actin genes; four encode alpha-actin, one beta- and one gamma-actin. Alpha-actin is found in muscle cells where it plays an important role in contracting the cell, whereas beta-actin is localized in the front of moving cells and gamma-actin forms stress fibers. Actin protein as a polymer without attached proteins is called filamentous actin (F-actin), while the globular actin monomers are called G-actin. The actin subunits are structured in two lobes with a cleft in between, where a magnesium ion (Mg+) and an ATP are located. After a G-actin is incorporated into a filament, the ATP is hydrolysed to ADP. There are a lot of proteins that regulate the actin assembly, filament length and stability. Microfilaments' association with the protein myosin is responsible for muscle contraction. Microfilaments can also carry out cellular movements including gliding, contraction, and cytokinesis. Myosin, which consists of an ATPase active head domain and a specific tail region, can move along microfilaments. These motor proteins can transport membrane vesicles or cause contractions not only in muscle cells but also in other cells.

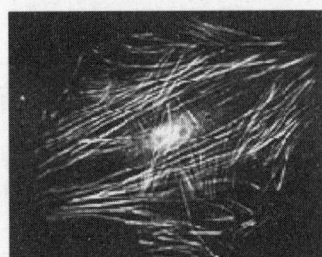

Figure 4.62: Micro filaments with fluorescent label

Actin Filaments

Actin filaments are 8 nm in diameter and consist of two strands of the protein actin that are bound around each other. They are especially prominent in muscle cells, where they provide for the contraction of muscle tissue, monomers of the protein actin polymerize to form long, thin fibers (Fig. 4.63). Some functions of actin filaments form a band just beneath the plasma membrane that provides mechanical strength to the cell, links trans-membrane proteins (e.g., cell surface receptors) to cytoplasmic proteins, anchors the centrosomes at opposite poles of the cell during mitosis and pinches dividing animal cells during cytokinesis. It generate cytoplasmic streaming in some cells, locomotion in cells such as white blood cells and the amoeba and interact with myosin ("thick") filaments in skeletal muscle fibers to provide the force of muscular contraction

Actin monomer has sub domains in which ATP binds, along with Mg^{++}. Actin can hydrolyze its bound ATP to ADP + P_i, releasing P_i. The actin monomer can exchange bound

ADP for ATP. The conformation of actin is different, depending on whether there is ATP or ADP in the nucleotide-binding site. G-actin (globular actin) with bound ATP can polymerize, to form F-actin (filamentous actin). F-actin may hydrolyze its bound ATP to ADP + P_i and release P_i. ADP release from the filament does not occur because the cleft opening is blocked. G-actin can release ADP and bind ATP, which is usually present in the cytosol at higher concentration than ADP.

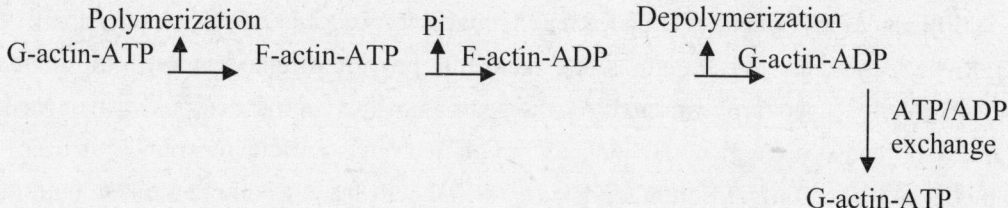

Actin filaments have polarity. The actin monomers all orient with their cleft towards the same end of the filament (designated the minus end). Capping proteins bind at the ends of actin filaments. Different capping proteins may either stabilize an actin filament or promote disassembly. They may have a role in determining the filament length. For example: Tropomodulins cap the minus end, preventing dissociation of actin monomers. Cap Z capping protein binds to the plus end, inhibiting polymerization. If actin monomers continue to dissociate from the minus end, the actin filament will shrink. Cross-linking proteins organize actin filaments into bundles or networks. Actin-binding domains of several of the cross-linking proteins (e.g., filamin, actinin, spectrin, dystrophin and fimbrin) are homologous. Most cross-linking proteins are dimeric or have 2 actin-binding domains.

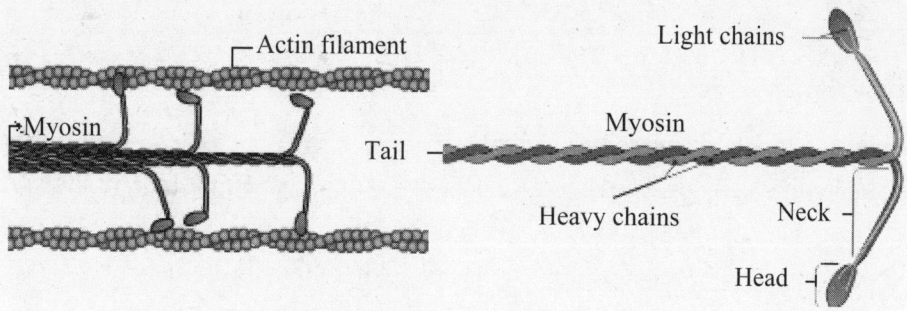

Figure 4.63: Muscle movements

4.12.2. Intermediate Filaments

Intermediate filaments (IFs) are tough and durable protein fibers in the cytoplasm of higher eukaryotic cells. In most animal cells, IFs form a 'basket' around the nucleus and extended out in gentle curving array to the cell periphery. They are constructed like woven ropes, about 10 nm in diameter (thus are "intermediate" in size between actin filaments (8 nm) and microtubules (25 nm) as well as of the thick filaments of skeletal muscle fibers) and provide tensile strength for the cell. Intermediate filaments are found resistant to chlchicine and cytochalasin B and are sensitive to proteolysis. Some intermediate filaments (IF) are homopolymeres of one protein, while some are hetero-polymeres of two or more proteins. All intermediate filament proteins (67 human genes known) have a common basic structure with main differences at both ends. They form a homogenous polar fiber with a diameter of 10-12 nm. Some IF proteins are ubiquitous (e.g. vimentin, provide mechanical strength to muscle and other cells) others are restricted, e.g. to neurons of the central nervous system (neuro-filament proteins, strengthen the long axons of neurons), muscle (desmin, syncoilin) or epithelial cells (keratin). Different kinds of epithelial cells use different keratins to built their intermediate filaments. Up to 85% of the dry weight of squamous epithelial cells can consist of keratins. As well as the expression the organization of the intermediate filaments is cell-type-dependent. In many epithelial cells, filaments are distributed all over the cytoplasm and attach to the nucleus, while in primary fibroblasts vimentin is orientated towards the periphery and spans neither the whole cytoplasm nor is it connected to cell-cell-adhesion sites. The intermediate filaments network is dynamically influenced by a bunch of other proteins. The IFs provide mechanical stability as well as they take part in the assembly of the nuclear envelope.

Intermediate filaments are not well-characterized in plants to date. In animals, these filaments are formed of polymers of keratin, vimentin, or lamin. In plants, filaments of these diameters (10–13 nm) are known, but the monomers that form the polymers are not well known. In one case, where a filament was identified in plants, its monomer turned out to be a glycolytic enzyme.

4.12.3. Microtubules

Microtubules are highly dynamic protein polymers that form a crucial part of the cytoskeleton in all eukaryotic cells. Robertis and Franchi (1953) observed first time in the axoplasm of the mylineated nerve fibres, which they called them neurotubules. Microtubules were first described in detail by Ledbetter and Porter (1963). Microtubules are conveyer belts inside the cells. Microtubules are cylindrical tubes, 20–25 nm in diameter and composed of protein tubulin subunits. These subunits are termed as alpha and beta. Each micro-tubule is composed of eleven pairs of these tubulin subunits arranged in a ring (Table 4.9). In animal cells, microtubules arise from a region of the cell called the microtubule organizing center (MTOC) located near the nucleus. From this center, microtubules come out across the cell, forming a network of "tracks" over which various organelles move within the cell and act as a scaffold to determine cell shape. Microtubules also form small, paired structures called centrioles within animal cells. In plant cells, microtubules are created at many sites scattered through the cell. In animal cells, the microtubules originate at the centrosome (Fig. 4.65). The relatively stiff microtubules play an important role as highway for transport of vesicles and organelles and in the separation of chromosomes during mitosis (karyo-kinesis).

Some eukaryotic cells move about by means of microtubules attached to the exterior of the plasma membrane. These microtubules are called flagella and cilia. Flagella and cilia both have the same structure: a ring of nine tubulin triplets arranged around two tubulin sub-units. The difference between flagella and cilia lies in their movement and numbers. Flagella are attached to the cell by a "crank"-like apparatus that allows the flagella to rotate. Cilia, on the other hand, are not attached with a "crank," and beat back and forth to provide move-ment. Ciliated cells usually have hundreds of these projections that cover their surfaces. For example, the protist **P**aramecium moves by means of a single flagellum, while the protist **D**idinium is covered with numerous cilia.

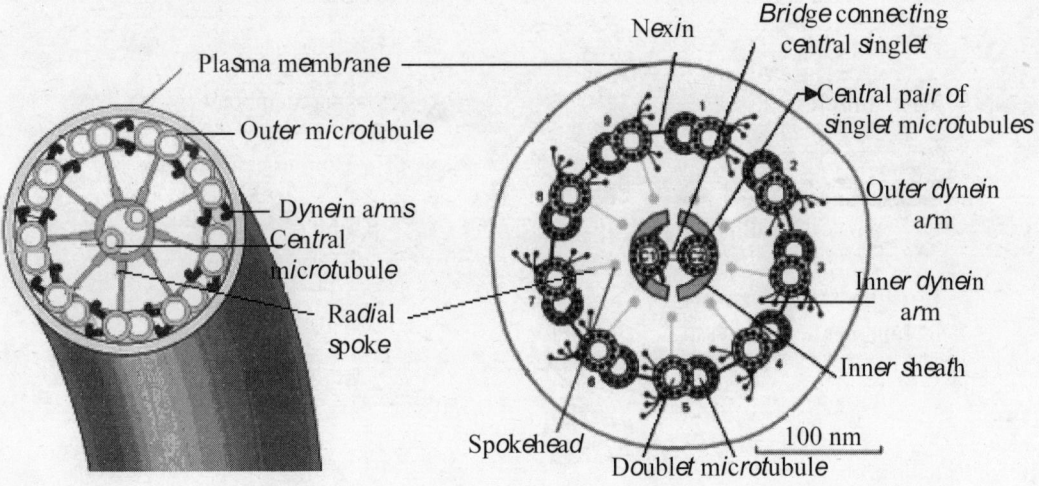

Figure 4.65: Structure of microtubules

In microtubules one alpha- and one beta-tubulin form a hetero-dimer. Long chains of these hetero-dimers composed of proto-filaments, wherein always an alpha-tubulin is fol-lowed by a beta-tubulin. Every microtubule has a (-) and a (+) end. At the (+) or beta-tubulin end new heterodimers are added faster and at lower tubulin concentrations than at the (-) or alpha-tubulin end. The alpha-tubulin as well as the beta-tubulin subunit binds a small guanosine tri-phosphate (GTP). The GTP bound to the alpha-tubulin faces the beta-tubulin subunit of the heterodimer, while the GTP of the beta-tubulin subunit directs away from the heterodimer. When a new dimer is incorporated into a microtubule the beta-tubulin bound GTP is hydrolysed to guanosine di-phosphate (GDP). If the polymerisation is faster than the hyrdolysation, a GTP-cap occupies the (+) end and causes the microtubule to de-polymerise faster than polymerise (Fig. 4.66).

In a cell the dynamics of microtubules are regulated by microtubule-associated proteins (MAPs). Some MAPs stabilize microtubules, while others destabilize microtubules. Stabilizing MAPs have a microtubule-binding domain and an acidic projection domain, which can bind to intermediate filaments or membranes and is suspected to determine the distance in between bundled microtubules. An important role of microtubules is providing a pathway for intracellular movements of organelles and proteins. This is done by motor proteins (kinesins and dyneins) under consumption of ATP. Most kinesins carry their cargo along microtubules in (+) direction, while dyneins do so in (-) direction. These proteins have two head-domains, and the tail domain of the kinesin appoints the kind of cargo that can be bound and transported. Dynein can bind its cargo not directly to its tail domain but needs the protein dynactin for mediation.

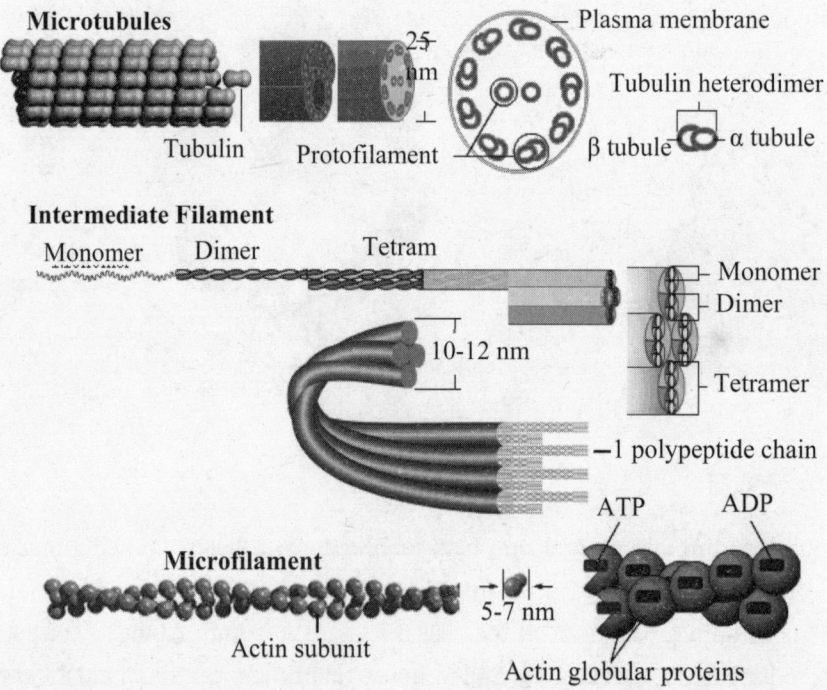

Figure 4.66: Structure of microtubules, intermediate filaments and microfilaments

Table 4.9: Difference between Microtubules, Intermediate filaments and Microfilaments

Property	Microtubules	Intermediate filaments	Microfilaments
Structure	Hollow with walls made up of 13 protofilaments	Hollow with walls made up of 4-5 protofilaments	Solid made up of polymerized actin (F-actin)
Diameter (nm)	24-25	10	7-9
Monomer units	α-and β- tubulin	Five types of protein defining five major classes	G-actin
ATPase activity	Present in dynein arms	None	None
Function	1. Motility of eukaryotes 2. Chromosome movement 3. Movements of intracellular materials 4. Contribute toward maintaining cell shape	1. Integrate contractile units in muscle 2. Cytoskeletal structural function in cytoplasm	1. Muscle contraction 2. Cell shape changes 3. Protoplasmic streaming 4. Cytokinesis.

4.12.4 Cellular Movement

Cellular movement is accomplished by cilia and flagella. Cilia are hair-like structures that can beat in synchrony causing the movement of unicellular *Paramecium*. Both cilia and flagella are constructed from microtubules, and both provide either locomotion for the cells (e.g., sperm) or move fluid (e.g., ciliated epithelial cells that line our air passages and move a film of mucus towards the throat). Each cilium or flagellum is made of a cylindrical array of 9 evenly-spaced microtubules, each with a partial microtubule attached to it. 2 single microtubules run up through the centre of the bundle, completing the so-called "9+2" pattern. The entire assembly is sheathed in a membrane that is simply an extension of the plasma membrane. Dynein "arms" attached to the microtubules serve as the molecular motors. Defective dynein arms cause male infertility and also lead to respiratory tract and sinus problems.

The bacterial flagellum is made up of the protein flagellin. It is a 20 nm thick hollow tube. It is helical and has a sharp bend just outside the outer membrane. A shaft runs between the hook and the basal body, passing through protein rings in the cell's membrane that act as bearings. Gram-positive organisms have 2 of these basal body rings, one in the peptidoglycan layer and other one in the plasma membrane. Gram-negative organisms have 4 such rings: the L ring associates with the lipo-polysaccharides, the P ring associates with peptidoglycan layer, the M ring is embedded in the plasma membrane, and the S ring is directly attached to the plasma membrane. The filament ends with a capping protein (Fig. 4.67).

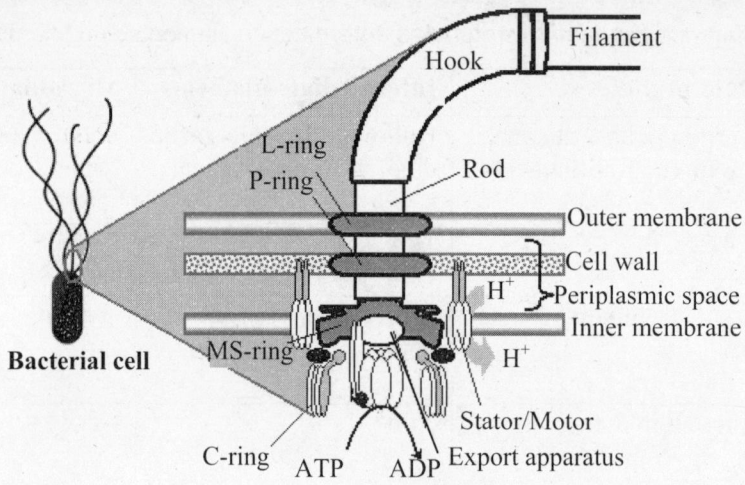

Figure 4.67: Structure of bacterial flagellum

*Each cilium or flagellum grows out from and remains attached to a basal body embed-ded in the cytoplasm. Motion of cilia and flagella is created by the microtubules sliding past one another. This requires motor molecules of dynein, which link adjacent microtubules to-gether, and the energy of ATP. At the flagellum's anchor point on the inner cell membrane there is a rotary engine made up of protein (Mot complex), which helps the flagellum in movements . The engine is powered by proton motive force, i.e., by the flow of protons (hydrogen ions) across the bacterial cell membrane due to a concentration gradient set up by the cell's metabolism. Flagella do not rotate at a constant speed but instead can increase or decrease their rotational speed in relation to the strength of the proton motive force. Flagellar rotation can move bacteria through liquid media at speeds of up to 60 cell lengths/second.

4.12.5. Cellular Motors

Cells have protein motors that bind two molecules, and using ATP as energy, cause one molecule to shift in relationship to the other. Two types of these protein motors are myosin and actin, and dynein or kinesin and microtubules. These families of proteins all have a mo-tor end, but may have several kinds of different molecular structures on the binding end. When these proteins bind the molecules they are moved to different organelles. When linked to other microtubules, protein motors can cause motion if the ends are fixed or extend the lengths of the fiber bundles if the ends are free.

4.12.6. Centrosome

The centrosome is located in the cytoplasm attached to the outside of the nucleus. It is dupli-cated during S phase of the cell cycle. Just before mitosis, the two centrosomes move apart until they are on opposite sides of the nucleus. As mitosis proceeds, microtubules grow out from each centrosome with their plus ends growing toward the metaphase plate. These clusters of microtubules are called spindle fibers.

4.12.7. Centrioles

Each centrosome contains a pair of centrioles. Centrioles are built from a cylindrical array of 9 microtubules, each of which has attached to it 2 partial microtubules. When a cell enters the cell cycle and passes through S phase, each centriole is duplicated. A "daughter" centriole grows out of the side of each parent centriole. Centrioles appear to be needed to organize the centrosome in which they are embedded. Sperm cells contain a pair of centrioles; eggs have none. The sperm's centrioles are absolutely essential for forming a centrosome which will form a spindle enabling the first division of the zygote to take place. Centrioles are also needed to make cilia and flagella.

Suggested Reading

- Molecular Cell Biology, J. Darnell. H. Lodish and D. Baltimore, Scientific American Book INC, USA.
- Molecular Biology of the Cell, B. Alberts, D. Bray, J. Lewis, M. Raff, K. Roberts and J.D. Watson Garland Publishing INC, New York.
- Bainton, D. 1981. The discovery of lysosomes. J. Cell Biol. 91:66s–76s. Cross, P. A and K L Mercer. 1993. Cell and Tissue Ultrastructure: A Functional Perspective. W. H. Freeman and Company.
- Bray D. 2001. Cell Movements: From Molecules to Motility. Garland. Excellent overview of the cytoskeleton and motility.
- Fawcett, D. W. 1993. Bloom and Fawcett: A Textbook of Histology, 12th ed. Chapman & Hall.
- Lamond and W. Earnshaw. 1998. Structure and function in the nucleus. Science 280:547–553.

CHAPTER 5

Cell Receptors and Cell Signaling

- Principle of Cell Signaling
- Communication through electrical signals
- Communication through chemical signals
- Signaling mechanisms
- Signaling via Hydrophobic Molecules
- Signaling via Ion Channels
- Signaling via G-protein-Coupled Receptors
- Intracellular Signaling
- Cell Surface Receptors
- Steroid Receptors
- Nitric Oxide (NO) Receptors
- G-Protein-coupled receptors (GPCRs)
- Frizzled Receptors and Wnt Signaling
- The Notch Signaling Pathway
- Cytokine Receptors
- Receptor Tyrosine Kinases (RTKs)
- JAK-STAT Pathways
- TGF-β Receptors
- TNF-αReceptors and the NF-κB Pathway
- The T-Cell Receptor for Antigen (TCR)
- Ras protein and MAPK pathway
- Apoptosis

Cells in organisms constantly communicate with each other. This cellular discourse occurs through both electrical and chemical signals. Communication through electrical signals is very fast and depends upon the presence of gap junctions, which allows information to pass directly from one cell to its neighbor. In case of chemical signals one cell releases a chemical stimulus (e.g. a neurotransmitter, hormone or growth factor), which then alters the activity of the target cells. Here the receptors are capable of detecting the incoming signal and transferring the information to the appropriate internal cell signaling pathway to bring about a change in cellular activity (Fig. 5.1). Different signals have different responses, e.g. the yeast Saccharomyces cerevisiae sends a peptide signal, the mating factor, into their environment, which may bind to a cell surface receptor expressed on other yeast cells and induce them to prepare for mating. Similarly, pheromones are the chemical signals released by the insect to contact with each other.

The nervous system and the endocrine system serve as the mode of intercellular, communication and there is a remarkable convergence of these regulatory systems. For example, neural regulation of the endocrine system is important in the production and secretion of some hormones; many neurotransmitters resemble hormones in their synthesis, transport, and mechanism of action; and many hormones are synthesized in the nervous system.

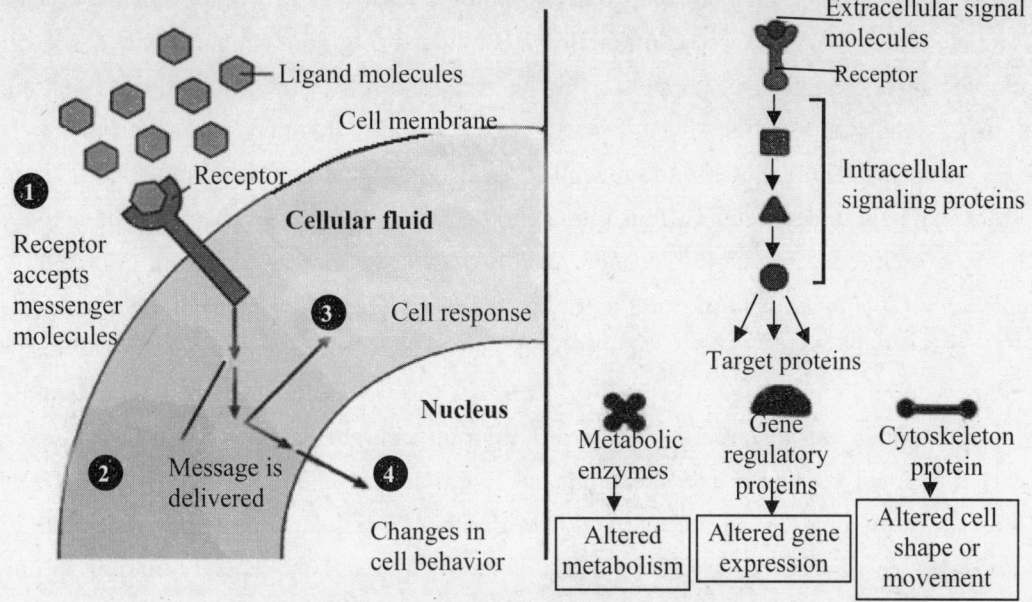

Figure 5.1: Cell signaling pathways

The word "hormone" is derived from a Greek term that means to arouse to activity. As classically defined, a hormone is a substance that is synthesized in one organ and transported by the circulatory system to act on another tissue. There are about 200 types of differentiated cells in humans. Only a few produce hormones, but virtually all of the 75 trillion cells in a human are targets of one or more of the over 50 known hormones. The concept of the target cell is a useful way of looking at hormone action. It was thought that hormones affected a single cell type or only a few kinds of cells and that a hormone elicited a unique biochemical or physiologic action. Cells must be ready to respond to essential signals in their environment. These are often chemicals in the extra cellular fluid (ECF) from distant locations in a multicellular organism - endocrine signaling by hormones or nearby cells - paracrine stimulation by cytokines; or even secretions by themselves - autocrine stimulation. They may also respond to molecules on the surface of adjacent cells (e.g. producing contact inhibition). Signaling molecules may trigger an immediate change in the metabolism of the cell (e.g., increased glycogenolysis when a liver cell detects adrenaline); an immediate change in the electrical charge across the plasma membrane (e.g., the source of action potentials) and a change in the gene expression or transcription within the nucleus (Fig. 5.2).

A target cell is defined by its ability to selectively bind a given hormone to its cognate receptor. Several biochemical features of this interaction are important for hormone-receptor interactions to be physiologically relevant: (1) binding should be specific, i.e., displaceable by agonist or antagonist; (2) binding should be saturable; and (3) binding should occur within the concentration range of the expected biologic response. All receptors have at least two functional domains. A recognition domain binds the hormone ligand and a second region generates a signal that couples hormone recognition to some intracellular function. Coupling (signal transduction) occurs in two general ways. Polypeptide and protein hormones and the catecholamine bind to receptors located in the plasma membrane and thereby generate a signal that regulates various intracellular functions, often by changing the activity of an enzyme. In contrast, steroid, retinoid, and thyroid hormones interact with intracellular receptors, and it is this ligand-receptor complex that directly provides the signal, generally to specific genes whose rate of transcription is thereby affected. The domains responsible for hormone recognition and signal generation have been identified in the protein polypeptide and catecholamine hormone receptors. Steroid, thyroid, and retinoid hormone receptors have several functional domains: one site binds the hormone; another binds to specific DNA regions; a third is involved in the interaction with other co-regulator proteins that results in the activation (or repression) of gene transcription; and a fourth may specify binding to one or more other proteins that influence the intracellular trafficking of the receptor.

5.1. Principle of Cell Signaling

Stimuli (e.g. hormones, neurotransmitters or growth factors) acting on cell-surface receptors relay information through intracellular signaling pathways that can have a number of components. They usually begin with the activation of transducers that use amplifiers to generate internal messengers that either act locally or can diffuse throughout the cell. These messengers then engage sensors that are coupled to the effectors that are responsible for activating cellular responses. The cell signaling is a dynamic process consisting of ON mechanisms during which information flows down the pathway, opposed by the OFF mechanisms that switch off the different steps of the signaling pathway (Fig. 5.2).

5.1.1. Communication through electrical signals

Communication through electrical signals is found mainly in excitable systems, particularly in the heart and brain. It is usually fast and requires the cells to be coupled together through low-resistance pathways such as the gap junctions. In addition to passing electrical charge, the pores in these gap junctions are large enough for low-molecular-mass molecules such as metabolites and second messengers to diffuse from one cell to another. Cells that are connected through the low-resistance gap junctions can communicate rapidly with each other by passing electrical current or through the diffusion of low-molecular-mass second messengers such as cyclic AMP and inositol 1,4,5-trisphosphate (InsP3).

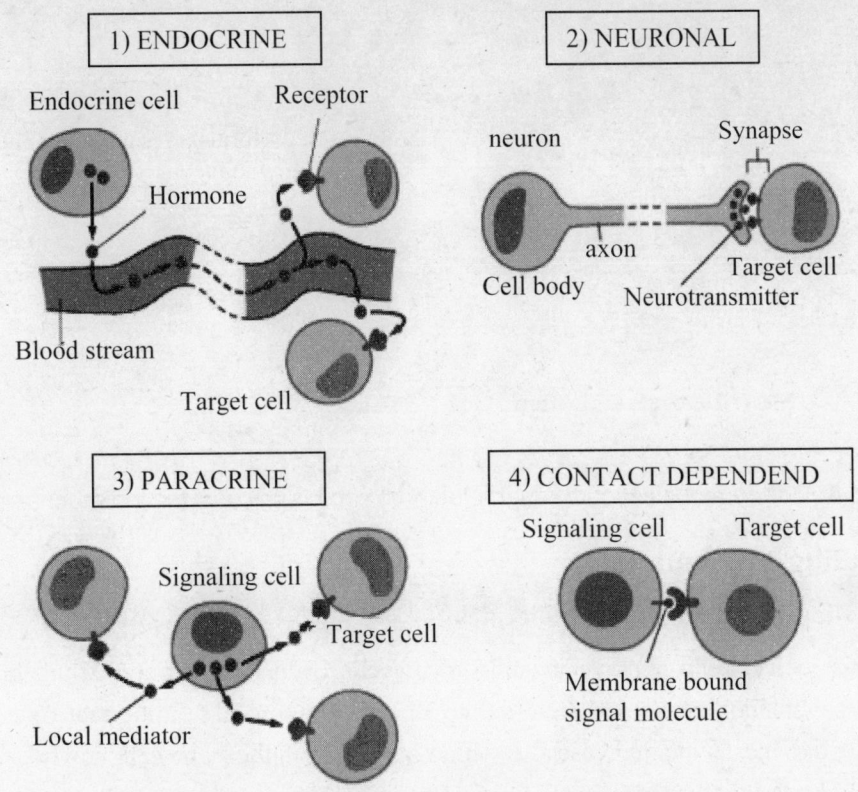

Figure 5.2: Different types of cell signaling

5.1.2. Communication through Chemical Signals

Cells are enclosed within a lipophilic plasma membrane, which represents a formidable barrier that has to be crossed by all incoming signals. Hydrophobic hormones, such as the steroid hormones, can simply diffuse across this cell surface barrier to gain an access to protein receptors located either in the cytoplasm or the nucleus. More elaborate mechanisms are required for the water-soluble stimuli (e.g. hormones, neurotransmitters and growth factors) that cannot cross the plasma membrane. The basic concept of a cell signaling pathway, therefore, concerns the mechanisms responsible for receiving this external information and relaying it through internal cell signaling pathways to activate the sensor and effecter mechanisms that bring about a change in cellular responses. In case of chemical communication one cell releases a stimulus, which diffuses to a target cell that has receptors to detect the stimulus and to relay information along various cell signaling pathways to activate effectors either in the nucleus or cytoplasm (Fig. 5.3).

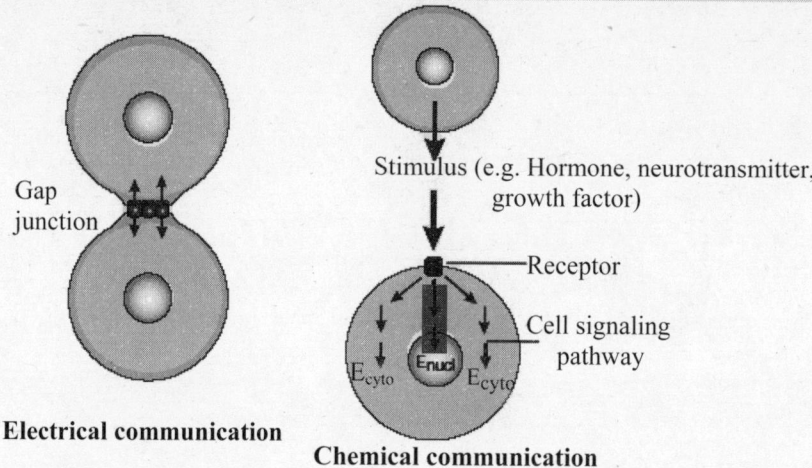

Figure 5.3: Cell communication through electrical and chemical signaling mechanisms.

5.2. Signaling Mechanisms

5.2.1. Signaling via Hydrophobic Molecules

Hydrophobic molecules can move in and out of cells by passing through lipid bilayers. Nitric oxide, arachidonic acid and steroids have been shown to play important roles in cell signaling. Unlike most signaling cascades which occur within the same cell, newly generated NO or arachidonic acid diffuses to act on target molecules in neighboring cells (Fig. 5.4).

Stimulus

Diffuse to
target cell

Exterior

Generate NO or
arachidonic acid

Cytosol

Figure 5.4: Signaling with NO or arachidonic acid

(a) Nitric oxide

Nitric oxide (NO) is produced from the following reaction:

$$L\text{-arginine} \xrightarrow{\text{NO synthase}} L\text{-citrulline} + NO$$

NO generated in a cell, diffuses to act on target molecules in neighboring cells. NO may stimulate soluble guanylyl cyclase to produce cGMP which regulates several enzymes and ion channels. In smooth muscle, an important action of cGMP is to induce muscle relaxation. Normally, cGMP will soon be converted into GMP by phosphodiesterase (Fig. 5.5). The well known drug for impotence, Viagra (sildenafil citrate), inhibits phosphodiesterase.

(b) Arachidonic acid

Arachidonic acid is generated from phospholipid hydrolysis catalyzed by phospholipase. Like NO, its target is usually not located in the cell where it was first generated. After diffusing to target cells, arachidonic acid may activate protein kinase, resulting in phosphorylation of target molecules (Fig. 5.6).

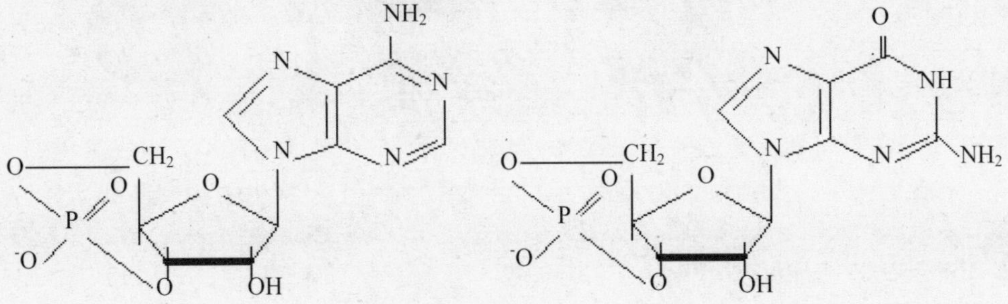

Figure 5.5: Structures of cAMP and cGMP

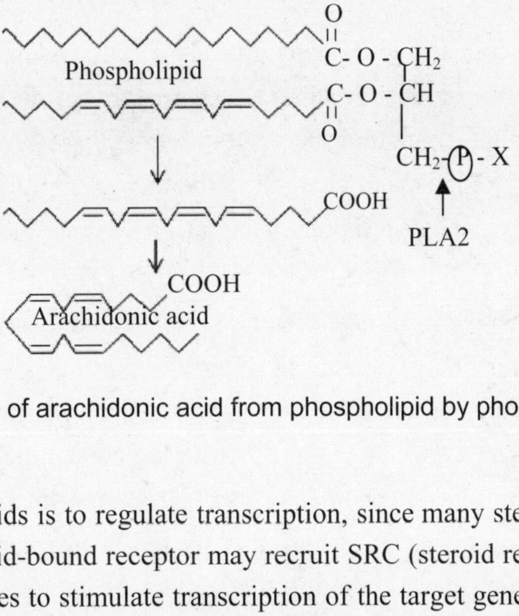

Figure 5.6: Generation of arachidonic acid from phospholipid by phospholipase A_2 (PLA$_2$)

(c) Steroids

The major role of steroids is to regulate transcription, since many steroid receptors are transcription factors. Steroid-bound receptor may recruit SRC (steroid receptor coactivator) and histone acetyltransferases to stimulate transcription of the target gene. In the absence of the steroid, several steroid receptors may recruit corepressors (e.g., SMRT and NCoR) and histone deacetylases to repress transcription (Fig. 5.7).

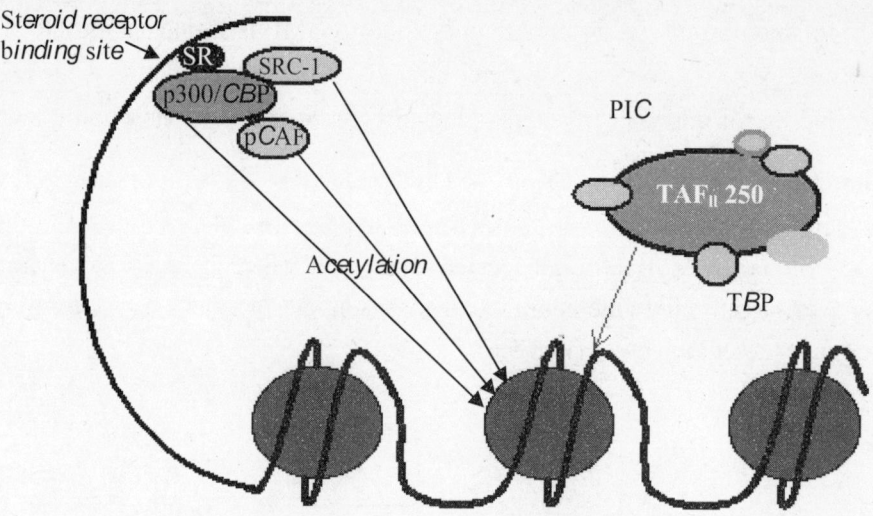

Figure 5.7: A transcriptional activation mechanism by steroid receptor (SR)

5.2.2. Signaling via Ion Channels

Ion channels are membrane proteins that allow ions to pass through. In terms of ion selectivity, they are classified as calcium channels, sodium channels, potassium channels, etc. In terms of gating (how channels are opened), they may be classified as voltage-gated channels, ligand-gated channels, etc.

Ion channels play a crucial role in many aspects of cell signaling such as to function as receptors for a number of external stimuli. These receptors are multifunctional in that they detect the incoming stimulus, they transduce the information into channel opening and, by virtue of conducting large amounts of charge they markedly amplify the signal. Such amplification is the reason for channel receptors being effective transducers of sensory information.

Ion channels are sensitive to a range of stimulus and can thus be considered to be receptors. Unlike other receptors, they combine all of the components of the signaling pathway in a single protein. When they detect the incoming stimulus (receptor function), they undergo a conformational change (transducer function) to gate large quantities of ions (amplification function). With regard to messenger function, those receptors that gate Ca^{2+} contribute to Ca^{2+} signaling pathways. The gating of ions also changes membrane potential (δV) and this can have a messenger function by altering the activity of voltage-operated Ca^{2+} channels (VOCs). Calmodulin is an important molecule that can bind to Ca^{2+} and modulate its activity (Fig. 5.8).

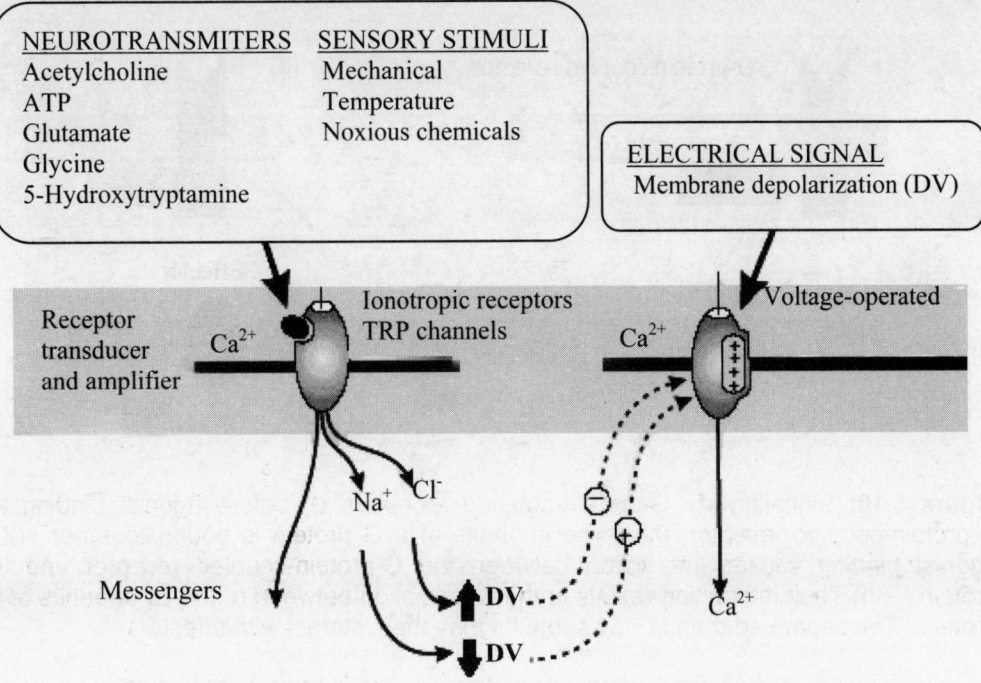

Figure 5.8: Function of ion channels as receptors for cell stimuli

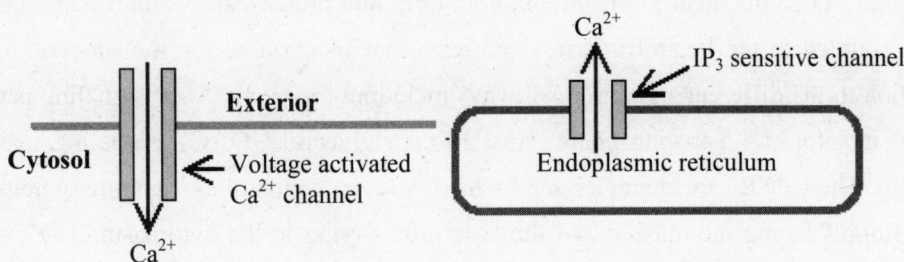

Figure 5.9: Two types of Ca^{2+} channels. (1) The voltage-activated Ca^{2+} channels located on the plasma membrane. (2) The IP_3-sensitive Ca^{2+} channels located on the membrane of endoplasmic reticulum

The major role of sodium and potassium ions is to regulate the membrane potential. However, the calcium ion also plays important roles in other cellular functions, since many enzymes are calcium-dependent. Fig. 5.9 shows the two pathways by which Ca^{2+} enters the cytosol.

5.2.3. Signaling via G-protein-Coupled Receptors

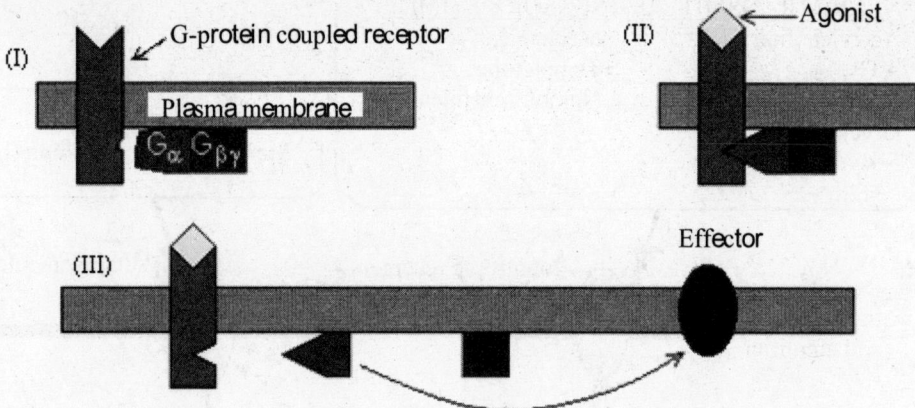

Figure 5.10: Signaling via G-protein-coupled receptors (I) before agonist binding to the G-protein-coupled receptor, the three subunits of a G protein is bound together (II) The agonist binding causes interaction between the G-protein-coupled receptor and the G protein.   (III) Their interaction results in the dissociation between α and βγ subunits of the G protein. The separated α and/or βγ subunits may then interact with effectors

The G protein-coupled receptors (GPCRs) represent a very large super family of receptors that are capable of responding to an enormous number and variety of extra cellular stimuli (light, odorants, neurotransmitters, hormones and proteases). As their name implies, they are coupled to the heterotrimeric G proteins that function as the transducers to relay information to the different signaling pathways including the cyclic AMP signaling pathway and the inositol 1,4,5-trisphosphate (InsP3)/diacylglycerol (DAG) signaling pathway (Fig. 5.10). The GPCRs are characterized by having seven membrane- spanning regions with the N-terminus facing the outside and the C-terminus lying in the cytoplasm. The external ligands, which usually bind to a pocket formed by the external regions of some of the trans-membrane domains, induce a conformational change in the receptor that is then transmitted through the membrane to activate the GTP-binding proteins (G proteins). These G proteins fall into two main groups: the heterotrimeric G proteins and the monomeric G proteins. It is the heterotrimeric G proteins that are the main transducers responsible for transferring information from the GPCRs to a number of signaling pathways. The receptor activates the G proteins by functioning as a guanine nucleotide exchange factor (GEF) to induce the exchange of GDP for GTP. When the G protein is bound to GTP it activates a variety of downstream effectors including adenylyl cyclase and phospholipase C.

(a) Ca^{2+}-sensing receptor (CaR)

The Ca^{2+} sensing receptor (CaR) belongs to the family of G protein-coupled receptors (GPCRs). The primary function of the CaR is to regulate parathyroid hormone (PTH) synthesis and release, but it is also expressed in many other cell types, such as bone cells, neurons, intestine, kidney, skin, pancreas and heart. It is a typical GPCR with the usual seven transmembrane domains, a large extracellular N terminal domain and a C-terminal domain of 216 amino acids, some of which have potential phosphorylation sites for protein kinase C (PKC) and protein kinase A (PKA). The CaR operates as a dimer, with the two subunits linked together by two disulfide bonds. In the parathyroid gland, the CaR dimers are located on caveolae where they appear to be linked to both caveolin and the scaffolding protein filamin. In addition to responding to Ca^{2+}, CaR is also sensitive to a number of other agonists that fall into three main groups. The first group consists of related inorganic ions (Mg^{2+} and Gd^{3+}) or organic polycations (neomycin and spermine) that act in much the same way as Ca^{2+} to directly activate the receptor. The other two groups function indirectly as allosteric regulators that alter the affinity of the receptor, either positively (calcimimetics) or negatively (calcilytics). In the parathyroid gland, CaR functions as a 'calciostat' in that it is very sensitive to small fluctuations in the plasma level of Ca^{2+}. It has the potential of relaying information to the parathyroid cell through different signaling pathways. The main mechanism appears to be through the inositol 1,4,5-trisphosphate (InsP3)/Ca^{2+} signaling cascade. It may also act to inhibit the Ca^{2+} inhibitable isoform of adenylyl cyclase (AC) via a pertussis-insensitive G protein (Gi). When expressed in other cell types, CaR has also been found to activate the mitogen-activated protein kinase (MAPK) signaling pathway and phospholipase A2 (PLA2). Various diseases characterized by an alteration in Ca^{2+} homoeostasis have been linked to inherited mutations in the CaR such as familial hypocalciuretic hypercalcaemia (FHH), neonatal severe hyperparathyroidism (NSHPT), autosomal dominant hypocalcaemia (ADH) and type V Bartter's disease.

5.2.4. Signaling enzymes which are cell-surface receptors

It involves receptor tyrosine kinases and serine/threonine kinases, details of which are discussed in the latter part of this chapter.

5.3. Intracellular Signaling

The role of intracellular messengers is to carry information generated at the cell surface to the internal sensors and effectors. These messengers can take many forms. The concept of an internal messenger first emerged in the cyclic AMP signaling pathway where the external stimulus was considered to be the first messenger, whereas the cyclic AMP formed during information transduction was referred to as the second messenger. Intracellular messengers can take many different forms such as Ca^{2+} is one of the major intracellular messengers that transmit information for the Ca^{2+} signaling pathways.

5.4. Cell Surface Receptors

Cell surface proteins that bind signaling molecules external to the cell with high affinity and convert this extracellular event into one or more intracellular signals that in turn alter the behavior of the target cell. Cell surface receptors, unlike enzymes, do not chemically alter their ligands. They are glycoproteins that are embedded or otherwise attached to the plasma membrane and have a binding site for specific ligands (cytokines, hormones, growth factors, neurotransmitters, adhesion molecules, etc.) exposed to the extracellular environment. Ligand binding to a cell surface receptor generally leads to a biological signal that is propagated from the receptor towards the cell interior, resulting in a cellular response such as prolifereation, differentiation, apoptosis, degranulation, etc. Cell surface receptors transduce ligand signals by a variety of mechanisms such as receptor clustering, activation of a hidden enzymatic activity, opening of ion channels, etc.

Activation of all cell surface receptors leads directly or indirectly to the changes in protein phosphorylation through the activation of protein kinases or protein phosphatases. Animal cells contain two types of protein kinases: those that add phosphate to the hydroxyl group on tyrosine residues and those that add phosphate to the hydroxyl group on serine or threonine (or both) residues. Phosphatases, which remove phosphate groups, can act in concert with kinases to switch the function of various proteins on or off. The human genome encodes about 500 protein kinases and 100 different phosphatases. In some signaling pathways, the receptor itself possesses intrinsic kinase or phosphatase activity; in other pathways, the receptor interacts with cytosolic or membraneassociated kinases.

5.4.1. Steroid Receptors

Steroids are small hydrophobic molecules that can freely diffuse across the plasma membrane, through the cytosol, and into the nucleus. Steroid receptors are dimers of zinc-finger proteins located within the nucleus (except for the glucocorticoid receptor which resides in the cytosol until it binds its ligand). Until their ligand finds them, some steroid receptors within the nucleus associate with histone deacetylases (HDACs), keeping gene expression repressed in those regions of the chromosome. Some steroids that regulate gene expression include glucocorticoids (e.g., cortisol), mineralocorticoids (e.g., aldosterone), sex hormones such as estradiol, progesterone and testosterone. The mechanism of action involves the steroid binds to its receptor and forms the complex, which releases the HDACs and recruits histone acetylases (HATs) relieving chromosome repression and binds to a specific DNA sequence called the Steroid Response Element (SRE) in the promoters of genes.

5.4.2. Nitric Oxide (NO) Receptors

NO diffuses freely across cell membranes and there are so many other molecules, with which it can interact, that it is quickly consumed close to where it is synthesized. Thus NO acts in a paracrine or even autocrine fashion i.e. affecting only cells near its point of synthesis. The signaling functions of NO begin with its binding to protein receptors in the cell. The binding sites can be either a metal ion in the protein or one of its sulfur atoms (e.g., on cysteine). In either case, binding triggers an allosteric change in the protein which, in turn, triggers the formation of a "second messenger" within the cell. The most common protein target for NO seems to be guanylyl cyclase, the enzyme that generates the second messenger i.e., cyclic GMP (cGMP).

5.4.3. G-Protein-coupled receptors (GPCRs)

G-protein-coupled receptors are transmembrane proteins that wind seven times back and forth through the plasma membrane. Their ligand-binding site is exposed outside the surface of the cell and their effector site extends into the cytosol. Some of the many ligands that alter gene expression by binding GPCRs include protein and peptide hormones such as thyroid-stimulating hormone (TSH) and ACTH and serotonin.

The mechanism of action involves the ligand binds to a site on the extracellular portion of the receptor. Binding of the ligand to the receptor activates a G protein associated with the cytoplasmic C-terminal. This initiates the production of a "second messenger". The most common of these are cyclic AMP, (cAMP) which is produced by adenylyl cyclase from ATP, and inositol 1,4,5-trisphosphate (IP_3). The second messenger, in turn, initiates a series of intracellular events such as phosphorylation and activation of enzymes responsible for release of Ca^{2+} into the cytosol from stores within the endoplasmic reticulum. In the case of cAMP, these enzymatic changes activate the transcription factor CREB (cAMP response element binding protein). Here it binds to its response element 5' TGACGTCA 3' in the promoters of genes that are able to respond to the ligand, activated CREB turns on gene transcription and the cell begins to produce the appropriate gene products in response (Fig. 5.11).

A cell must also be able to stop responding to a signal, i.e., to turn off GPCRs. When activated, the Gα subunit of the G protein swaps GDP for GTP. However, the Gα subunit is a GTPase and quickly converts GTP back into GDP restoring the inactive state of the receptor. The receptor itself is phosphorylated by a kinase, which not only reduces the ability of the receptor to respond to its ligand but recruits a protein, β-arrestin, which further desensitizes the receptor, and triggers the breakdown of the second messengers of the GPCRs such as cAMP for some GPCRs.

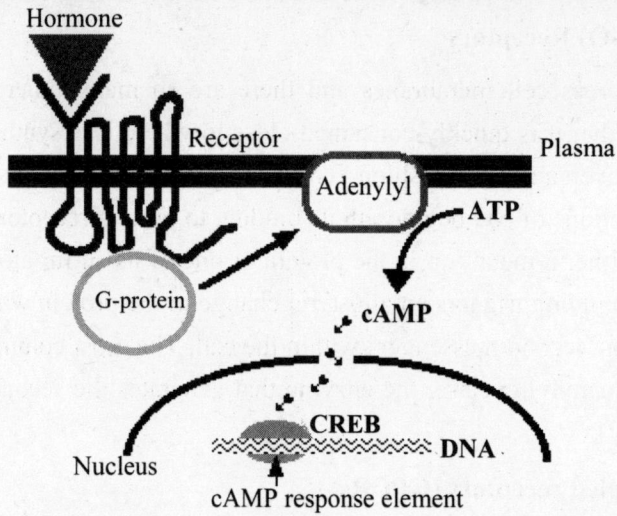

Figure 5.11: Mechanism of action of G-Protein-Coupled Receptors (GPCRs)

5.4.4. Frizzled Receptors and Wnt Signaling

Frizzled receptors, like GPCRs, are transmembrane proteins, their ligand-binding site is exposed outside the surface of the cell and their effector site extends into the cytosol. The ligands of the receptors are Wnt proteins. The name derived from two of the first discovered, proteins encoded by *wingless* (*wg*) in Drosophila and its homolog *Int-1* in mice.

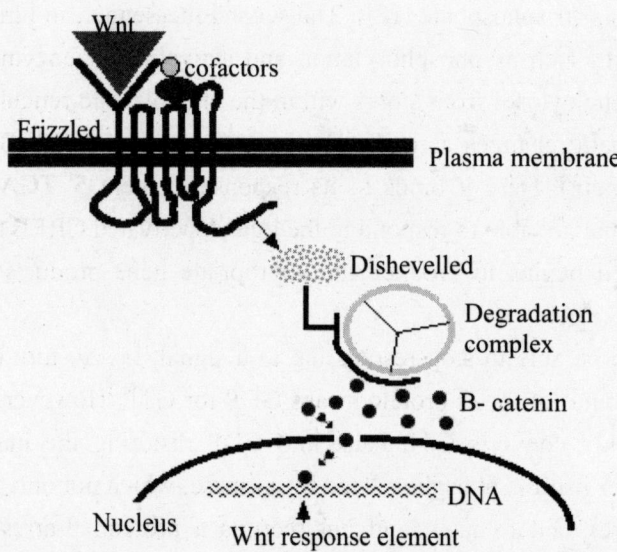

Figure 5.12: Mechanism of cation of Frizzled Receptors and Wnt Signaling

The binding of a Wnt ligand to Frizzled activates Frizzled, which in turn, activates a cytosolic protein called Dishevelled. Activated Dishevelled inhibits the β-catenin degradation complex so β-catenin (β-catenin molecules connect actin filaments to the cadherins that make up adherens junctions that bind cells together) escapes destruction by proteasomes and is free to enter the nucleus where it binds to the promoters and/or enhancers of its target genes (Fig. 5.12).

Wnt-controlled gene expression plays many roles in embryonic development (e.g., a gradient from low at the future head to high at the future tail establishes the anterior-posterior axis through out the metazoa), it guides regeneration as well as regulatory activities in the adult body.

5.4.5. The Notch Signaling Pathway

This pathway differs from many of the other signaling pathways in that the ligands as well as their receptors are transmembrane proteins embedded in the plasma membrane of cells. Thus, signaling in this pathway requires direct cell-to-cell contact. Notch proteins are single -pass transmembrane glycoproteins. They are encoded by four genes in vertebrates. However, the first notch gene was discovered in Drosophila where its mutation produced notches in the wings.

The mechanism of action involves when a cell bearing the ligand comes in contact with a cell displaying the notch receptor, the external portion of notch is cleaved away from the cell surface and engulfed by the ligand-bearing cell by endocytosis. The internal portion of the notch receptor is cut away from the interior of the plasma membrane and travels into the nucleus where it activates transcription factors that turn the appropriate genes on (and off). Proper development of virtually all organs such as brain, pancreas, GI tract, heart, blood vessels, mammary glands etc., depends on notch signaling. Notch signaling appears to be a mechanism by which one cell informs an adjacent cell as to which path of differentiation to take (or not take). Defects in notch signaling have been implicated in some cancers, e.g. melanoma.

5.4.6. Cytokine Receptors

The cytokines form a family of relatively small, secreted proteins (generally containing about 160 amino acids) that control many aspects of growth and differentiation of specific types of cells. During pregnancy prolactin, for example, induces epithelial cells lining the immature ductules of the mammary gland to differentiate into the acinar cells which produce milk proteins and secrete them into the ducts. Another cytokine, interleukin 2 (IL-2), is essential for proliferation and functioning of the T cells of the immune system; its close relative IL-4 is essential for the formation of functional antibody-producing B cells.

Cytokine receptors are important class of cell-surface receptors, whose cytosolic domains are closely associated with a member of a family of cytosolic protein tyrosine kinases, the JAK kinases. The mechanisms by which cytokine receptors and receptor tyrosine kinases become activated by ligands are very similar, and there is considerable overlap in the intracellular signal-transduction pathways triggered by activation of receptors in both classes. Dozens of cytokine receptors have been discovered. Most of these fall into one or the other of two major families: Receptor Tyrosine Kinases (RTKs) and Receptors that trigger a JAK-STAT pathway.

5.4.6.1. Receptor Tyrosine Kinases (RTKs)

The receptors are transmembrane proteins that span the plasma membrane just once. Some ligands that trigger RTKs includes insulin, vascular endothelial growth factor (VEGF), platelet-derived growth factor (PDGF), epidermal growth factor (EGF), fibroblast growth factor (FGF) and macrophage colony-stimulating factor (M-CSF)

The mechanism of action of RTKs involves the binding of the ligand to two adjacent receptors forming an active dimer. This activated dimer is a tyrosine kinase; an enzyme that attaches phosphate groups to certain tyrosine (Tyr) residues — first on itself, then on other proteins converting them into an active state. Many of these (the human genome encode 90 different tyrosine kinases) in this way activate a cascade of expanding phosphorylations within the cytosol. Some of these cytosolic tyrosine kinases act directly on gene transcription by entering the nucleus and transferring their phosphate to transcription factors thus activating them. Others act indirectly through the production of second messengers. In this case the RTKs, stop responding to a signal (off mechanism) by quickly engulfing and destroying the ligand-receptor complex by receptor-mediated endocytosis. For growth factor receptors, failure to do so could lead to uncontrolled mitosis or cancer.

5.4.6.2. JAK-STAT Pathways

The receptor consists of two identical single-pass transmembrane proteins (homodimers) embedded in the plasma membrane. Each of their cytoplasmic ends binds a molecule of a Janus kinase ("JAK"). The ligands which trigger JAK-STAT pathway includes interferons, most of the interleukins (IL-2, IL-3, IL-4, etc.), Growth hormone, Erythropoietin (EPO), Thrombopoietin and Granulocyte-Macrophage Colony-Stimulating Factor (GM-CSF).

The mechanism of action involves the binding of the ligand that activates the JAK molecules which phosphorylate certain tyrosine (Tyr) residues on each other as well as on one or another of several STAT ("Signal Transducer and Activator of Transcription) proteins. These, in turn, form dimers which enter the nucleus and bind to specific DNA sequences in the promoters of genes that begin the transcription. The JAK-STAT pathways are much shorter and simpler than the pathways triggered by RTKs and so the response of cells to these ligands tends to be much more rapid.

5.4.7. Transforming Growth Factor-beta (TGF-β) Receptors

Here the receptor, single-pass transmembrane proteins that, when they bind to their ligand, become kinases that attach phosphate groups to serine and/or threonine residues of their target proteins. Ligands for these receptors include Transforming Growth Factor-beta, activins, Bone Morphogenic Proteins (BMPs) and Myostatin, an inhibitor of skeletal muscle growth.

The mechanism of action involves the binding of the ligand to the extracellular portion of the receptors, results in gaining kinases activity which phosphorylate one or more SMAD proteins in the cytosol. The SMAD proteins move into the nucleus where they form dimers with another SMAD protein designated SMAD4. These dimers bind to a DNA sequence (CAGAC) in the promoters of target genes and with the aid of other transcription factors they enhance, or repress gene the transcription.

5.4.8. Tumor Necrosis Factor-alpha (TNF-α) Receptors and the NF-κB Pathway

TNF-α is synthesized and secreted by macrophages and other cells of the immune system. Receptor consists of trimers of three identical cell-surface transmembrane proteins. The ligands consist of TNF-α and Lymphotoxin.

NF-κB resides in the cytosol bound to an inhibitor called IκB. Binding of ligand to the receptor triggers phosphorylation of IκB, IκB then becomes ubiquinated and destroyed by proteasomes. This liberates NF-κB so that it is now free to move into the nucleus where it acts as a transcription factor binding to the promoters and/or enhancers of more than 60 genes NF-κB got its name from its discovery as a transcription factor bound to the enhancer of the kappa light chain antibody gene. However, it also turns on the genes encoding IL-1 and other cytokines that promote inflammation.

5.4.9. The T-Cell Receptor for Antigen (TCR)

T cells use a trans-membrane dimeric protein as a receptor for a particular combination of antigen fragment nestled in the cleft of a glycoprotein encoded by genes in the major histocompatibility complex.

Activation of the TCR causes a rise in intracellular Ca^{2+} which activates calcineurin, a phosphatase which removes phosphate from NF-AT ("Nuclear Factor of Activated T cells"). Dephosphorylated NF-AT enters the nucleus, and with the help of accessory transcription factors (designated AP-1), binds to the promoters of some 100 genes expressed in activated T cells. The immunosuppressant drugs tacrolimus and cyclosporine inhibit calcineurin thus reducing the threat of transplant rejection by T cells.

5.5. Ras Protein and MAPK Pathway

The gene family *ras* encodes small GTPases that are involved in cellular signal transduction. Ras the super-family of proteins regulates diverse cell behaviors such as cell growth, differentiation and survival. Since Ras communicates signals from outside the cell to the nucleus, mutations in *ras* genes can permanently activate it and cause inappropriate transmission inside the cell even in the absence of extracellular signals. Because these signals result in cell growth and division, disregulated Ras signaling can ultimately lead to oncogenesis and cancer.

Ras proteins function as binary molecular switches that control intracellular signaling networks. Ras-regulated signal pathways control processes such as actin- cytoskeletal integrity, proliferation, differentiation, cell adhesion, apoptosis, and cell migration. Ras and ras-related proteins are often deregulated in cancers, leading to increased invasion and metastasis, and decreased apoptosis. Activated Ras activates the protein kinase activity of RAF kinase. RAF kinase phosphorylates and activates MEK. MEK phosphorylates and activates a mitogen-activated protein kinase (MAPK).

Mitogen-activated protein (MAP) kinases are serine/threonine-specific protein kinases that respond to extracellular stimuli (mitogens, osmotic stress, heat shock and proinflammatory cytokines) and regulate various cellular activities, such as gene expression, mitosis, differentiation, proliferation, and cell survival/apoptosis. MAPK pathways are activated within the protein kinase cascades called "MAPK cascade". Each one consists of three enzymes, MAP kinase, MAP kinase kinase (MKK, MEKK, or MAP2K) and MAP kinase kinase kinase (MKKK or MAP3K) that are activated in series. A MAP3K that is activated by extracellular stimuli, which phosphorylates a MAP2K on its serine and threonine residues and this MAP2K activates a MAP kinase through phosphorylation on its serine and tyrosine residues. The phosphorylation of tyrosine precedes to the phosphorylation of threonine, although phosphorylation of either residue can occur in the absence of the other. Because both tyrosine and threonine phosphorylations are required to activate the MAP kinases, phosphatases that remove phosphate from either sites will inactivate them. This MAP kinase signaling cascade has been evolutionary well-conserved from yeast to mammals. Cascades convey information to effectors, coordinates incoming information from other signaling pathways, amplify signals, and allow for a variety of response patterns.

Down-regulation of MAP kinase pathways may occur through dephosphorylation by serine/threonine phosphatases, tyrosine phosphatases, or dual-specificity phosphatases and through feedback inhibitory mechanisms that involve the phosphorylation of upstream kinases. Drugs that selectively down-regulate MAP kinase cascades could prove to be valuable as therapeutic agents in the control of malignant disease.

5.5. Apoptosis

Apoptosis, the programmed cell death is characterized by chromatin condensation and cell shrinkage in the early stage and then the nucleus and cytoplasm fragment, forming membrane-bound apoptotic bodies which can be engulfed by phagocytes. In contrast, cells undergo another form of cell death, necrosis, swell and rupture. The released intracellular contents can damage surrounding cells and often cause inflammation. Apoptosis is an important process during normal development. It also involved in aging and various diseases such as cancer, AIDS, Alzheimer's disease and Parkinson's disease.

Programmed cell death, or apoptosis, is mediated by proteolytic enzymes called caspases, which are synthesized in the precursor forms as procaspases. When activated by various signals, caspases function to cause cell death in most organisms, ranging from *C. elegans* to human beings. Apoptosis provides a means deciding the shapes of body parts in the course of development and a means of eliminating cells producing anti-self antibodies or infected with pathogens as well as cells containing large amounts of damaged DNA. Cytotoxic T cells initiate apoptosis in cells to which they bind through T-cell receptor–class I MHC-peptide interactions aided by interactions with the coreceptor molecule CD8.

Under some circumstances, such as when DNA damage is extensive, p53 also activates expression of genes that lead to apoptosis, the process of programmed cell death that normally occurs in specific cells during the development of multicellular animals. In vertebrates, the p53 response evolved to induce apoptosis in the face of extensive DNA damage, presumably to prevent the accumulation of multiple mutations that might convert a normal cell into a cancer cell.

During apoptosis, the cell is digested by a class of proteases called caspases. More than 10 caspases have been identified. Some of them (e.g., caspase 8 and 10) are involved in the initiation of apoptosis, others (caspase 3, 6, and 7) execute the death order by destroying essential proteins in the cell (Fig. 5.13). The apoptotic process can be summarized as follows:

- Activation of initiating caspases by specific signals.
- Activation of executing caspases by the initiating caspases which can cleave inactive caspases at specific sites.
- Degradation of essential cellular proteins by the executing caspases with their protease

activ-   ity.

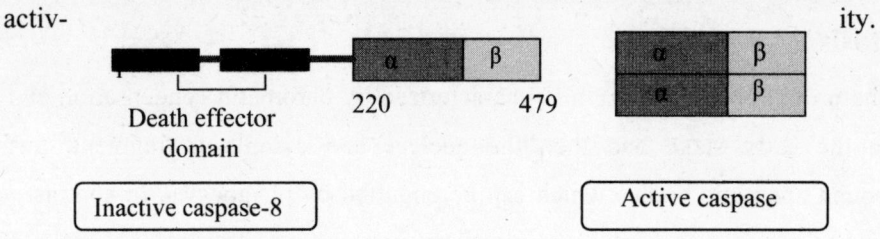

Inactive caspase-8   Active caspase

Figure 5.13: Comparison between active and inactive forms of caspases. Newly produced caspases are inactive. Specifically cleaved caspases will dimerize and become active

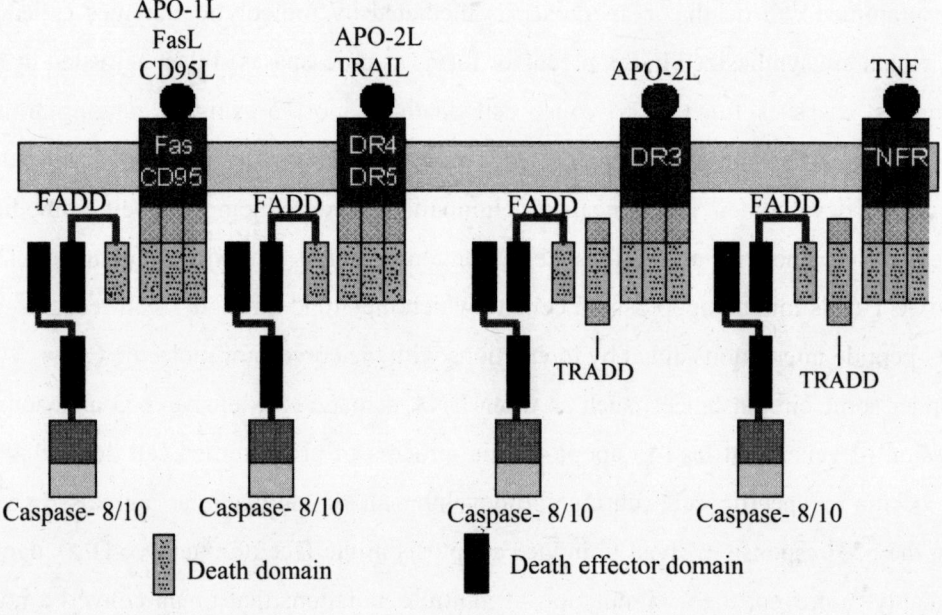

Figure 5.14: Coupling of caspase 8 or 10 to death receptors

- **Death receptors:** Fas/CD95, DR4/DR5, DR3, and TNFR (Tumor Necrosis Factor Receptor).

- **Adaptors:** FADD (Fas-associated death domain protein) and TRADD (TNFR-associated death domain protein).

- **Activation:** Binding of death ligands (FasL/CD95L, TRAIL/APO-2L, APO-3L and TNF) induces trimerization of their receptors, which then recruit adaptors and subsequently activate the caspases (Fig. 5.14).

Suggested Readings

- Molecular Cell Biology, J. Darnell. H. Lodish and D. Baltimore, Scientific American Book INC, USA.
- Molecular Biology of the Cell, B. Alberts, D. Bray, J. Lewis, M. Raff, K. Roberts and J.D. Watson Garland Publishing INC, New York.
- Benedict, C. A., P. S. Norris, and C F Ware. 2002. To kill or be killed: viral evasion of apoptosis. Nature Immunol. 3:1013–1018.
- Calcium, Calcineurin, and the Control of Transcription - J. Biol. Chem., 2001.
- Cellular Signaling through Multifunctional Ca^{2+}/Calmodulin-dependent Protein Kinase II - J. Biol. Chem., 2001.
- G Protein-Coupled Receptor Dimerization: Function and Ligand Pharmacology - Mol. Pharma., 2004.
- Oxygen Reduction by Nitric-oxide Synthases - J. Biol. Chem., 2001.
- Regulation of Nitric Oxide-Sensitive Guanylyl Cyclase - Circulation Research, 2003.

CHAPTER 6

Genetics: Study of Genes

- What are genes?
- Mendelian Genetics
- Mendelian Principles
  - law of dominance
  - Principle of Segregation
  - Principle of Independent Assortment
- The Punnett square
- Test Cross
- Backcrossing
- Chromosomal Disorders

- Limitations of the Mendelian System
- Polygenic or quantitative inheritance
- Multiple Alleles
- Chromosomal theory of inheritance
- Sex-linked Characteristics
- Linkage and Crossing-Over
- Mutations
- Autosomal Mutations
- Recessive Disorders
- Dominant Disorders

"We have found the secret of life……..." Nobel laureate James Watson

6.1. What are genes?

The term 'gene' was coined by Danish botanist Wilhelm Johannsen in 1909. It is the basic physical and functional unit of heredity. Heredity is the transfer of characters from parents to their offspring, that is why children resemble their parents.   A hereditary unit consists of a sequence of DNA (except in some viruses that contain RNA, instead) that occupies a specific location on a chromosome and determines a particular characteristic in an organism. DNA is a vast chemical information database that carries the complete set of instructions for making all the proteins that a cell will ever need. Each gene contains a particular set of instructions, usually coding for a particular protein. Genes achieve their effects by directing protein synthesis. The sequence of nitrogenous bases along a strand of DNA determines the genetic code. When the product of a particular gene is needed, the portion of the DNA molecule that contains that gene splits, and a complementary strand of RNA, called messenger RNA (mRNA), forms and then passes to ribosomes, where proteins are synthesized. A second type of RNA, transfer RNA (tRNA), matches up the mRNA with specific amino acids, which combine in series to form polypeptide chains, the building blocks of proteins. Experiments have shown that many of the genes within a cell are inactive much or even all of the time, but they can be switched on and off.

DNA resides in the core, or nucleus, of each of the body's trillions of cells. Every human cell (with the exception of mature red blood cells, which have no nucleus) contains the same DNA. Each human cell has 46 molecules of double-stranded DNA. Human cells contain two sets of chromosomes, one set inherited from the mother and one from the father. (Mature sperm and egg cells carry a single set of chromosomes). Each set has 23 single chromosomes - 22 autosomes and an X or Y sex chromosome. (Females inherit an X from each parent, while males get an X from the mother and a Y from the father.) In humans, genes vary in size from a few hundred DNA bases to more than 2 million bases.   The Human Genome Project has estimated that humans have between 20,000 and 25,000 genes. Every person has two copies of each gene, one inherited from each parent. Most genes are the same in all people, but a small number of genes (less than 1 percent of the total) are slightly different between people. Alleles are forms of the same gene with small differences in their sequence of DNA bases. These small differences contribute to each person's unique physical features. Genes carry information that determines the traits, the characteristics we inherit from our parents. The branch of biology that deals with heredity, especially the mechanisms of hereditary transmission and the variation of inherited characteristics among similar or related organisms is known as genetics.

6.2. Mendelian Genetics

Sir Gregor Johann Mendel (1822 to 1884) was Austrian monk who used garden pea (*Pisum sativum*) for his experiments and published his results in 1865. His work, however, was rediscovered in 1900, long after Mendel's death, by Tschermak, Correns and DeVries. Mendel was the first to suggest principles underlying inheritance. He is regarded as the founder or father of genetics. He developed the concept of the factors to explain results obtained while cross breeding strains of garden peas. He identified physical characteristics (phenotypes), such as plant height and seed colour, which could be passed on, unchanged, from one generation to another. The hereditary factor that predicted the phenotype was later termed a "gene." The genetic constitution of an organism is known as genotype. Mendel hypothesized that genes were inherited in pairs, one from the male and one from the female parent. Plants that bred true had inherited identical genes (homozygotes) from their parents, whereas plants that did not breed true inherited alternative copies (hybrids, or heterozygotes) of the genes (alleles) from one parent that were similar, but not identical, to those from the other parent. Alleles are the alternative forms of the same gene which determine contrasting characters. One chromosome might contain a version of the eye colour gene that produces blue eyes, and other chromosome might contain a version that produces brown eyes. If an individual has both versions of the gene, the individual is heterozygous for the eye colour trait. If an individual has the same version of the eye colour gene on both chromosomes, the individual is homozygous for the eye colour trait. In case plants the allelic character of height are the tall (T) and dwarf (t).

Alleles are one alternative of a pair or group of genes that could occupy a specific position on a chromosome. Genes are composed of sequences of nucleotides, and a variation in this sequence can affect the protein made from that gene. A change in the manufacture of a protein in an organism often leads to an observable result. There are many different alleles for the gene that manufactures protein to give humans their unique eye colour. There are two alleles for flower colour in the common garden pea.

Some of these alleles had a greater effect on the phenotypes of hybrids than others. For example, if a single copy of a given allele was sufficient to produce the same phenotype seen in homozygous organisms, that gene is termed a "dominant." Conversely, if the allele could only be detected in the minority of the offspring of hybrid parents that were homozygous for that "weaker" allele, the gene is termed a "recessive." Dominant and recessive are relative terms. Consider a plant with a gene for red flower colour and a gene for blue flower colour. This plant bears red flowers, although it has a gene for blue flower colour, too. Red flower colour is the dominant trait, while blue flower colour is the recessive trait. The red colour gene in a sense overpowers the blue colour gene. In order for the plant to have blue flowers, it would need to completely lack the gene for red flower colour. Dominant traits are normally represented by uppercase letters, such as R. The corresponding recessive trait would be represented by a lowercase letter, r. A plant with genotype Rr will have red flowers, as would a plant with genotype RR. But a plant with genotype rr would have blue flowers.

Mendelian genetics, also known as classical genetics, is the study of the transmission of inherited characteristics from parent to offspring. Gregor Mendel actually calculated the ratios of observable characteristics in the common garden pea plant *Pisum sativum*. Mendel studied seven characteristics in peas including seed texture, seed colour, flower colour, flower position; stem length, pod shape and pod colour (Fig. 6.1). Peas were a good model system, because he could easily control their fertilization by transferring pollen with a small paintbrush. This pollen could come from the same flower (self-fertilization), or it could come from another plant's flowers (cross-fertilization). Because the seven pea plant characteristics tracked by Mendel were consistent in generation after generation of self-fertilization. These parental lines of peas could be considered pure-breeders (or, in modern terminology, homozygous for the traits of interest). Mendel and his assistants eventually developed 22 varieties of pea plants with combinations of these consistent characteristics. He applied mathematics and statistics to analyze the results obtained by him.

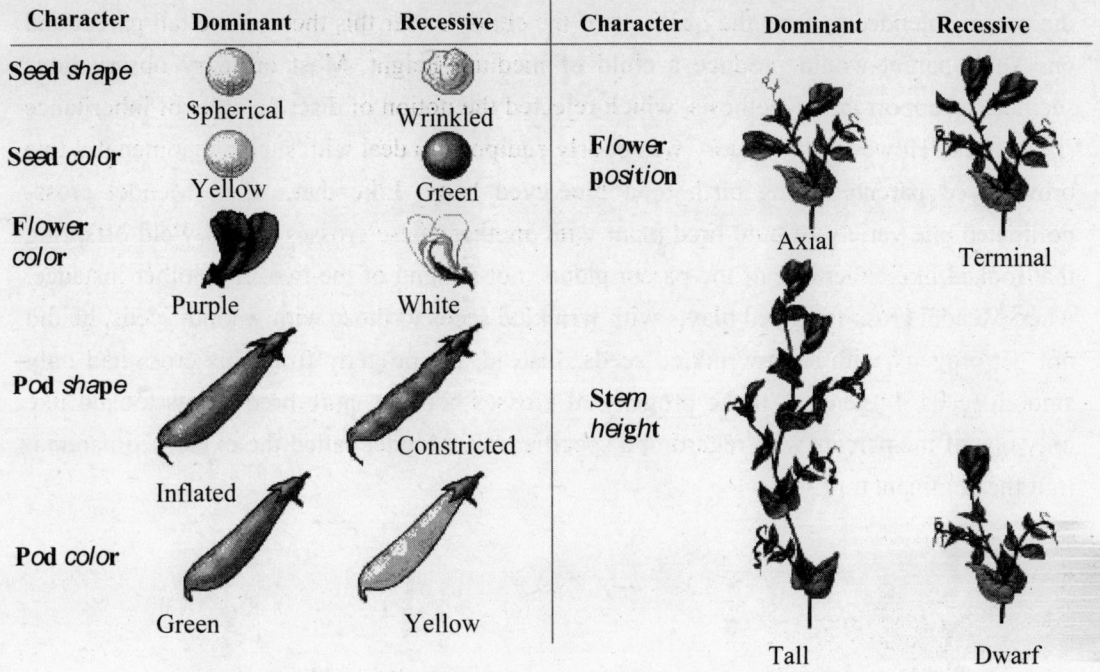

Figure 6.1: The seven pairs characters used by Mendel in his work

Mendel started his pea breeding program by allowing certain pea plants to repeatedly self-fertilize. Peas are able to fertilize their own flowers which are called selfing. If pea selfing continues over many generations the pea plants will be homozygous or have an identical pair of genes for a certain characteristic. These plants will contain either two identical recessive genes (homozygous recessive) for a characteristic or two identical dominant genes (homozygous dominant) for the same characteristic and are considered pure-breeding for those characteristics. For example, purple flower colour in peas is dominant and white flower colour in peas is recessive. When a white flowered (homozygous recessive) pea plant is crossed with a purple flowered (homozygous dominant) pea plant, the resulting offspring all has purple flower colour. The gene composition (genotype) for the flower genes in each of these types of pea plants is represented as shown below.

Genetic organization	Genotype	Phenotype
Homozygous recessive	pp	white flower
Homozygous dominant	PP	purple flower
Heterozygous (one of each gene type)	Pp	purple flower

Before Mendel's work, the most popular theory of inheritance stated that the qualities of the parents blended to form the qualities of the child. Under this theory, one tall parent and one short parent would produce a child of medium height. Most ordinary observations seemed to support this hypothesis, which rejected the notion of discrete units of inheritance (i.e., genes). However, this theory was poorly equipped to deal with such phenomena as two brown-eyed parents giving birth to a blue-eyed baby. Like that, when Mendel cross-pollinated one variety of pure bred plant with another, these crosses would yield offspring that looked like either one of the parent plants, not a blend of the two. In another instance, when Mendel cross-fertilized plants with wrinkled seeds to those with smooth seeds, he did not get progeny with semi-wrinkled seeds. Instead, the progeny from this cross had only smooth seeds. In general, if the progeny of crosses between pure bred plants looked like only one of the parents with regard to a specific trait, Mendel called the expressed parental trait the dominant trait.

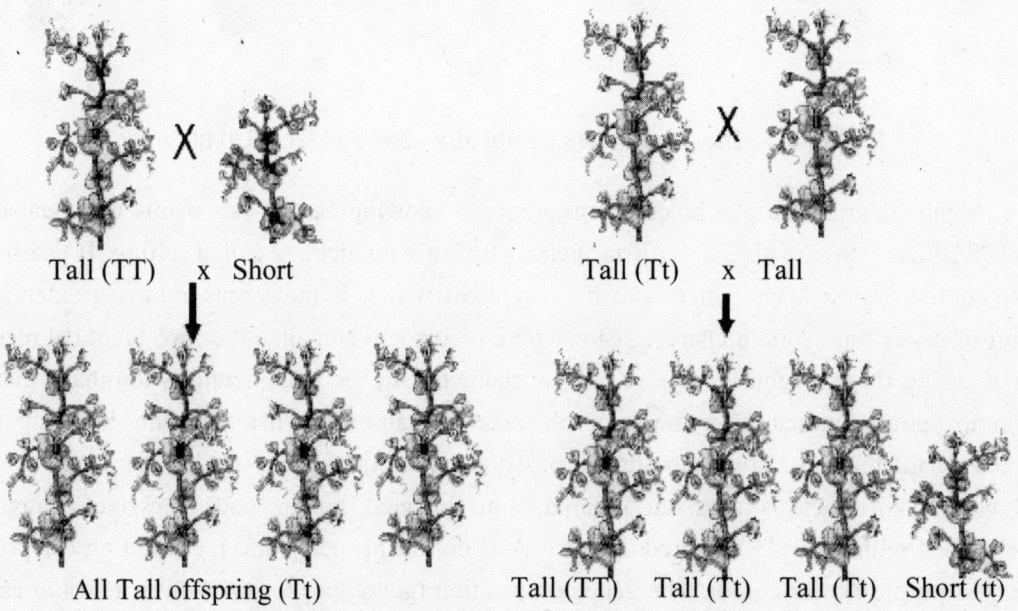

Figure 6.2: Mendel's experiment on pea plant

Mendel used characteristics of pea plants and four o'clock flowers (*Mirabilis jalapa*) to analyze the hereditary patterns of these traits. His historic experiments led him to the conclusion that inherited characteristics were carried in discrete, independent units (later named genes). In Mendel's interpretation, hereditary characteristics occurred in pairs of factors that had specific relationships. Mendel first crossbred one tall, true-breeding plant with one short, true-breeding plant. Contrary to the blending theory, all the offspring were tall. In terms of genotype, the original tall plant was TT (two dominant alleles; homozygous), the short plant was tt (two recessive alleles; homozygous), and the second-generation plants were Tt (one dominant and one recessive allele; heterozygous). When Mendel next allowed these plants to self-fertilize, he found that the short trait reappeared in the third generation. The ratio of short to tall plants was almost exactly 3:1. Their genotypes were as follows - 1 short (tt) : 2 tall (Tt) : 1 tall (TT). Based on these observations (Fig. 6.2), Mendel formulated a series of laws that are the basis of what we now term "Mendelian" inheritance patterns.

6.3. The Punnett Square

Mendel worked by observing characteristics (phenotypes) and calculating the ratios of each type to form his principles of inheritance. However we can predict the ratios of phenotypes by using Mendel's principles. One of the most common methods of determining the possible outcome of a cross between two parents is called a Punnett square. To perform a Punnett square one must first figure out all the possible combinations of the alleles to be studied for each parent. The possible gametes for one parent go on the X axis and the possible gametes for the other parent go on the Y axis (one allele in each cell of the upper row (traditionally the mother) and rightmost column (traditionally the father). The gamete combinations are then paired in the squares below and to the side of each type, i.e. the offspring's genotypes are then calculated by observing the intersection of the mother's and father's individual alleles (much like a multiplication table).

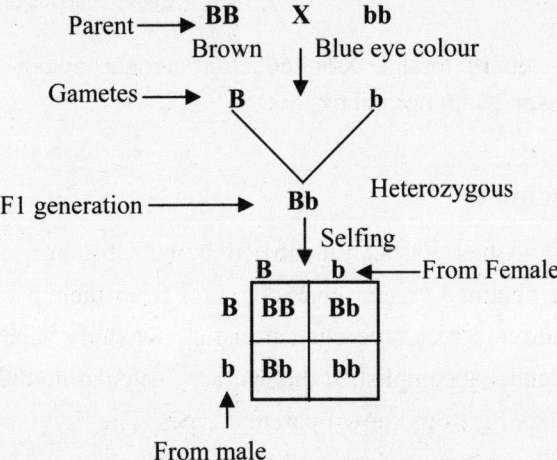

Figure 6.3: A Punnett square for a monohybrid cross between two heterozygous individuals

Example 1: Eye colour in human is much more complex. A mother and father, both having the brown eye phenotype, have a child. We know that both parents carry the gene for blue eye colour and therefore are heterozygous for this trait. These parents can either donate a dominant B to the gamete or a recessive b to the gamete (Fig.6.3).

The outcome of this cross shows that 3 times out of 4 (75%) the child will have brown eyes and 1 out of 4 times the child will have blue eyes (25%). The probability that the child's genotype will be heterozygous, for eye colour alleles, is 50%. The probability is 25% for either the homozygous recessive or dominant genotype.

Example 2: **X**-linked characteristic: colour blindness in human

There are several known X-linked characteristics in humans but few, if any, Y-linked characteristics are usually reported. Females have two X chromosomes with one or the other X chromosome remaining active in a mosaic pattern in a tissue. Males have only one X chromosome so if the X chromosome of a male has a defective allele there is no companion X chromosome to compensate for the deficiency. A female must have the same defective allele on both her X chromosomes to demonstrate any deficiencies (Fig. 6.4).

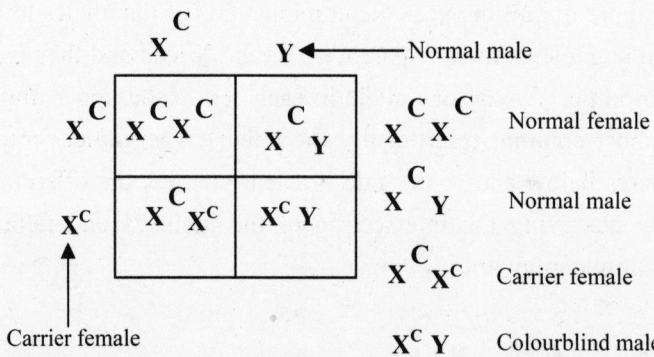

Figure 6.4: A punnett square for the X-linked characteristic colour blindness in human (Female carrier $X^C X^c$ crossed with normal male $X^C Y$)

6.4 Mendelian Principles

During Mendel's time DNA had not been identified as the substance of heredity and it was unknown how offspring obtained certain characteristics from their parents. Since Mendel's work elucidated dominant and recessive characteristics his study supported the particulate theory of inheritance. Mendel accomplished this work by calculating the ratios of observable characteristics of the offspring from known parental types. The first parental types were homozygous recessive and homozygous dominant pure breeding types. The parental generation or P generation, by definition, is always homozygous recessive and homozygous dominant for the traits to be studied. The offspring which results from the mating of parental types (P generation) will always be heterozygous for the characteristic.

6.4.1. Mendel's law of Dominance

The first law of Mendel states that "In a cross of parents that are pure for contrasting traits, only one form of the trait will appear in the progeny, in other words factors retain their identity from generation to generation and do not blend in the hybrid. In other words it says that, if two plants that differ in just one trait are crossed, then the resulting hybrids will be uniform in the chosen trait. Depending on the traits is the uniform features either one of the parents' traits (a dominant-recessive pair of characteristics) or it is intermediate. When two pure breeding organisms of contrasting characters are crossed, only one character of the pair appears in the F1 generation, known as the dominant character (example: tallness) and the other unexpressed or hidden character is known as the recessive character (example: dwarfness). When Mendel crossed a true breeding red flowered plant with a true breeding white flowered one, the progeny was found to be red coloured. The white colour suppressed and the red colour dominated.

Mendel's law of dominance is generally true, but there are many exceptions to the law. For each of the seven pairs of characters examined, it was observed that one allelomorph dominated over the other, so that F1 exhibits one or the other alternative phenotypes represented in the parents. Some inherited traits do not exhibit strict Mendelian dominant/recessive relationships. The simplest example of this phenomenon is called codominance, or incomplete dominance. This pattern is displayed in the colours of four o'clock flowers. When a white and a red flower are cross-fertilized, the second generation is all pink. However, when a pink flower is allowed to self-fertilize, the white and red attributes return. The colour ratios for this third-generation cross are - 1 white: 2 pink: 1 red. This pattern is due to the fact that three alleles, instead of the usual two, determine colour in four o'clock flowers. If red colour is designated R and white colour r, then pink colour (not red or white) is the phenotypic effect of genotype Rr. (This is one type of pattern formerly used in support of the blending theory of inheritance). Thus in certain cases the hybrid offsprings resemble one parent much more closely than the other but does not resemble it exactly, so the dominance is incomplete. This is termed as incomplete dominance (Fig. 6.5).

Another example of codominance is the ABO blood typing system used to determine the type of human blood. It is common knowledge that a blood transfusion can only take place between two people who have compatible types of blood. Human blood is separated into different classifications on the basis of presence and absence of specific antigens or proteins in the red blood cells. The protein's structure is controlled by three alleles; i, IA and IB. The first allele is, i, the recessive of the three, and IA and IB are both codominant when paired together. If the recessive allele i is paired with IB or IA, it's expression is hidden and is not shown. When the IB and IA are together in a pair, both proteins A and B are present and expressed.

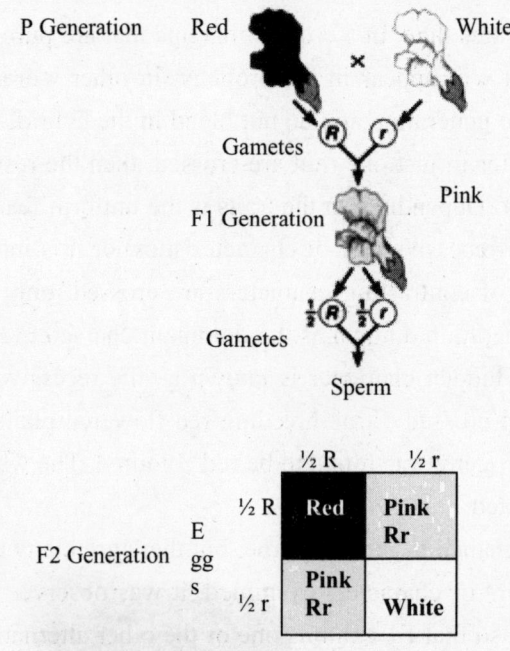

Figure 6.5: Incomplete dominance

The ABO system is called a multiple allele system for there are more than two possible allele pairs for the locus. The individual's blood type is determined by which combination of alleles he/she has. There are four possible blood types in order from most common to most rare: O, A, B and AB. The O blood type represents an individual who is homozygous recessive (ii) and does not have an allele for A or B (Table 6.2).

Table 6.2: Blood grouping

Parent 1	Parent 2	Child
Type O (i i)	Type O	Type O (i i)
Type A (IA)	Type A (IA)	Type A (IAIA)
Type B (IB)	Type B (IB)	Type B (IBIB)
Type A (IA)	Type O (i i)	Type A (IAi)
Type B (IB)	Type O (i i)	Type B (IBi)
Type A (IA)	Type B (IB)	Type AB (IAIB)

Blood types A and B are codominant alleles. Codominant alleles are expressed even if only one is present. The recessive allele i for blood type O is only expressed when two recessive alleles are present. Blood type O is not apparent if the individual has an allele for A or B. Individuals who have blood type A have a genotype of IAIA or IAi and those with blood type B, IBIB or IBi, but an individual who is IAIB has blood type AB.

6.4.2. Mendel's Law of Segregation

The law of segregations is a law of inheritance proposed by Mendel in 1866. According to this law, "each organism is formed of a bundle of characters. Each character is controlled by a pair of factors (genes). During gamete formation, the two factors of a character separate and enter different gametes". This law is also called law of purity of gametes. At formation of gametes, the two chromosomes of each pair separate (segregate) into two different cell which form the gametes. This is a universal law and always during gamete formation in all sexually reproducing organisms, the two factors of a pair pass into different gametes. Each gamete receives one member of a pair of factors and the gametes are pure. That is two members (alleles) of a single pair of genes are never found in the same mature sperm or ovum (gamete) but always separate out (segregate).The factors of inheritance (genes) normally are paired, but are separated or segregated in the formation of gametes (eggs and sperm), i.e., it states that the individuals of the F_2 generation are not uniform, but that the traits segregate. Depending on a dominant-recessive crossing or an intermediate crossing are the resulting ratios 3:1 or 1:2:1. This concept of independent traits explains how a trait can persist from generation to generation without blending with other traits. It explains, too, how the trait can seemingly disappear and then reappear in a later generation. The principle of segregation was consequently of the utmost importance for understanding both genetics and evolution.

6.4.2.1. Monohybrid Cross

The crossing of two plants differing in one character is called monohybrid cross. Mendel carried out monohybrid experiments on pea plants and based on the results of monohybrid experiment, he formulated the law of segregation. Mendel selected two pea plants, one with a tall stem and the other with a dwarf or short stem. These plants were considered as parental plants (P) and were pure breed. A pure plant is one that breeds true in respect of a particular character for a number of generations. The pure-bred tall and dwarf plants were treated as parents and were crossed. Seeds were collected from these plants. These seeds were sown and a group of plants were raised. These plants constituted the first filial generation (F1 generation). All the F1 plants were tall and were inbred. The seeds were collected and the next generation (F2) was raised. In the F2 generation, two types of plants were found. They were tall and dwarf. Mendel counted the number of tall and dwarf plants. Of the 1064 plants of F2 generation, 787 plants were tall and 277 plants were dwarf (75% were tall plants and 25% were dwarf plants). Thus the tall plants occurred in the ratio 3: 1 (Fig. 6.6).

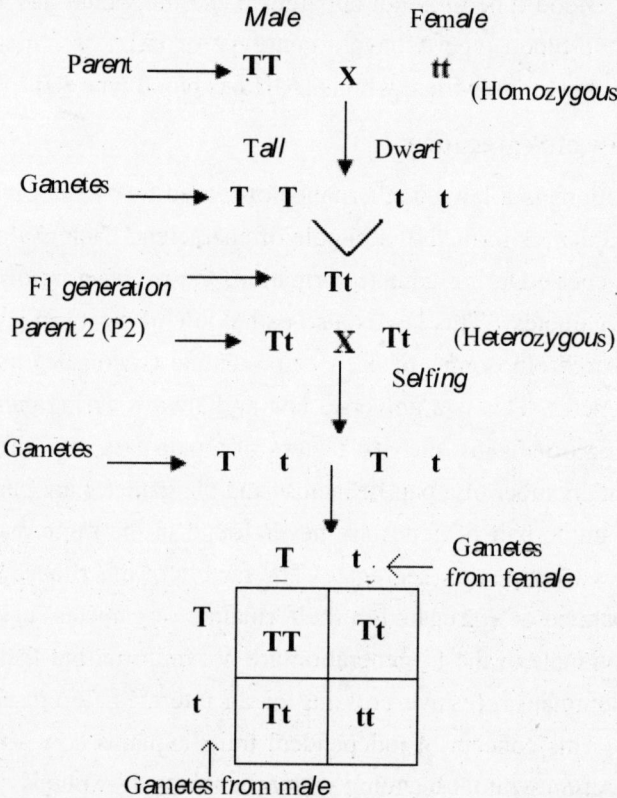

Figure 6.6: Diagram of a cross between two parental types for one trait (monohybrid cross). TT x tt P generation monohybrid crosses. All offspring in the F1 generation are heterozygous for the dominant (T) or the recessive (t) trait

6.4.3. Mendel's Principle of Independent Assortment

The Principle of Independent Assortment describes how different genes independently separate from one another when reproductive cells develop. Mendel formulated the Principle of Independent Assortment from the observations he got from the dihybrid crosses, which are crosses between organisms that differ with regard to two traits.

It is now known that this independent assortment of genes occurs during meiosis in eukaryotes. Meiosis is a type of cell division that reduces the number of chromosomes in a parent cell by half to produce four reproductive cells called gametes. In humans, diploid cells contain 46 chromosomes, with 23 chromosomes inherited from the mother, while a second similar set of 23 chromosomes inherited from the father. Pairs of similar chromosomes are called homologous chromosomes. During meiosis, the pairs of homologous chromosome are divided in half to form haploid cells, and this separation, or assortment of homologous chromosomes is random. This means that all the maternal chromosomes will not be separated into one cell, while all the paternal chromosomes are separated into another. Instead, after meiosis occurs, each haploid cell contains a mixture of genes from the organism's mother and father.

Another feature of independent assortment is recombination. Recombination occurs during meiosis and is a process that breaks and recombines the pieces of DNA to produce new combinations of genes. Recombination scrambles pieces of maternal and paternal genes, which ensures that genes assort independently from one another. It is important to note that there is an exception to the law of independent assortment for genes that are located very close to one another on the same chromosome because of genetic linkage.

6.4.3.1. Dihybrids cross between two heterozygous individuals

A dihybrid cross is a breeding experiment between P generation (parental generation) organisms that differ in two traits. Mendel determined what happens when two plants that are each hybrid for two traits are crossed. Mendel therefore decided to examine the inheritance of two characteristics at once. Based on the concept of segregation, he predicted that traits must sort into gametes separately. By extrapolating from his earlier data, Mendel also predicted that the inheritance of one characteristic did not affect the inheritance of a different characteristic.

Mendel tested the idea of trait independence with more complex crosses. First, he generated plants that were pure bred for two characteristics, such as seed colour (yellow and green) and seed shape (round and wrinkled). These plants would serve as the P_1 generation for the experiment. In this case, Mendel crossed the plants with Round and Yellow seeds (RRYY) with plants with wrinkled and green seeds (rryy). From his earlier monohybrid crosses, Mendel knew which traits were dominant: round and yellow. So, in the F_1 generation, he expected all round, yellow seeds from crossing these pure bred varieties, and that is exactly what he observed. Mendel knew that each of the F_1 progeny were dihybrids; in other words, they contained both alleles for each characteristic (RrYy). He then crossed individual F_1 plants (with genotypes RrYy) with one another. This is called a dihybrid cross. Mendel's results from this cross were present in a 9:3:3:1 ratio. The outcome shows a phenotypic ratio of 9 of the offspring having yellow round peas, 3 having yellow wrinkled peas, 3 having green round peas and 1 having green wrinkled peas. This is a classic 9:3:3:1 phenotypic ratio which is always the result in a dihybrid cross between two heterozygotes with unlinked traits.

The proportion of each trait was still approximately 3:1 for both seed shape and seed colour. In other words, the resulting seed shape and seed colour looked as if they had come from two parallel monohybrid crosses; even though two characteristics were involved in one cross, these traits behaved as though they had segregated independently. From these data, Mendel developed the third principle of inheritance: the principle of independent assortment i.e. alleles at one locus segregate into gametes independently of alleles at other loci. Such gametes are formed in equal frequencies (Fig. 6.7).

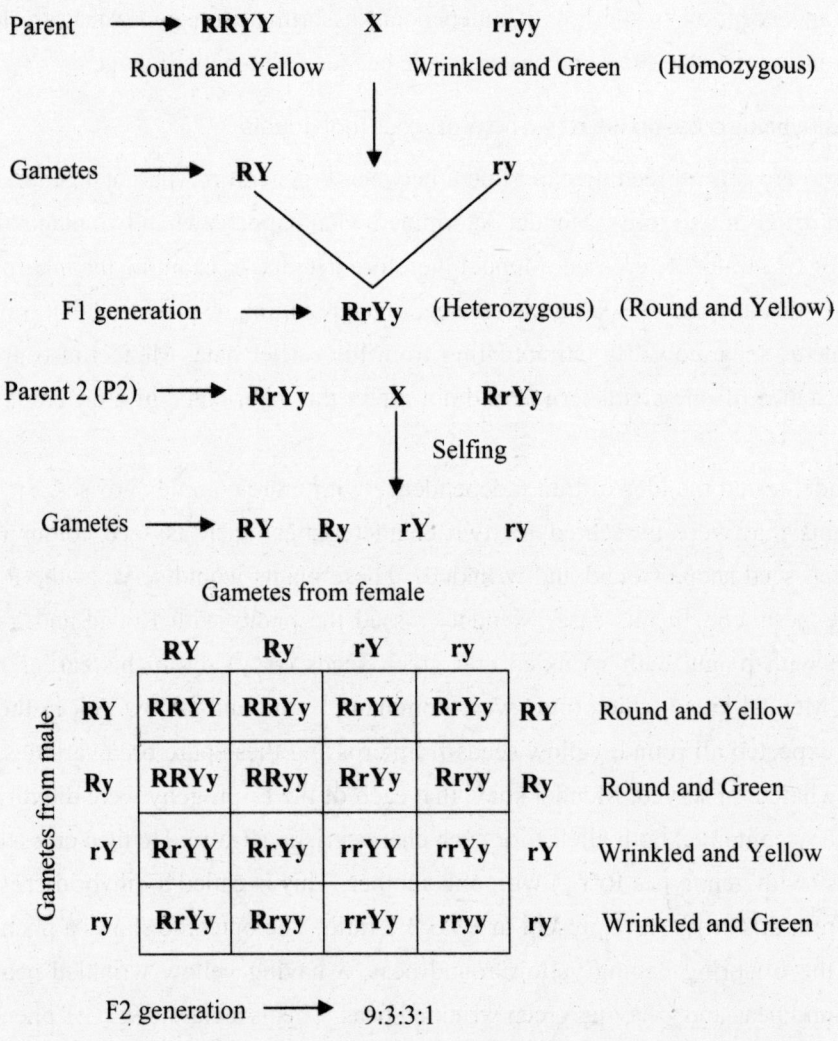

Figure 6.7: Dihybrid crosses between two heterozygous individuals

6.4.3.2. Trihybrid Cross

A trihybrid cross is a breeding experiment between P generation (parental generation) organisms that differ in three traits (Fig. 6.8).

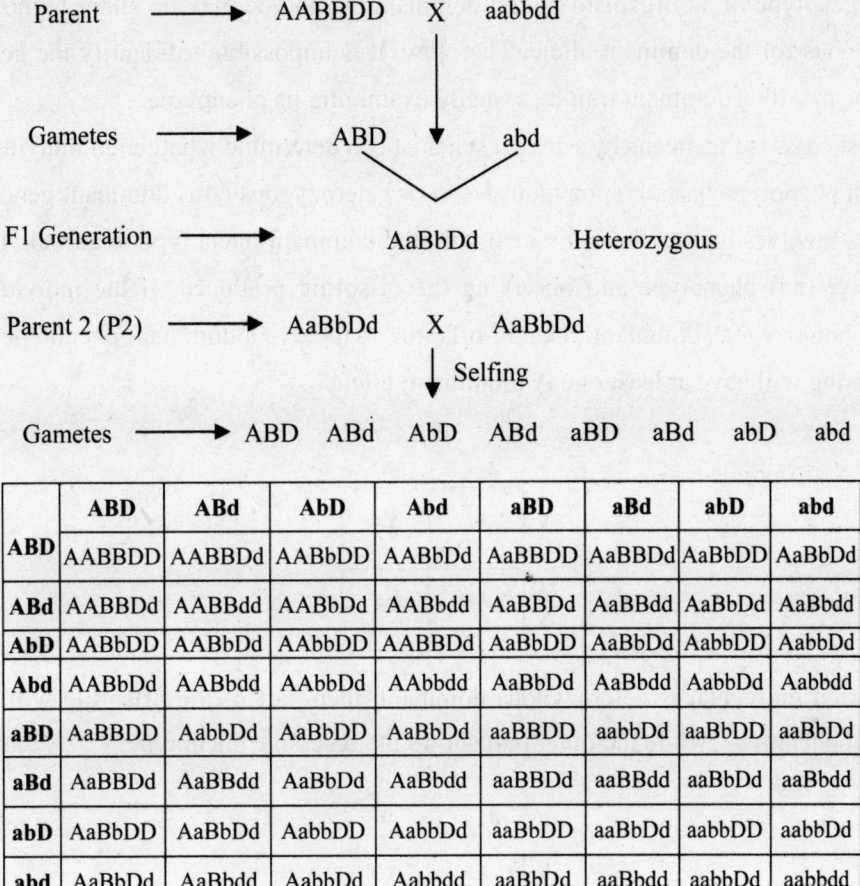

Phenotypic ratio: 27:9:9:9:3:3:3:1

Figure 6.8: Trihybrid (three different characteristics) crosses

6.5. Test Cross

A test cross is a way to explore the genotype, the genetic makeup of an organism. Early use of the test cross was as an experimental mating test used to determine what alleles are present in the genotype. Consequently, a test cross can help to determine whether a dominant phenotype is homozygous or heterozygous for a specific allele.

Diploid organisms, like humans, have two alleles at each genetic locus, or position, and one allele is inherited from each parent. Different alleles do not always produce equal outward effects or phenotypes. One allele can be dominant and mask the effect of a second recessive allele in a heterozygous organism that carries two different alleles at a specific locus. Recessive alleles only express their phenotype if an organism carries two identical copies of the recessive allele, meaning it is homozygous for the recessive allele. This means that the genotype of an organism with a dominant phenotype may be either homozygous or heterozygous for the dominant allele. Therefore, it is impossible to identify the genotype of an organism with a dominant trait by visually examining its phenotype.

A test cross is the means by which a scientist can determine whether an individual with a dominant phenotype has a homozygous (AA) or heterozygous (Aa) dominant genotype. The test cross involves mating the individual with the dominant phenotype to an individual with a recessive (aa) phenotype and observing the offspring produced. If the individual being tested is homozygous dominant, then all offspring will have a dominant phenotype, since all the offspring will have at least one A (dominant) allele.

	a	a
A	A*a*	A*a*
A	A*a*	A*a*

If the tested individual is heterozygous dominant, then half of the offspring will show the dominant phenotype, while the other half shows the recessive phenotype.

	a	a
A	A*a*	A*a*
a	*aa*	*aa*

6.6. Backcrossing

It is the crossing of a hybrid with one of its parents or an individual genetically similar to its parent, in order to achieve offspring with a genetic identity which is closer to that of the parent or it is the crossing of a heterozygous organism and one of its homozygous parents. It is used in horticulture, animal breeding and in production of gene knockout organisms (Fig. 6.9).

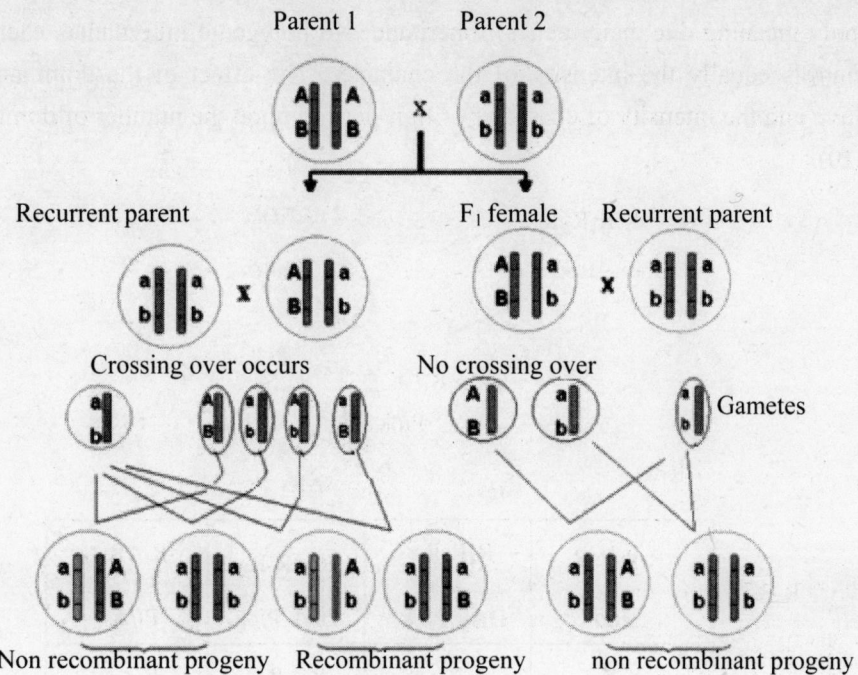

Figure 6.9: Back crossing

6.7. Limitations of the Mendelian System

The simple system of Mendelian genetics is very powerful and serves to explain the inheritance patterns of numerous traits. However, many traits are controlled by many genes acting in tandem, and thus do not obey strict Mendelian patterns (although their constituent genes may). Furthermore, many human traits are strongly influenced by the environment as well, and therefore their phenotypes cannot be said to be Mendelian (though the genetic components may be). In sum, Mendelian patterns are important, but cannot be applied universally. Individual traits must be researched to find out if they obey typical Mendelian patterns.

6.8. Polygenic or Quantitative Inheritance

When a trait (feature or character) is controlled by a single gene it is termed monogenic inheritance. Many traits or features are controlled by a number of different genes. For example, the skin colour of humans and the kernel colour of wheat results from the combined effect of several genes, none of which are singly dominant. Polygenes affecting a particular trait are found on many chromosomes. Each of these genes has equal contribution and cumulative the total effect. Three to four genes contribute towards formation of the pigment in the skin of humans. So there is a continuous variation in skin colour from very fair to very dark. Such inheritance controlled by many genes is termed quantitative inheritance or polygenic (poly meaning due many genes) inheritance. In polygenic inheritance, each dominant gene controls equally the intensity of the character. The effect of the dominant genes in cumulative and the intensity of character or trait depend upon the number of dominant genes (Fig. 6.10).

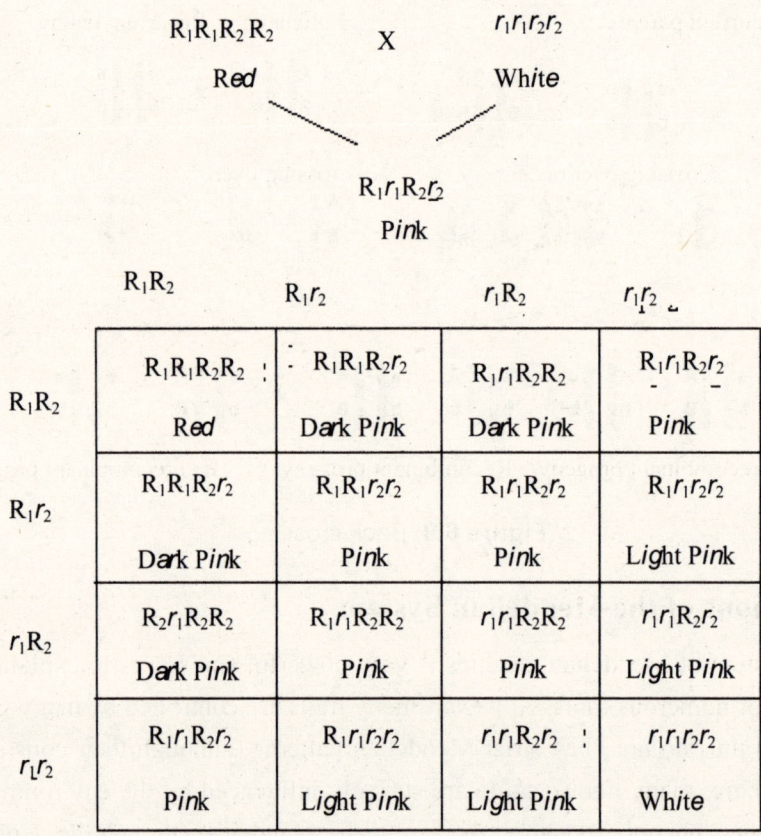

1 Red : 4 Dark pink : 6 Pink : 1 White

Figure 6.10: Polygenic or quantitative inheritance

6.9. Multiple Alleles

Alleles are located in corresponding parts of homologous chromosomes, only one member of a pair can be present in a given chromosome and only two are present in a cell of a diploid. Alleles are genes that are members of the same gene pair, each kind of allele affecting a trait differently than the other. A diploid organism has, by its definition, only two alleles at one time, yet exceptions to the rules do appear. Many examples were found where more than two alternative alleles, also called multiple alleles, are present. In these cases two or more different mutations must have taken place at the same locus but in different individuals or at different times. Multiple alleles are alternative states at the same locus. The different alleles of a series are usually represented by the same symbol. Subscripts and superscripts are used to identify different members of a series of alleles. Most alleles produce variations of the same trait, but some produce very different phenotypes.

The most famous example of multiple alleles was discovered in rabbits. It was known that Albino rabbits were produced on occasion in variously coloured rabbit populations. After conducting a monohybrid cross between a coloured and Albino rabbit, it was discovered that the members of a pair of alternative genes, either c^a or C, must be responsible for coloured or albino rabbits. A cross of homozygous coloured (CC) and albino ($c^a c^a$) rabbits were made and the F1 generation was all coloured, while the F2 generation had three coloured and one albino. This showed that one pair of alleles was involved, the wild C and the mutant

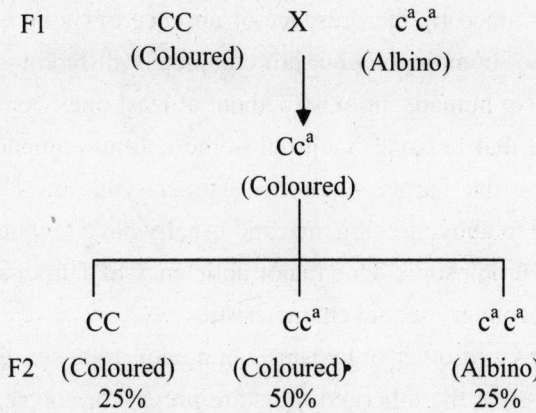

allele c^a. It was determined that C was dominant over c^a (Fig. 6.11).

Figure 6.11: *Inheritance of skin colour*

6.10. Chromosomal Theory of Inheritance

Sutton and Boveri in 1902 observed by that maternal (from mother) and paternal (from father) characters come together in the progeny which is diploid or 2n and has chromosomes in pairs and later on segregate during the formation of gametes. The gametes have a single chromosome from each pair and are haploid or n. Chromosomes from two parents come together in the same zygote as a result of the fusion of two gametes and again separate out during the formation of gametes. Chromosomes are filamentous bodies present in the nucleus and seen only during cell division. The above two observations proved that there is a remarkable similarity between the behavior of characters during inheritance and that of chromosomes during meiosis. This led Sutton and Boveri to propose 'chromosomal theory of inheritance' and its salient features are as follows:

1. The somatic (body) cells of an organism, which are derived by the repeated division of zygote have two identical sets of chromosomes, i.e., they are diploid. Out of these, one set of chromosomes is received from the mother (maternal chromosomes) and one set from the father (paternal chromosomes). Two chromosomes of one type (carrying same genes) constitute a homologous pair. Humans have 23 pairs of chromosomes.

2. The chromosomes of homologous pair separate out during meiosis at the time of gamete formation.

3. The behavior of chromosomes during meiosis indicates that Mendelian factors or genes are located linearly on the chromosomes. With progress in molecular biology it is now known that a chromosome is made up of a molecule of DNA and segments of DNA are the genes.

6.11. Sex-linked Characteristics

In animals the sex is determined by the presence or absence of the Y chromosome. The X and Y chromosomes are not homologous but are completely different chromosomes which carry unique information. No human can exist without at least one X chromosome. There is a viable human phenotype that has one X chromosome and no companion X or Y. These individuals are said to have the Turner syndrome. Turner syndrome (X 0) individuals are females who are of normal to above intelligence and usually have few deficiencies considering their lack of an entire chromosome. One major deficiency of Turner syndrome is sterility and non-development of secondary sexual characteristics.

Certain traits in humans and other organisms can demonstrate sex-linked inheritance of characteristics. This means that the inherited traits are present on the sex determining chromosomes the X or the Y. Since there appears to be more information on the X chromosome than on the Y chromosome of humans, most known sex-linked characteristics are actually X-linked characteristics.

In sex-linked traits, such as colour-blindness, the gene for the trait is found on the X chromosome (a sex chromosome). Sex-linked traits affect primarily males, since they have only one copy of the X chromosome (male genotype: XY). Females, who have two copies of the X chromosome, are affected only if they are homozygous for the trait. Females can, however, be carriers for sex-linked traits, passing their X chromosomes on to their sons. Sex-linked inheritance works as follows: if a female carrier and a normal male give birth to a daughter, she has a 1 in 2 chance of being a carrier of the trait (like her mother). If the child is a son, he has a 1 in 2 chance of being affected by the trait . If a female carrier and an affected male give birth to a daughter, she will either be affected or be a carrier. If the child is a son, he will either be affected or be entirely free of the gene.

Another example of a sex-linked trait is haemophilia, made famous by the "Queen Victoria pedigree" of the European nobility. Beginning with Queen Victoria of England (in whom it was probably a spontaneous mutation), the haemophilia gene spread quickly throughout the European rulers (who intermarried as a matter of course). The disease, which prevents blood from clotting properly and renders a minor injury a life-threatening event, claimed several young men of the royal line. Especially since male heirs were pre-ferred over female as successors to the thrones of Europe, the spread of such a debilitating disease was a major problem.

6.12 Linkage and Crossing over

The fact behind Mendel's success was the genes encoding his selected traits did not reside close together on the same chromosome. If they had, his dihybrid cross results would have been much more confusing, and he might not have discovered the law of independent assort-ment. The law of independent assortment holds true as long as two different genes are on separate chromosomes. When the genes are on separate chromosomes, the two alleles of one gene (A and a) will segregate into gametes independently of the two alleles of the other gene (B and b). Equal numbers of four different gametes will result: AB, aB, Ab, ab. But if the two genes are on the same chromosome, then they will be linked and will segregate together during meiosis, producing only two kinds of gametes.

For instance, if the genes for seed shape and seed colour were on the same chromosome and a homozygous double dominant (yellow and round, RRYY) plant was crossed with a homozygous double recessive (green and wrinkled, rryy), the F_1 hybrid offspring, as usual, would be double heterozygous dominant (yellow and round, RrYy). However, since in this example the R and Y are linked together on the chromosome inherited from the dominant parent, with r and y linked together on the other chromosome, only two different gametes can be formed: RY and ry. Therefore, instead of 16 different genotypes in the F_2 offspring, only three are possible: RRYY, RrYy, rryy and instead of four different phenotypes, only the original two will exist. Notice that the inheritance pattern now resembles that seen in a monohybrid cross, with a 3:1 phenotypic ratio, rather than the 9:3:3:1 ratio expected from the dihybrid cross. If physically linked on a single chromosome, the round and yellow alleles would segregate together, and the wrinkled and green alleles would segregate together, no round green seeds or wrinkled yellow seeds would ever appear.

The above explanation, however, neglects the influence of the crossing over of genetic material that occurs during meiosis. The farther away two genes are from one another, the more likely an exchange point for crossing over will form between them. At these exchange points, the alleles of one gene switch to the opposite homologous chromosome, while the other gene alleles remain with their original chromosomes. When alleles switch places like this, the resulting gametes are called recombinant. In the example above, the original parental gametes would be RY and ry, while the recombinant gametes would be Ry and rY. Thus four different kinds of gametes will be formed, instead of only two formed when the genes were linked (Fig. 6.12).

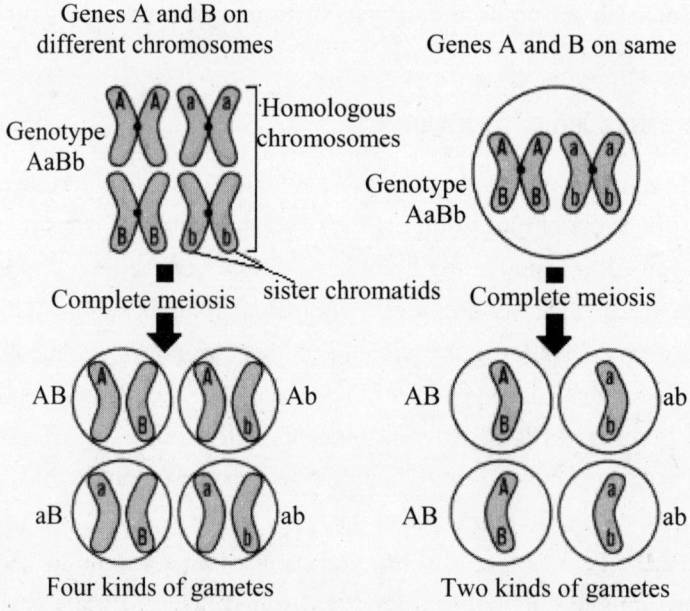

Figure 6.12: Gamete formation: when genes are on the same and different chromosome

If two genes are extremely close together, crossing over will almost never occur between them, and the recombinant gametes will almost never form. If they are very far apart on the chromosome, crossing over will almost certainly occur between them, and recombinant gametes will form just as often as if the genes were on different chromosomes (50 percent of recombinant). If the genes are at an intermediate distance from each other, crossing over may sometimes occur between them and sometimes not (Fig. 6.13). Therefore, the percentage of recombinant gametes (reflected in the percentage of recombinant offspring) correlates with the distance between two genes on a chromosome. By comparing the recombination rates of multiple different pairs of genes on the same chromosome, the relative position of each gene along the chromosome can be determined. This method of ordering genes on a chromosome is called a linkage map.

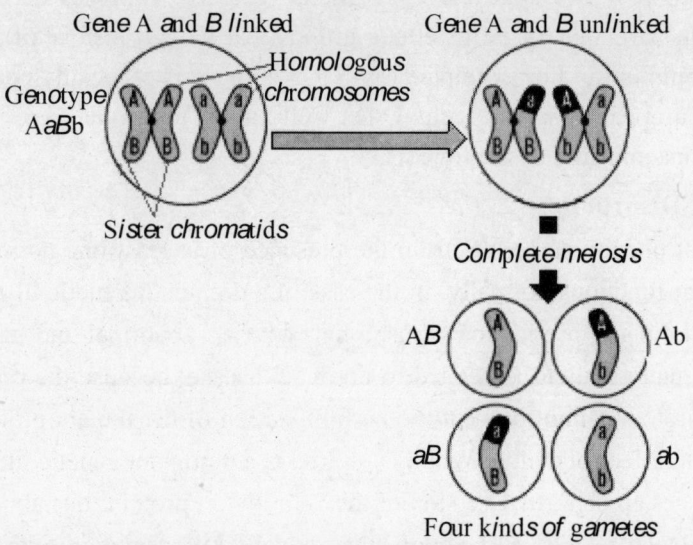

Figure 6.13: Gamete formation when genes are linked and unlinked

6.13. Mutations

Mutations are errors in the genotype that create new alleles and can result in a variety of genetic disorders. In order for a mutation to be inherited from one generation to another, it must occur in sex cells, such as eggs and sperm, rather than in somatic cells. The best way to detect a genetic disorder is karyotyping.

6.13.1. Autosomal Mutations

There are certain human genetic diseases which are inherited in a Mendelian fashion such as disease phenotype will have either a clearly dominant or clearly recessive pattern of inheritance, similar to the traits in Mendel's peas. Such a pattern will usually only occur if the disease is caused by an abnormality in a single gene. The mutations that cause these diseases occur in genes on the autosomal chromosomes, the chromosomes that determine bodily characteristics and exist in all cells, both sex and somatic, as opposed to sex-linked diseases.

6.13.2. Recessive Disorders

Genetic disorders are initially arises as a new mutation that changes a single gene so that it no longer produces a protein that functions normally. A disease resulting from a mutation that an allele which produces a non-functional protein will be inherited in a recessive fashion so that the disease phenotype will only appear when both copies of the gene carry the mutation, resulting in a total absence of the necessary protein. If only one copy of the mutated allele is present, the individual is a heterozygous carrier, showing no signs of the disease but able to transmit the disease gene to the next generation. Albinism is an example of a recessive illness, resulting from a mutation in a gene that normally encodes a protein needed for pigment production in the skin and eyes. Many recessive illnesses occur with much greater frequency in particular racial or ethnic groups that have a history of intermarrying within their own community. For example, Tay-Sachs disease is especially common among people of Eastern European Jewish descent. Other well-known autosomal recessive disorders include sickle-cell anaemia and cystic fibrosis.

6.13.3. Dominant Disorders

Usually, a dominant phenotype results from the presence of at least one normal allele producing a protein that functions normally. In the case of a dominant genetic illness, there is a mutation that results in the production of a protein with an abnormal and harmful action. Only one copy of such an allele is needed to produce disease, because the presence of the normal allele and protein cannot prevent the harmful action of the mutant protein. Huntington's disease, which killed folksinger Woody Guthrie, is a dominant genetic illness. A single mutant allele produces an abnormal version of the Huntington protein; this abnormal protein accumulates in particular regions of the brain and gradually kills the brain cells.

6.13.4. Chromosomal Disorders

Mutation of a single gene results in recessive and dominant characteristics. Some genetic disorders result from the gain or loss of an entire chromosome. Normally, paired homologous chromosomes separate from each other during the first division of meiosis. If one pair fails to separate, an event called non-disjunction, then one daughter cell will receive both chromosomes and the other daughter cell will receive none. When one of these gametes joins with a normal gamete from the other parent, the resulting offspring will have either one or three copies of the affected chromosome, rather than the usual two.

(a) **Trisomy:** A single chromosome contains hundreds to thousands of genes. A zygote with three copies of a chromosome (trisomy), instead of the usual two, generally cannot survive embryonic development. Chromosome 21 is a major exception to this rule; individuals with three copies of this small chromosome (trisomy 21) develop the genetic disorder called Down syndrome. People with Down syndrome show at least mild mental disabilities and have unusual physical features including a flat face, large tongue, and distinctive creases on their palms. They are also at a much greater risk for various health problems such as heart defects and early Alzheimer's disease.

(b) **Monosomy:** The absence of one copy of a chromosome (monosomy) causes even more problems than the presence of an extra copy. Only monosomy of the X chromosome is compatible with life.

(c) **Polyploidy:** Polyploidy occurs when a failure occurs during the formation of the gametes during meiosis. The gametes produced in this instance are diploid rather than haploid. If fertilization occurs with these gametes, the offspring receive an entire extra set of chromosomes. In humans, polyploidy is always fatal, though in many plants and fish it is not.

Suggested Readings

- Alberts B (1994). Molecular Biology of the Cell, 3rd edition. New York: Garland Publishing.
- Atherly A.G., J.R. Girton and J.F. McDonald. The Science of Genetics. Saunders College Publishing. Harcourt Brace College Publishers, NY.
- Brooker, R.J. Genetics : Analysis and Principles. Benjamin / Cummings, Longman Inc.
- Fairbanks, D.J. and W.R. Anderson. Genetics – The continuity of life. Brooks / Cole Publishing Company, TTP, NY, Toronto.
- Gardner, E.J., M.J. Simmons and D.P. Snustads. Principles of Genetics, John Wiley and Sons Inc., NY.
- Griffith, A.J.F., J.H. Miller, D.T. Suziki, R.C. Lewontin and W.M. Gellbart. An introduction to genetic analysis. W.H. Freeman and Company, New York.
- Lewin, B. Genes. VI Oxford University Press, Oxford, New York, Tokyo.
- Snustad, D.P. and M. Simmons. Principles of Genetics. John Wiley and Sons Inc., NY.
- Macfarlane WM (2000). "Demystified Transcription." Molecular Pathology 53(1):1–7.
- Monk M (1995). "Epigenetic Programming of Differential Gene Expression in Development and Evolution." Developmental Genetics 17(3):188–197.
- Watson JD. (1998). The Double Helix: A Personal Account of the Discovery of the Structure of DNA. New York: Scribners.

CHAPTER 7

Replication of Genetic Material

- Genetic Material: DNA not Protein
- DNA replication
- Meselson and Stahl Experiment
- The Replisome
- Features of DNA Replication
- Prokaryotic Replication
- Eukaryotic DNA replication
- Telomeres and Telomerase
- Post-Replicative Modification of DNA
- Mutations
- Mechanisms of Mutation
  - Deamination
  - Mutation by UV light
- Mutation by Chemical Agents
  - Acridines
  - Alkylating agents
  - Nitrous acid (HNO_2)
- Mutation by Replication Errors
- DNA Repair Mechanisms
  - Base excision
  - Nucleotide excision
  - Mismatch repair
- DNA Recombination
  - Homologous Recombination
  - Site-specific Recombination
  - Transpositional Recombination

Amazing the six billion nucleotides of the diploid human genome are replicated in only a few hours while generating so few errors that the spontaneous mutation rate may be less than 1 mutation per genome per cell division!!!! This incredible accuracy results from three major error avoidance processes: the high selectivity of DNA polymerases, exonucleolytic proofreading, and post replication mismatch repair (Loeb 1991).

7.1. Genetic Material: DNA not Protein

As early as 1848, Wilhelm Hofmeister, a German botanist, has observed that cell nuclei resolve themselves into small, rod-like bodies during mitosis. Later, these structures were found to absorb certain dyes and so came to be called chromosomes (colored bodies). In 1869, Friedrich Miescher, a Swiss physician, isolated a substance from cell nuclei that he called nuclein - now known as DNA.

The chromosomes of eukaryotes contain a variety of proteins in addition to DNA. Until the early 1950s most biologists were inclined to believe that the proteins were the chief carriers if heredity. Nucleic acids contain only four different unitary building blocks, but proteins are made up of 20 different amino acids. Proteins therefore appeared to have a greater diversity structure, and the diversity of the genes seemed first likely to rest on the diversity of the proteins.

In 1928, Frederick Griffith, an English army doctor, wanted to make a vaccine against *Streptococcus pneumoniae*, which caused pneumonia. Since the time of Pasteur, about 50 years before, vaccines had been made using killed microorganisms which could be injected into patients to elicit the immune response of live cells without risk of disease. Though, he failed in making the vaccine he stumbled on a demonstration of the transmission of genetic instructions by a process we now call the "transformation principle".

In his experiments, Griffith used two strains that are distinguishable by the appearance of their colonies when grown in laboratory cultures. In one strain, a normal virulent type, the cells are enclosed in a polysaccharide capsule, giving colonies a smooth appearance; hence, this strain is labeled '*S*'. In Griffith's other strain, a mutant non-virulent type that grows in mice but is not lethal, the polysaccharide coat is absent, giving colonies a rough appearance; this strain is called '*R*'. The R bacteria were harmless, but the S bacteria were lethal when injected into mice. Heat-killed S cells were also harmless - the same effect seen by Pasteur. However, surprisingly when live R cells were mixed with killed S cells and injected into mice, the mice died, and the bacteria rescued from the mice had been "transformed" into the S type (Fig. 7.1). Griffith announced that it was because of a phenomenon other than mutation, which he called transformation. This experiment strongly implied that genetic material had been transferred from the dead to the live cell. It was hard to be certain of this, or to know what exactly genetic material was transferred and was responsible for the transformation process.

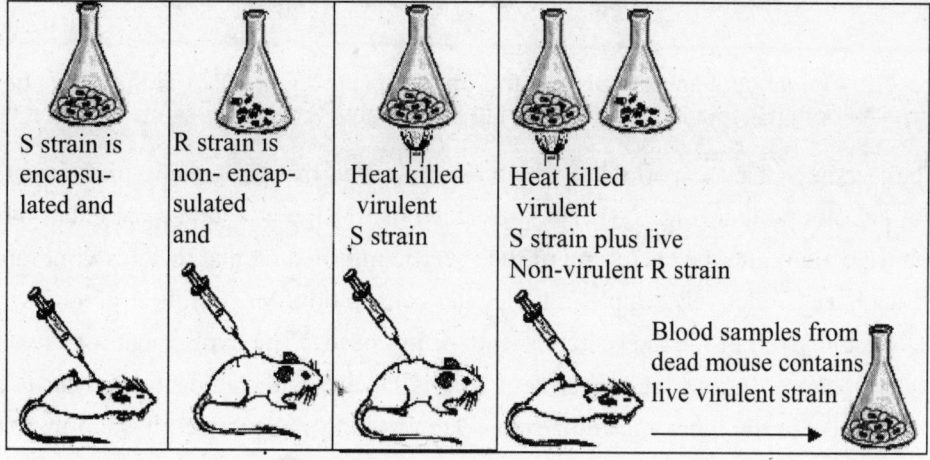

S strain is encapsulated and

R strain is non- encapsulated and

Heat killed virulent S strain

Heat killed virulent S strain plus live Non-virulent R strain

Blood samples from dead mouse contains live virulent strain

Figure 7.1: Griffith experiment: Demonstration of DNA as genetic material

In 1944, the team of Avery, MacLeod and McCarty revised the above experiment. They extracted and purified DNA, proteins and other materials from *Streptococcus pneumoniae* S bacteria, they mixed R bacteria with these different materials. Only those mixed with DNA were transformed into S bacteria (Fig.7.2). This led to the conclusion that the chromosome of S-bacteria causes the transformation and not the capsule. So they announced that bacterial transformation involves transfer of a part of DNA from the dead bacterium (donor) to the active living bacterium (recipient), which expresses the character of the donor cell, and so is called a recombinant. This experiment strongly implied that DNA is the "transforming factor" and not proteins or other materials and this demonstrated what is known to us as the transforming principle - that genes are made of DNA. Amazingly, not everyone was convinced by the experiments of Avery's, MacLeod's and McCarty's. It was the experiments of Hershey and Chase (1952) that finally proved that DNA was the genetic material and not protein.

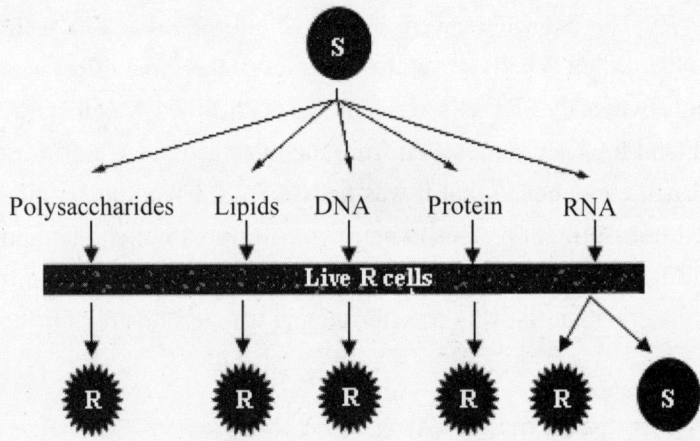

Figure 7.2: Demonstration that DNA is the transforming agent. DNA is the only agent that produces smooth (S) colonies when added to live rough (R) cells

The Hershey-Chase experiment, which demonstrated that the genetic material of phage is DNA and not protein (Fig. 7.3). They reasoned that phage infection must entail the introduction (injection) into the bacterium of the specific information that dictates viral reproduction. The phage is relatively simple in molecular constitution. Most of its structure is protein, with DNA contained inside the protein sheath of its "head." The experiment uses two sets of T2 bacteriophages. In one set, the protein coat is labeled with radioactive sulfur (^{35}S), not found in DNA. In the other set, the DNA is labeled with radioactive phosphorus (^{32}P), not found in protein. When the ^{32}P-labeled phages were used, most of the radioactivity ended up inside the bacterial cells, indicating that the phage DNA entered the cells. ^{32}P can also be recovered from phage progeny. When the ^{35}S-labeled phages were used, most of the radioactive material ended up in the phage ghosts, indicating that the phage protein never entered the bacterial cell. Only the ^{32}P is injected into the *E. coli,* indicating that DNA is the agent necessary for the production of new phages.

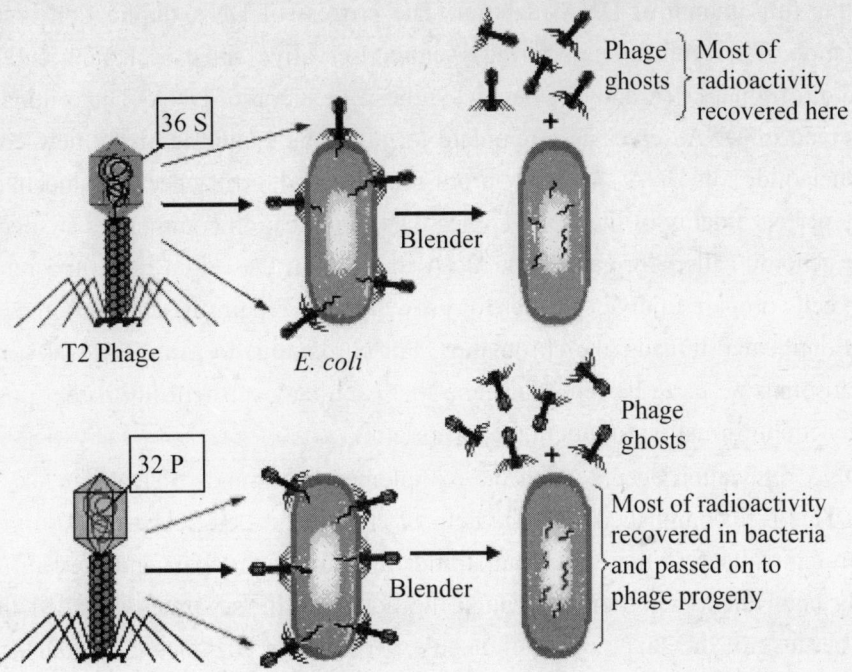

Figure 7.3: The Hershey-Chase experiment, which demonstrated that DNA is the hereditary material; the phage proteins are mere structural packaging that is discarded after delivering the viral DNA to the bacterial cell

7.2. DNA Replication

Chromosomes are structures within a cell which contain the genetic information that is passed on from one generation to the next. Specific regions, called genes, on each chromosome contain the hereditary information which distinguishes individuals from each other. The genes also contain the coded information required for the synthesis of proteins and enzymes needed for the normal functions of the cells. Bacterial cells may have 1000 genes, while the human cell contains more than a million genes. In prokaryotes, there is usually a large circular chromosome. In addition, there may be several smaller circular chromosomes called plasmids. None of these is enclosed in a membrane; they merely drift around within the cytoplasm of the prokaryote cell. A single *E. coli* (bacteria) chromosome of double helical DNA consists of 3.4 million base pairs. In eukaryotes, most chromosomes are located in the cell nucleus and are composed of protein and DNA. Smaller chromosomes exist in mitochondria and chloroplasts - these tend to regulate activity solely within the organelle in which they occur.

DNA replication is the basis for biological inheritance. Prior to cell division, the DNA material in the original cell must be duplicated so that after cell division, each new cell contains the full amount of DNA material. The process of DNA duplication is usually called replication. The replication is termed semiconservative since each new cell contains one strand of original DNA and one newly synthesized strand of DNA. The original polynucleotide strand of DNA serves as a template to guide the synthesis of the new complementary polynucleotide of DNA. Cellular proof-reading and error-checking mechanisms ensure nearly perfect fidelity of the DNA copies. DNA replication commences at specific locations in the genome called "origins." The DNA unwinds at the origin to form a replication fork. When cells prepare to divide, either for growth or for repair, the chromosomes become visible as duplicated threads, the chromatids. For chromatids to form, the DNA of the original chromosomes needs to be reproduced so that each new cell will ultimately possess the correct genetic information to function appropriately.

DNA replication occurs when the complementary strands of DNA break apart and unwind. This is accomplished with the help of enzymes called helicases. Additional enzymes and proteins attach to the individual strands, holding them apart and preventing them from coiling upon them. The point at which the double helix separates is called the replication fork, because of the shape of the molecule. At this site enzymes called DNA polymerases move along each of the separated DNA strands, adding nucleotides to the exposed bases according to the base pairing rules. The ribose-phosphate bonds form between the new nucleotides to hold the new strand together. The process continues until the original double helix is completely unwound and two new double helices have been formed. Each new double helix is composed of one old DNA strand and one new strand. This is described as semiconservative replication

For heredity, biological information must be accurately copied and transmitted from each cell to all of its progeny. Three ways for DNA molecules to replicate may be considered, each obeying the rules of complementary base pairing (Fig.7.4).

- **Conservative replication** would leave intact the original DNA molecule and generate a completely new molecule.
- **Dispersive replication** would produce two DNA molecules with sections of both old and new DNA interspersed along each strand.
- **Semiconservative replication** would produce molecules with both old and new DNA, but each molecule would be composed of one old strand and one new one. The replication is semiconservative. Each strand acts as a template for the synthesis of a new DNA molecule by the sequential addition of complementary base pairs, thereby generating a new DNA strand that is the complementary sequence to the parental DNA. Each daughter DNA molecule ends up with one of the original strands and one newly synthesized strand (Fig. 7.4).

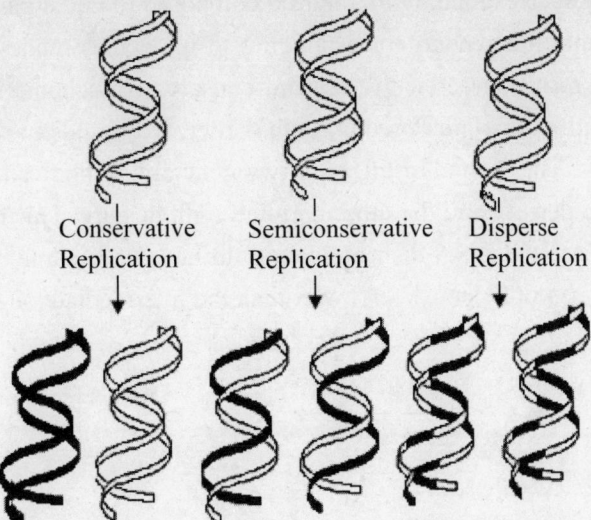

Figure 7.4: Possible models of replication: The two original strands of DNA are shown in light colour; newly synthesized DNA is dark

7.3. Meselson and Stahl Experiment

The Meselson-Stahl experiment was an important step in developmental biology research. Two scientists, Matthew Meselson and Franklin Stahl carried out their experiment in 1958 to prove the semiconservative DNA replication hypothesis proposed by James Watson and Francis Crick.

The experiment carried out by Meselson and Stahl involved growing a culture of *Escherichia coli* in a medium containing $^{15}NH_4Cl$ (ammonium chloride labeled with the heavy isotope of nitrogen). Cells were then transferred to normal medium (containing $^{14}NH_4Cl$) and samples taken after 20 minutes (one cell division) and 40 minutes (two cell divisions). DNA was extracted from each sample and the molecules analyzed by density gradient centrifugation. After 20 minutes the entire DNA contained similar amounts of ^{14}N and ^{15}N, but after 40 minutes two bands were seen, one corresponding to hybrid ^{14}N-^{15}N-DNA, and the other to DNA molecules made entirely of ^{14}N. The banding pattern seen after 20 minutes enables conservative replication to be discounted because this scheme predicts that after one round of replication there will be two different types of double helix, one containing just ^{15}N and the other containing just ^{14}N. The single ^{14}N-^{15}N-DNA band that was actually seen after 20 minutes is compatible with both dispersive and semiconservative replication, but the two bands seen after 40 minutes are consistent only with semiconservative replication. Dispersive replication continues to give hybrid ^{14}N-^{15}N molecules after two rounds of replication, whereas the granddaughter molecules produced at this stage by semiconservative replication include two that are made entirely of ^{14}N-DNA. Now the density gradient revealed two bands of DNA, the first corresponding to a hybrid composed of equal parts of newly synthesized and old DNA, and the second corresponding to molecules made up entirely of new DNA (Fig. 7.5). This result agrees with the semi-conservative scheme but is incompatible with dispersive replication; the latter predicting that after two rounds of replication all molecules would be hybrids. The second result, after two generations, showed that one part of the DNA had intermediate density and the other part had light density. This ruled out dispersive replication as in that case the DNA distribution would have been same between the strands and the resulting density would have been lower than the intermediate one.

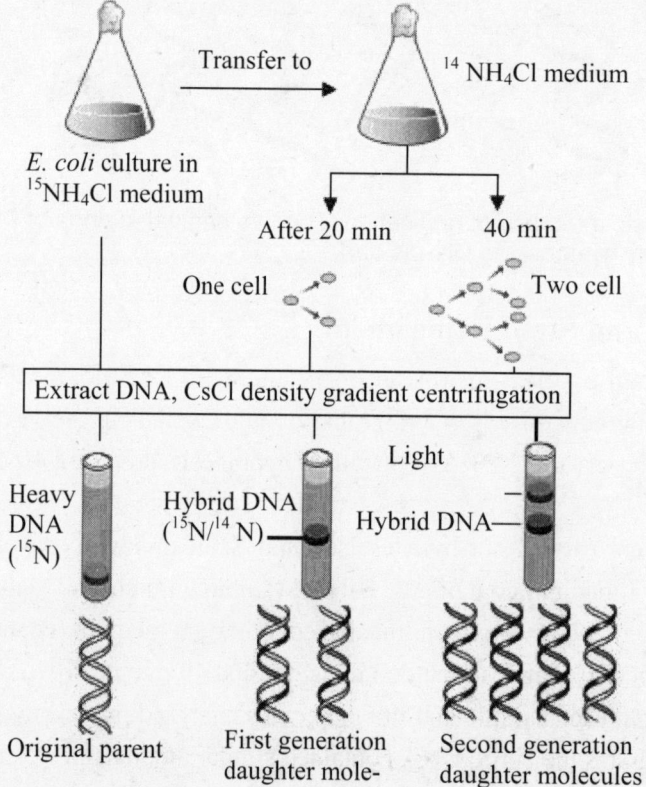

Figure 7.5: Meselson and Stahl experiment

7.4. The Replisome

The replisome is a complex molecular machine that carries out replication of DNA. It is comprised of a number of subcomponents, each performing a specific function during the process of replication.

(a) Helicase is an enzyme which breaks the hydrogen bonds between the two strands of DNA, thus separating the strands ahead of DNA synthesis. As helicase unwinds the double helix, it induces the formation of supercoils in other areas of the DNA.

(b) Gyrase relaxes and removes the supercoiling which has been caused by the helicase by cutting the DNA strands, allowing it to rotate and release the supercoil, and then rejoining the strands. Gyrase is most commonly located upstream of the replication fork - where the supercoils are being formed.

(c) Primase adds complementary RNA primers to a DNA strand to begin Okazaki fragments as well as leading strand since DNA polymerase can only continue (but not begin) a strand.

(d) DNA polymerases: All DNA polymerases, whether from prokaryotic or eukaryotic sources, share the following properties: (a) The incoming base is selected within the DNA polymerase active site, as determined by Watson-Crick geometric interactions with its corresponding base in the template strand, (b) chain growth is in the 5' →3' direction and is antiparallel to the template strand, and (c) DNA polymerases cannot initiate DNA synthesis de novo—all require a primer oligonucleotide with a free 3'-OH to build upon. DNA polymerase enzymes are numbered I, II, and III, in order of their discovery. DNA polymerases I and II function principally in DNA repair; DNA polymerase III is the chief DNA-replicating enzyme of *E. coli*. Only 10 to 20 copies of this enzyme are present per cell (Table 7.1).

One mechanism intrinsic to virtually all DNA polymerases is a separate 3'→5' exonuclease activity that serves to double-check each nucleotide after it is added. This nuclease activity permits the enzyme to remove a nucleotide just added and is highly specific for mismatched base pairs. If the wrong nucleotide has been added, translocation of the polymerase to the position where the next nucleotide is to be added is inhibited. The 3'→5' exonuclease activity removes the mispaired nucleotide, and the polymerase begins again. This activity, called proofreading, is not simply the reverse of the polymerization reaction, because pyrophosphate is not involved.

The mechanics of DNA replication was originally characterized in the bacterium, *E. coli* which contains 3 distinct enzymes capable of catalyzing the replication of DNA. These have been identified as DNA polymerase (pol) I, II, and III. Pol I is the most abundant replicating activity in *E. coli* but has as its primary role to ensure the fidelity of replication through the repair of damaged and mismatched DNA. Replication of the *E. coli* genome is the job of pol III. This enzyme is much less abundant than pol I, however, its activity is nearly 100 times that of pol I. The DNA polymerase I is used to fill the gap between DNA fragments of the lagging strand. It is also the major enzyme for gap filling during DNA repair. The DNA polymerase II is encoded by the *PolB* gene, which is involved in the SOS response to DNA damage. DNA replication is mainly carried out by the DNA pol III.

Table 7.1: Properties of the DNA polymerases of *E. coli*

Property	Pol I	Pol II	Pol III (core)
Mass (kD)	103	90	130, 27.5, 8.6
Molecules/cell	400	?	40
Turnover number[†]	600	30	1200
Structural gene	*polA*	*polB*	*dnaE* (a subunit) *dnaQ* (esubunit) *holE* (q subunit)
Polymerization 5′ → 3′	Yes	Yes	Yes
Exonuclease 3′ → 5′	Yes	Yes	Yes
Exonuclease 5′ → 3′	Yes	No	No
Mass (kD)	103	90	130, 27.5, 8.6
Molecules/cell	400	?	40
Turnover number[†]	600	30	1200
Structural gene	*polA*	*polB*	*dnaE* (a subunit) *dnaQ* (esubunit) *holE* (q subunit)
Polymerization 5′ → 3′	Yes	Yes	Yes
Exonuclease 3′ → 5′	Yes	Yes	Yes
Exonuclease 5′ → 3′	Yes	No	No

(i) DNA polymerase I: In 1957, Arthur Kornberg and his colleagues discovered the first DNA polymerase, DNA polymerase I, awarded the Nobel Prize in physiology in 1959. DNA polymerase I catalyzed the synthesis of DNA *in vitro,* if provided with all four deoxynucleoside-5′-triphosphates (dATP, dTTP, dCTP, dGTP), a template DNA strand to copy, and a primer. A primer is essential because DNA polymerases can elongate only pre-existing chains; they cannot join two deoxyribonucleoside-5′-phosphates together to make the initial phosphodiester bond. The primer base-pairs with the template DNA, forming a short, double-stranded region. This primer must possess a free 3′-OH end to which an incoming deoxynucleoside monophosphate is added. All four dNTPs are substrates to polymerase, while pyrophosphate (PPi) is released following the formation of the bond, and the dNMP is linked to the 3′-OH of the primer chain through formation of a phosphodiester bond. The deoxynucleoside monophosphate to be incorporated is chosen through its geometric fit with the template base to form a Watson-Crick base pair. The reaction can be written as

$$(DNA)_n + dNTP \leftrightarrow (DNA)_{n+1} + PP_i$$

As DNA polymerase I catalyzes the successive addition of deoxynucleotide units to the 3'-end of the primer, the chain is elongated in the 5' → 3' direction, forming a polynucleotide sequence that runs antiparallel to the template but complementary to it. DNA polymerase I can precede along the template strand, synthesizing a complementary strand of about 20 bases before it dissociates from the template. The degree to which the enzyme remains associated with the template through successive cycles of nucleotide addition is referred to as its processivity.

DNA polymerase I remove the RNA primers set by primase and completes the Okazaki fragments. As there is such a small gap remaining after the action of DNA polymerase I has continued the strand of the Okazaki fragment, ligases is required to fill in the gap. The two ends of the Okazaki fragments are subsequently connected by covalent bonds. Single-strand binding proteins bind to the exposed bases in an effort to counteract their instability and prevent the single-strand DNA from hydrogen-bonding to itself to form dangerous hairpin structures. DNA polymerases contain a 'proofreading' mechanism, commonly referred to as 'exonuclease activity'. This removes nucleotides that have been mistakenly added.

E. *coli* DNA polymerase I is a 109-kD protein consisting of a single polypeptide of 928 amino acid residues. In addition to its 5' → 3' polymerase activity, DNA polymerase I has two other catalytic functions, a 3' → 5' exonuclease (3'-exonuclease) activity and a 5' –› 3' exonuclease (5'-exonuclease) activity. The three distinct catalytic activities of DNA polymerase I reside in separate active sites in the enzyme. As shown by Hans Klenow, the DNA polymerase I polypeptide chain can be cleaved into two fragments by limited proteolysis with subtilisin or trypsin. The smaller fragment (residues 1 through 323) contains the 5'-exonuclease activity, whereas the larger fragment (residues 324 through 928, the so-called Klenow fragment) has the polymerase and 3'-exonuclease activities.

The exonuclease activities of E. *coli* DNA polymerase I serve proofreading and editing functions that enhance the accuracy of DNA replication. The 3'-exonuclease activity removes nucleotides from the 3'-end of the growing chain an action that apparently negates the effects of the polymerase activity. Its purpose, however, is to remove incorrect (mismatched) bases.

(ii) DNA polymerase II: The enzyme is 90 kDa in size and is coded by the polB gene. It has 3'-5' exonuclease activity and involved in repair of damaged DNA. It is unable to replicate long single strands with short complementary primer. Strains of *E. coli* with mutations in polymerase II were found to grow and otherwise behave normally, so the role of this enzyme in the cell is unknown. Pol II has a low error rate but it is too much slow to be of any use in normal DNA synthesis. Pol II differs from Pol I in that it lacks a 5'→3' exonuclease activity, and cannot use a nicked duplex template.

(iii) DNA polymerase III: DNA polymerase III is comprised of two catalytic cores-one for replication of the leading strand and one for the lagging strand. DNA polymerase III, however, cannot stay on the DNA strand long enough to efficiently replicate a daughter strand. Hence, DNA polymerase III stays on the strands via a dimer beta clamp which contains three subunits that come together to enclose the strand. It is the main polymerase in bacteria (elongates in DNA replication); has 3'→5' exonuclease proofreading ability. It is 15 times more active than DNA Pol I and 300 times than DNA Pol II. DNA Polymerase III (pol III) from *E. coli* is a single protein of molecular weight 130 kDa (130,000 grams per mole). It is also referred to as polC, dnaE, or the alpha subunit. DNA pol III works to replicate DNA in the bacterial cell in conjunction with other proteins. This multi-protein complex is referred to as the pol III holoenzyme.

The DNA polymerase III consists of several subunits, among them α, ε, and θ subunits constitute the core polymerase. The major role of other subunits is to keep the enzyme from falling off the template strand. Two β subunits can form a donut-shaped structure to clamp a DNA molecule in its center, and slide with the core polymerase along the DNA molecule. By acting as a sliding clamp, beta helps the holoenzyme to replicate long stretches of DNA without falling off the strand. Pol III holoenzyme directs both leading and lagging strand synthesis simultaneously by virtue of having two polymerase subunits (Fig. 7.6). This allows continuous polymerization of up to 5×10^5 nucleotides. In the absence of β-subunits, the core polymerase would fall off the template strand after synthesizing 10-50 nucleotides.

The α subunit carries out the catalytic polymerase function. The e subunit performs the $3' \to 5'$ exonuclease activity and contributes proofreading ability to the "core" polymerase. The role of subunit θ is unknown. The γ complex is responsible for assembly of the DNA polymerase III holoenzyme complex onto DNA. The γ complex of the holoenzyme acts as a clamp loader by catalyzing the ATP-dependent transfer of a pair of β- subunits to each strand of the DNA template. Epsilon functions as 3'-to-5' exonuclease (editing exonuclease). Theta subunit stimulates 3'-to-5' exonuclease while Tau dimerizes cores and activates DnaB helicase activity. These are sub-assembled in core enzyme.

The beta subunit can be loaded onto DNA by the clamp loader (gamma complex) in an ATP-dependent reaction. Beta cannot be loaded onto linear DNA , covalently closed circular DNA, or single-stranded circular DNA, but it can be loaded onto nicked circles, gapped circles, and primed single-stranded circles; that is, clamp loader requires and recognizes a 3'-hydroxyl-terminus (primer-terminus). Once loaded onto a nicked circle, beta stays associated with the DNA. However, linearization of the nicked circle with a restriction endonuclease releases beta from the DNA; that is, beta is a sliding clamp. It can slide along double-stranded DNA (or DNA-RNA in double-stranded form), but cannot slide on single-stranded DNA or single-stranded DNA coated with SSB.

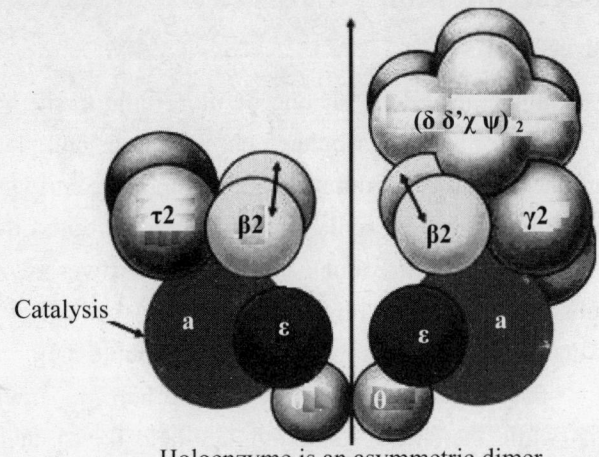

Holoenzyme is an asymmetric dimer

Figure 7.6: DNA polymerase III holoenzyme

(e) Eukaryotic DNA polymerase: Eukaryotic cells contain five DNA polymerases: α, β, γ, δ, and ϵ. Polymerase γ is located in mitochondria and is responsible for replication of mitochondrial DNA. The other four enzymes are located in the nucleus and are therefore candidates for involvement in nuclear DNA replication. Polymerases α, δ, and ϵ are most active in dividing cells, suggesting that they function in replication. In contrast, polymerase β is active in nondividing and dividing cells, indicating that it may function primarily in the repair of DNA damage.

Two types of experiments have provided evidence to the roles of polymerases α, δ, and ϵ in DNA replication. First, replication of the DNAs of some animal viruses, such as SV40, can be studied in cell-free extracts. The ability to study replication *in vitro* has allowed direct identification of the enzymes involved, and analysis of such cell-free systems has shown that polymerases α and δ are required for SV40 DNA replication. Second, polymerases α, δ, and ϵ are found in yeasts as well as in mammalian cells, enabling the use of the powerful approaches of yeast genetics to test their biological roles directly. Such studies indicate that yeast mutants lacking any of these three DNA polymerases are unable to proliferate, implying a critical role for polymerase ϵ as well as for α and δ. However, further studies have shown that the essential function of polymerase ϵ in yeast does not require its activity as a replicative DNA polymerase.

(f) DNA ligase forms new bonds between adjacent nucleotides by forming phosphodiester bond, cooperates with DNA polymerase, repairs single strand nicks in the duplex DNA, joins fragments of DNA in the process of recombination which occurs during genetic transformation and transduction in bacteria.

7.5. Features of DNA Replication

(a) **Replication is Bidirectional**

(b) Replication of DNA molecules begins at one or more unique sites called origin(s) of replication and, except in certain bacteriophage chromosomes and plasmids, proceeds in both directions from the origin. For example, replication of E. coli DNA begins at ori*C*, a unique 245-bp site. From this site, replication advances in both directions around the circular chromosome. That is, bidirectional replication involves two replication forks, which move in opposite directions by unwinding the DNA helix (Fig. 7.7). Semiconservative replication depends on unwinding the DNA double helix to expose single-stranded templates to polymerase action. For a double helix to unwind, it must either rotate about its axis (while the end of its strands are held fixed), or positive supercoils must be introduced, one for each turn of the helix unwound. If the chromosome is circular, as in E. coli, only the latter alternative is available, because DNA replication in E. coli proceeds at a rate approaching 1000 nucleotides per second, and there are about 10 bp per helical turn, the chromosome would accumulate 100 positive supercoils per second, as result the DNA would become too tightly supercoiled to allow unwinding of the strands.

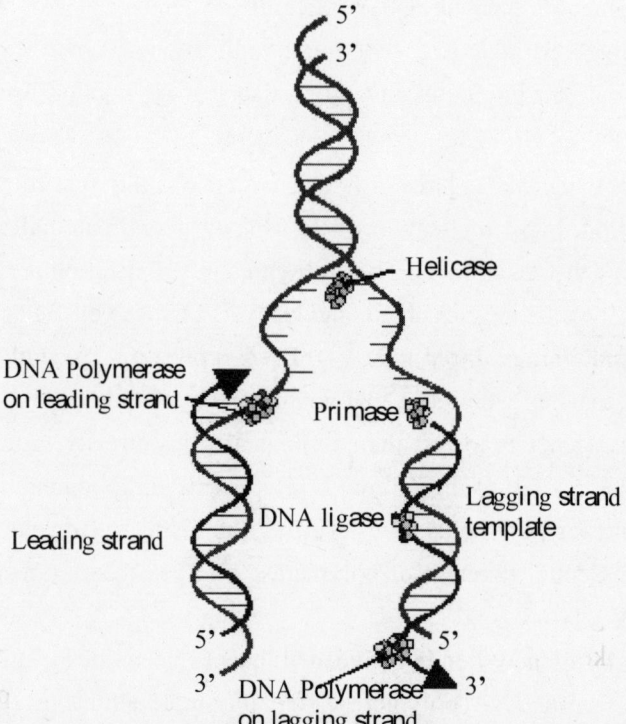

Figure 7.7: DNA replication: formation of leading and lagging strand

DNA gyrase, a Type II topoisomerase, acts to overcome the torsional stress imposed upon unwinding by introducing negative supercoils at the expense of ATP hydrolysis. The unwinding reaction is driven by helicases, a class of proteins that catalyze the ATP-dependent unwinding of DNA double helices. Unlike topoisomerases that alter the linking number of dsDNA through phosphodiester bond breakage and reunion, helicases simply disrupt the hydrogen bonds that hold the two strands of duplex DNA together. A helicase molecule requires a single-stranded region for binding. It then moves along the DNA strand, its translocation coupled to ATP hydrolysis and to strand unwinding. SSB (ssDNA-binding protein), binds to the unwound strands, preventing their re-annealing. At least 10 distinct DNA helicases involved in different aspects of DNA and RNA metabolism have been found in *E. coli* alone.

Unidirectional versus bidirectional replication can be resolved if cells grown several generations in the presence of low amounts of radioactive ^{3}H-thymidine to lightly label the chromosome. They are then exposed briefly to high amount of ^{3}H-thymidine to cause heavy labeling in newly synthesized regions of DNA. If replication is unidirectional, only one advancing replication fork is present and only the DNA adjacent to it should be heavily labeled. If replication is bidirectional, autoradiograms of replicating chromosomes should show two replication forks heavily labeled with radioactive thymidine (Fig. 7.8).

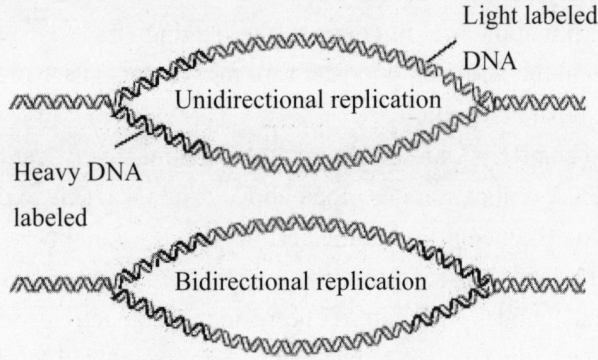

Figure 7.8: Bidirectional replication of the *E. coli* chromosome

(b) Replication is Semi-discontinuous

The autoradiographic results indicate that the two strands of duplex DNA are both replicated at each advancing replication fork by DNA polymerase. DNA polymerase uses ssDNA as a template and makes a complementary strand by polymerizing deoxynucleotides in the order specified by their base-pairing with bases in the template. DNA polymerases synthesize DNA only in a 5' → 3' direction, reading the antiparallel template strand in a 3' → 5' sense. A dilemma arises: How does DNA polymerase copy the parent strand that runs in the 5' → 3' direction at the replication fork? It turns out that the two daughter strands are synthesized in different ways so that replication is semidiscontinuous (Fig. 7.9). As the DNA helix is unwound during its replication, the 3' → 5' strand (as defined by the direction that the replication fork is moving) can be copied continuously by DNA polymerase proceeding in the 5' → 3' direction behind the replication fork. The other parental strand is copied only when a sufficient stretch of its sequence has been exposed for DNA polymerase to move along it in the 5' → 3' mode. Thus, one parental strand is copied continuously to give a newly synthesized copy, the leading strand; the other parental strand is copied in an intermittent, or discontinuous, mode to yield a set of fragments. These fragments are then joined to form an intact lagging strand.

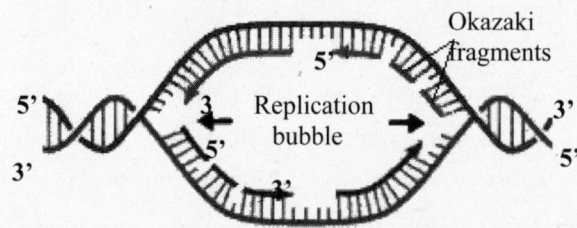

Figure 7.9: The semidiscontinuous model for DNA replication

(c) The Lagging strand is formed from Okazaki fragments

The leading strand is synthesized as one continuous polynucleotide, beginning at the origin and ending at the termination site. In contrast, the lagging strand is synthesized discontinuously in short pieces in the direction opposite fork movement. These pieces of lagging strand are then joined by a separate reaction.

In 1968, Tuneko and Reiji Okazaki provided biochemical verification of the semidiscontinuous pattern of DNA replication described above. The Okazakis exposed a rapidly dividing *E. coli* culture to ^{3}H-labeled thymidine for 30 seconds, quickly collected the cells, and found that half of the label incorporated into nucleic acid appeared in short ssDNA chains just 1000 to 2000 nucleotides in length. (The residual radioactivity was recovered in very large DNA molecules). Subsequent experiments demonstrated that, with time, the newly synthesized short ssDNA Okazaki fragments became covalently joined to form longer polynucleotide chains, in accord with a semidiscontinuous mode of replication. This semidiscontinuous mode of replication has been established with the help of electron micrographs of DNA undergoing replication in eukaryotic cells.

(d) Speed of Replication

The single molecule of DNA that is the *E. coli* genome contains 4.7×10^6 nucleotide pairs. DNA replication begins at a single, fixed location in this molecule, the replication origin, proceeds at about 1000 nucleotides per second, and thus is done in no more than 40 minutes.

The average human chromosome contains 150×10^6 nucleotide pairs which are copied at about 50 base pairs per second. The process would take a month (rather than the hour it actually does) but for the fact that there are many places on the eukaryotic chromosome where replication can begin. Replication begins at some replication origins earlier in S phase than at others, but the process is completed for all by the end of S phase. As replication nears completion, "bubbles" of newly replicated DNA meet and fuse, finally forming two new molecules.

7.6. Prokaryotic Replication

Replication of the prokaryotic chromosome begins at a single replication origin and proceeds bidirectionally until the two replication forks meet. At each replication fork, both leading and lagging strand synthesis are catalyzed by a single multiprotein replication machine, the so-called replisome, which consists of DNA-unwinding proteins; the priming apparatus, or primosome, which is needed to initiate, or prime DNA replication; and DNA polymerase III holoenzyme with two equivalents of "core" polymerase, one for the leading strand and one for the lagging strand. As this replisome follows the replication fork, the template for lagging strand synthesis (the strand running 5' → 3' in the direction of fork movement) must be looped around so that it can be read in the 3' → 5' direction (Fig. 7.10).

(a) Initiation

In the initiation step, origin of replication is unwound, and the partially unwound strands form a replication bubble, with one replication fork on either end. Each group of enzymes at the replication fork (pre-replication complex) moves away from the origin, unwinding and replicating the original DNA strands as they proceed. The pre-replication complex consists of helicase, single-strand binding proteins (SSB) and a primase, which generates an RNA primer to be used in DNA replication.

Replication of the E. *coli* chromosome is initiated at a unique site, *oriC*. Within *oriC* are four 9-bp repeats. DnaA protein, a 52-kD polypeptide, is the initiation factor, which recognizes and binds to these repeats. DnaA protein binding is cooperative; once the four 9-bp repeats are occupied, 20 to 40 additional DnaA monomers bind so that the entire *oriC* region is complexed with DnaA protein. HU, a histone-like protein, prevents nonspecific initiation at sites other than *oriC*. The resulting complex resembles a nucleosome, with negatively supercoiled *oriC* DNA wrapped around a DnaA core. The DnaA protein then mediates the separation of the strands of the DNA duplex by acting on three AT-rich tandem repeats located at the 5'-end of the sequence defining *oriC*.

Formation of this open complex by DnaA protein is ATP-dependent. Next, DnaB protein binds to the open *oriC*. DnaB protein is delivered to *oriC* by DnaC protein, but DnaC protein does not enter the protein assemblage at *oriC*. Delivery of DnaB protein by DnaC protein is assisted by DnaT protein. The addition of DnaB protein completes assembly of the pre-priming complex. ATP hydrolysis drives the formation of this complex. DnaB protein has helicase activity and it further unwinds the DNA in the pre-priming complex in both directions, assisted by DNA gyrase. SSB tetramers coat single-stranded regions as they arise. Unwinding exposes the base sequence of the strands so that RNA primers can be synthesized by primase, and the strands can be read as templates by the replicative polymerase.

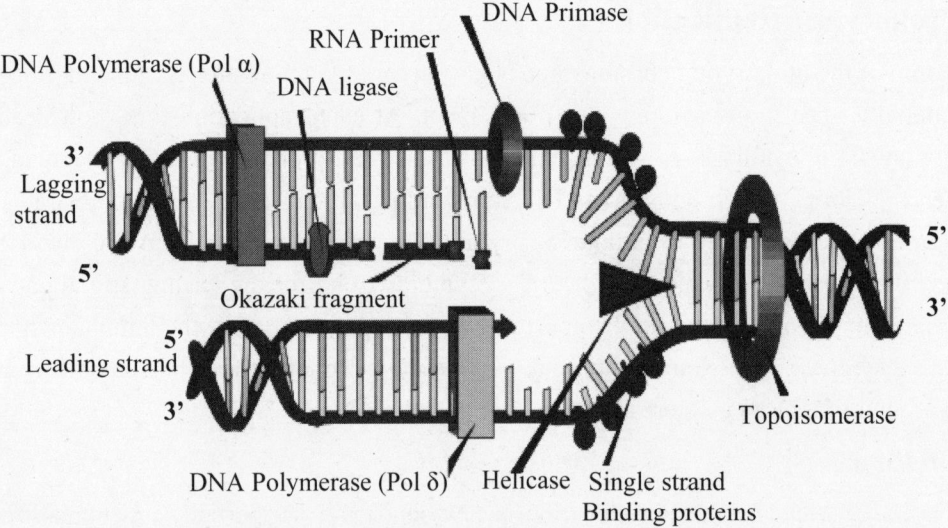

Figure 7.10: Events involved in DNA replication

(b) Elongation

After the helicase unwinds the DNA, single-strand binding protein is used to hold the DNA strands apart. RNA primase is then bound to the starting DNA site. At the beginning of replication, an enzyme called DNA polymerase binds to the RNA primase, which indicates the starting point for the replication. DNA polymerase can only synthesize new DNA from the 5' → 3' (of the new DNA), because of this, the DNA polymerase can only travel on one side of the original strand without any interruption. This original strand, which goes from 3'→5', is called the leading strand. The complement of the leading strand, from 5'→3', is the lagging strand. Each time the helicase unwinds additional DNA, a (potentially) new DNA polymerase needs to be added. As a result, the DNA of the lagging strand is replicated in a piece-meal fashion. Another enzyme, DNA ligase, is used to connect the so-called Okazaki fragments. Coupled leading strand and lagging strand synthesis is achieved by the action of the pol III holoenzyme.

Two "core" DNA polymerase III units are present. One is synthesizing the leading strand, using the parental 3' → 5' strand as template. The other synthesizes the lagging strand using the 5' → 3' parental strand as template. The lagging strand template must be looped out so that it can be copied in the 3' → 5' direction. The "core" pol III on this lagging strand has completed the synthesis of an RNA-primed Okazaki fragment when it encounters the 5'-end of the previous fragment. Synthesis of the next RNA primer by the primosome triggers the γ complex to disassemble the β_2-sliding clamp, releasing the lagging strand from the DNA polymerase III holoenzyme. The γ complex assembles a new β_2-sliding clamp at the 3'-OH end of the next RNA primer, re-attaching the lagging strand "core" polymerase III to begin a new round of lagging strand synthesis (Fig. 7.11).

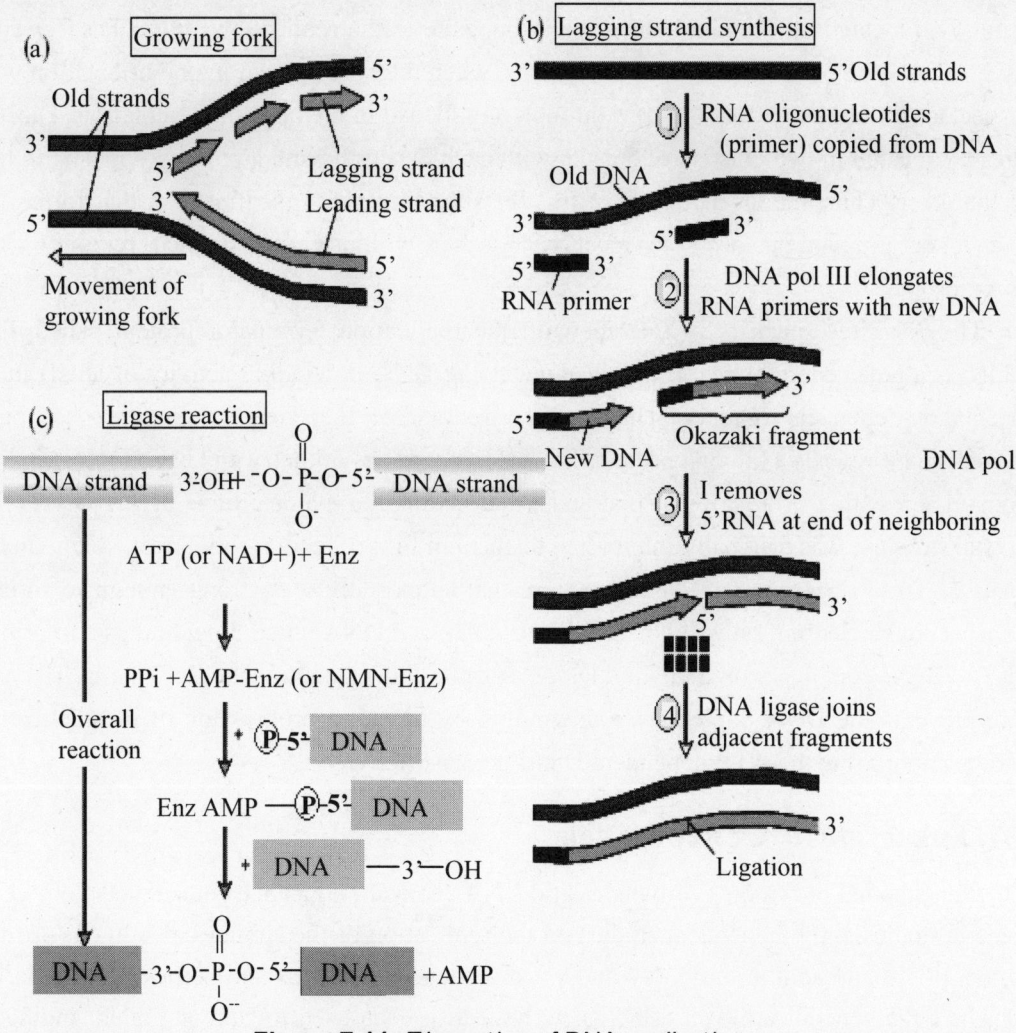

Figure 7.11: *Elongation of DNA replication*

The double helix must be unwound ahead of the advancing replication fork. Unwinding is driven by ATP hydrolysis; DnaB protein has the helicase activity associated with the primosome. DnaB moves in the 5' → 3' direction along the leading strand template, hydrolyzing 2 ATPs for each base pair that it separates. Protein-protein interaction between a *t* subunit of the DNA polymerase III holoenzyme and DnaB is essential for rapid replication fork progression. PriA protein is, like DnaB, a helicase associated with the primosome, but PriA moves 3' → 5' along the lagging strand. The binding of SSB protein to the single-stranded regions created behind these proteins prevents re-annealing.

(c) Termination

Replication termination of prokaryotic and of some eukaryotic chromosomes occurs at specific sequences called replication termini. In *Escherichia coli*, there are 10 replication termini (*Ter*) located in a region diametrically opposite to the replication origin. The *Ter* sites have polarity, i.e., they arrest replication forks, when they are present in one orientation with respect to *ori*, but allow forks to pass through unimpeded in the opposite orientation. The *Ter* sites are located in two clusters of 5 each, with each cluster having a polarity opposite to that of the other. Thus, the arrangement of the *Ter* sites forms a replication trap that forces the two forks, initiated at *oriC*, to meet each other within a well-defined region of the chromosome

The *Ter* sites specifically interact with the replication terminator protein called Tus, which is a polar contrahelicase, i.e., it impedes the DNA unwinding activity of DnaB in an orientation-dependent manner. The crystal structure of the Tus–*Ter* complex has been solved, and it reveals a bilobed protein that has structural asymmetry and has a DNA-binding domain, consisting of a series of β-strands, that invade the major groove of *Ter* DNA. The crystal structure was originally interpreted to account for replication fork arrest, solely on the basis of Tus–*Ter*, protein–DNA interaction, that supposedly was strong enough to form a nonspecific barrier, not only to DnaB helicase-catalyzed DNA unwinding, but also, in principle, to any protein that would unwind DNA. Tus protein is a contrahelicase. That is, Tus protein prevents the DNA duplex from unwinding by blocking progression of the replication fork and inhibiting the ATP-dependent DnaB helicase activity.

7.7. Eukaryotic DNA Replication

The fundamental enzymology of eukaryotic DNA replication has been elucidated from yeast genetic studies and biochemical studies on the replication of the simian virus 40 (SV40) genome *in vitro*. In addition to SV40 and yeast models, adenovirus and herpes simplex virus, of which the genetics are well established, have also been used to gain an understanding of the protein machinery that functions at the replication fork during duplication of cellular DNA in eukaryotes.

DNA replication requires the coordinated action of several proteins and enzymes to ensure efficient and accurate duplication of the genome. DNA replication is initiated from chromosomal sites termed origins, where two replication forks are established which proceed in opposite directions until the next replication unit is reached. At least two DNA polymerases, Pols α and δ, function at the replication fork. Processive DNA synthesis is guaranteed by their accessory proteins: proliferating cell nuclear antigen (PCNA), which forms a clamp structure around DNA, and a clamp-loader protein, replication factor C (RFC). DNA primase, single stranded DNA binding protein RPA (replication protein A), DNA topoisomerases, DNA helicases, RNase H, DNA ligases, and other factors are needed for efficient replication of the genome. The structure of these proteins appears to be conserved in all the eukaryotic organisms analyzed so far, and their function in DNA replication has been established by reconstitution experiments *in vitro* with purified proteins.

The mechanism of DNA replication in eukaryotic cells shows strong parallels with prokaryotic DNA replication, but the situation in eukaryotes is vastly more complex. For example, in a growing human cell, some 6 billion bp of DNA must be duplicated with high fidelity once in each cell cycle. The events associated with cell growth and division in eukaryotic cells fall into a general sequence having four distinct phases, M, G_1, S, and G_2 .Eukaryotic cells have solved the problem of replicating their enormous genomes in the few hours allotted to the S phase by initiating DNA replication at multiple origins of replication distributed along each chromosome. Depending on the organism and cell type, replication origins, also called replicators, occur every 3 to 300 kbp (for example, an average human chromosome has several hundred replication origins). In lower eukaryotes such as yeast, replicators are small discrete chromosomal regions (100-200 bp), but in mammalian chromosomes, the zones where initiation of DNA replication occurs may span 500 to 50,000 bp. So that eukaryotic DNA replication can proceed concomitantly throughout the genome, each eukaryotic chromosome contains many units of replication, so-called replicons.

(a) Initiation of eukaryotic DNA replication

Saccharomyces cerevisiae is an excellent model system to study the initiation of chromosome replication, since the origins exist as short, well-defined sequences of about 150 bp. These origins, termed autonomously replicating sequences (ARSs). In mammalian cells the replication origin apparently consists of a large chromosomal region permissive for initiation, within which some regions are more frequently used than others.

DNA synthesis is initiated by the binding of initiator proteins to the origins of replication. In *S. cerevisiae* a multi-subunit protein called the origin recognition complex (ORC) binds specifically to ARS sequences. This complex consists of six proteins, Orc1p-Orc 6p, which are all essential for viability and initiation of DNA replication. In *S. cerevisiae*, the ORC complex is bound to origins in all stages of the cell cycle and forms the core of the origin complex to which other components are loaded in a step-wise manner.

The binding of Cdc6 protein to the ORC is essential for the next step in initiation, which is loading of MCM (mini chromosome maintenance) proteins onto origins. A complex of ORC, Cdc6 and MCMs forms a pre-replicative complex called the pre-RC, which is established at the end of mitosis, after separation of sister chromatids. Recently, a novel loading factor for MCM proteins, Cdt1, was identified in both *S. pombe* and *Xenopus*, which appears to function co-ordinately with Cdc6. At the onset of S-phase, the pre-RC has to be converted into an initiation complex that leads to initiation of DNA synthesis. This activation of pre-RC is accomplished by the action of S-phase specific cyclin-dependent kinases (CDKs) and Dbf4-dependent kinases (DDKs), which activate the firing of replication origins.

(b) Assembly of replicative complexes on to origins

Initiation requires a stepwise association of proteins with replication origins before DNA synthesis can begin. The origin recognition complex (ORC) binds to DNA and provides a site on the chromosome where additional replication factors can associate (Fig. 7.12). An early step leading to initiation, called licensing or pre-replicative complex formation, involves the association of Mcm2-7 complex with DNA at ORC, in a process requiring Cdt1 and Cdc6. Mcm2-7 proteins provide helicase activity for DNA synthesis and loading of these proteins confers competence on the origin to fire in S phase. Onset of DNA synthesis requires the action of two protein kinases (cyclin dependent kinase (CDK) and Cdc7), which trigger the association of additional proteins with the origin, such as Cdc45 and GINS (Go, Ichi, Nii, and San; five, one, two, and three in Japanese). During the process of initiation, DNA polymerases are also recruited and DNA synthesis starts. During replication, Mcm2-7 proteins move away from the origin and further assembly of pre-replicative complexes is blocked. This ensures that origins can only fire a single time per cell cycle.

In the conversion of the pre-RC complex into an initiation complex, Cdc6 and MCM proteins are released from the pre-RC complex and DNA polymerases are recruited onto origins to assemble a replicative complex. This assembly process takes place in a step-wise manner and the loading of Cdc45 is required for the loading of other replication proteins, such as the eukaryotic single-stranded DNA binding protein RPA. The ability of RPA to bind single-stranded DNA is essential for the first step of DNA replication, unwinding of

DNA at the origin of DNA replication. RPA binding precedes loading of Pol α-primase and Pol α is bound after origin unwinding. Recruitment of DNA polymerases onto origins is also controlled by the Dpb11 protein, which apparently associates with the origins after the pre-RC assembly, since loading of Dpb11 is dependent on MCM and RPA. Loading of Pol α and Pol ε onto replication origins is dependent on Dpb11, suggesting that the association of Dpb11 with origins is a prerequisite for the assembly of a replicative complex in order to initiate cellular DNA replication.

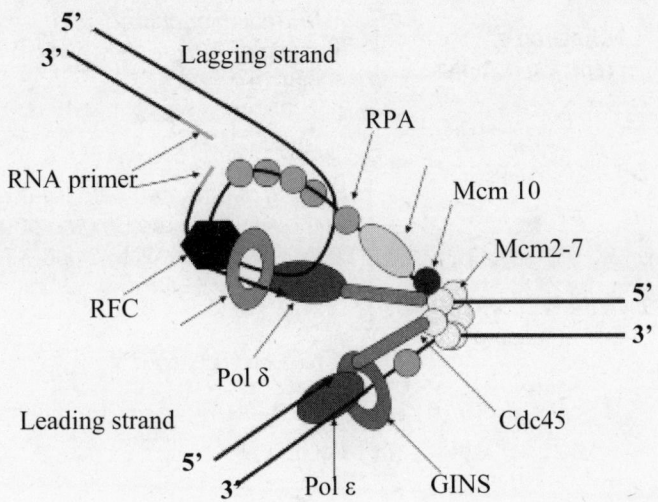

Figure 7.12: SV40 DNA replication *in vitro* as a model of the eukaryotic replication fork

(c) Elongation

The elongation process is different for the 5'-3' and 3'-5' template. The 3'-5' proceeding daughter strand that uses a 5'-3' template- is called leading strand because DNA polymerase delta can read the template and continuously adds nucleotides complementary to the nucleotides of the template.

Lagging strand synthesis of Okazaki fragments is initiated in essentially the same way as leading strand synthesis: synthesis is primed by DNA polymerase α, a deoxynucleotide stretch is added by DNA polymerase α, and then switching to DNA polymerase δ takes place. Priming is a frequent event in lagging strand synthesis, with RNA primers placed every 50 or so nucleotides. About 10-nucleotide lengths of RNA primer are extended through addition of 10 to 20 deoxynucleotides by DNA polymerase α before DNA polymerase δ (or ε) enters. All but one of the ribonucleotides in the RNA primer are removed by RNase H1; then the exonuclease activity of the FEN1/RTH1 complex removes the one remaining ribonucleotide, and DNA ligase joins the Okazaki fragment to the growing DNA strand. Each new double helix is consisted of one old and one new chain. This is what we call semi-conservative replication (Fig. 7.13).

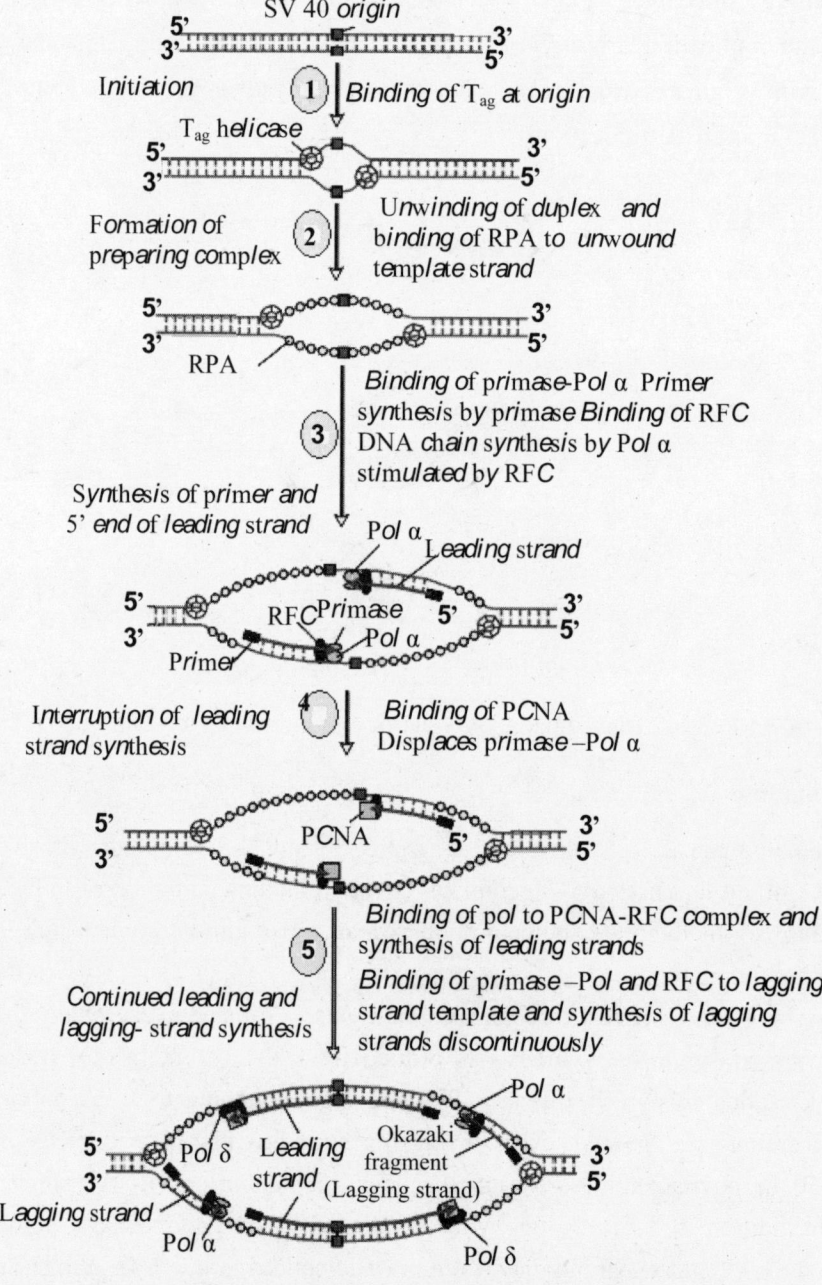

Figure 7.13: Events involved in eukaryotic replication

(d) Termination

The last step of DNA replication is the termination. This process happens when the DNA polymerase reaches to an end of the strands. In the last section of the lagging strand, when the RNA primer is removed, it is not possible for the DNA polymerase to seal the gap (because there is no primer). So, the end of the parental strand where the last primer binds isn't replicated. These ends of linear (chromosomal) DNA consist of noncoding DNA that contains repeat sequences and are called telomeres. As a result, a part of the telomere is removed in every cycle of DNA replication. The DNA replication is not completed before a mechanism of repair fixes possible errors caused during the replication. Enzymes like nucleases remove the wrong nucleotides and the DNA polymerase fills the gaps.

7.8. Replicating the ends of Chromosomes—Telomeres and Telomerase

Telomeres are short (5-8 bp), tandemly repeated, G-rich nucleotide sequences that form protective caps 1-12 kbp long on the ends of chromosomes. Vertebrate telomeres have a TTAGGG consensus sequence. Telomeres are necessary for chromosome maintenance and stability. DNA polymerases cannot replicate the extreme 5'-ends of chromosomes because these enzymes require a template and a primer and replicate only in the 5' → 3' direction. Thus, lagging strand synthesis at the 3'-ends of chromosomes is primed by RNA primase to form Okazaki fragments, but these RNA primers are subsequently removed, resulting in gaps in the progeny 5'-terminal strands at each end of the chromosome. Telomerase, an RNA-dependent DNA polymerase (126 kD) whose catalytic subunit show substantial homology to other reverse transcriptases, maintains telomere length by restoring telomeres at the 3'-ends of chromosomes. Telomerase is a ribonucleoprotein, and its RNA component contains a 9- to 30-nucleotide-long region that serves as a template for the synthesis of telomeric repeats at DNA ends. The telomerase contains an essential RNA component which is complementary to the telomere repeat sequence. Hence, the internal RNA can serve as the template for synthesizing DNA. Through telomerase translocation, a telomere may be extended by many repeats. The human telomerase RNA component is 450 nucleotides long; its template sequence is CUAACCCUAAC. Telomerase uses the 3'-end of the DNA as a primer and adds successive TTAGGG repeats to it, employing its RNA as template over and over again. Bacteria do not have the end-replication problem, because its DNA is circular. In eukaryotes, telomeres help to protect chromosomes from fusing with each other and to solve the end-replication problem. In the absence of telomerase, the telomere will become shorter after each cell division. When it reaches a certain length, the cell may cease to divide and die. Therefore, telomerase plays a critical role in the aging process.

When the polymerase reaches the end of replication, there is another problem due to the antiparallel structure. The RNA primer on the leading strand occupies a small portion of the

DNA, which is not exposed to polymerase and therefore is not copied. As a result, there would be a gap on the newly duplicated DNA at the original leading strand on the 5' end of non-circular (viz. eukaryotic) chromosomes. The sticking out 3' end consists of noncoding DNA called the telomere, which can be simply cut off (Fig. 7.14). Before the DNA replication is finally complete, enzymes are used to proofread the sequences to make sure the nucleotides are paired up correctly. If mistake or damage occurs, an enzyme called nuclease will remove the incorrect DNA. DNA polymerase will then fill in the gap.

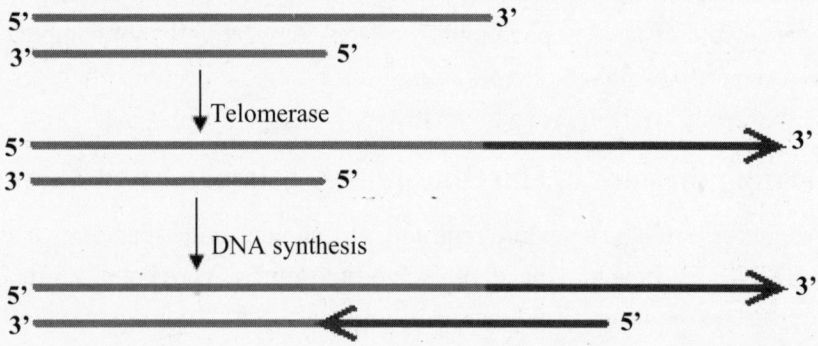

Figure 7.14: Telomerase and telomere extension. To extend the length of a telomere, the telomerase first extends its longer strand. Then, using the same mechanism as synthesizing the lagging strand, the shorter strand is extended

7.9. Post-replicative Modification of DNA: Methylation

One of the major post-replicative reactions that modify the DNA is methylation. DNA methylation is universal in bacteria, plant, and animal. DNA methylation is a type of chemical modification of DNA that are stable over rounds of cell division but do not involve changes in the underlying DNA sequence of the organism. Chromatin and DNA modifications are two important features of Epigenetics and play a role in the process of cellular differentiation, allowing cells to stably maintain different characteristics despite containing the same genomic material. However, the DNA methylation level is dynamic over the course of development in multicellular organisms.

Methylation of DNA in prokaryotic cells also occurs. The function of this methylation is to prevent degradation of host DNA in the presence of enzymatic activities synthesized by bacteria called restriction endonucleases. In prokaryotic organisms, DNA methylation occurs at the number 5 carbon of the cytosine pyrimidine ring and the number 6 nitrogen of the adenine purine ring. However, in eukaryotic organisms DNA methylation occurs only at the number 5 carbon of the cytosine pyrimidine ring. In mammalian, DNA methylation occurs most at the number 5 carbon of the cytosine of a CpG dinucleotide. "CpG" is shorthand for

"—C—phosphate —G—", that is, cytosine and guanine separated by a phosphate, which links the two nucleosides together in DNA.

The role of methylation in eukaryotic DNA serves two clearly defined and overlapping functions. The methylation of CpG dinucleotides affects the overall structure of chromatin which in turn broadly alters the availability of the chromatin to the transcriptional machinery. This effect of methylation is one mechanism of epigenesis. Epigenetics is defined as the study of the mechanism that produces phenotypic effects from gene activity during differentiation and development, or heritable changes in gene expression that do not involve changes in gene sequence.

CpG dinucleotide is only 1% in human genome, which is great fewer than expected. Between 70-80% of all CpGs are methylated. Unmethylated CpGs are grouped in clusters called "CpG islands" that are present in the 5' regulatory regions of many genes. In many disease processes such as cancer, gene promoter CpG islands acquire abnormal hypermethylation, which results in heritable transcriptional silencing. DNA methylation may impact the transcription of genes in two ways. First, the methylation of DNA may itself physically impede the binding of transcriptional proteins to the gene, thus blocking transcription. Second, and likely more important, methylated DNA may be bound by proteins known as Methyl-CpG-binding domain proteins (MBDs). MBD proteins then recruit additional proteins to the locus, such as histone deacetylases and other chromatin remodelling proteins that can modify histones, thereby forming compact, inactive chromatin termed silent chromatin. This link between DNA methylation and chromatin structure is very important. In particular, loss of Methyl-CpG-binding Protein 2 (MeCP2) has been implicated in Rett syndrome and Methyl-CpG binding domain protein 2 (MBD2) mediates the transcriptional silencing of hypermethylated genes in cancer.

7.10. Mutations

A mutation is a permanent change in the DNA sequence of a gene. Since the DNA sequence is interpreted in groups of three nucleotide bases, called codons. Each codon specifies a single amino acid in a protein. Mutations in a gene's DNA sequence can alter the amino acid sequence of the protein encoded by the gene.

(a) Substitution

In the substitution mutation, one or more nucleotides are substituted by the same number of different nucleotides. In most cases, only one nucleotide is changed. Based on the change in the nucleotide type, the substitution mutation may be divided into transition and transversion mutations. Based on the consequence of mutation, the substitution mutation may be grouped into silent, missense and nonsense mutations (Fig. 7.15).

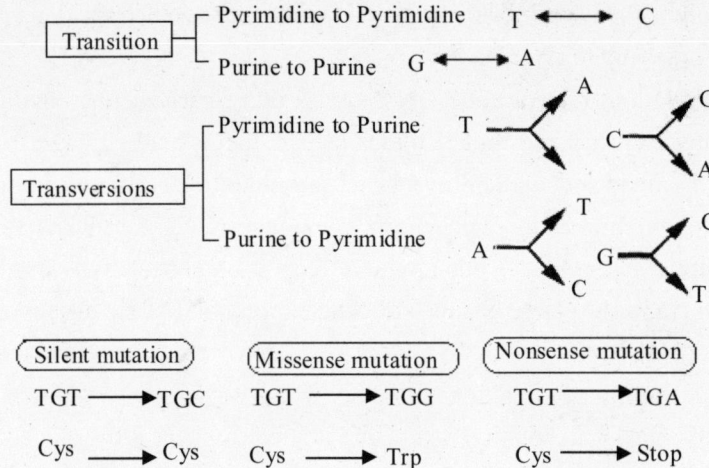

Figure 7.15: The substitution mutation : (a) Illustration of transition and transversion mutations. In the transition mutation, a pyrimidine (C or T) is substituted by another pyrimidine, or a purine (A or G) is substituted by another purine. The transversion mutation involves the change from a pyrimidine to a purine, or vice versa

(b) Deletion

The deletion mutation involves elimination of one or more nucleotides from a DNA sequence. It may cause frame shift, producing a non-functional protein (Fig. 7.16).

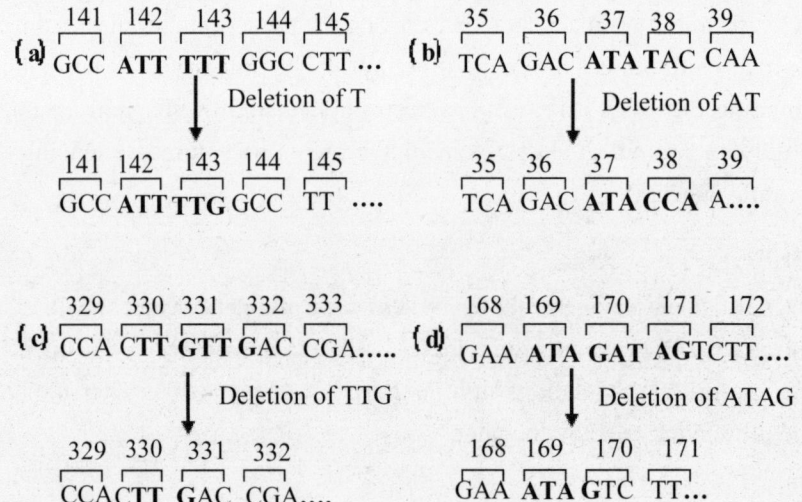

Figure 7.16: Real examples of deletion mutations which cause diseases

(a) Deletion of "T" from the sequence "TTTTT" in the *CFTR* gene.
(b) Deletion of "AT" from the sequence "ATAT" in the *CFTR* gene.
(c) Deletion of "TTG" from the sequence "TTGTTG" in the *FIX* gene.
(d) Deletion of "ATAG" from the sequence "ATAGATAG" in the AP*C* gene.

(c) Insertion

In the insertion mutation, one or more nucleotides are inserted into a sequence. If the number of inserted bases is not a multiple of 3, it will cause frame shift, resulting in serious consequences (Fig 7.17). As shown in the following Table 7.2, non-frame shift insertions may also cause diseases.

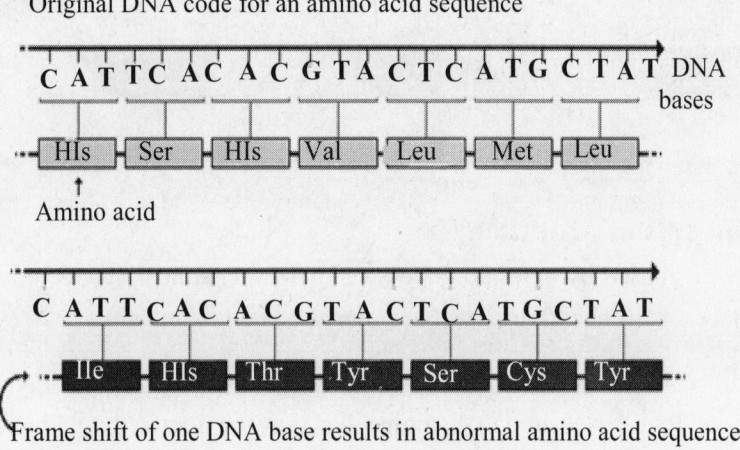

Figure 7.17: Frame shift mutation: A frame shift mutation changes the amino acid sequence from the site of the mutation

Table 7.2: Examples of diseases caused by insertion mutation

Disease	Gene Location	Repeat Sequence	Normal Repeat Number	Mutated Repeat Number
Huntington Disease	4p 16.3	CAG	9-35	37-100
Kennedy Diseases	Xq21	CAG	17-24	40-55
SCA1	6p23	CAG	19-36	43-81
DRPLA	12p	CAG	7-23	> 49
Fragile X site A	Xq27.3	CGG	6-54	> 200

(d) Exon skipping

Splicing of an intron requires an essential signal: "GT........AG". If the splice acceptor site AG is mutated (e.g., A to C in this figure), the splicing machinery will look for the next acceptor site. As a result, the exon between two introns is also removed (Fig. 7.18).

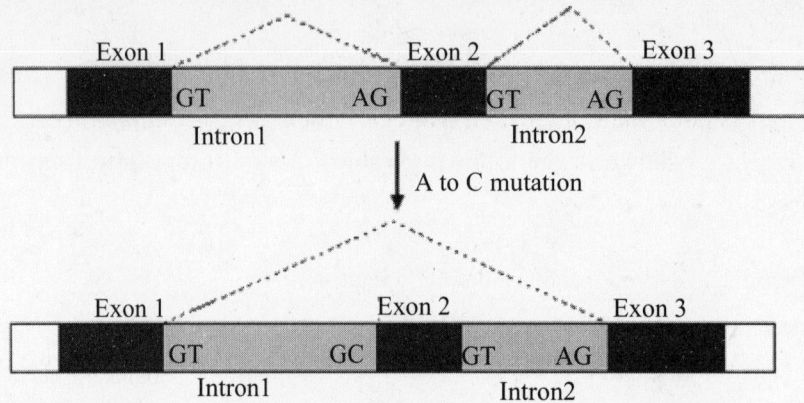

Figure 7.18: Example of exon skipping

7.11. Mechanisms of Mutation

Mutations may be caused by external factors (UV light, chemical agents, etc.) or spontaneous cellular processes (replication errors, accidental deamination, etc).

(a) Deamination

Cytosine, one of four bases in DNA molecules may be mutated to uracil by deamination. Since uracil is not part of DNA, this mutation can easily be detected and repaired by base excision. Suppose DNA, like RNA was made up of uracil, then the cytosine to uracil mutation could be corrected only by mismatch repair which is very inefficient. This may explain why DNA chooses thymine, instead of uracil, even though the chemical structure of uracil is simpler than thymine (Fig. 7.19).

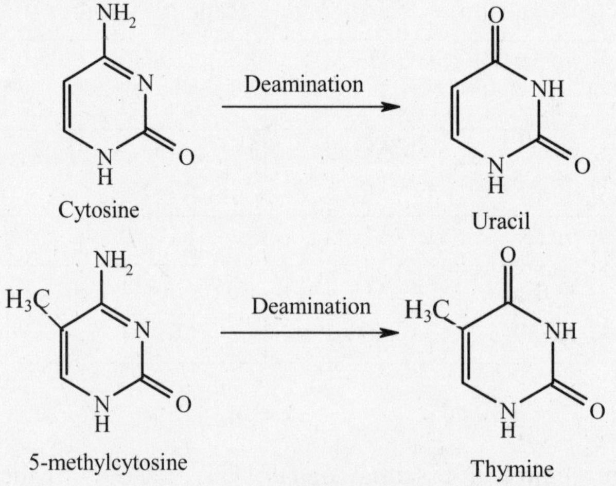

Cytosine →(Deamination)→ Uracil

5-methylcytosine →(Deamination)→ Thymine

Figure 7.19: Examples of deamination which involves the removal of an amino group. Accidental deamination may change the cytosine to uracil, or the methylated cytosine to thymine

(b) Mutation by UV light

UV light may cause two adjacent pyrimidine residues (cytosine or thymine) to form a dimer. In a normal cell, the dimer can be detected by p53, which then triggers the repairing process. However, if p53 itself is mutated and become non-functional, the pyrimidine dimer may lead to mutation (Fig. 7.20).

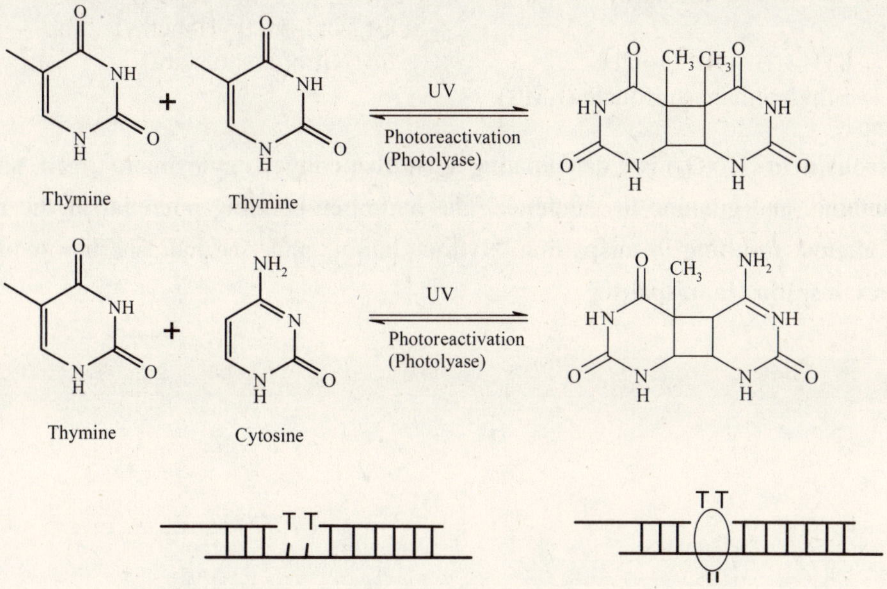

Figure 7.20: Pyrimidine dimmer induced by UV light

(c) Mutation by Chemical Agents

The chemical agents which may cause mutation are called mutagens. Most of them are also carcinogens. The following figure shows the chemical structures of a few potent mutagens.

(i) Acridines (e.g., proflavin) are positively charged molecules. They may be inserted between two DNA strands, thereby altering DNA's structure and rigidity. As a result, DNA replication will not be faithful.

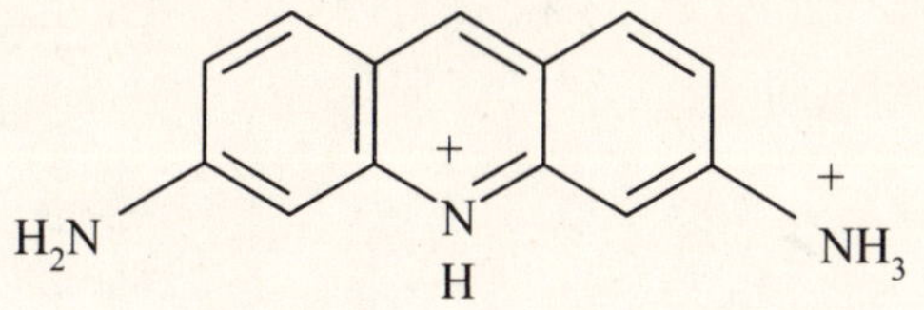

2,8-Diamino acridine (Proflavin)

(ii) Alkylating agents are chemicals that add an alkyl group (C_nH_{2n+1}) to another molecule. Alkylation of a base may change the normal base pairing. For example, the alkylating agent ethylmethanesulphonate (EMS) converts guanine to 7-ethylguanine which pairs with thymine. The mispairing will lead to mutation. Some alkylating agents may also cross-link DNA, resulting in chromosome breaks.

$Cl\text{-}CH_2\text{-}CH_2\text{-}S\text{-}CH_2\text{-}CH_2\text{-}Cl$
Di-(2-chloroethyl) sulfide
(Sulfer mustard)

CH_3
|
$Cl\text{-}CH_2\text{-}CH_2\text{-}N\text{-}CH_2\text{-}CH_2\text{-}Cl$
Di-(2-chloroethyl) methylamine
(Nitrogen mustard)

$CH_3\text{-}CH_2\text{-}O\text{-}\text{-}SO_2\text{-}CH_3$
Ethylmethane sulfonate (EMS)

(iii) Nitrous acid (HNO_2) is a deaminating agent that converts cytosine to uracil, adenine to hypoxanthine, and guanine to xanthine. The hydrogen-bonding potential of the modified base is altered, resulting in mispairing. Hydroxylamine and free radicals may modify base structures, resulting in mispairing

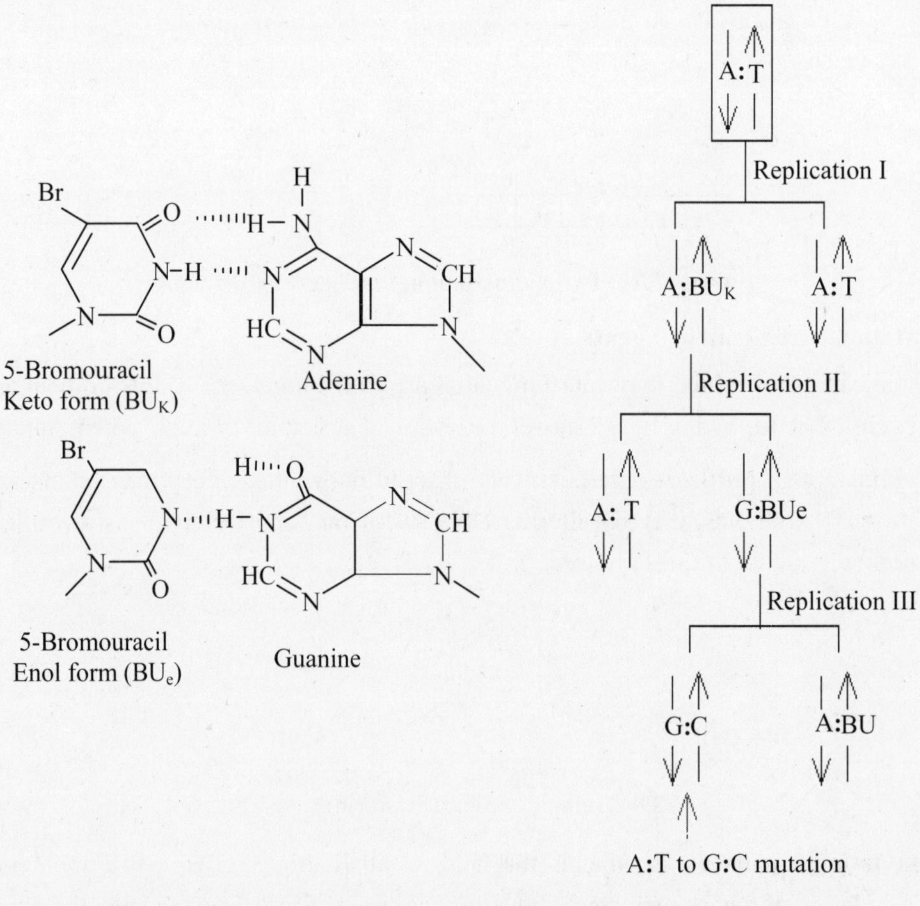

Figure 7.21: Mechanism of mutation induced by 5-bromouracil

5-bromouracil molecule has two tautomeric isoforms. Its keto form (BU_k) pairs with adenine whereas its enol form (BU_e) pairs with guanine. Suppose in the first replication the keto form was incorporated into a new DNA strand. During the second replication, if the keto form undergoes a tautomeric shift to the enol form, it will cause A: T to G: C mutation (Fig. 7.21).

(d) Mutation by Replication Errors

Replication errors are the main source of mutations. It has been estimated that uncorrected replication errors occur with a frequency of 10^{-9} - 10^{-11} for each nucleotide added by DNA polymerases (Fig. 7.22). Since a cell division requires synthesis of 6×10^9 nucleotides, the mutation rate is about one per cell division.

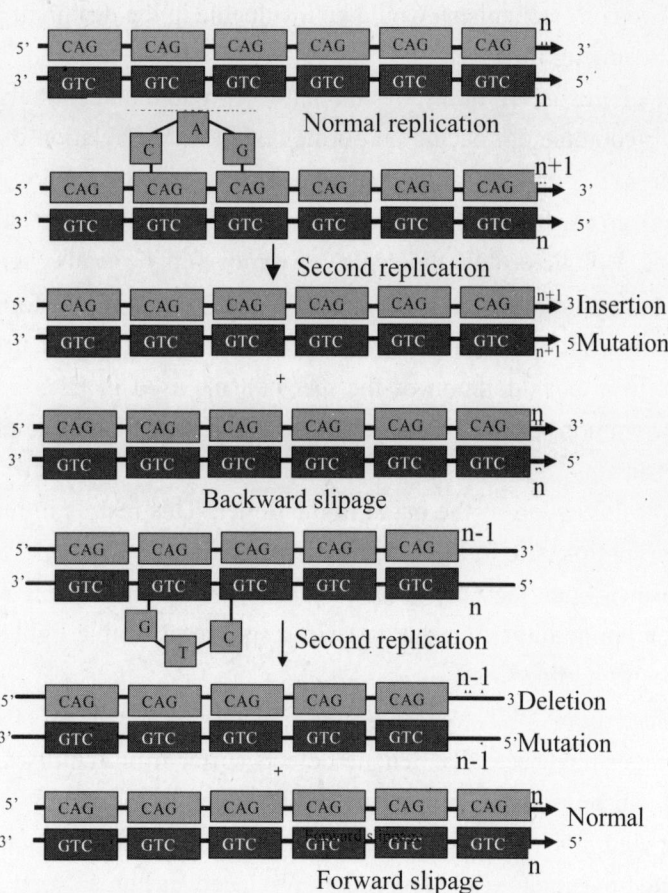

Figure 7.22: The mutation caused by replication slippage. In this figure, mispairing involves only one repeat. In fact, the slippage could cause several repeats to become unpaired. **(a)** Normal replication. **(b)** Backward slippage, resulting in the insertion mutation. **(c)** Forward slippage, resulting in the deletion mutation

A commonly observed replication error is the replication slippage, which occurs at the repetitive sequences when the new strand mispairs with the template strand. The microsatellite polymorphism is mainly caused by the replication slippage. If the mutation occurs in a coding region, it could produce abnormal proteins, leading to diseases. The Huntington's disease is a well known example.

7.12. DNA Repair Mechanisms

Deoxyribonucleic acid (DNA) can be damaged by a variety of factors and this damage must be repaired quickly and efficiently to sustain the integrity of the genome. Cancer, in most non-viral induced cases, is the severe medically relevant consequence of the inability to repair damaged DNA. It is clear that multiple somatic cell mutations in DNA can lead to the genesis of the transformed phenotype. Therefore, it should be obvious that complete understanding of DNA repair mechanisms would be invaluable in the design of potential therapeutic agents in the treatment of cancer.

Modification of the DNA bases by alkylation (predominately the incorporation of – $CHCH_3$ groups) predominately occurs on purine residues. Methylation of G residues allows them to base pair with T instead of C. A unique activity called O^6-alkylguanine transferase removes the alkyl group from G residues. The protein itself becomes alkylated and is no longer active, thus, a single protein molecule can remove only one alkyl group.

The prominent by-product from UV irradiation of DNA is the formation of thymine dimers. These form from two adjacent T residues in the DNA. Repair of thymine dimers is most understood from consideration of the mechanisms used in E. coli. However, several mechanisms are common to both prokaryotes and eukaryotes. Thymine dimers are removed by several mechanisms. Specific glycohydrolases recognize the dimer as abnormal and cleave the N-glycosidic bond of the bases in the dimer. This results in the base leaving and generates an apyrimidinic site in the DNA. This is repaired by DNA polymerase and ligase. Another, widely distributed activity is DNA photolyase or photoreactivating enzyme. This protein binds to thymine dimers in the dark. In response to visible light stimulation the enzyme cleaves the pyrimidine rings.

Humans defective in DNA repair, (in particular the repair of UV-induced thymine dimers), due to autosomal recessive genetic defects suffer from the disease Xeroderma pigmentosum (XP). Nucleotide excision repair (NER) involves the removal of a wide array of structurally unrelated DNA lesions including cyclobutane thymine dimers, other pyrimidine dimers, pyrimidine-pyrimidone photoproducts produced in human skin by shortwave UV, and helix-distorting chemical adducts induced by carcinogens.

In addition to DNA polymerase 3'→5' exonuclease proof-reading at the replicating fork, mammalian cells utilize five major DNA repair pathways: Homologous recombination

(HRR); Non homologous End Joining (NHEJ); Nucleotide Excision Repair (NER); Base Excision Repair (BER) and Mismatch repair (MMR). There are three major DNA repairing mechanisms: base excision, nucleotide excision and mismatch repair.

(a) Base excision

Deamination or alkylation may leads to modification or damage of DNA's bases. The position of the modified (damaged) base is called the "abasic site" or "AP site (apurinic/apyrimidinic site) ". In *E. coli*, the DNA glycosylase can recognize the AP site and remove its base. Then, the AP endonuclease removes the AP site and neighboring nucleotides. The gap is filled by DNA polymerase I and DNA ligase. The enzymes DNA glycosylase, DNA polymerase beta, and DNA ligase are capable of removing, inserting, and patching the DNA strand, respectively, in the event of oxidative damage. A common point mutation is the alteration of cytosine to thymine by the addition of a methyl group followed by deamination. DNA glycosylase actually belong to a family of several proteins that recognize specific mutations, with a number that are specific for uracil recognition and removal. Mutations in the genes of the base excision pathway have been associated with accumulated DNA damage and the occurrence of some cancers (Fig. 7.23).

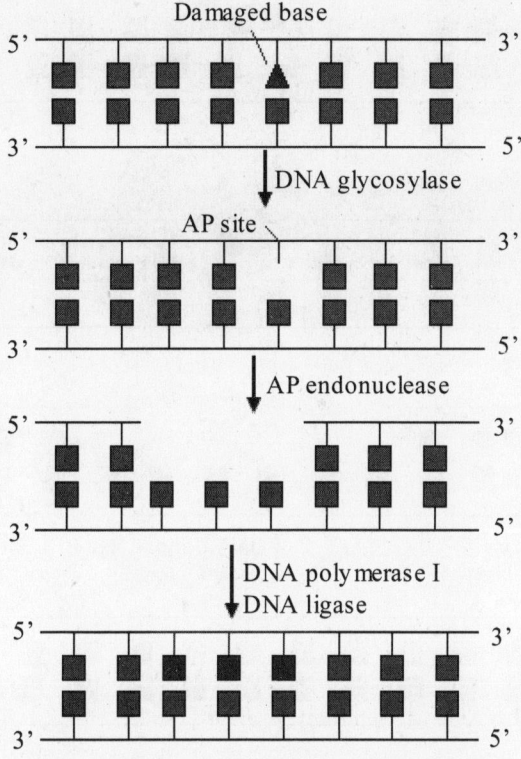

Figure 7.23: DNA repair by base excision

(b) Nucleotide excision

Nucleotide excision repair system removes a patch of nucleotides that includes the damaged base and proceeds rapidly in cells actively undergoing transcription. An important gene in this process is *XP* (Xeroderma Pigmentosum), which is also the name of a rare genetic disorder caused by an impaired repair process.

Repair has been linked to RNA polymerase II, the enzyme that builds the RNA strand during transcription. This indicated that there is potential for correcting errors as the transcription machinery runs into chemically altered bases that are not binding correctly. In this context, nucleotide excision allows transcription to correct the code before mutations occur. The entire process requires approximately 20 genes. The various steps involved in nucleotide excision repair consists of recognition of the damaged base, and the damaged nucleotide(s) will be removed by making incisions on the damaged strand on both sides of the lesion. A patch will be synthesized by DNA polymerase using the other strand as a template and DNA ligase seals off any remaining cut via ligation (Fig. 7. 24).

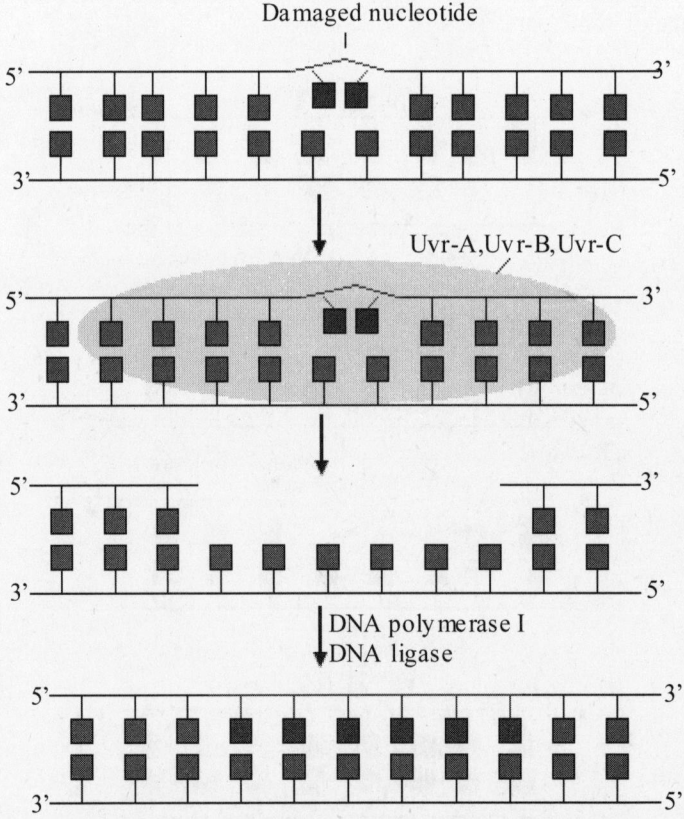

Figure 7.24: DNA repair by nucleotide excision

Mismatch repair

The insertion of a wrong nucleotide by the replication machinery results in mismatched base pairs. Repair of the mismatch requires recognition and removal of the wrongly inserted base. The mismatch repair mechanism was first seen and studied in *E. coli*. If the cell does not correct mismatches, future generations of DNA will have the mutation incorporated, possibly altering the protein product and cell function.

Mismatch repair involves a protein encoded by the MSH genes recognizes mismatched bases. An enzyme encoded by the MLH (or PMS) genes takes the lead in removing the base. The DNA is then patched by DNA polymerase in a process similar to DNA replication (Fig. 7.25). Mutations in these genes have been associated with colon cancer

To repair mismatched bases, the system has to know which base is the correct one. In *E. coli*, this is achieved by a special methylase called the "Dam methylase", which can methylate all adenines that occur within (5')GATC sequences. Immediately after DNA replication, the template strand has been methylated, but the newly synthesized strand is not methylated yet. Thus, the template strand and the new strand can be distinguished.

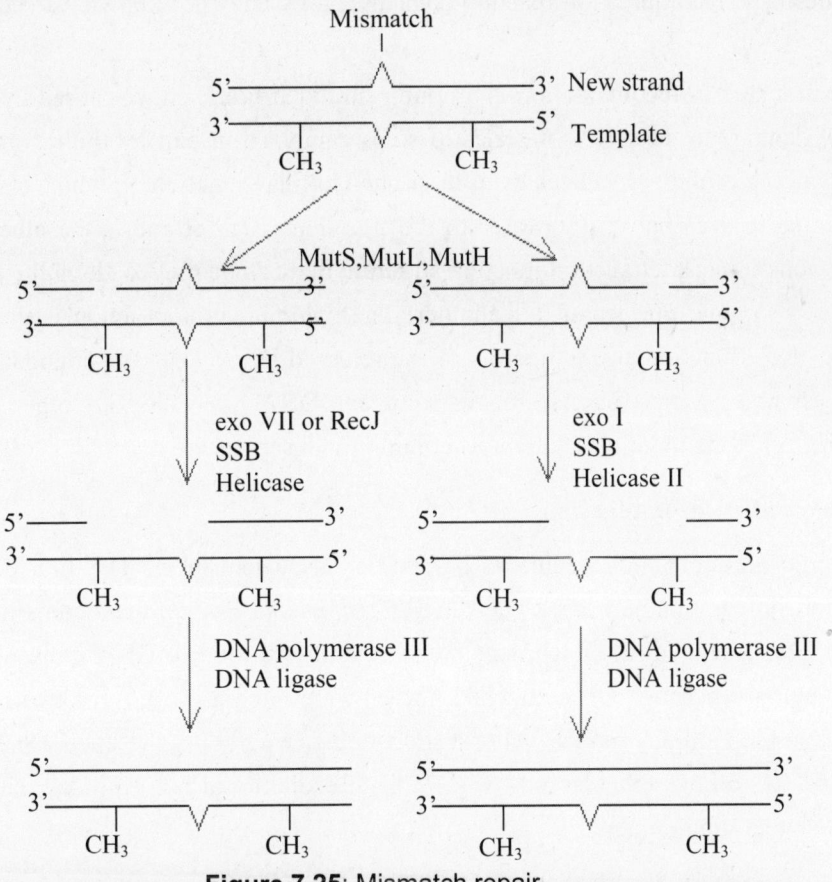

Figure 7.25: Mismatch repair

7.13. DNA Recombination

A DNA helix usually does not interact with other segments of DNA, and in human cells the different chromosomes even occupy separate areas in the nucleus called "chromosome territories". This physical separation of different chromosomes is important for the ability of DNA to function as a stable repository for information, as one of the few times chromosomes interact during chromosomal crossover when they recombine. Chromosomal crossover is when two DNA helices break, swap a section and then rejoin.

Recombination allows chromosomes to exchange genetic information and produces new combinations of genes, which increases the efficiency of natural selection and can be important in the rapid evolution of new proteins. Genetic recombination can also be involved in DNA repair, particularly in the cell's response to double-strand breaks.

The most common form of chromosomal crossover is homologous recombination, where the two chromosomes involved share very similar sequences. Non-homologous recombination can be damaging to cells, as it can produce chromosomal translocations and genetic abnormalities. The recombination reaction is catalyzed by enzymes known as "recombinases", such as RAD51.

The first step in recombination is a double-stranded break either caused by an endonuclease or damage to the DNA. A series of steps catalyzed in part by the recombinase then leads to joining of the two helices by at least one Holliday junction, in which a segment of a single strand in each helix is annealed to the complementary strand in the other helix. The Holliday junction is a tetrahedral junction structure that can be moved along the pair of chromosomes, swapping one strand for another. The recombination reaction is then halted by cleavage of the junction and re-ligation of the released DNA. DNA recombination refers to the process that a DNA segment moves from one DNA molecule to another DNA molecule. The following three types are most commonly observed.

- **Site-specific Recombination**

Site-specific recombination occurs at a specific DNA sequence. The first example was found in the integration between λ DNA and *E. coli* DNA. Both of them contain a sequence, 5'-TTTATAC-3', called the attachment site, which allows the two DNA molecules to attach together by base pairing. Once attached, the enzyme integrase catalyzes two single strand breaks as in the Holliday model. After a short branch migration, the integrase exerts a second strand cuts on two other strands (Fig. 7.26). Resolution of two Holliday junctions completes the integration process.

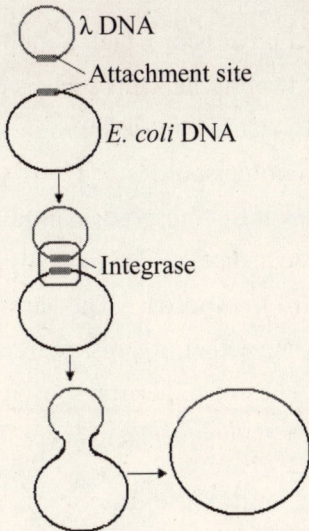

Figure 7.26: Site-specific recombination between λ DNA and *E. coli*

- **Homologous Recombination**

Homologous recombination occurs between two homologous DNA molecules. It is also called DNA crossover. During meiosis, two homologous pairs of sister chromatids align side by side (Fig. 7.27). The DNA crossover is very likely to occur. It could be as often as several times per meiosis. The mechanism of DNA crossover was first explained by Robin Holliday in 1964

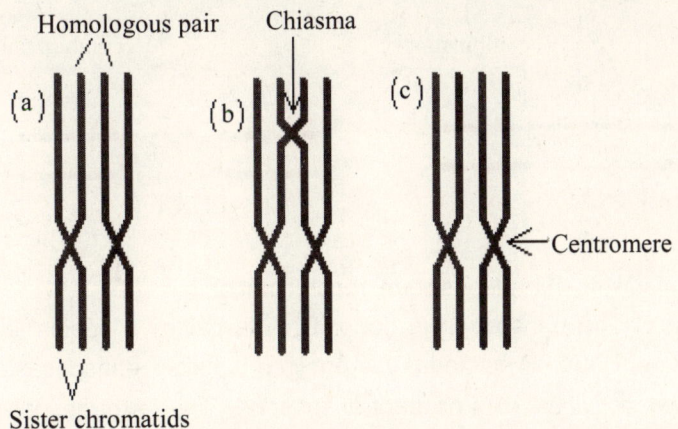

Figure 7.27: DNA crossover. (a) Two homologous pairs of sister chromatids align side by side. (b) The two homologs are connected at a certain point called chiasma. (c) The two homologs exchange the DNA segment from the chiasma to the end of chromosomes

- **Transpositional Recombination**

Transpositional recombination is a process in which a mobile element is inserted into a target DNA. It may occur by one of two mechanisms such as directly as DNA or through RNA (Fig. 7.28). The mobile elements that transpose through DNA are called transposons and those via RNA are referred to as retrotransposons.

In bacteria, the target DNA is cut by transposase, producing sticky ends (single strands, easy to pair with complementary sequences). The transposase also has ligase activity which may ligate the intermediate DNA of transposons. The gaps at sticky ends are filled by DNA polymerase, generating direct repeats. Other organisms are expected to use the same mechanism to insert the DNA intermediates of either transposons or retrotransposons into target DNA. The direct repeats generated by this mechanism are found in all mobile elements.

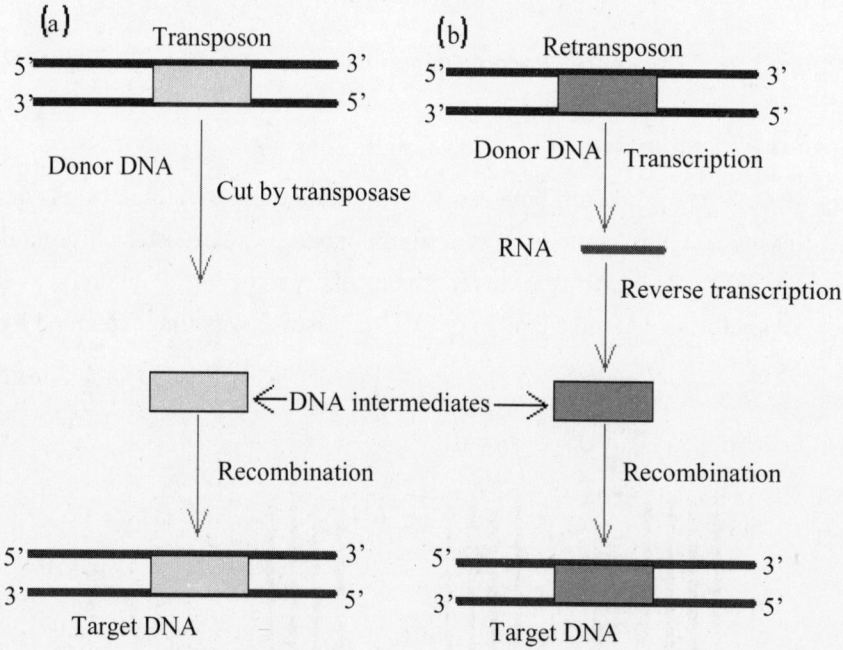

Figure 7.28: Mechanisms of transpositional recombination
(a) For trasposons. The transposon in donor DNA is cut by a special enzyme and then inserted into a target DNA. In bacteria, this enzyme is called transposase which has both nuclease and ligase activities. **(b)** For retrotransposons. The retrotransposon in donor DNA is first transcribed into RNA and then reverse-transcribed into DNA, which is inserted into a target DNA by the same recombination mechanism as the DNA intermediates of transposons.

Suggested Readings

- Alberts B (1994). Molecular Biology of the Cell, 3rd edition. New York: Garland Publishing.
- Fairbanks, D.J. and W.R. Anderson. Genetics – The continuity of life. Brooks / Cole Publishing Company, TTP, NY, Toronto.
- Gardner, E.J., M.J. Simmons and D.P. Snustads. Principles of Genetics, John Wiley and Sons Inc., NY.
- Griffith, A.J.F., J.H. Miller, D.T. Suziki, R.C. Lewontin and W.M. Gellbart. An introduction to genetic analysis. W.H. Freeman and Company, New York.
- Lewin, B. Genes. VI Oxford University Press, Oxford, New York, Tokyo.
- Mechanisms in Eukaryotic Mismatch Repair - J. Biol. Chem., 2006.
- Cellular machineries for chromosomal DNA repair - Genes and Development, 2004.

Gene Expression

Beadle and Tatum proposed the "one gene one *enzyme hypothesis*" for which they won the Nobel Prize in 1958. *Since the chemical reactions occurring in the body are mediated by enzymes, which are proteins hence they are essentially heritable traits, because there exists always a relationship between the genes and proteins. George Beadle, during the 1940s, proposed that mutant eye colors in* **Drosophila** *were caused by a change in one protein in a biosynthetic pathway. Biosynthesis of amino acids (the building blocks of proteins) is a complex process with many chemical reactions mediated by enzymes, which if mutated would shut down the pathway, resulting in no-growth. One gene codes for the production of one protein. "One gene one enzyme" has since been modified to "one gene one polypeptide" since many proteins (such as hemoglobin) is made up of more than one polypeptide. Genes are nothing but segments of* DNA.

8.1. Crick's Central Dogma

DNA, *deoxyribonucleic acid, carries the information necessary for an organism to grow and develop. This information is housed deep within the nucleus of a cell in genes – highly-specific sequences of nucleotides, the building blocks of DNA. Information flow (with the exception of reverse transcription) is from DNA to RNA via the process of transcription, and then to protein via translation (Fig 8.1). Transcription is the making of an RNA molecule of* a DNA template. Translation is the construction of an amino acid sequence (polypeptide) from an RNA molecule. Although originally called dogma, this idea has been tested repeatedly with almost no exceptions to the rule being found.

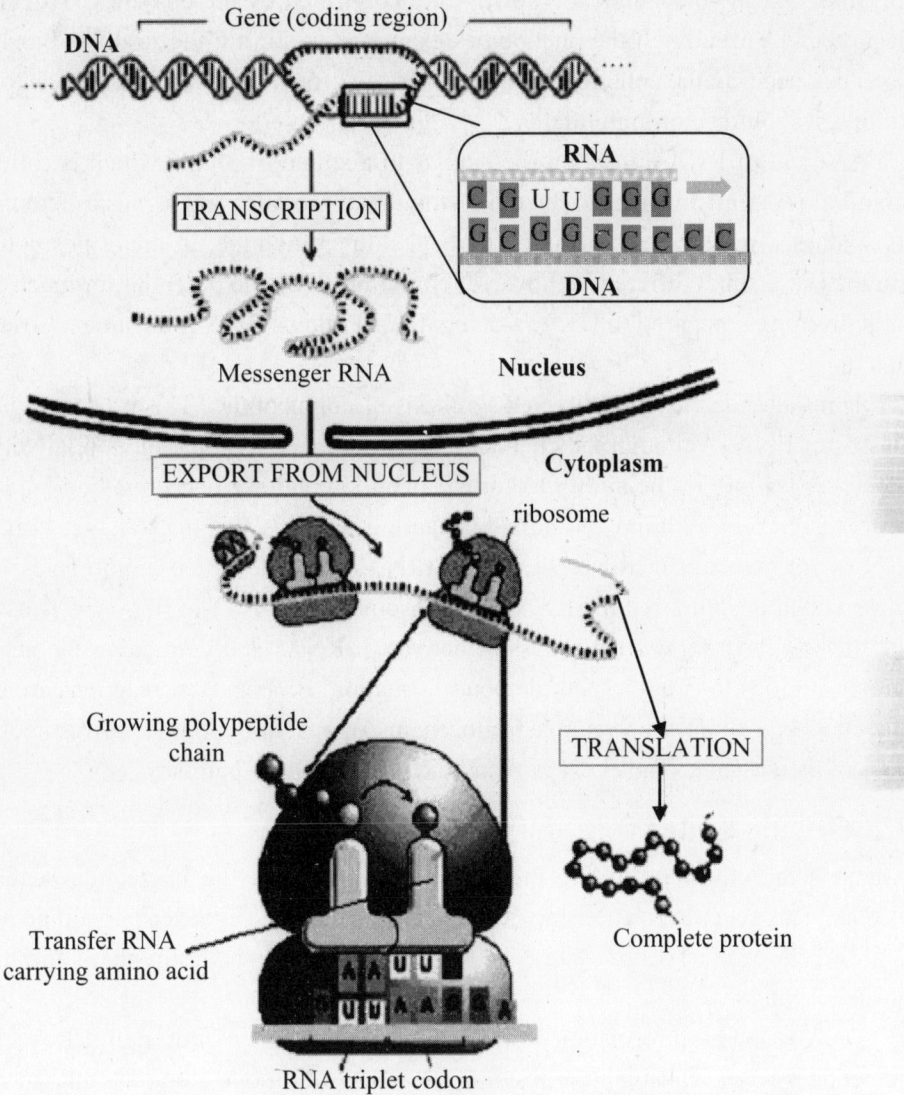

Figure 8.1: Central dogma of molecular biology

Proteins are one of the most important structural and functional units of cell. They are organic compounds made up of amino acids arranged in a linear chain. The amino acids are joined together by the peptide bonds between the carboxyl and amino groups of adjacent amino acid residues. Proteins are the information impregnated in the DNA, the blue print of life. They are synthesized through the intermediate mRNA, transcribed product of DNA. The sequence of amino acids in a protein is defined by the sequence of a gene, which is encoded in the genetic code. In general, the genetic code specifies 20 standard amino acids, however in certain organisms the genetic code can include selenocysteine and in certain archaea pyrrolysine. All the biochemical pathways are controlled by the enzymes, basically composed of proteins. Virtually all the phenotypes examined so far are the result of biochemical reactions that occur in the cell. Since any error in the protein synthesis may leads to disease conditions, it should be of high fidelity.

A strand of RNA appears to be similar to a strand of DNA, which is called the coding strand. It is complementary to the other strand that provides and serves as template strand for its synthesis, only except for uracil that substitutes thymine, in the 2' position of hydroxyl group. These small differences however confer on RNA the potential for much greater structural diversity compared to DNA, a diversity that allows RNA to assume a variety of cellular functions.

Translation is the RNA directed synthesis of polypeptides. This process requires all three classes of RNA. Although the chemistry of peptide bond formation is relatively simple; the processes leading to the ability to form a peptide bond are exceedingly complex. The template for correct addition of individual amino acids is the mRNA, yet both tRNAs and rRNAs are involved in the process. The tRNAs carry activated amino acids into the ribosome which is composed of rRNA and ribosomal proteins. The ribosome is associated with the mRNA ensuring correct access of activated tRNAs and containing the necessary enzymatic activities to catalyze peptide bond formation. Biochemical reactions are controlled by enzymes, and often are organized into chains of reactions known as metabolic pathways. Loss of activity in a single enzyme can inactivate an entire pathway.

8.2. Genetic Code

Amino acid sequences of the protein are governed by the nucleotide sequences of the mRNA. This specific relationship between the nucleotide sequence and amino acid sequence is known as genetic code, which was deciphered by Marshall Nirenberg and his colleagues in early 1960s.

DNA transfers information to mRNA in the form of a code defined by a sequence of nucleotides bases. During protein synthesis, ribosomes move along the mRNA molecule and "read" its sequence three nucleotides at a time (codon) from the 5' end to the 3' end. Each amino acid is specified by the mRNA's codon and then pairs with a sequence of three complementary nucleotides carried by a particular tRNA (anticodon). The genetic code consists of 64 triplets of nucleotides (Fig. 8.2). These triplets are called codons.

Since RNA is constructed from four types of nucleotides, there are 64 possible triplet sequences or codons (4x4x4=64). With three exceptions, each codon encodes for one of the

20 amino acids used in the synthesis of proteins, that produces some redundancy in the code: most of the amino acids being encoded by more than one codon. Three of these possible codons specify the termination of the polypeptide chain, called "stop codons", that leaves 61 codons to specify only 20 different amino acids. Therefore, most of the amino acids are represented by more than one codon. The genetic code is said to be degenerate.

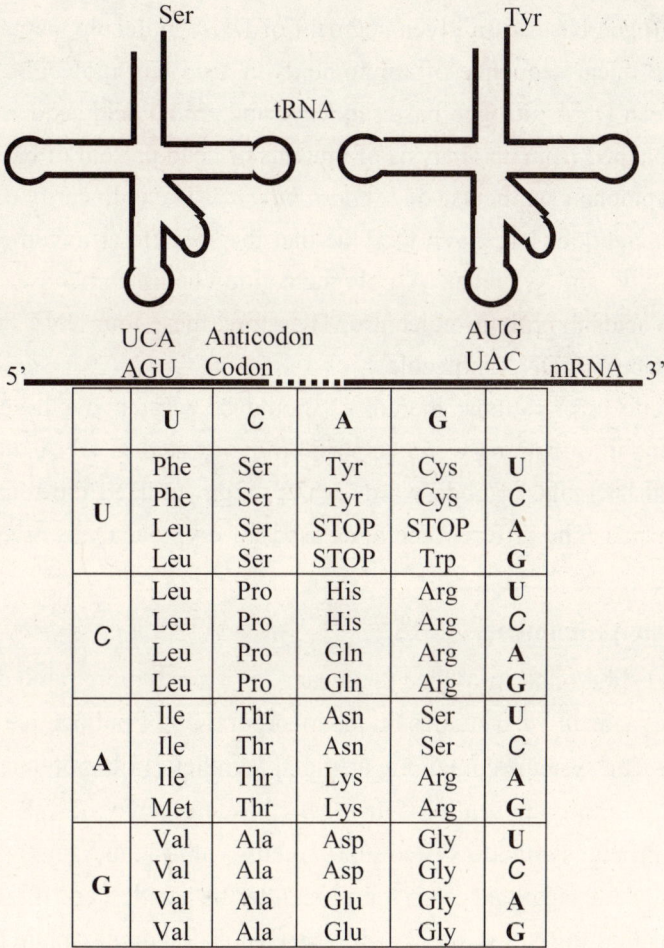

		U	C	A	G	
		Phe	Ser	Tyr	Cys	U
		Phe	Ser	Tyr	Cys	C
	U	Leu	Ser	STOP	STOP	A
		Leu	Ser	STOP	Trp	G
		Leu	Pro	His	Arg	U
		Leu	Pro	His	Arg	C
	C	Leu	Pro	Gln	Arg	A
		Leu	Pro	Gln	Arg	G
		Ile	Thr	Asn	Ser	U
		Ile	Thr	Asn	Ser	C
	A	Ile	Thr	Lys	Arg	A
		Met	Thr	Lys	Arg	G
		Val	Ala	Asp	Gly	U
		Val	Ala	Asp	Gly	C
	G	Val	Ala	Glu	Gly	A
		Val	Ala	Glu	Gly	G

Figure 8.2: Concept of codon, anticodon and genetic code

The genetic code can be expressed as either RNA codons or DNA codons. RNA codons occur in messenger RNA (mRNA) and are the codons that are actually "read" during the synthesis of polypeptides (the process called translation). But each mRNA molecule acquires its sequence of nucleotides by transcription from the corresponding gene.

8.3. Cracking of Genetic Code

DNA is a genetic material, which carries genetic information from cell to cell and from generation to generation. The genetic information may be written in any one of the three moieties of DNA, phosphoric acid, deoxyribose sugar, and nitrogen bases. But the poly-sugar-phosphate backbone is always the same, and it is therefore, unlikely that these moieties of DNA molecule carry the genetic information. The nitrogen bases, however vary from one segment of DNA to another, so the informations might well depend on their sequences. The sequences of nitrogen bases of a given segment of DNA molecule, actually has been found to be identical to linear sequence of amino acids in a protein molecule. The proof of such colinearity between DNA nitrogen base sequence and amino acid sequence in protein molecules has first obtained from an analysis of mutants of head protein of bacteriophage T4, and the A-protein tryptophan synthetase of *Escherichia coli*. The colinearity of protein molecules and DNA polynucleotides has given the clue that the specific arrangement of four nitrogen bases (e.g., A, T, C and G) in DNA polynucleotide chains somehow, determines the sequence of amino acids in protein-molecules. Therefore, these four DNA bases can be considered as four alphabets of DNA molecule.

All the genetic informations, therefore, should be written by these four alphabets of DNA. The genetic informations were supposed to be existed in DNA molecule in the form of certain special language of code words which might utilized the four nitrogen bases of DNA for its symbols. The different methods used for cryptoanalysis or cracking the genetic code are:

a. *In Vitro* Codon Assignments

Nirenberg in1961, first of all, provided the means for a much more rapid decipherment of the genetic code. He made *in vitro* studies on the incorporation of radioactive amino acids in cell free protein synthetic systems containing artificial (synthetic) ribopolynucleotides or mRNA. A cell free system for protein synthesis includes ribosomes, enzymes, tRNA, etc. To produce such a cell free protein synthetic system the protein synthesizing components of broken cell (usually *E. coli*) were separated from the remainder by gentle centrifugation. During these manipulations natural mRNA is subjected to mechanical and enzymatic break down. Artificial messenger RNAs were then introduced.

The artificial mRNA was prepared for each nitrogen base with the aid of a polynucleotide phosphorylase enzyme obtained from *Azobacter vinelandii* or *Micrococcus lysodeikticus*. The enzyme differed from RNA polymerase enzyme in not requiring the presence of DNA as a primer or template for the synthesis of RNA. Thus, Nirenberg prepared a polyuridylic acid (UUUU ...), poly cytidylic acid (CCCCC ...), polyadenylic acid (AAAAA ...)

and guanylic acid (GGGGG ...) from uracil, cytosine, adenine and guanine respectively. When he introduced these artificial homopolymeric polyribonucleotides or mRNA (e.g., poly D, poly C, poly A and poly G acids) in different cell free protein synthetic systems of *E. coli* containing radioactive amino acids, he found that each artificial mRNA stimulated the synthesis of polypeptides of single kind of amino acids. For example, poly U acid stimulates the *in vitro* synthesis of monotonus polypeptide-namely polyphenylalanine whose amino acid residues were phenylalanine. Therefore, he concluded that a sequence of UUU coded for phenylalanine. Likewise, because polycytidylic acid was found to direct synthesis of polyproline hence, the sequence of CCC codes designates proline and because, polyadenylic acid directs synthesis of poly lysine, so the sequence of AAA designates lysine. Later on, the sequence of GGG was found to specify glycine.

In this way four of 64 codons were easily accounted for. In order to gain some insight into the meaning of the remaining 60 codons, containing more than one kind of nucleotide Nirenberg continued these experiments by using artificially synthesized random ribopolynucleotides (mixed copolymers) containing two, three or four different nucleotide constituents. By using artificial mRNAs, viz., poly-UA, poly UC, and poly UG, he cracked the codes for arginine, alanine, serine, proline, tyrosine, isoleucine, valine, leucine, cysteine, tryptophan, glycine, methionine and glutamic acid. Further, when mixed copolymers are made, one can calculate all the possible triplets they contain assuming that the bases are incorporated randomly into the molecule; for example, when poly AC is synthesized from a mixture containing equal proportions of A and C, six triplets should occur with equal frequency: AAA, ACA, ACC, CCC, CCA and CAA. Using poly AC it was found that six amino acids were incorporated into polypeptides: aspargine, glutamine, histidine, lysine, threonine and proline.

The next step was to vary the ratio of A and C, and it was found that when the copolymer contained more A than C the ratio of aspargine to histidine in the polypeptide increased, By such experiments the composition of the bases in certain triplets could often be deduced.

After learning of Nirenberg's first success with poly U, Ochoa and his collaborators carried out entirely analogous sets of decoding experiments in which they used artificial random ribopolynucleotides. Through the parallel efforts of these two research groups the empirical formula of many amino acid codes or codons became known within a year or so. But this work could not establish the actual sequence of the nucleotides within any codon, except for, UUU, CCC, AAA and GGG.

In order to ascertain that which structural isomer of a codon of a given empirical formula designates which amino acid, artificial mRNAs of known sequences were employed. H. G. Khorana first of all succeeded in synthesizing polyribonucleotides or mRNA of known sequences and be synthesized an alternating copolymer such as-UGU-GUG-UGU-. Use of this particular alternating polynucleotide as a mRNA in the *in vitro* protein-synthesizing system gave rise to the formation of the alternating polypeptide (e.g. valine-cysteine valine-cysteine) evidently directed by the codon sequence-UGU-GUG-UGU-GUG. This result established that the UUG (Iucine) codon is not UGU, and that neither the UUG (tryptophan) nor the UGG (glycine) codon is GUG, but, UUG (valine) is UGU, and GUG is a cysteine synonym, or that UUG (cysteine) is UGU nor GUG is a valine synonym. Thus, Khorana determined the exact sequence of nucleotides in various genetic codons which discovered either by Nirenberg or by himself.

In all of these *in vitro* experiments magnesium concentrations were kept artificially high in order to facilitate the translation of artificial messengers. High magnesium concentrations allowed initiation without an initiation codon, and an AUG codon is, of course, absent from most of the artificial polyribonucleotides that might be synthesized *in vitro*.

In 1964, while Khorana was just completing the difficult synthesis of the first artificial ribopolynucleotides of defined sequence, Nirenberg made a second discovery that made possible a rapid culmination of the code-breaking efforts. He found that addition of simple trinucleotides of known base sequences to ribosomes would cause these ribosomes to bind that, and only that, aminoacyl-tRNA which carries the anticodon complementary to the trinucleotide added to the reaction mixture. For example, the trinucleotide GCC was found to be active in promoting the binding of alanyl-tRNAala but not of any other aminoacyl-tRNA and it was therefore concluded that GCC is a codon for alanine. These studies enabled the preparation of the complete genetic code dictionary.

b. *In vivo* Codon Assignment

The cell free protein synthetic systems, though have proved of great significance in decipherment of the genetic code, but, they could not tell us whether the genetic code so decipherd is used in the living systems of all organisms also. Three kinds of techniques are used by different molecular biologists to determine whether the same code is also used *in vivo* (a) amino acid replacement studies (e.g., tryptophan synthetase synthesis in *E. coli* (Yanofsky *et al*, 1963) and haemoglobin synthesis in man), (b) frame shift mutations (e.g., investigations of Terzaghi *et.al*., 1966), on lysozyme enzyme of T4, bacteriophages, and (c), comparison of a DNA or mRNA polynucleotide cryptogram with its corresponding polypeptide clear text (e.g., comparison of amino acid sequence of the R17 bacteriophage coat protein with the nucleotide sequence of the R17 mRNA in the region of the molecule that dictates coat-protein synthesis (Cory *et al*., 1970). Thus, *in vitro* and *in vivo* studies gave the way to formulate a code table for twenty amino acids. In genetic dictionary, each codon is written as it would appear in RNA reading in a 5'→3' direction; the corresponding codons in DNA will of course, be both complementary to them and written in the reverse order on a 5'→3' strand.

Similarly, the bases in the corresponding tRNA anticodons will be both complementary and anti polar to the mRNA codons.

8.4. Characteristics of Triplet Codon

The genetic dictionary of mRNA codons reveals following important features of triplet codons:

• **Codon is triplet** - Twenty different amino acids are incorporated during translation. Thus, at least 20 different codons must be formed using the four symbols (bases) available in the mRNA. Two bases per codon would yield only 4^2 or 16 possible codons which are clearly not enough. Three bases per codon yield 4^3 or 64 possible codons apparently excess. It is now known that each codon consists of a sequence of three nucleotides, i.e., it is a triplet code. The deciphering of the genetic code depended heavily on the chemical synthesis of nucleotide polymer, particularly triplets in repeated sequence.

• **Degeneracy**-The code contains many synonyms, in that almost all amino acids are represented by more than one codon. The occurrence of more than one codon per amino acid is called degeneracy. All amino acids except methionine and tryptophan have more than one codon, so that all the possible triplets have a meaning, despite there being 64 triplets and only 20 amino acids. Leucine, serine and arginine have six different codons. Isoleucine has three codons. The degeneracy in the genetic code is not at random: instead, it is highly ordered. Usually multiple codons specifying an amino acid differ by only one base, the third or 3 base of codon. For example, the three amino acids-arginine, serine and leucine-each have six synonymous codons. However, for many of the synonym codons specifying the same amino acid the first two bases of the triplet are constant, whereas the third can vary; for example, all codons starting with CC specify proline (CCU, CCC, CCA and CCG) and all codons starting with AC specify threonine. This flexibility in the third nucleotide of a codon may well help to minimize the consequences of errors.

The degeneracy can be either partial or complete. A complete degeneracy is a condition in which the third base position is of less significance. Any base present in this position will lead to same amino acid, but if the third position is occupied by one type of purine/ pyrimidine, then they code for one type of amino acid and if the position is occupied by another type of purine/ pyrimidines, without any change in the first two positions, they code for another amino acid. Such a condition is called as partial degeneracy, e.g. CAU or CAC code for His whereas CAA and CAG code for Gly. Because of the degeneracy of the genetic code there must either be several different tRNAs that recognize the different codons specifying a given amino acid or the anticodon of a given tRNA must be able to base-pair with several different codons. Actually both of these occur. Several tRNAs exist for certain amino acids and some tRNAs recognize more than one codon. The hydrogen bonding between the bases in the anticodon of tRNA and the codon of mRNA appears to follow strict base pairing rules only for the first two bases of the codon and is apparently less stringent, allowing what Crick has called wobble at this site.

- **Non-overlapping:** The code is non-overlapping, meaning that no single base can take part in the formation of more than one codon. This means that successive triplets are read in order. Each nucleotide is part of only one triplet codon.

- **Ambiguity:** The genetic code is ambiguous, that is, same codon may specify more than one amino acid. For example, UUU codon usually code for phenylalanine but in the presence of streptomycin, may also code for isoleucine, leucine or serine.

- **Commaless:** The genetic code is commaless, which means that no codon is reserved for punctuations. There are no commas or some specific nucleotide sequences to separate the codons, i.e., CCCAAAUUUGGG have four code words and upon translation we have a tetrapeptide chain of pro-lys-phen-gly. So all the letters are used to code for one or other amino acid.

- **Starting codons:** AUG codon is called starting or chain initiation codon, because, it initiates, the synthesis of polypeptide chain.

- **Stop codons/ Non-sense codons:** There are 3 codons (UAA, UAG, and UGA) that are stop codons. When any one of these codons is reached during transcription, transcription stops. The UAA (also called ochre), UAG (also called amber because an investigator who studied the properties of this codon belonged to the Bernstein family, and Bernstein means "amber" in German) and UGA codons do not specify any amino acid, and so, are called non-sense codons. They are also called termination codons, because, these codons are used by the cell to signal the natural end of translation of a particular polypeptide. However, their inclusion in any mRNA results in the abrupt termination of the message at the point of their location even though the polypeptide chain has not been-completed.

- **Universality:** The genetic code has been found to be universal, because, same code applies in all kinds of living systems. It was postulated that the genetic code must be frozen and unable to evolve because a change in a codon meaning would cause almost every protein in the cell to be altered. The genetic codes are indeed universal and can be demonstrated quite directly by presenting an *E. coli* in *in vitro* protein synthesizing system with, for example, purified mRNA from polio virus (which is normally translated by human cells) and observing the synthesis of virus protein. Experiments with cell free system with mammalian extract yielded same results as that of *E. coli*. The major exception to the universality of the code occurs in mitochondria of humans, yeast and several other species where UGA is a tryptophan codon. UGA is a termination codon in the non mitochondrial system.

Also, in yeast mitochondria, CUA specifies threonine instead of the usual leucine and in mammalian mitochondria; AUA specifies methionine instead of isoleucine. Still more surprising is the discovery that the meaning of a codon can vary from gene to gene in the same organism. In human nuclear genes UGA is frequently used as a termination codon in accordance with its standard meaning. However, in at least two human genes, for the enzymes glutathione peroxidase and iodothyronine-5-deiodinase, UGA specifies the unusual amino acid called selenocysteine (a cysteine in which the sulphur atom is replaced by selenium). It appears that the mRNA transcribed from these genes have special stem loop structures in their trailer regions, and these stem loops play some role during translation, ensuring that the UGA triplet is recognized as a selenocysteine codon rather than a termination signal.

8.5. Wobble Hypothesis

The triplet code is a degenerate one with many more codons than the number of amino acid types coded. An explanation for this degeneracy is provided by the 'wobble hypothesis' proposed by Crick (1966). Since there are 61 codons specifying amino acids, the cell should contain 61 different tRNA molecules, each with a different anticodon. Actually, however, the number of tRNA molecule types discovered is much less than 61. This implies that the anticodons of some tRNAs read more than one codon on mRNA. According to the wobble hypothesis only the first two positions of a triplet codon on mRNA have a precise pairing with the bases of the tRNA anticodon.

The pairing of the third position bases of the codon may be ambiguous, and varies according to the nucleotide present in this position. Thus a single tRNA type is able to recognize two or more codons differing only in the third base. The anticodon UCG of serine tRNA recognizes two codons, AGC and AGU. The bonding between UCG and AGC follows the usual Watson-Crick pairing pattern. In UCG-AGU pairing, however, hydrogen bonding takes place between G and U. This is a departure from the usual Watson-Crick pairing mechanism where G pairs with C and A with U. Such interaction between the third bases is referred to as 'wobble pairing'.

The degeneracy of the code is not random. Mostly, the different codons for a particular amino acid have the same first two letters (leucine, serine and arginine are exceptions). Thus the first two letters of all the four codons for valine are GU and for alanine GC.

8.6. Codon Bias

All but two of the amino acids (Met and Trp) can be encoded by from 2 to 6 different codons. However, the genome of most organisms reveals that certain codons are preferred over others. In humans, for example, alanine is encoded by GCC four times as often as by GCG. Why this is uncertain? It probably reflects a greater translation efficiency by the translation apparatus (e.g., ribosomes) for certain codons over their synonyms.

Codon bias even extends to pairs of codons: wherever a human protein contains the amino acids Ala-Glu, the gene encoding those amino acids is seven times as likely to use the codons GCAGAG rather than the synonymous GCCGAA. Codon bias is exploited by the biotechnology industry to improve the yield of the desired product. The ability to manipulate codon bias may also usher in an era of safer vaccines.

8.7. Protein Synthesis

Proteins are widely used in cells to serve diverse functions. Some proteins provide the structural support for cells while others act as enzymes to catalyze certain reactions. To manufacture proteins, cells follow a very systematic procedure that first transcribes DNA into mRNA and then translates the mRNA into chains of amino acids. The amino acid chain then folds into specific proteins.

8.8. Transcription (DNA to mRNA in nucleus)

In transcription, a section of DNA (a gene), carrying the genetic code for the synthesis of a specific protein molecule, is copied into mRNA. Messenger RNA then migrates to the cytoplasm where ribosomes are then translating the code to construct the protein.

Transcription has similarities to DNA replication but only involves a small portion of the DNA molecule. In transcription, the DNA will unzip between the nitrogenous bases and expose the sequence of a gene that codes for a specific protein. RNA nucleotides, present in the nucleus, will then move in and complementary base pair with one side of the unzipped DNA. The complementary base pairing is the same with the exception of Uracil which replaces Thymine (e.g. an adenine nucleotide in DNA will transcribe a uracil nucleotide in the mRNA). The RNA nucleotides are joined together by an enzyme called RNA polymerase. The mRNA then moves out of the nucleus through nuclear pores to deliver the coded message to the ribosomes in the cytoplasm. Transcription also produces ribosomal RNA (rRNA) and transfer RNA (tRNA) that are used in protein synthesis. rRNA is a component of ribosomes and tRNA delivers amino acids to the ribosome during translation.

DNA sequence is enzymatically copied by RNA polymerase, RNA polymerase binds to a special region called promoter region. This the start point surrounds the first base pair that is transcribed into RNA, from this point RNA polymerase moves along the template, synthesizing RNA until it reaches a terminator sequence. This action defines a complete transcription unit that extends from the promoter to the terminator. The stretch of DNA that is transcribed into an RNA molecule is called a transcription unit. A DNA transcription unit that is translated into protein contains sequences that direct and regulate protein synthesis (Fig. 8.3). In addition to the coding sequence that is translated into protein, there is a regulatory sequence located before (towards the 5' DNA end) the coding sequence, it is called 5' untranslated region (5'UTR) and sequence found towards the 3' DNA end.

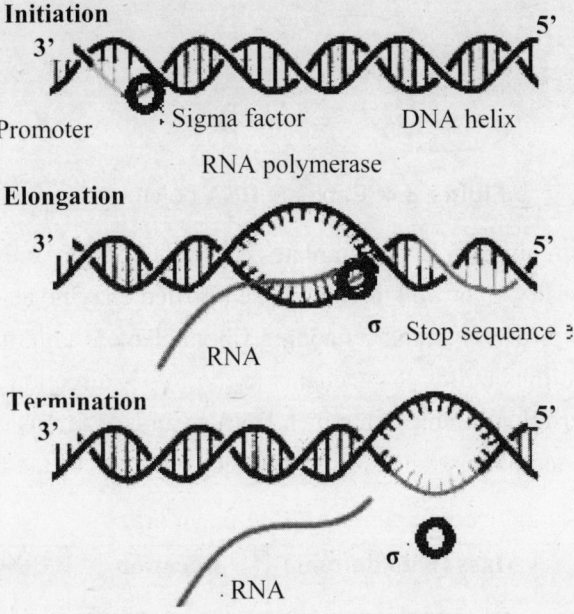

Figure 8.3: Steps involved in transcription

8.8.1. RNA Polymerases

RNA Polymerases are DNA-directed RNA polymerase. They are essential to life and are found in all organisms and many viruses. In chemical terms, they are nucleotidyl transferase that polymerizes ribonucleotides at the 3' end of an RNA transcript.

(a) Prokaryotic RNA polymerase

E. coli has a single DNA-directed RNA polymerase that synthesizes all types of RNA. It is a large and complex enzyme, containing five core subunits and a sixth subunit, called Sigma factor (σ) that binds transiently to the core enzyme and directs the enzyme to for initiation sites on the DNA (Sigma factor (σ) binds to the initiation site). These six subunits constitute the RNA polymerase holoenzyme (Holoenzyme = Core enzyme + Sigma factor). The σ subunit is weakly bound and can be separated from the other subunits, yielding a core polymerase consisting of two α, one β, one β' and one ω subunits ($\alpha_2\beta\beta\omega$; MW. 390,000) (Table 8.1). The core polymerase is fully capable of catalyzing the polymerization of NTPs into RNA, indicating that σ is not required for the basic catalytic activity of the enzyme. The core polymerase does not bind specifically to the DNA sequences that signal the normal initiation of transcription; therefore, the σ subunit is required to identify the correct sites for initiation of transcription. Sigma factor will be released after initiation (Fig. 8.4).

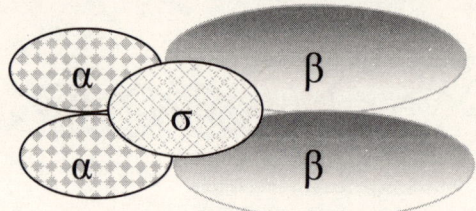

Figure 8.4: Bacterial RNA polymerase

RNA polymerase requires a DNA template, ATP, GTP, UTP, and CTP as precursors of the nucleotide units of RNA, as well as Mg^{2+}. The purified enzyme also contains Zn^{2+}. RNA polymerase elongates an RNA strand by adding ribonucleotide units to the 3'-hydroxyl end of the RNA chain and thus builds RNA chains in the 5'→3' direction. RNA synthesis takes place within a "transcription bubble," in which DNA strands are transiently separated into its single strands and the template strand is used to direct synthesis of the RNA strand.

Table 8.1: Subunits and coding genes of RNA polymerase

Subunit and gene	Mass (Kilo daltons)	Location	Possible function
α (rpo A)	40 each	Core enzyme	RNAP assembly
β (rpo B)	155	Core enzyme	Catalysis
β' (rpo C)	160	Core enzyme	Catalysis
ω (rpo -)	-	Core enzyme	RNAP assembly
σ (rpo D)	32-90	Holoenzyme	Initiation

(b) Eukaryotic RNA polymerase

There are three classes of eukaryotic RNA polymerases: I, II and III, each comprising of two large subunits and 12-15 smaller subunits. The two large subunits are homologous to the *E. **coli*** β and β' subunits. Two smaller subunits are similar to the *E. **coli*** α sub-unit. However, the eukaryotic RNA polymerase does not contain any subunit similar to the *E. **coli*** Sigma factor. Therefore, in eukaryotes, transcriptional initiation should be mediated by other proteins (Table 8.2).

Table 8.2: Eukaryotic RNA polymerase

Enzyme and location	Sub-units	Product and abundance	Sensitivity to α – amanitin*
RNAP I (nucleolus)	RPAs	rRNA (50-70%)	Not sensitive
RNAP II (nucleoplasm)	RPBs	hnRNA (20-40%)	Sensitive
RNAP III (nucleoplasm)	RPCs	tRNA (approx. 10%)	Inhibited in animals at high level; not in yeast and insect

* The three RNAPs are distinguished on the basis of their sensitivity towards transcription inhibitors like α – amanitin

8.9. Promoters

A promoter is a regulatory region of DNA located upstream (towards the 5' region) of a gene, providing a control point for regulated gene transcription. The promoter contains specific DNA sequences that are recognized by proteins known as transcription factors. These factors bind to the promoter sequences, recruiting RNA polymerase, the enzyme that synthesizes the RNA from the coding region of the gene (Fig. 8.5).

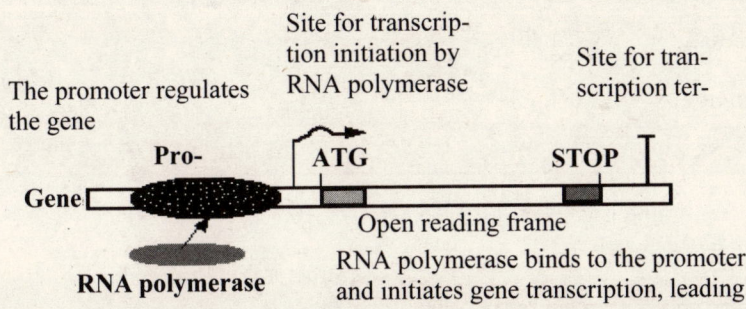

Figure 8.5: Promoters

8.10. Difference between Eukaryotic and Prokaryotic Promoters

(a) Prokaryotic promoters

In prokaryotes, the promoter consists of two short sequences at -10 and -35 positions upstream from the transcription start site.

● The sequence at -10 is called the Pribnow box, or the -10 element, and usually consists of the six nucleotides TATAAT. The Pribnow box is absolutely essential to start transcription in prokaryotes (Fig. 8.6).

● The other sequence at -35 (the -35 element) usually consists of the six nucleotides TTGACA. Its presence allows a very high transcription rate.

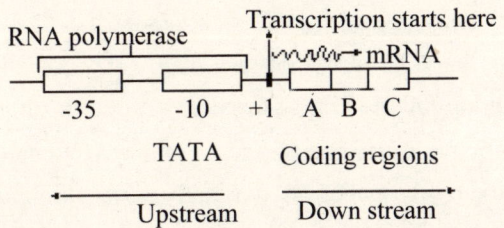

Figure 8.6: TATA Box (-10) and -35 regions

(b) Eukaryotic promoters

Eukaryotic promoters are extremely diverse and are difficult to characterize. They typically lie upstream of the gene and can have regulatory elements several kilobases away from the transcriptional start site. In eukaryotes, the transcriptional complex can cause the DNA to bend back on itself, which allows for placement of regulatory sequences far from the actual site of transcription. Many eukaryotic promoters, contain a TATA box (sequence TA-TAAA), which in turn binds a TATA binding protein which assists in the formation of the RNA polymerase transcriptional complex. The TATA box typically lies very close (Fig. 8.7) to the transcriptional start site (often within 50 bases).

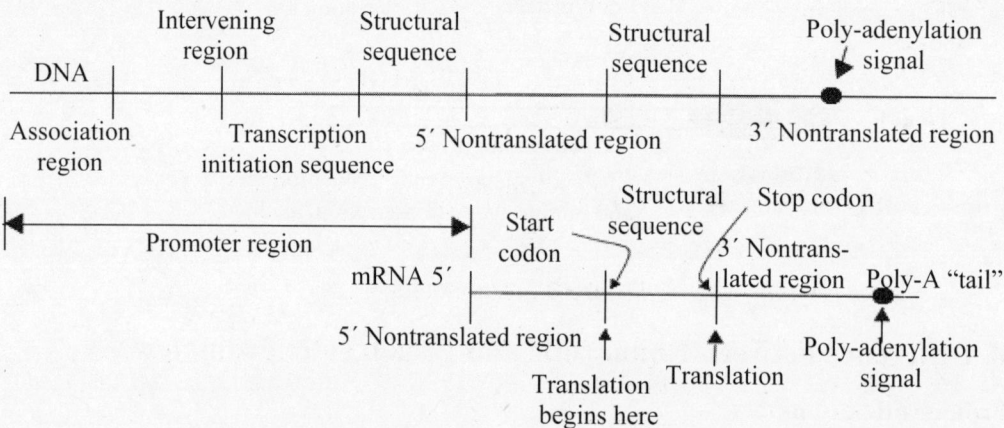

Figure 8.7: *Structure of a typical gene*

Promoters in eukaryotic organisms- e.g. plants, animals- comprise multiple elements, some of which are found in nearly all promoters (Table 8.3). These include:

- **CAAT box**. A consensus sequence close to -80 bp from the start point (+1). It plays an important role in promoter efficiency, by increasing its strength, and it seems to function in either orientation. This box is replaced in plants by a consensus sequence called the **AGGA box**.

- **TATA box**. A sequence usually located around 25 bp upstream of the start point. The TATA box tends to be surrounded by GC rich sequences. The TATA box binds RNA polymerase II and a series of transcription factors [TFIIX, X being a letter that identifies an individual transcription factor (TF)] to form an initiation complex.

- **GC box**. A sequence rich in guanidine (G) and cytidine (C) nucleotides, is usually found in multiple copies in the promoter region, normally surrounding the TATA box.

- **CAP site**. A transcription initiation sequence or start point defined as +1, at which the transcription process actually starts.

Table 8.3: Promoters in eukaryotic organisms

Conserved eukaryotic promoter elements	Consensus sequence
CAAT box	GGCCAATCT
TATA box	TATAA
GC box	GGGCGG
CAP site	TAC

RNA polymerase II is the enzyme that transcribes a gene into RNA. It works in conjunction with other transcription factors that recognize signals embodied in the promoter region. RNA polymerase II starts its "journey" at the TATA region where it binds and travels along the DNA until it reaches the CAP site where the actual synthesis of RNA starts. The transcription process only takes place in the downstream direction, from 5' (left) to 3' (right).

8.11. Enhancers

Enhancers act to stimulate the activity of certain promoters. In common with upstream promoter elements they can be active in all tissues or can display tissue-specificity. They are modular in structure and can act co-operatively. Many enhancers seem to contain multiple binding sites for transcription factors which interact and often these are sites which are also found in promoter sequences. Enhancers are thought to act by binding transcription factors, to form an enhanceosome (a protein complex that binds to the "enhancer" region of a gene, found upstream or downstream, of the promoter, or within a gene) and looping out the DNA between the enhancer and the promoter thus bringing factor binding sites together, increasing efficiency of recruitment of transcription factors to the promoter and therefore transcription initiation.

8.12. Prokaryotic Transcription

Much of the pioneering work on transcription was carried out in prokaryotes, most notably in the bacterium *E. coli*. These studies laid the foundation for work that was later carried out in the more complex eukaryotes. Transcription can be divided into three phases: initiation, elongation, and termination.

8.12.1. Initiation

Initiation describes the formation of the first nucleotide bonds in RNA. It starts with template recognition which begins with the binding of RNA polymerase holoenzyme to the double-stranded DNA at a promoter to form a "closed complex". Then the strands of DNA are separated to form the "open complex" that makes the template strand available for base pairing with ribonucleosides. The transcription bubble is created by localized unwinding that begins at the site where RNA polymerase binds. RNA polymerase binds to the promoter in at least two distinguishable steps. The holoenzyme first binds the DNA and migrates to the - 35 region, forming the "closed complex." The DNA is then unwound for about 17 base pairs beginning at the -10 region, exposing the template strand at the initiation site. The RNA polymerase binds more tightly to this unwound region; forming an "open complex" for RNA synthesis, to begin. The initiation phase ends when the enzyme succeeds in extending the chain and clears the promoter. The sigma factor eventually dissociates from the holoenzyme after recognizing the initiation site and elongation proceeds. Promoters can differ in "strength," or how actively they promote transcription of their adjacent DNA sequence. Promoter strength is in many (but not all) cases, a matter of how tightly RNA polymerase and its associated accessory proteins bind to their respective DNA sequences (Fig. 8.8). Most transcripts originate using adenosine-5'-triphosphate (ATP) and, to a lesser extent, guanosine -5'-triphosphate (GTP) (purine nucleoside triphosphates) at the +1 site.

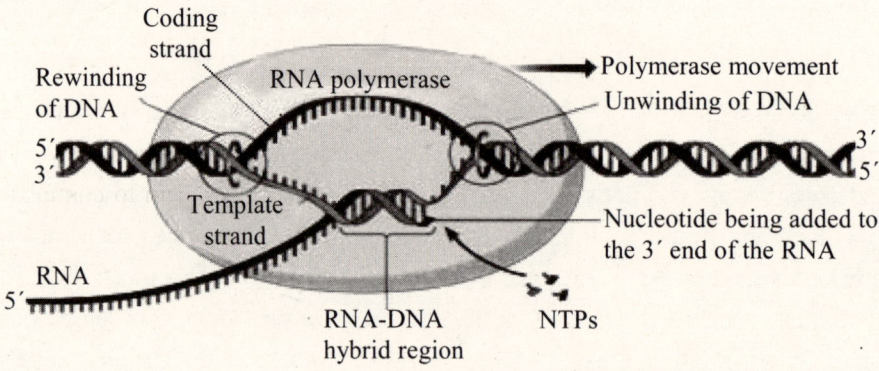

Figure 8.8: Initiation of protein synthesis

8.12.2. Elongation

Elongation is the function of the RNA polymerase core enzyme. RNA polymerase moves along the template, locally "unzipping" the DNA double helix. This allows a transient base pairing between the incoming nucleotide and newly-synthesized RNA and the DNA template strand. As it is made, the RNA transcript forms secondary structure through intra-strand base pairing. The average speed of transcription is about 40 nucleotides per second, much slower than DNA polymerase. Other protein factors may bind to polymerase and alter the rate of transcription and some specific sequences are transcribed more slowly than others. Eventually, RNA polymerase comes to the end of the region under transcription.

8.12.3. Termination

Termination depends on the protein factor. Rho factor is a protein involved in assisting *E. coli* RNA polymerase to terminate transcription at certain terminators (called rho-dependent terminators). Rho-dependent terminators are sequences that terminate transcription by bacterial RNA polymerase in the presence of the rho factor. Rho-independent terminators have a characteristic structure, which features (a) a strong G-C rich stem and loop, (b) a sequence of 4–6 U residues in the RNA, which are transcribed from a corresponding stretch of A in the template. Intrinsic terminators are able to terminate transcription by bacterial RNA polymerase in the absence of any additional factors. Core enzyme can terminate *in vitro* at certain sites in the absence of any other factor. There are ~1100 sequences in the *E. coli* genome that fit these criteria, suggesting that about half of the genes have intrinsic terminators. All hairpins that form in the RNA product cause the polymerase to slow (and perhaps to pause) in RNA synthesis. Pausing occurs at sites that resemble terminators but have an increased separation (typically 10-11 bases) between the hairpin and the U-run. If the pause site does not correspond to a terminator, usually the enzyme moves on again to continue transcription. The length of the pause varies, but at a typical terminator lasts ~60S.

8.13. Eukaryotic Transcription

Most of the eukaryotic protein-coding genes contain segments called introns, which break up the amino acid coding sequence into segments called exons. The transcript of these genes is resulted as pre-mRNA (precursor-mRNA). The pre-mRNA is then processed in the nucleus where the introns are removed and the exons are spliced together into a translatable mRNA. The mRNA subsequently released from the nucleus and are translated in to proteins in the cytoplasm by ribosomes (Fig. 8.9).

8.13.1. RNA Polymerase

Although transcription in eukaryotes is similar to that in prokaryotes, the process appears to be complex. Instead of one RNA polymerase, there are three (RNA polymerases I, II, and III) involved in eukaryotic transcription. RNA polymerase I (localized to the nucleolus) transcribes the rRNA precursor molecules. RNA polymerase II produces most mRNAs and snRNAs. RNA polymerase III is responsible for the production of pre-tRNAs, 5SrRNA and other small RNAs. The mitochondria and chloroplasts have their own RNA polymerases. There is considerable relatedness between the three eukaryotic RNA polymerases and to the prokaryotic *E. coli* RNA polymerase, especially between the largest and second largest subunits. RNA polymerase II differs from the others in that the largest subunit has a carboxy terminal extension called the carboxy terminal domain (CTD). The CTD contains a highly repeated heptapeptide Tyr-Ser-Pro-Thr-Ser-Pro-Ser, which can be heavily phosphorylated. This phosphorylated domain is essential for transcription by RNA polymerase II in most eukaryotes, and it also links the processes of transcription and RNA processing.

(a) RNA polymerase I

RNA polymerase I is a complex of 13 subunits. Promoters for RNA polymerase I contain two important regulatory elements, a core promoter located from around 20 nucleotides downstream of the transcription initiation site to around 40 nucleotides upstream, and an up-stream control element (UCE) situated some 100 nucleotides upstream of the transcription initiation site. The first step in formation of the polymerase I transcription initiation complex is binding of two molecules of Upstream Binding Factor (UBF), one to the UCE and the other to the core promoter element. Interaction between the two UBFs bound to the pro-moter result in looping out of the intervening promoter DNA and provision of a promoter structure that can be recognized, and bound by, in humans, the core promoter element-binding factor, selectivity factor 1 (SL1). SL1 is a multi-subunit protein composed of TATA-binding protein (TBP) and three TBP-associated factors to which RNA polymerase I binds to complete the transcription initiation complex.

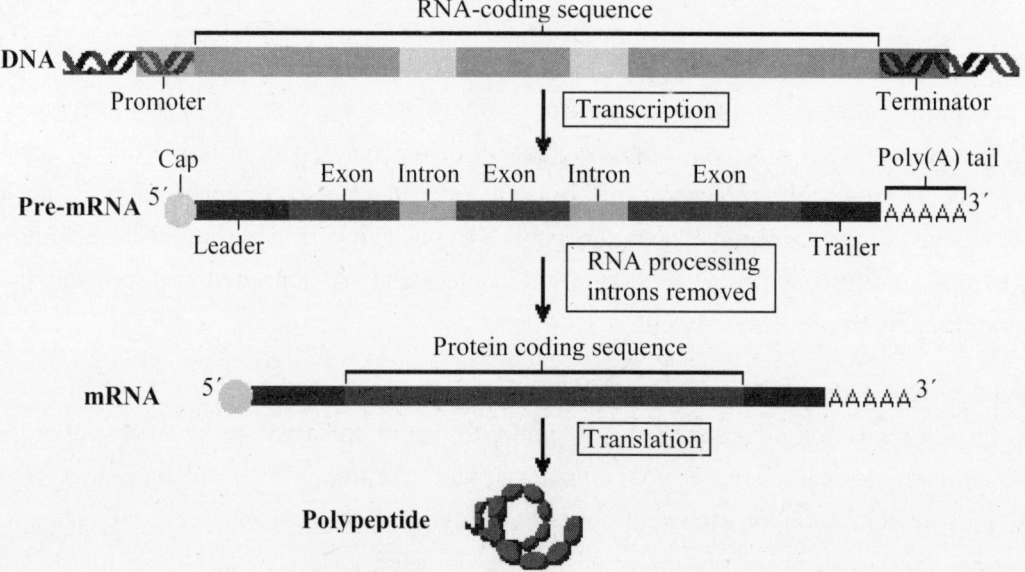

Figure 8.9: Eukaryotic gene expression

(b) RNA polymerase II

Formation of the stable transcription initiation complex on the promoter of a gene is directed by a DNA sequence with the consensus TATA/TAA/T, around 30 nucleotides upstream of the transcription initiation site of the gene, the so-called TATA box. Mutations in the TATA box sequence have a striking effect on transcription; few mutations are tolerated, demon-strating that this is a crucial sequence. The primary transcription complex, TFIID, consisting of up to 12 different TAFs, forms on TBP bound to the TATA box, and acts to direct RNA polymerase II to the correct transcription initiation site that serves as a focus for formation of the stable transcription initiation complex. A huge multi-protein structure is thus assembled in a highly ordered manner on TFIID.

(c) **RNA polymerase III**

(d) The promoters for genes transcribed by RNA polymerase III are located downstream of the transcription initiation site, within the coding region of the gene. For tRNA genes a large multi-subunit protein, TFIIIC, binds with high affinity to the so-called "B-box" within the gene, and with lower affinity to the "A-box" upstream. TFIIIC acts as an assembly site for recruitment of the TFIIIB trimeric complex (containing TBP), which has no distinct sequence requirement for binding. The TFIIIB/C complex is capable of binding RNA polymerase III and initiating transcription. For 5S RNA there is only one promoter box within the gene, the "C-box", which binds TFIIIA. This factor binds TFIIIC, as for the tRNA genes and positions it at a similar distance with respect to the transcription initiation site. TFIIIB can then bind followed by RNA polymerase III as before.

8.13.2. The Promoter

Eukaryotic nuclear genes have three classes of promoters which are specific for the three types of RNA polymerases. The promoter for RNA polymerase I has two components: 1) a core promoter (surrounding the start point) and 2) an upstream control element. The core promoter region is located from -31 to +6 around the transcription start point. Another sequence further upstream, called the upstream control element (UCE), located from -187 to -107 is also required for efficient transcription. Both elements are closely related; there is approximately 85% sequence identity between them. These elements are also unusual in that they are GC-rich. In general, sequences around the start-point of transcription tend to be AT-rich so that melting of the DNA duplex is easier.

After the binding of appropriate transcription factors to both sites, RNA polymerase I binds to the core promoter. The typical promoter for RNA polymerase II has a short initiator sequence, consisting mostly of pyrimidines and usually a TATA box about 25 bases upstream from the start point. This type of promoter (with or without the TATA box) is often called a polymerase II core promoter, because for most genes a variety of upstream control elements also play important role in the initiation of transcription. The promoters for RNA polymerase III vary in structure but the ones for tRNA genes and 5S rRNA genes are located entirely downstream of the start point, within the transcribed sequence.

General transcription factors and the polymerase undergo a pattern of sequential binding to initiate transcription of nuclear genes. TFIID binds to the TATA box followed by the binding of TFIIA and TFIIB. The resulting complex is now bound by the polymerase, to which TFIIF has already attached. The initiation complex is completed by the addition of

TFIIE, TFIIJ, and TFIIH. After an activation step requiring ATP-dependent phosphorylation of the RNA polymerase molecule, the polymerase can initiate transcription at the start point (Fig. 8.10).

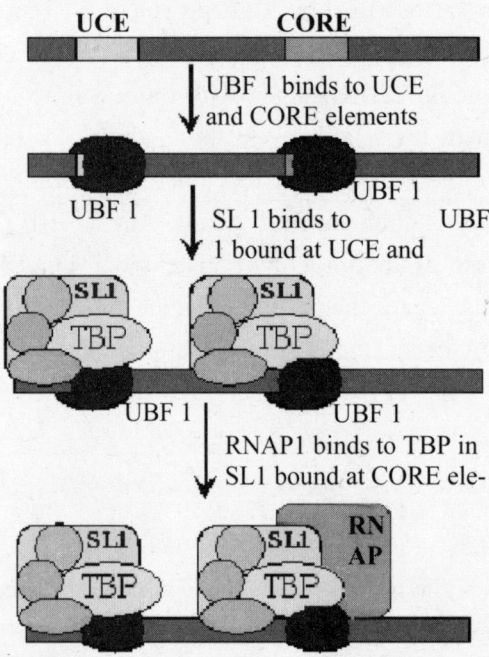

Figure 8.10: Binding of transcription factors and RNA polymerase

The TATA-binding protein (TBP) is a subunit of the TFIID and plays a role in the activity of both RNA polymerase I and RNA polymerase III transcription. TBP is also essential for transcription of TATA-less genes. TBP differs from most DNA-binding proteins in that it interacts with the minor groove of DNA, rather than the major groove and imparts a sharp bend to the DNA. The TBP has been highly conserved during evolution. When TBP is bound to DNA, other transcription-factor proteins can interact with the convex surface of the TBP saddle. TBP is required for transcription initiation on all types of eukaryotic promoters.

Termination signals end the transcription of RNA by RNA polymerase I and RNA polymerase III without the activity of hairpin structures as seen in prokaryotes. mRNA is cleaved 10 to 35 base-pairs downstream of a AAUAAA sequence (which acts as a poly-A tail addition signal). Ribosomal RNA processing involves cleavage of multiple rRNAs from a common precursor. The eukaryotic transcription unit that includes the genes for the three largest rRNAs occurs in multiple copies and arranged in tandem arrays with non-transcribed spacers separate the units. Each transcription unit includes the genes for the three rRNAs and transcribed spacer regions. The transcription unit is transcribed by RNA polymerase I into a single long transcript (pre-rRNA) with a sedimentation coefficient of about 45S. RNA processing yields mature rRNA molecules (Fig. 8.11). RNA cleavage actually occurs in a series of steps which varies in order with the species and cell type but the final products are always the same three types of rRNA molecules.

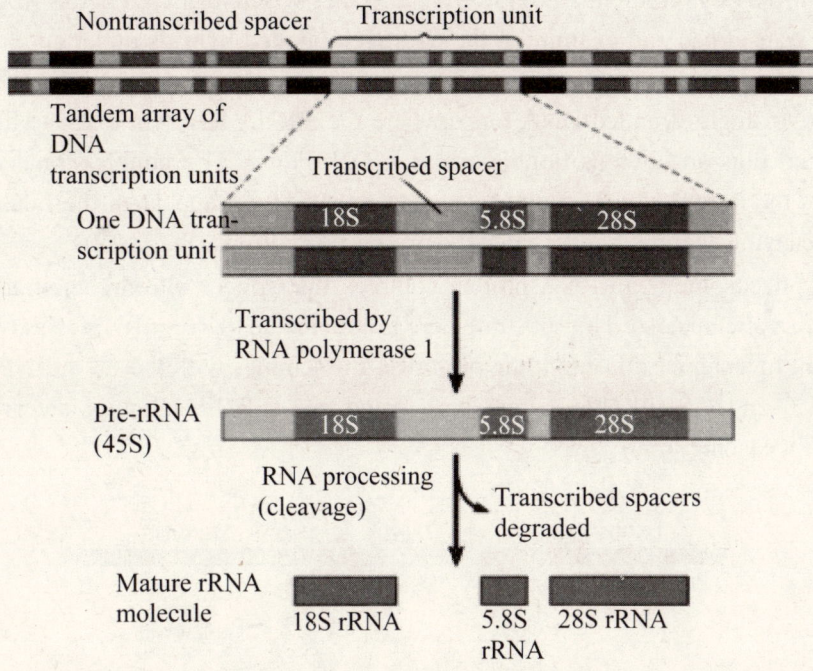

Figure 8.11: rRNA synthesis

Every tRNA gene is transcribed as a precursor that must be processed into a mature tRNA molecule by the removal, addition and chemical modification of nucleotides. Processing for some tRNA involves removal of the leader sequence at the 5' end, replacement of two nucleotides at the 3' end by the sequence CCA (with which all mature tRNA molecules terminate), chemical modification of certain bases and excision of an intron. The mature tRNA is often diagrammed as a flattened cloverleaf which clearly shows the base pairing between self-complementary stretches in the molecule.

Messenger RNA in eukaryotes is first made as heterogeneous nuclear mRNA (or pre-mRNA) then processed into mature mRNA through the addition of a 5' cap structure, addition of poly-A tails and the splicing out of introns. To give the mRNA stability, a 5' "cap" (a guanosine nucleotide methylated at the 7th position) is joined to the first nucleotide in an unusual 5' to 5' linkage (sort of "backwards"). During the capping process, the first two nucleotides of the message may also become methylated.

Transcription of eukaryotic pre-mRNAs often proceeds beyond the 3' end of the mature mRNA. An AAUAAA sequence located slightly upstream from the proper 3' end then signals that the RNA chain should be cleaved about 10—35 nucleotides downstream from the signal site, followed by addition of a poly-A tail catalyzed by poly(A) polymerase.

Spliceosomes remove introns from pre-mRNA. Introns were discovered to exist in eukaryotic mRNA by mixing mature mRNA molecules with the genes (DNA) from which they had been transcribed and examining the hydrogen bonded hybrids under an electron microscope. Hybridization of a eukaryotic mRNA molecule with a gene which has one intron will produce two single-stranded DNA loops where the mRNA has hybridized to the DNA template strand plus an obvious double-stranded DNA loop. The double-stranded DNA loop represents the intron, which contains sequences that do not appear in the final mRNA. Restriction enzyme analysis has revealed the presence of introns (Fig. 8.12).

The spliceosome is an RNA-protein complex that splices intron-containing pre-mRNA in the eukaryotic nucleus. The substrate here is a molecule of pre-mRNA with two exons and one intron. In a stepwise fashion, the pre-mRNA assembles with the U1 snRNP, U2 snRNP, and U4/U6 and U5 snRNPs (along with some non-snRNP splicing factors), forming a mature spliceosome.

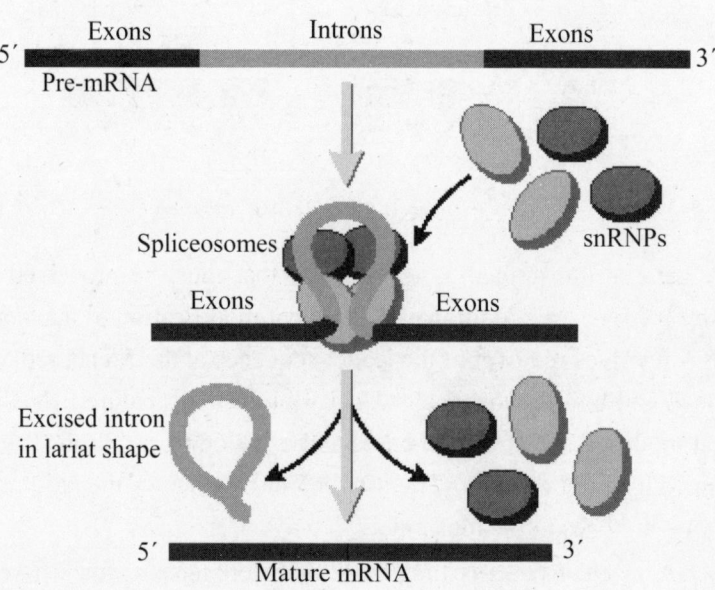

Figure 8.12: Post transcriptional modification of eukaryotic mRNA

The pre-mRNA is cleaved at the 5' splice site and the newly released 5' end is linked to an adenine (A) nucleotide located at the branch-point sequence, creating a looped lariat structure. Next the 3' splice site is cleaved and the two ends of the exon are joined together, releasing the intron for subsequent degradation. Alternative splicing may results in the formation of alternate forms of mRNA. Most mRNA molecules have a high turn over rate as the molecules are rapidly degraded and replaced. tRNA and rRNAs are relatively stable. Bacterial mRNAs have half-lives of a few minutes, while eukaryotic mRNA range from hours to days. Transcription allows amplification of the genetic information because many copies of the mRNA can be produced to direct a great deal of protein synthesis.

8.13.3. TATA binding protein (TBP)

TATA binding protein (TBP) is the general transcription factor common to all 3 RNA polymerase complexes. TBP is a 38 kDa saddle-shaped monomer which can contact and bend severely TATA-containing DNA in the minor groove. TBP therefore changes the conformation of the DNA and this is thought to facilitate transcription factor binding. It is highly conserved from yeast to mammals and is evolutionarily ancient, a related protein being found in archebacteria. TBP presents a wide outer surface for simultaneous binding of a number of TBP-associated factors (TAFs) and the complexes these form are the positioning factors for RNA polymerase. TAFs appear to regulate the activity of TBP and together they determine the specificity of polymerase binding to promoters.

8.14. Types of Promoters used to Regulate Gene Expression

Promoters used in biotechnology are of different types, according to the intended type of control of gene expression. Eukaryotic promoters are usually larger than just the TATA box and initiation site. They tend to be modular in architecture and can be very complex, if they are regulated in response to tissue type, differentiation stage, or cellular signals. Other transcription factor binding sites are generally found upstream of the TATA box and act through binding of different transcriptional activators and/or repressors to increase or decrease the level of transcription (i.e. increase or decrease the rate of loading of the RNA polymerase complex on the promoter). They can be generally divided into:

- **Constitutive promoters:** Constitutive factors interact with the basal transcription initiation complex to increase levels of transcription in all tissues. In the absence of these factors the basal promoter can provide only low levels of transcription initiation and binding of one or more of these factors is necessary for significant levels of transcription to occur. All these elements are essential for full transcriptional activity in promoters where they are present. The CCAAT box, at least, may be recognized by a variety of proteins that can activate or repress gene expression. These promoters direct expression in virtually all tissues and are largely, if not entirely, independent of environmental and developmental factors. As their expression is normally not conditioned by endogenous factors, constitutive promoters are usually active across species and even across kingdoms.

- **Tissue-specific or development-stage-specific promoters**. These direct the expression of a gene in specific tissue(s) or at certain stages of development. For plants, promoter elements that are expressed or affect the expression of genes in the vascular system, photosynthetic tissues, tubers, roots and other vegetative organs, or seeds and other reproductive organs can be found in heterologous systems (e.g. distantly related species or even other kingdoms) but the most specificity is generally achieved with homologous promoters (*i.e.* from the same species, genus or family). This is probably because the coordinate expression of transcription factors is necessary for regulation of the promoter's activity.

- **Inducible promoters**: Inducible factors are produced in response to specific cellular signals, e.g. stress, growth stimulation, metabolite concentrations etc. They interact with their appropriate promoter binding sites to modulate gene expression. Some examples are hormone receptors, metal ions, heat shock proteins, and cAMP. The performance inducible factors are not conditioned to endogenous factors but to environmental conditions and external stimuli that can be artificially controlled. Within this group, there are promoters modulated by abiotic factors such as light, oxygen levels, heat, cold and wounding. Since some of these factors are difficult to control outside an experimental setting, promoters that respond to chemical compounds, not found naturally in the organism of interest, are of particular interest. Along those lines, promoters that respond to antibiotics, copper, alcohol, steroids, and herbicides, among other compounds, have been adapted and refined to allow the induction of gene activity independent of other biotic or abiotic factors.

- **Synthetic promoters**. Promoters are synthesized by bringing together the primary elements of a promoter region from diverse origins in a molecule.

8.15. Translation

Translation is a process where genetic information is translated from a "nucleic acid language" in to an "amino acid language". It is catalyzed by ribosome, which contains proteins and ribosomal RNA (rRNA). Translation is a RNA directed synthesis of polypeptides. This process requires all three classes of RNA, mRNA, rRNA and transfer RNA (t-RNA) which can bind to three base pair codons on a messenger RNA (mRNA) and also carry the appropriate amino acid encoded by the codon. The chemistry of peptide bond formation is relatively simple; the processes leading to the formation of a peptide bond are exceedingly complex. The tRNAs carry activated amino acids into the ribosome which is composed of rRNA and ribosomal proteins. The ribosome is associated with the mRNA ensuring correct access of activated tRNAs and containing the necessary enzymatic activities to catalyze peptide bond formation. The ribosome is inactive when it exists as two subunits (a large one and a small one) before it contacts an mRNA. The small unit of the ribosome initiates the process of translation when it encounters an mRNA in the cytoplasm.

Translation proceeds in an ordered process. First accurate and efficient initiation occurs, and then chain elongation and finally accurate and efficient termination must occur. All these three processes require specific proteins, some of which are ribosome associated and many others are separate from the ribosome, but may be temporarily associated with it. The first A-U-G codon on the 5' end of the mRNA acts as a "start" signal for the translation machinery and codes for the introduction of a methionine amino acid. Initiation is completed when the methionine tRNA occupies one of the two binding sites on the ribosome. First site is the site where the growing peptide will reside, it is known as the P site and another site just to the 3' direction of the P site; it is known as the A site where the incoming tRNA is attached. Every protein begins with the methionine amino acid, not all proteins will ultimately have methionine at one end. If the "start" methionine is not needed, it is removed before the new protein goes to work

The ribosome binds to the mRNA at the start codon (AUG) that is recognized only by the initiator tRNA. The ribosome proceeds to the elongation phase of protein synthesis. During this stage, complexes, composed of an amino acid linked to tRNA, sequentially bind to the appropriate codon in mRNA by forming complementary base pairs with the tRNA anticodon. The ribosome moves from codon to codon along the mRNA. Amino acids are added one by one, translated into polypeptidic sequences dictated by DNA and represented by mRNA. At the end, a release factor binds to the stop codon, terminating translation and releasing the complete polypeptide from the ribosome.

8.15.1. Activation of Amino Acids

It is the step in which each of the participating amino acid reacts with ATP to form amino acid AMP complex and pyrophosphate. The reaction is catalyzed by a specific amino acid activating enzyme called aminoacyl-tRNA synthetase in the presence of Mg^{2+}. There is a separate aminoacyl tRNA synthetase enzyme for each kind of amino acid. Much of the energy released by the separation of phosphate groups from ATP is trapped in the amino acid AMP complex. The complex remains temporarily associated with the enzyme. The amino acid AMP enzyme complex is called an activated amino acid. The pyrophosphate is hydrolyzed to two inorganic phosphates (2pi). Each tRNA and the amino acid it carries, is recognized by individual aminoacyl-tRNA synthetases. Activation of amino acids requires energy in the form of ATP. First the enzyme attaches the amino acid to the α-phosphate of ATP with the concomitant release of pyrophosphate. This is termed an aminoacyl-adenylate intermediate. Then the enzyme catalyzes transfer of the amino acid to either the 2'– or 3'–OH of the ribose portion of the 3'-terminal adenosine residue of the tRNA generating the activated aminoacyl-tRNA, this is the reversible reaction. Accurate recognition of the correct amino acid as well as the correct tRNA is different for each aminoacyl-tRNA synthetase. Different amino acids have different R groups; the enzyme for each amino acid has a different binding pocket for its specific amino acid. It is absolutely necessary that the discrimination of correct amino acid and correct tRNA be made by a given synthetase prior to release of the aminoacyl-tRNA from the enzyme. After the product is released; there is no means thus proof-read whether a given tRNA is coupled to its corresponding tRNA (Fig. 8.13).

8.15.2. Charging of tRNA

Here the amino acid AMP-enzyme complex joins with the amino acid binding site of its specific tRNA, where its COOH group bonds with the OH group of the terminal base triplet CCA. The reaction is catalyzed by the same enzyme, aminoacyl tRNA synthetase. The resulting tRNA-amino acid complex is called a charged tRNA. AMP and enzyme are released. The released enzyme can activate and attach another amino acid molecule to another tRNA molecule. The energy released by change of ATP to AMP is retained in the amino acid-tRNA complex. This energy is later used to drive the formation of peptide bond when amino acids link together and form a polypeptide. The tRNA amino acid complex moves to the ribosomes, the site of protein synthesis.

$$\text{Amino acid AMP— enzyme complex} \atop + \atop \text{tRNA} \xrightarrow[\text{Synthetase}]{\text{Aminoacyl — tRNA}} \text{tRNA- amino acid complex} \atop + \atop \text{AMP + Enzyme}$$

8.15.3. Activation of Ribosome

It is the step in which the smaller and the larger subunits of ribosome are joined together. This is brought about by mRNA chain. The mRNA joins the smaller ribosomal subunit with the help of the first codon by a base pairing with an appropriate sequence on rRNA. The combination of the two is called initiation complex. The larger subunit later joins the small subunit, forming active ribosome. Activation of ribosome by mRNA requires proper concentration of Mg^{++}.

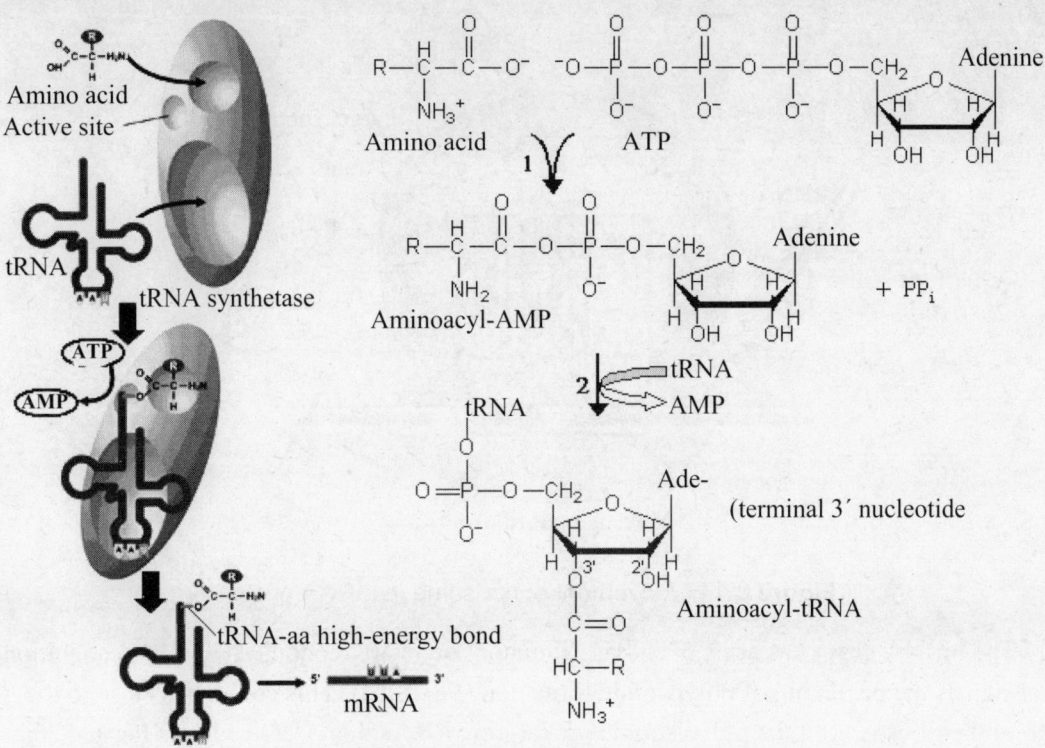

Figure 8.13: Activation of amino acids

8.15.4. Polypeptide Formation in Prokaryotes

It involves three events: initiation, elongation and termination of polypeptide chain.

(a) Initiation

Translation in prokaryotes involves the assembly of the components of the translation system which are the two ribosomal subunits (small and large), the mRNA to be translated, the first (formyl) aminoacyl tRNA (the tRNA charged with the first amino acid), GTP (as a source of energy), and three initiation factors (IF1, IF2, and IF3) which help the assembly of the initiation complex.

The ribosome has three sites: the A site, the P site, and the E site. The A site is the point of entry for the aminoacyl tRNA (except for the first aminoacyl tRNA, fMet-tRNA$_f^{Met}$, which enters at the P site). The P site is where the peptidyl tRNA is formed in the ribosome, while in E site which is the exit site of the now uncharged tRNA after it supplies its amino acid to the growing peptide chain.

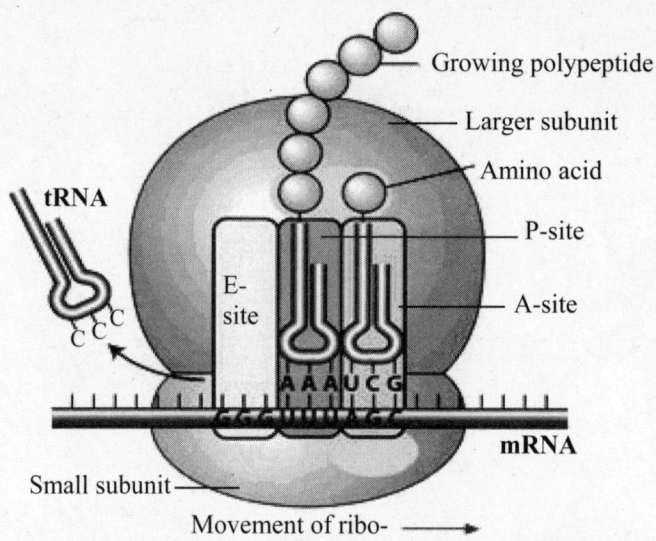

Figure 8.14: Movement of ribosome in mRNA chain

The mRNA chain has at its 5' end an "initiator" or "start" codon (AUG), its recognition that signals the beginning of polypeptide formation (Fig. 8.14). This codon lies close to the P site of the ribosome. In the polycistronic prokaryotic RNAs this AUG codon is located adjacent to a Shine-Delgarno element in the mRNA. The Shine-Delgarno element (Fig. 8.15) is recognized by complimentary sequences in the small subunit rRNA (16*S* in *E. coli*).

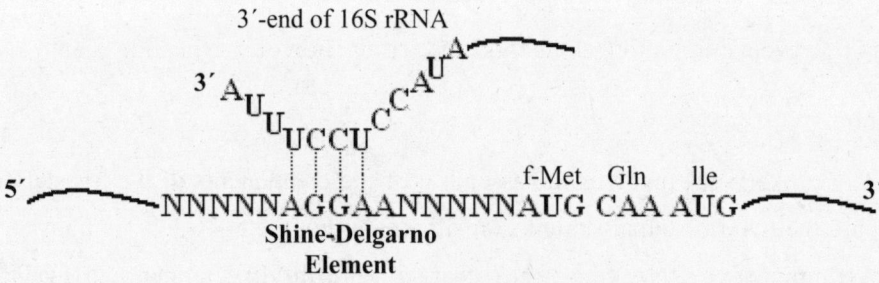

Figure 8.15: Shine-Delgarno sequences

The amino acid formylmethionine (methionine in eukaryotes) initiates the process. It is carried by tRNA having an anticodon UAC which bonds with the initiator codon AUG of mRNA. Initiation factors (IF1, IF2 and IF3) and GTP promote the initiation process. The large ribosomal subunit now joins the small subunit to complete the ribosome. At this stage, GTP is hydrolysed to GDP. The ribosome has formylmethionine bearing tRNA at the P site. Later, the formylmethionine is changed to normal methionine by the enzyme deformylase in prokaryotes. If not required, methionine is later separated from the polypeptide chain by a proteolytic enzyme aminopeptidase (Fig. 8.16).

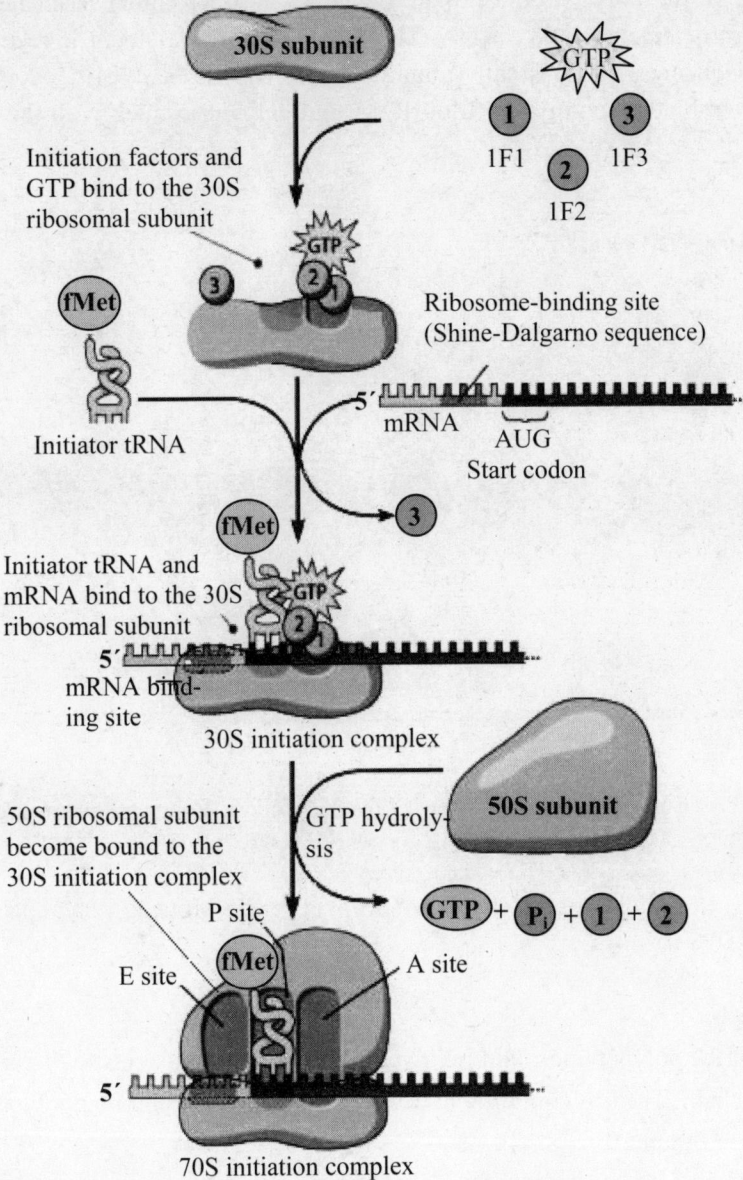

Figure 8.16: The process of initiation of translation in prokaryotes

In the initiation process of protein synthesis first Initiation factors IF-1 and IF-3 bind to the 30S ribosomal subunit, prevents 30S and 50S subunits combining prematurely. Binding of the mRNA to the 30S subunit takes place in such a way that the initiation codon (AUG) binds to a precise location on the 30S subunit. The prevention of subunit re-association allows the pre-initiation complex to form. Binding of IF-1 helping to insure that the initiation aminoacyl-tRNA, fMet-tRNA^{fMet} can bind only in the P site and other aminoacyl-tRNA can bind in the A site during initiation. The initiation of translation requires recognition of an AUG codon. In the polycistronic prokaryotic RNAs, AUG codon is located adjacent to a Shine-Delgarno element in the mRNA. The Shine-Delgarno element is recognized by complimentary sequences in the small subunit rRNA (16S in *E. coli*). IF-2 is a small GTP-binding protein binds the initiator fMet-tRNA and helps it to dock with the small ribosome subunit.

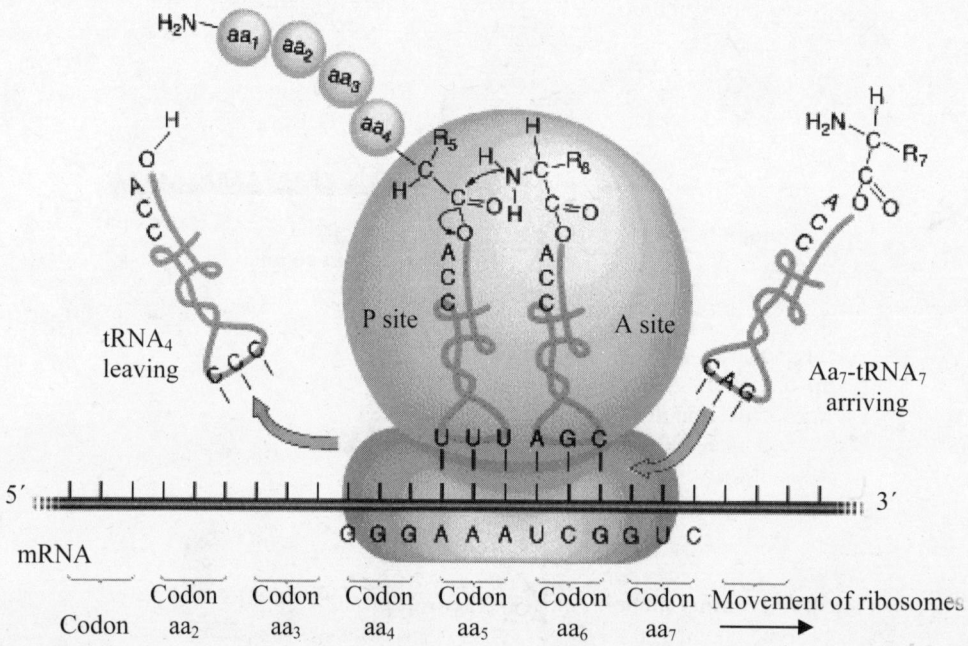

Figure 8.17: The addition of a single amino acid to the growing polypeptide chain during translation of mRNA

(b) Elongation

Elongation of the polypeptide chain involves addition of amino acids to the carboxyl end of the growing chain. The growing protein exits the ribosome through the polypeptide exit tunnel in the large subunit (Fig. 8.17).

Three elongation factors (EF Tu, EF Ts and EF G) assist in the elongation of the polypeptide chain. Elongation starts when the fmet-tRNA enters the P site, causing a conformational change which opens the A site for the new aminoacyl-tRNA to bind. This binding is facilitated by elongation factor-Tu (EF-Tu), a small GTPase. Now the P site contains the beginning of the peptide chain of the protein to be encoded and the A site has the next amino acid to be added to the peptide chain. The growing polypeptide connected to the tRNA in the P site is detached from the tRNA in the P site and a peptide bond is formed between the last amino acids of the polypeptide and the amino acid still attached to the tRNA in the A site. This process, known as peptide bond formation, is catalyzed by a ribozyme peptidyltransferase, an activity intrinsic to the 23S ribosomal RNA in the 50S ribosomal subunit. A charged tRNA molecule along with its amino acid, proline, for example, enters the ribosome at the A site. Its anticodon GGA locates and binds with the complementary codon CCU of mRNA chain by hydrogen bonds. The amino acid methionine is transferred from its tRNA onto the newly arrived proline tRNA complex where the two amino acids join by a peptide bond. The process is catalyzed by the enzyme peptidyl transferase located on the ribosome. In this process, the linkage between the first amino acid and its tRNA is broken, and the -COOH group now forms a peptide bond with the free $-NH_2$ group of the second amino acid. Thus, the second tRNA carries a dipeptide, formylmethionineproline. The energy required for the formation of a peptide bond comes from the free energy released by separation of amino acid (formylmethionine or methionine) from its tRNA.

The first tRNA, now uncharged, separates from mRNA chain at the P site of the ribosome and returns to the mixed pool of tRNAs in the cytoplasm. Here, it is now available to transport another molecule of its specific amino acid. Now the ribosome moves one codon along the mRNA in the 3' direction. With this, tRNAdipeptide complex at the A site is pulled to the P site. This process is called translocation. It requires GTP and a translocase protein called EF-G factor. The GTP is hydrolysed to GDP and inorganic phosphate to release energy for the process.

At this stage, a third tRNA molecule with its own specific amino acid, arginine, for example arrives at the A site of the ribosome and binds with the help of anticodon AGA to the complementary codon UCU of the mRNA chain. The dipeptide formylmethionineproline is shifted from the preceding tRNA on the third tRNA where it joins the amino acid arginine again with the help of peptidyl transferase enzyme. The dipeptide, thus, becomes a tripeptide, formyl-methionine-proline-arginine. The second tRNA being now uncharged, leaves the mRNA chain, vacating the P site. The tRNAtripeptide complex is translocated from A site to P site.

The entire process involving arrival of tRNA-amino acid complex, peptide bond formation and translocation is repeated. As the ribosome moves over the mRNA, all the codons of mRNA arrive at the A site one after another, and the peptide chain grows. Thus, the amino acids are linked up into a polypeptide in a sequence communicated by the DNA through the mRNA. A polypeptide chain which is in the process of synthesis is often called a nascent polypeptide. Since tRNAs are linked to mRNA by codon-anticodon base-pairing, tRNAs move relative to the ribosome taking the nascent polypeptide from the A site to the P site and moving the uncharged tRNA to the E exit site. This process is catalyzed by elongation factor G (EF-G). The ribosome continues to translate the remaining codons on the mRNA as more aminoacyl-tRNA bind to the A site, until the ribosome reaches a stop codon on mRNA (UAA, UGA, or UAG). The growing polypeptide chain always remains attached to its original ribosome, and is not transferred from one ribosome to another. Only one polypeptide chain can be synthesized at a time on a given ribosome.

(C) Termination

Termination occurs when one of the three termination codons moves into the A site. These codons are not recognized by any tRNAs. It is not joined by the anticodon of any tRNA amino acid complex. Hence, there can be no further addition of amino acids to the polypeptide chain. Instead, they are recognized by proteins called release factors, namely RF1 (recognizing the UAA and UAG stop codons) or RF2 (recognizing the UAA and UGA stop codons). These factors trigger the hydrolysis of the ester bond in peptidyl-tRNA and the release of the newly synthesized protein from the ribosome. A third release factor RF-3 catalyzes the release of RF-1 and RF-2 at the end of the termination process. The release is catalyzed by the peptidyl transferase enzyme, the same enzyme that forms the peptide bonds. The ribosome jumps off the mRNA chain at the stop codon and dissociates into its two subunits. The completed polypeptide (amino acid chain) becomes free in the cytoplasm. The ribosomes and the tRNAs on release from the mRNA can function again in the same manner and result in the formation of another polypeptide of the same protein.

8.16. Eukaryotic translation of mRNA

Initiation of translation in both prokaryotes and eukaryotes requires a specific initiator tRNA, tRNA^{met}, that is used to incorporate the initial methionine residue into all proteins but tRNA^{met} is specific for initiation in eukaryotes.

8.16.1. Eukaryotic Initiation Factors and Their Functions

The specific non-ribosomally associated proteins required for accurate translational initiation are termed initiation factors. In *E. coli* they are called Ifs, while in eukaryotes they are denoted as eIFs. Numerous eIFs have been identified as shown in Table 8.4.

(a) Initiation

Initiation of translation requires four basic specific steps: The ribosome must dissociate into its' 40S and 60S subunits. A ternary complex i.e. the preinitiation complex is formed involving the initiator, GTP, eIF-2 and the 40S subunit. The mRNA is bound to the preinitiation complex. The 60S subunit associates with the preinitiation complex in order to form the 80S

Table 8.4: Eukaryotic initiation factors and their functions

Initiation Factor	Activity
eIF-1	repositioning of met-tRNA to facilitate mRNA binding
eIF-2	ternary complex formation
eIF-2A	AUG-dependent met-tRNA$_{met}^{i}$ binding to 40S ribosome
eIF-2B (also called GEF) guanine nucleotide exchange factor	GTP/GDP exchange during eIF-2 recycling
eIF-3, composed of 13 subunits	ribosome subunit antiassociation by binding to 40S subunit; eIF-3e and eIF-3i subunits transform normal cells when overexpressed, eIF-3A (also called eIF3 p170) overexpression has been shown to be associated with several human cancers
Initiation factor complex often referred to as eIF-4F composed of 3 primary subunits: eIF-4E, eIF-4A, eIF-4G and at least 2 additional factors: PABP, Mnk1 (or Mnk2)	mRNA binding to 40S subunit, ATPase-dependent RNA helicase activity, interaction between polyA tail and cap structure
PABP: polyA-binding protein	binds to the polyA tail of mRNAs and provides a link to eIF-4G
Mnk1 and Mnk2 eIF-4E kinases	phosphorylate eIF-4E increasing association with cap structure
eIF-4A	ATPase-dependent RNA helicase
eIF-4E	5' cap recognition; frequently found overexpressed in human cancers, inhibition of eIF4E is currently a target for anti-cancer therapies
4E-BP (also called PHAS) 3 known forms	when de-phosphorylated 4E-BP binds eIF-4E and represses its' activity, phosphorylation of 4E-BP occurs in response to many growth stimuli leading to release of eIF-4E and increased translational initiation
eIF-4G	acts as a scaffold for the assembly of eIF-4E and -4A in the eIF-4F complex, interaction with PABP allows 5'-end and 3'-ends of mRNAs to interact
eIF-4B	stimulates helicase, binds simultaneously with eIF-4F
eIF-5	release of eIF-2 and eIF-3, ribosome-dependent GTPase
eIF-6	ribosome subunit antiassociation

initiation complex. The initiation factors eIF-1 and eIF-3 bind to the 40*S* ribosomal subunit favoring anti-association to the 60*S* subunit. The prevention of subunit re-association thus allows the pre-initiation complex to form (Fig. 8.18).

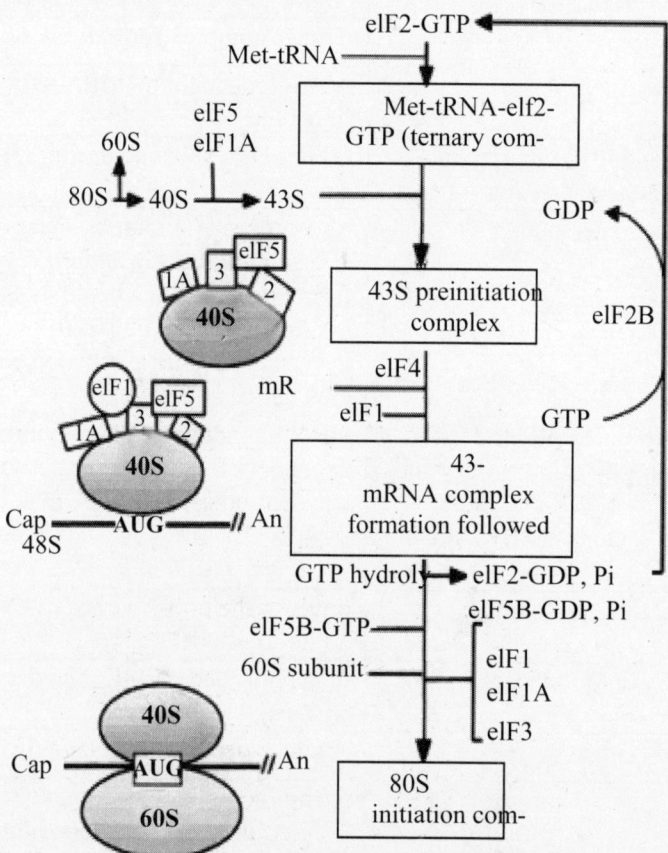

Figure 8.18: Formation of initiation complex

The first step in the formation of the preinitiation complex is the binding of GTP to eIF-2 to form a binary complex. eIF-2 is composed of three subunits, α, β and γ. The binary complex then binds to the activated initiator tRNA, i.e. met-tRNA^{met} forming a ternary complex that then binds to the 40S subunit forming the 43S preinitiation complex. The preinitiation complex is stabilized by an earlier association of eIF-3 and eIF-1 to the 40S subunit. The cap structure of eukaryotic mRNAs is bound by specific eIFs prior to association with the preinitiation complex. Cap binding is accomplished by the initiation factor eIF-4F. This factor is actually a complex of 3 proteins; eIF-4E, A and G. The protein eIF-4E is a 24 kDa protein which physically recognizes and binds to the cap structure. eIF-4A is a 46 kDa protein which binds and hydrolyzes ATP and exhibits RNA helicase activity. Unwinding of mRNA secondary structure is necessary to allow an access of the ribosomal subunits. eIF-4G aids in binding of the mRNA to the 43S preinitiation complex.

Once the mRNA is properly aligned onto the preinitiation complex and the initiator met-tRNA^{met} is bound to the initiator AUG codon (a process facilitated by eIF-1) the 60S subunit associates with the complex. The association of the 60S subunit requires the activity of eIF-5 which is already bound to the preinitiation complex. The energy needed to bring about the formation of the 80S initiation complex from the hydrolysis of the GTP bound to eIF-2. The GDP bound form of eIF-2 then binds to eIF-2B which stimulates the exchange of GTP for GDP on eIF-2. When GTP is exchanged eIF-2B dissociates from eIF-2. This is termed as eIF -2 cycle. This cycle is absolutely required for eukaryotic translational initiation to occur. The GTP exchange reaction can be affected by phosphorylation of the α-subunit of eIF-2.

At this stage the initiator met-tRNA is bound to the mRNA within a site of the ribosome P-site. The other site within the ribosome to which incoming charged tRNAs bind is the A-site for amino acid site. The eIF-2 cycle involves the regeneration of GTP-bound eIF-2 following the hydrolysis of GTP during translational initiation. When the 40S preinitiation complex is engaged with the 60S ribosome to form the 80S initiation complex, the GTP bound to eIF-2 is hydrolyzed providing energy for the process of association. In order to undergo additional rounds of translational initiation to occur, the GDP bound to eIF-2 must be exchanged for GTP. This is the function of eIF-2B which is also called guanine nucleotide exchange factor (GEF).

(b) Elongation

The process of elongation too requires specific non-ribosomal proteins. In *E. coli* these are EFs and in eukaryotes eEFs. Elongation of polypeptides occurs in a cyclic manner such that at the end of one complete round of amino acid addition the A site is available empty and ready to accept the incoming aminoacyl-tRNA as dictated by the next codon of the mRNA. This means that not only does the incoming amino acid need to be attached to the peptide chain but the ribosome must also move down the mRNA to the next codon. Each incoming aminoacyl-tRNA is brought to the ribosome by an eEF-1α-GTP complex. When the correct tRNA is registered into the A site the GTP is hydrolyzed and the eEF-1α-GDP complex dissociates. For additional translocation events the GDP must be exchanged with GTP. This is carried out by eEF-1βγ similarly to the GTP exchange that occurs with eIF-2 catalyzed by eIF-2B.

The peptide attached to the tRNA in the P site is transferred to the amino group at the aminoacyl-tRNA in the A site. This reaction is catalyzed by peptidyltransferase. This process is termed transpeptidation. The elongated peptide now resides on a tRNA in the A site.

The A site needs to be free in order to accept the next aminoacyl-tRNA (Fig. 8.19). The process of moving the peptidyl-tRNA from the A site to the P site is termed, translocation. Translocation is catalyzed by eEF-2 coupled to GTP hydrolysis. In the process of translocation the ribosome is moved along the mRNA such that the next codon of the mRNA resides under the A site. Following the translocation eEF-2 is released from the ribosome. The cycle can now begin again. The ability of eEF-2 to carry out translocation is regulated by the state of phosphorylation of the enzyme, when phosphorylated the enzyme is inhibited. Phosphorylation of eEF-2 is catalyzed by the enzyme eEF2 kinase (eEF2K).

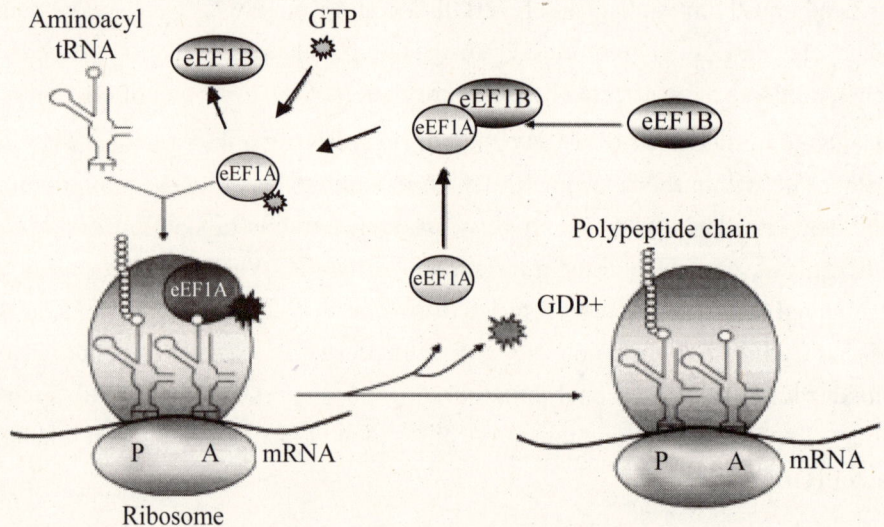

Figure 8.19: Translational elongation

(c) Termination

Similar to initiation and elongation, translational termination requires specific protein factors identified as releasing factors, RFs in *E. coli* and eRFs in eukaryotes. There is one eRFs in eukaryotes. The signals for termination are the same in both prokaryotes and eukaryotes. These signals are termination codons present in the mRNA. There are 3 termination codons, UAG, UAA and UGA.

In *E. coli* the termination codons UAA and UAG are recognized by RF-1, whereas RF-2 recognizes the termination codons UAA and UGA. The eRF binds to the A site of the ribosome in conjunction with GTP. The binding of eRF to the ribosome stimulates the peptidy-transferase activity to transfer the peptidyl group to water instead of an aminoacyl-tRNA. The resulting uncharged tRNA left in the P site is expelled with concomitant hydrolysis of GTP. The inactive ribosome then releases its mRNA and the 80S complex dissociates into the 40S and 60S subunits ready for another round of translation.

8.17. Energy Used for Protein Synthesis

One GTP is hydrolysed to GDP as each successive amino acid-tRNA complex attaches to the A site of the ribosome. A second GTP is broken down to GDP as the ribosome moves to each new codon in the mRNA. One ATP is hydrolysed to AMP during amino acid activation. Thus, the formation of each peptide bond uses 3 high-energy molecules, one ATP and two GTP.

$$ATP + 2\ GTP \xrightarrow[\text{peptide bond}]{\text{Formation of}} AMP + 2GDP + 4H_2PO_4^{2-}$$

An interesting aspect of protein synthesis is that the DNA and ribosomes are located at different sites in the cell. Location of instruction centre (DNA) and manufacturing centre (ribosomes) at different sites in a cell is advantageous. If both were in the nucleus, the manufacturing centre would be far away from the energy sources and raw materials; and if both were in the cytoplasm, the information centre would be exposed to respiratory breakdown. The nuclear envelope preserves the stability of the DNA by protecting it from respiratory destruction. The message in the DNA in the form of genes (codes) are permanent, authentic master documents from which working copies are prepared in the form of mRNAs, as and when required by the cell.

8.18. Modification of Released Polypeptide

The just released polypeptide is a straight, linear exhibiting a primary molecule structure. It may lose some amino acids from the end with the help of a peptidase enzyme, and then coil and fold on itself to acquire secondary and tertiary structure. It may even combine with other polypeptides, to have quaternary structure. The proteins synthesized on free polysomes are released into the cytoplasm and function as structural and enzymatic proteins. The proteins formed on the polysomes attached to ER pass into the ER channels and are exported as cell secretions by exocytosis after packaging in the Golgi apparatus.

8.19. Polysome Formation

When the ribosome moves sufficiently down the mRNA chain towards 3' end, another ribosome takes up position at the initiator codon of mRNA, and starts synthesis of a second molecule of the same polypeptide chain. At any given time, the mRNA chain will, therefore, carry many ribosomes over which are similar polypeptide chains of varying length, shortest near the initiator codon and longest near the terminator codon. A row of ribosomes joined to the mRNA molecule, is called a polyribosome, or a polysome. Synthesis of many molecules of the same polypeptide simultaneously from one mRNA molecule by a polysome is called translational amplification.

8.20. Post-translational Processing of Proteins

Post-translational modifications are the chemical modifications that most of the proteins which undergo before becoming functional in different body cells. It plays a crucial role in generating the heterogeneity in proteins and also helps in utilizing identical proteins for different cellular functions in different cell types. The modifications occurring at the peptide terminus of the amino acid chain play an important role in translocating them across biological membranes. Translocated proteins carry an N-terminal extension of about twenty amino acids, termed a signal peptide; it binds to a receptor in the membrane as soon as it is synthesized and emerges from the ribosome. The signal peptide is recognized by a multi-protein complex termed the signal recognition particle (SRP). This signal peptide is removed following passage through the endoplasmic reticulum membrane. These include secretory proteins in prokaryotes and eukaryotes and also proteins that are intended to be incorporated in various cellular and organelle membranes such as lysosomes, chloroplast, mitochondria and plasma membranes. Sometimes in eukaryotes different types of functional proteins are produced by proteolytic cleavage at multiple points in the protein chain, in which one gene codes for multiple products. The best studied example is the complex of polypeptide hormones produced by the pituitary gland. The major post translational modifications are:

I. Proteolytic cleavage: Most proteins undergo proteolytic cleavage following translation. The simplest form of this is the removal of the initiation methionine. Many proteins are synthesized as inactive precursors that are activated under proper physiological conditions by limited proteolysis. Inactive precursor proteins that are activated by removal of polypeptides are termed proproteins. Certain proteins particularly of the enzyme class are synthesized as inactive precursors called zymogens. Zymogens are activated by proteolytic cleavage such as is the situation for several proteins of the blood clotting cascade.

The preproprotein insulin secreted from the pancreas has a prepeptide. After cleavage of the 24 amino acid signal peptide the protein folds into proinsulin, which is further cleaved yielding active insulin, composed of two peptide chains linked together through disulfide bonds.

II. Chemical modification: The chemical modification mainly includes methylation, sulfation, phosphorylation, lipid addition, and glycosylation.

(a) Glycosylation: Many proteins, particularly in eukaryotic cells, are modified by the addition of carbohydrates, a process called glycosylation. Glycosylation in proteins results in addition of a glycosyl group to asparagine, hydroxylysine, serine, or threonine.

(b) Acylation: Acylation involves of the addition of an acyl group, usually at the N-terminus of the protein. In most cases the initiator methionine is hydrolyzed and an acetyl group is added to the new N-terminal amino acid. Acetyl-CoA is the acetyl donor for these reactions.

(c) Methylation: The most common methylations are on the ε-amine of lysine residues, occurs on nitrogen and oxygen. The activated methyl donor is S-adenosylmethionine (SAM). Methylation of the oxygen of the R-group carboxylates of gutamate and aspartate also takes place and forms methyl esters. Proteins can also be methylated on the thiol R-group of cysteine. Methylation of histones in DNA is an important regulator of chromatin structure and consequently of transcriptional activity.

(d) Phosphorylation: Post-translational phosphorylation occurs as a mechanism to regulate the biological activity of a protein in animal cells. In animal cells, serine, threonine and tyrosine are the amino acids subject to phosphorylation. As an example, the activity of numerous growth factor receptors is controlled by tyrosine phosphorylation. Other relevant examples are the phosphorylations that occur in glycogen synthase and glycogen phosphorylase in hepatocytes in response to glucagon release from the pancreas. Phosphorylation of synthase inhibits its activity, whereas, the activity of phosphorylase is increased. These two events lead to increased hepatic glucose delivery to the blood.

(e) Sulfation: Sulfate modification of proteins occurs at tyrosine residues such as in fibrinogen and in some secreted proteins (e.g.: gastrin). The universal sulfate donor is 3'-phosphoadenosyl-5'-phosphosulphate (PAPS). Since sulfate is added permanently it is necessary for the biological activity and not used as a regulatory modification like that of tyrosine phosphorylation.

(f) Vitamin C-Dependent Modifications: Modifications of proteins that depend upon vitamin C as a cofactor include proline and lysine hydroxylations and carboxy terminal amidation. The hydroxylating enzymes are identified as prolyl hydroxylase and lysyl hydroxylase. The donor of the amide for C-terminal amidation is glycine. The most important hydroxylated proteins are the collagens. Several peptide hormones such as oxytocin and vasopressin have C-terminal amidation.

(g) Vitamin K-Dependent Modifications: Vitamin K is a cofactor in the carboxylation of glutamic acid residues. The result of this type of reaction is the formation of a γ-carboxyglutamate (gamma-carboxyglutamate), referred to as a gla residue. The formation of gla residues within several proteins of the blood clotting cascade is critical for their normal function. The presence of gla residues allows the protein to chelate calcium ions and thereby render an altered conformation and biological activity to the protein. The coumarin-based anticoagulants, warfarin and dicumarol function by inhibiting the carboxylation reaction.

(h) Selenoproteins: Selenium is a trace element and is found as a component of several prokaryotic and eukaryotic enzymes that are involved in redox reactions. The selenium in these selenoproteins is incorporated as a unique amino acid, selenocysteine, during translation. A particularly important eukaryotic selenoenzyme is glutathione peroxidase. This enzyme is required during the oxidation of glutathione by hydrogen peroxide (H_2O_2) and organic hydroperoxides.

8.21. Chaperons: The Protein Folding Machinery

There are more than 100,000 proteins in our bodies, which are produced from a set of only 20 building blocks, known as amino acids. All amino acids have the same basic structure- an amino group, a carboxyl group and a hydrogen atom, but differ due to the presence of a side-chain. This side-chain varies dramatically between amino acids, from a simple hydrogen atom in the amino acid glycine to a complex structure found in tryptophan. Depending on the nature of the side-chain, an amino acid can be hydrophilic (water-attracting) or hydrophobic (water-repelling), acidic or basic; and it is this diversity in side-chain properties that gives each protein its specific character. Details of protein chemistry are already explained in Chapter 3.

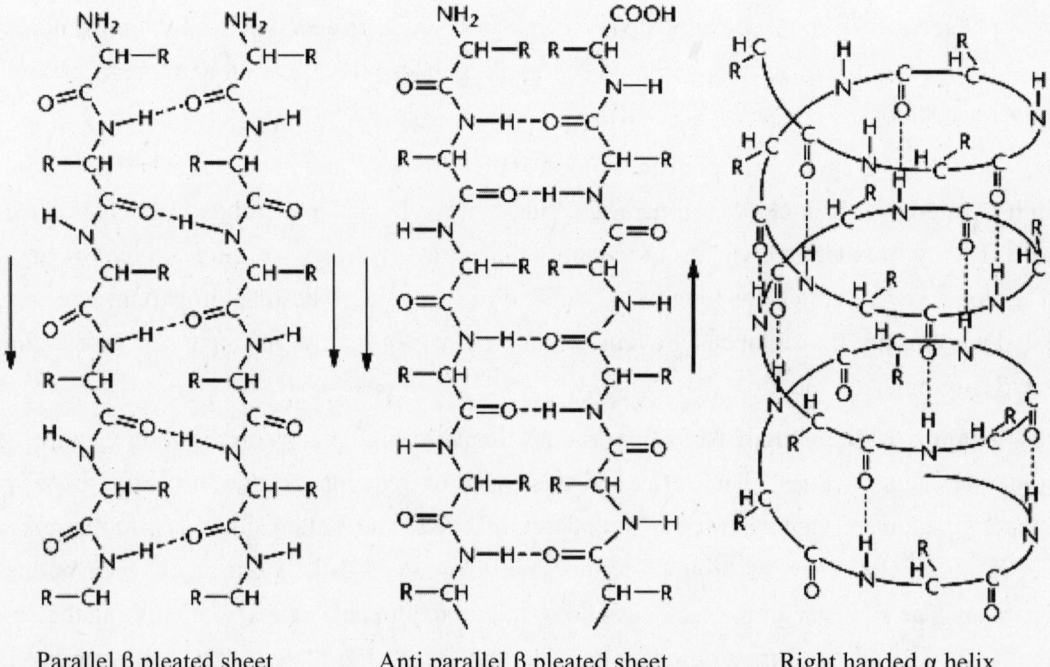

Parallel β pleated sheet   Anti parallel β pleated sheet   Right handed α helix

Figure 8.20: *Secondary structures of proteins: Major periodic elements of protein secondary structure*

The sequence of amino acids in a protein defines its primary structure, which is determined by triplet codons in the coding regions of genes. These base triplets are recognized by ribosomes, the protein building sites of the cell, which create and successively join the amino acids together. This is a remarkably quick process, a protein of 300 amino acids will be made in little more than a minute. The result is a linear chain of amino acids, but this only becomes a functional protein when it folds into its three-dimensional (tertiary structure) form. This occurs through an intermediate form, known as secondary structure, the most common of which are the rod-like α-helix and the plate-like β-pleated sheet (Fig.8.20). These secondary structures are formed by a small number of amino acids that are close together, which then, in turn, interact, fold and coil to produce the tertiary structure that contains its functional regions (domains). Although, it is possible to deduce the primary structure of a protein from a gene sequence, its tertiary structure cannot be determined.

The experiment carried out by Christian Anfinsen and colleagues in the early 1960s shed light in to the understanding of the process of protein folding. They investigated a protein called ribonuclease, isolated from the pancreatic tissue of cattle. This enzyme, made up of 124 amino acids, cleaves any ribonucleic acid (RNA) that could be harmful to the cell, such as truncated RNA that would not make a fully operational protein. Although, this was not known in Anfinsens time it briefly binds RNA in a binding site and requires several sulphur-containing amino-acid cysteine residues in the protein, which form bonds with each other (called disulphide bridges) and hold the protein structure together (Fig. 8.21).

Chemical agents such as beta-mercaptoethanol (β-ME), a disulfide reducing agent can covalently interact with specific protein functional groups. Other reagents, like urea, acting through generalized solvent changes or nonspecific interactions with the protein, can alter protein folding. Anfinsen used two different reagents, 8 M urea and beta-mercaptoethanol, in combination to unfold, or denature, RNase to the non-native or denatured state. He then removed the β-ME using dialysis, allowing the disulfides to reform. Next, he removed the denaturing reagent, urea. To monitor if the protein was correctly refolded or renatured, he tested the activity of the protein compared to native protein. He found that the "refolded" protein retained only 1% of its initial activity. If, however, he added catalytic amounts of β-ME, the protein soon retained 100% of its initial activity. In various studies, Anfinsen showed that this denaturation process could be completely reversed by removing these denaturing chemicals or by lowering the temperature. The ribonuclease then folds back to its natural functional state on its own. So, Anfinsen concluded that the amino-acid sequence determines the shape of a protein, a finding for which Anfinsen received the Nobel prize in Chemistry in 1972.

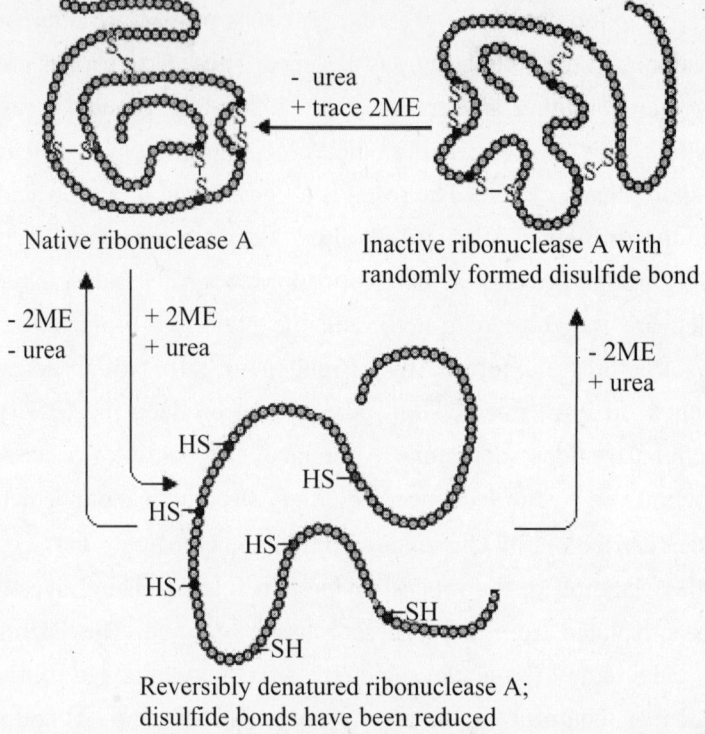

Native ribonuclease A   Inactive ribonuclease A with
                                          randomly formed disulfide bond

Reversibly denatured ribonuclease A;
disulfide bonds have been reduced

F*igure* 8.21: Anfinsen's experiment

8.22. Role of Chaperones in Protein Folding

Now we know protein molecules such as enzymes to be active, it must be molded into a particular three-dimensional form. This is achieved by help of certain molecules, called chaperones, a series of proteins present in the endoplasmic reticulum which guide the proper folding of secreted proteins through a complex series of binding and release reactions. These chaperones prevent molecules from folding wrongly or having elicited contact with other molecules, causing them to clump.

Molecular chaperones comprise several highly conserved families of unrelated proteins; many chaperones are also heat shock (stress) proteins. In the context of **in** *vivo* protein folding, chaperones prevent irreversible aggregation of non-native conformations and keep proteins on the productive folding pathway. In addition, they may maintain newly synthesized proteins in an unfolded conformation suitable for translocation across membranes and bind to nonnative proteins during cellular stress, among other functions.

The central dogma of **in** *vitro* protein folding has been the primary work of Anfinsen, which demonstrated that formation of the native protein from the unfolded state is a spontaneous process determined by the minimum global free energy. In contrast, most cells operate at ambient or homeothermically set temperatures (e.g., 37°C) where the hydrophobic effect will be stronger and thus protein denaturation and aggregation will be bigger problems, and the time-frame available for successful folding is short (Fig. 8.22). Chaperones helps to prevent aggregation and misfolding during the folding of newly synthesized chains, prevent nonproductive interactions with other cell components and direct the assembly of larger proteins and multiprotein complexes.

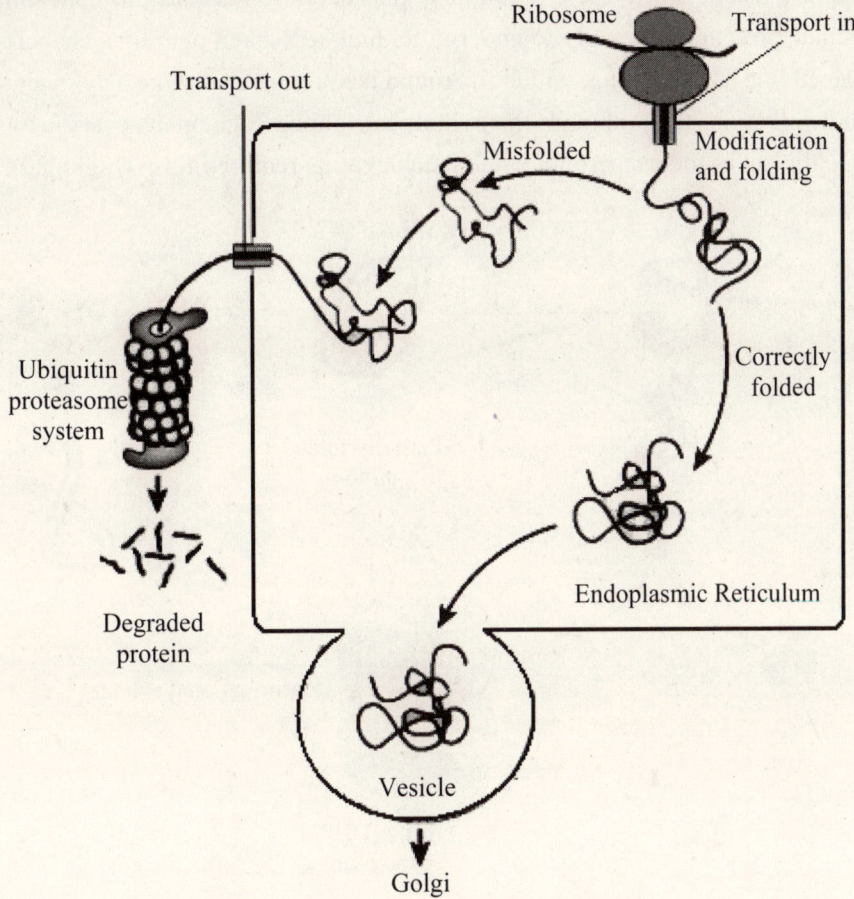

Figure 8.22: Modification of proteins

The above figure depicts how a protein gets in to its proper folding. Many newly synthesized proteins are translocated into the ER, where they fold into their three-dimensional structures with the help of a series of molecular chaperones and folding catalysts. Correctly folded proteins are then transported to the Golgi complex and then delivered to the extracellular environment. However, incorrectly folded proteins are detected by a quality-control mechanism and sent along another pathway (the unfolded protein response) in which they are ubiquitinated and then degraded in the cytoplasm by proteasomes.

Chaperones do not merely perform the folding of the protein, they also protect its tertiary structure in situations in which the cell is under stress; for example, elevated body temperature, so these chaperones have also been classified as heat-shock proteins (HSPs). The HSP70s, so called because they have a molecular weight of 70 kilodaltons, they represent the most important class of chaperones. They bind to the developing protein chain and protect those parts of the newly formed protein that are particularly sensitive and susceptible to premature reaction with the environment and therefore may lead to malformation. When there is new protein chain ready to undergo folding, it is taken over by a chaperonin, a molecule shaped like a double ring, which fits round the protein chain like a cylinder so that it can fold undisturbed inside. Although the cylindrical folding cage opens every ~10 seconds, the protein only leaves the chaperonin when it achieves its required form (Fig. 8.20).

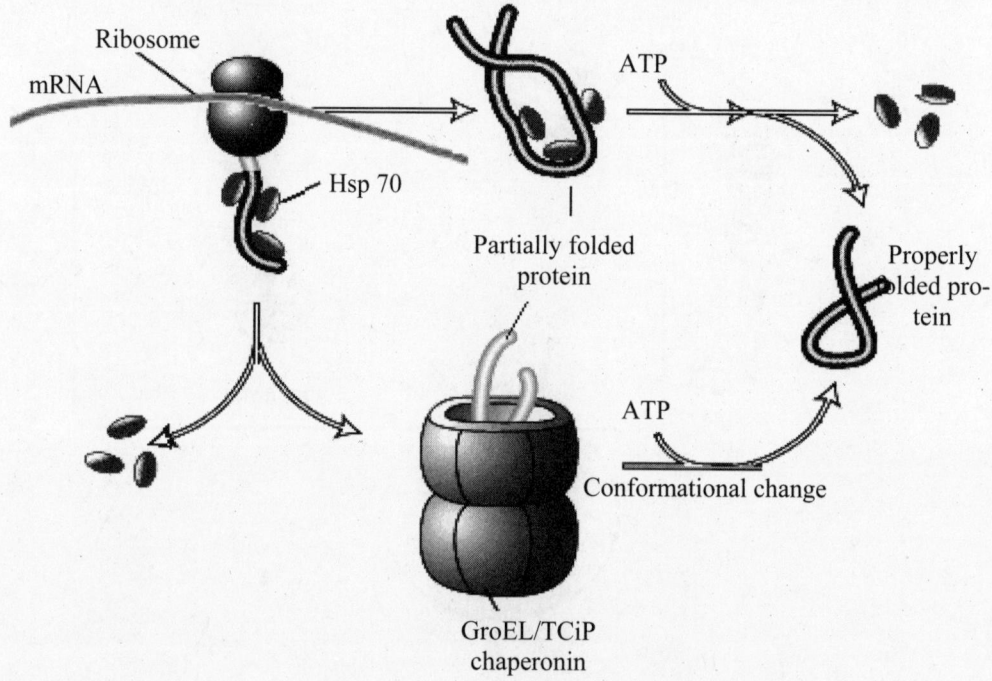

Figure 8.23: Chaperones modifier of protein

The molecular chaperones involved in the folding of newly synthesized proteins recognize nonnative substrate proteins predominantly via their exposed hydrophobic residues (Fig. 8.23). The major chaperone classes are 40-kDa heat shock protein (HSP40; the DnaJ family), 60-kDa heat shock protein [HSP60; including GroEL and the T-complex polypeptide 1 (TCP -1) ring complexes], 70-kDa heat shock protein (HSP70), and 90-kDa heat shock protein (HSP90). All these chaperones can prevent the aggregation of at least some unfolded proteins. In addition to aggregation prevention it has been suggested that HSP60 may permit misfolded structures to unfold and refold. The HSP90 are associated with a number of proteins and play important role in modulating their activity, most notably the steroid receptors. A number of other proteins involved in the folding of many newly synthesized proteins are often considered to be molecular chaperones; these include protein disulfide isomerase and peptidyl prolyl isomerase.

8.23. Diseases Associated with Protein Misfolding

It has long been known that the amino-acid sequence dictates the biologically active conformation of a protein. It is apparent that the stringent quality-control systems that come into play if the folding process fails, ensuring that the misfolded products are targeted for degradation before they cause harm. Those that escape this cellular surveillance are prone to forming aggregates that can damage or kill cells. Abnormal protein aggregation and deposition, caused by misfolding, have been shown to play important role in the pathogenesis of a wide range of important ageing-related neurodegenerative disorders. Neurons are vulnerable to the toxic effects of mutant or misfolded protein as they are not subject to somatic maintenance and turnover. Dysfunction of the systems involved in detection and elimination of misfolded proteins, such as the HSPs and the ubiquitin-proteosome system (UPS) play a role in the pathogenesis of neurodegenerative diseases.

A number of aetiologically distinct neurodegenerative disorders associated with ageing, *e.g.*, Alzheimer's disease (AD), Parkinson's disease (PD), Huntington's disease (HD), the tauopathies, and prion-related transmissible spongiform encephalopathies (TPE) such as Creutzfeldt-Jacob disease (CJD), show characteristic patterns of neuron damage due to deposition of protein aggregates in the brain. These neurodegenerative diseases primarily involve the central nervous system (CNS) and show toxic abnormal protein deposition leading to neuronal cell death. The deposits are generally comprised of dense intra- or extracellularly located fibrils or plaques in which the protein molecules have a high percentage of β-pleated sheet secondary structure. The deposits are generally ubiquitinated but have survived proteosome targeting and often consist of a number of different cellular proteins. Neuronal cell death that occurs due to these deposits and the resultant neuro-inflammatory response has a variety of pathological consequences in patients, including dementia (AD), Parkinsonism, memory loss, and eventually death. A huge variety of previously unrelated diseases, such as prion diseases, diabetes and cancer, share the pathological features of aggregated misfolded protein deposits.

8.24. Protein Targeting in Eukaryotes

Protein targeting is the mechanism by which a cell transports proteins to the appropriate positions in the cell or outside of it. Sorting targets can be the inner space of an organelle, any of several interior membranes, the cell's outer membrane, or its exterior via secretion. This delivery process is carried out on the basis of information contained in the protein itself. Correct sorting is crucial for the cell; while errors can lead to diseases.

Synthesis of all polypeptides encoded by nuclear genes begins in the cytosol. In cotranslational import, if the newly forming polypeptide is destined for any of the compartments of the endomembrane system, it becomes associated with the ER membrane and is transferred across the membrane into the lumen (cisternal space) of the ER as synthesis continues. The completed polypeptide then either remains in the ER or is transported via various vesicles and the Golgi complex to another final destination. Integral membrane proteins are inserted into the ER membrane as they are made, rather than into the lumen (Fig. 8.24).

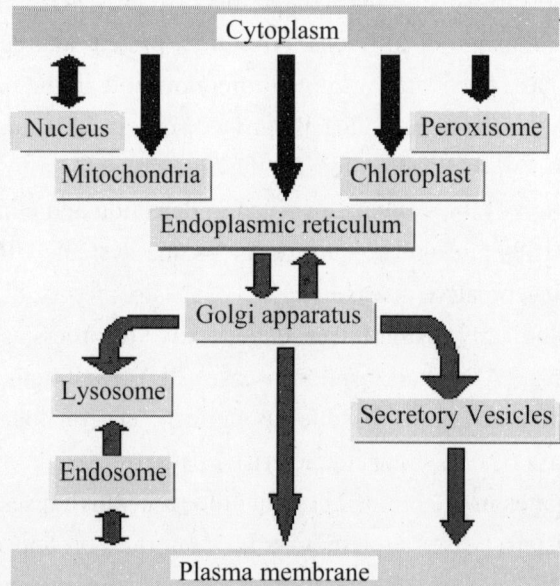

F*igure* 8.24: Protein targeting

In cotranslational import, proteins to be targeted to the endoplasmic reticulum initially have an N-terminal peptide, the ER signal sequence, translated by a cytosolic ribosome. The ER signal sequence is bound by a signal-recognition particle (SRP), a ribonucleoprotein complex composed of 6 peptides and a 300 nucleotide RNA molecule. The SRP binds to the SRP receptor to dock the ribosome on the ER membrane. When the SRP receptor binds GTP, the nascent polypeptide enters the pore. The SRP is released with hydrolysis of the GTP. The growing polypeptide translocates through a hydrophilic pore created by one or more membrane proteins called the translocon. The most recent evidence suggests that the ribosome fits tightly across the cytoplasmic side of the pore and that the ER-lumen side is somehow closed off until the polypeptide is about 70 amino acids long. When the polypepide is complete, the signal peptidase cleaves the signal to release the protein into the ER lumen while retaining the signal peptide, for a time, in the membrane. Afterwards the ribosome is released and the pore closes completely.

If the polypeptide is destined for the cytosol or for import into the nucleus, mitochondria, chloroplasts, or peroxisomes, its synthesis continues in the cytosol. When the polypeptide is complete, it is released from the ribosome and either remains in the cytosol or is transported into the appropriate organelle by posttranslational import. Polypeptide uptake by the nucleus occurs via the nuclear pores, using a mechanism different from that involved in posttranslational uptake by other organelles.

There are two possible mechanisms for the insertion of integral membrane proteins having a single transmembrane segment. Type I: Insertion of a polypeptide with both a terminal ER signal sequence and an internal stop-transfer sequence. The terminal peptide is eventually cut off, leaving a transmembrane protein with its N-terminus in the ER lumen and it's C-terminus in the cytosol. Type II: Insertion of a polypeptide with only a single, internal start transfer sequence, which both starts polypeptide transfer and anchors itself permanently in the membrane. The amino-carboxyl orientation of the completed protein depends on the orientation of the start-transfer sequence when it first inserts into the translocation apparatus.

Polypeptides synthesized on cytosolic ribosomes but destined for either the inter-membrane space or the inner membrane of the mitochondrion require two separate targeting sequences (both located at the N-terminus). The polypeptide is directed to a contact (translocation) site on the mitochondrion by a positively charged or amphipathic transit sequence. Cleavage of the transit sequence by a peptidase in the mitochondrial matrix uncovers a highly hydrophobic second signal sequence. This second signal sequence causes the polypeptide to be inserted into the inner membrane in the same way that mitochondrially encoded polypeptides are targeted to this membrane. The remainder of the polypeptide is then moved across the membrane into the inter-membrane space (or into the inner membrane for integral inner membrane proteins). Cleavage by a second peptidase can release the polypeptide into the inter-membrane space leaving the signal sequence behind in the inner membrane.

Suggested Readings

- Lehninger: Principles of Biochemistry, 4th edition, by David L. Nelson and M.M. Cox (2005) Maxmillan/ Worth publishers/ W.H. Freeman & Company.
- Biochemistry (2004) by J.David Rawn, Panima Publishing Corporation, New Delhi.
- Biochemistry, 2nd edition, by R H.Garrett and C.M. Grisham (1999). Saunders College Publishing, N.Y. Sons, NY.

- Biochemistry, 6th edition, by Jeremy M. Berg (2007). W. H. Freeman & Co., N.Y.

- Fundamentals of Biochemistry, 2nd ed., by Donald Voet, Judith G. Voet and Charlotte W. Pratt (2006) , John Wiley & Sons, INC.

- Biochemistry: The chemical reactions of living cells, 2nd edition, Volumes I & II by David E. Metzler (2001), Harcourt Academic Press.

- Principles of Peptide synthesis (1984), Miklos, Bodansky, Springer-Verlag Berlin, Heidelberg.

Cell Cycle

"omnis cellula e cellula"--every cell originates from another existing cell like it.

Rudolph Vichrow

Growth and development is one of the main characteristics of life. It is the process of an in-dividual organism growing organically; a purely biological unfolding of events involved in an organism changing gradually from a simple to a more complex level, while death is the permanent termination of all vital functions or life processes in an organism or cell. In general in growing condition a higher rate of anabolism is maintained than catabolism. A growing organism increases in size in all of its parts, rather than simply accumulating matter. Growth of an organism is characterized by an increase in the size of its body. In case of bacteria and other single celled organisms growth is meant by increase in number of individual cells. In biological systems growth is controlled by cell cycle systems involving mitosis and meiosis.

Cell cycle is an essential means through which a living cell divides, proliferates and propagates. In unicellular species, such as bacteria and yeasts, each cell division produces an additional organism. In multicellular species, multiple continuous cell divisions are needed to constitute living new individual. An adult human requires many millions of new cells each second in order to maintain the healthy state of the body. The duration of the cell cycle may vary, however certain requirements are universal. First and foremost, to produce a pair of genetically identical daughter cells, the DNA must be replicated, and the replicated chromosomes must be segregated into two separate cells. The duration of the cell cycle varies greatly from one cell type to another. Fly embryos have the shortest known cell cycles, each lasting as little as 8 minutes, while the cell cycle of a mammalian liver cell can last longer than a year.

9.1. Cell Cycle

In 1858 the pathologist Rudolph Virchow coined the cell doctrine which states that "When a cell arises, there must have been a previous cell, just as animals can only arise from animals and plants from plants." This doctrine is founded on the understanding that whether one is examining a single-celled organism or an animal as complex as man, the product is a result of repeated rounds of cell growth and division. Most eukaryotic cells will proceed through an ordered series of events in which the cell duplicates its contents and then divides into two cells (Fig. 9.1). This cycle of duplication and division is called the cell cycle. In order to maintain the fidelity of the developing organism, this process of cell division in multicellular organisms must be highly ordered and tightly regulated. The loss of control will lead to abnormal development and is the cause of cancer.

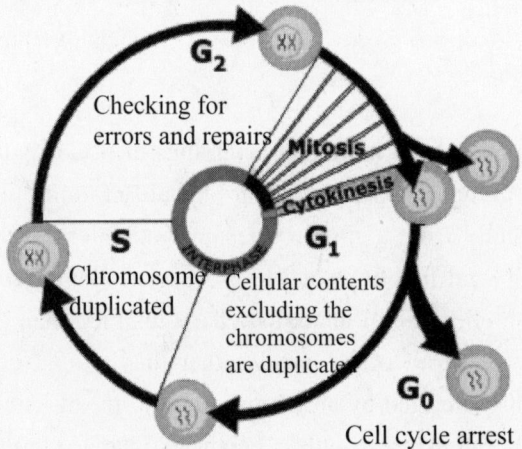

Figure 9.1: Overview of Cell cycle

The eukaryotic cell cycle is composed of five steps, or phases:

G_0 **phase:** It is also known as quiescent stage or the resting phase. Often a cell leaves the cell cycle, temporarily or permanently at G_1 stage and enters G_0 phase. In general G_0 cells do not reenter the cell cycle however instead continues to carry out their function in the organism until they die. For cells like lymphocyte, G_0 can be followed by reentry into the cell cycle.

Most of the lymphocytes in human blood are in G_0 phase. After stimulation by an antigen, they reenter the cell cycle (at G_1) and proceed on to expand through new rounds of alternating S phases and mitosis. The cancerous cells never enter G_0 phase and are destined to repeat the cell cycle indefinitely.

G_1 phase: The first gap in the normal cell cycle is called G_1 and is the period when the necessary proteins for DNA replication are synthesized. This is the first sub phase of interphase that depends in between the end of the M phase until the S phase. However, this phase of the cell cycle is not only characterized by synthesis of replication machinery. During this period the cell must monitor both the internal and external environments to ensure that all the preparations for DNA synthesis have been completed and that overall conditions for cell division are favorable. During this phase the biosynthetic activities of the cell, which were considerably slowed down during M phase, resume activity at a high rate. During this phase various enzymes that are required in S phase, mainly those needed for DNA replication are synthesized. Here, cells increase in size and G_1 associated checkpoint control mechanism and govern conditions which are appropriate favorable for DNA synthesis.

S phase: S phase is referred as synthesis phase where specifically DNA synthesis, chromosome duplication and histone proteins production takes place. Thus, the amount of DNA in the cell becomes quantitatively doubled. However, the rates of RNA transcription and protein synthesis are very low during this phase. This phase of the cell cycle is the longest taking 10–12 hours of a typical 24 hr eukaryotic cell cycle.

G_2 phase: During the second gap phase of the cell cycle the cell undertakes the synthesis of the proteins required to assemble the machinery required for separation of the duplicated chromosomes (the process called mitosis) and ultimately division of the parental cell into two daughter cells (the process termed cytokinesis). Maximum protein synthesis does take place during this phase, mainly involving the production of microtubules, which are required during the process of mitosis. Like the G_1 phase, the G_2 phase is also a stage when the internal and external environments are monitored to ensure that faithful replication of the DNA has occurred and that conditions are favorable for cytokinesis. The cell will continues to grow and the G_2 checkpoint control mechanism ensures that cellular conditions are appropriate to enter the M (mitosis) phase and divide. Inhibition of protein synthesis during G_2 phase moreover prevents the cell from undergoing mitosis.

M phase: A brief period of M phase is devoid of nuclear division, the Karyokinesis and cytoplasmic division known as cytokinesis. During M-phase there is an ordered series of events that leads to the alignment and separation of the duplicated chromosomes (called sister chromatids). This process is divided into distinct steps that were originally identified and characterized through light microscopic observations of dividing cells. The steps of mitosis are termed prophase, prometaphase, metaphase, anaphase and telophase. Although cytokinesis is the process by which the parental cell is physically separated into two new daughter cells, it actually begins during anaphase. The processes that occur during M-phase require much less time than those of S-phase, generally lasting only 1–2 hrs.

9.2. Cell Division

The cell, the basic unit of all living systems, has to maintain the integrity from generation to generation for that the heredity material has to be copied accurately, i.e. the cell division must result in two daughter cells similar to each other and resembles the parental cell from which they are produced. However, in cell divisions of sex cells, the daughter cells may be different from parent cell but they possess most of the essential features in common. There are two kinds of cell division in eukaryotes. Mitosis is a division involved in the development of an adult organism from a single fertilized egg, in growth and repair of tissues, in regeneration of body parts, and in asexual reproduction. In mitosis, the parent cell produces two "daughter cells" (The term "daughter cell" is conventional, but does not indicate the sex of the offspring cell.),which are genetically identical. Mitosis can occur in both diploid (2n) and haploid (n) cells. Mitosis and meiosis are similar processes in that they both result in the separation of existing cells into new ones. They differ, however, in their specific processes as well as in their products. The reason for these differences lies in the difference in the class of cells that each process creates. Mitosis is responsible for reproducing somatic cells, while meiosis is responsible for reproducing germ cells.

9.2.1. Mitosis

Mitosis, involves karyokinesis and cytokinesis, produces two identical daughter cells during prophase, prometaphase, metaphase, anaphase, and telophase. Mitosis is the process that facilitates the equal partitioning of replicated chromosomes into two identical groups. The daughter cells are identical to one another and to the original parent cell. The process of mitosis is complex and highly regulated. In single-cell organisms, mitosis is the only form of cellular reproduction. One round of mitosis yields two genetically identical cells. In bacteria, this process results in an entirely new, independent organism. This is classified as asexual reproduction because it does not require sex for the creation of new organisms. In multicellular organisms, like us, mitosis only occurs in somatic cells, which comprise all cells in an organism excluding germ cells (Fig. 9.2).

During mitosis the pairs of chromosomes condense and attach to fibers that pull the sister chromatids to the opposite sides of the cell. The cell then divides through cytokinesis, to produce two identical daughter cells. Both the alignment and separation processes are the consequence of the chromosomes interaction with filamentous proteinaceous structures, known as microtubules. The microtubules become organized into a biconical array known as a spindles, which are formed early in mitosis, and then disassemble as mitosis approaches completion. Some of the spindle microtubules become attached to the chromosomes at sites known as kinetochores. There are two kinetochores on each replicated chromosome (one on each chromatid), and when the replicated chromosomes split apart at the centromere at the onset of anaphase, each daughter chromosome possesses one centromere and one kinetochore. The linkages between kinetochores and microtubules are thought to be important in controlling both the positioning of the replicated chromosome in the central of the spindle during the alignment phase, and in separation of the daughter chromosomes apart after they split at their centromeres. The process of separation of daughter cells is known as cytokinesis, and is considered to be independent from mitosis. In cytokinesis, animal and plant cells differ considerably from each other. These differences are the consequence of having or not having a cell wall.

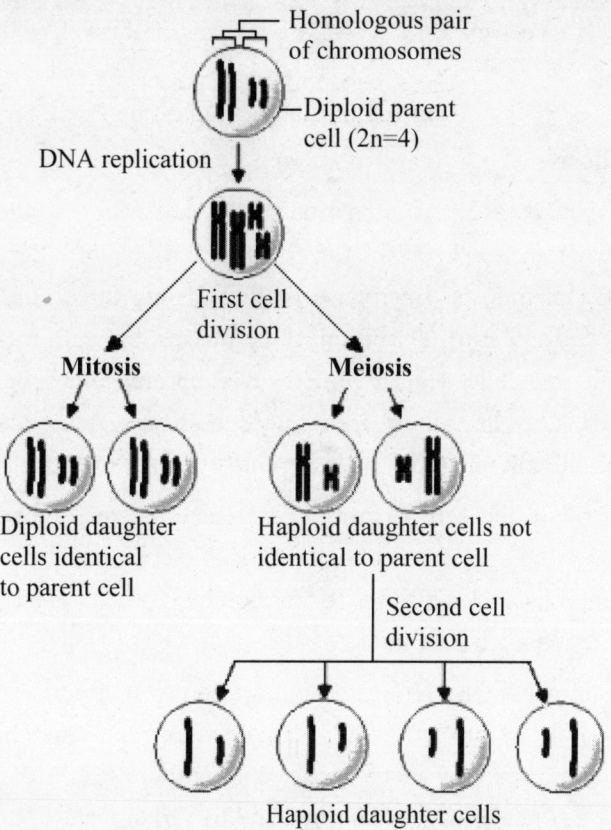

Figure 9.2: Comparative representations of mitosis and meiosis

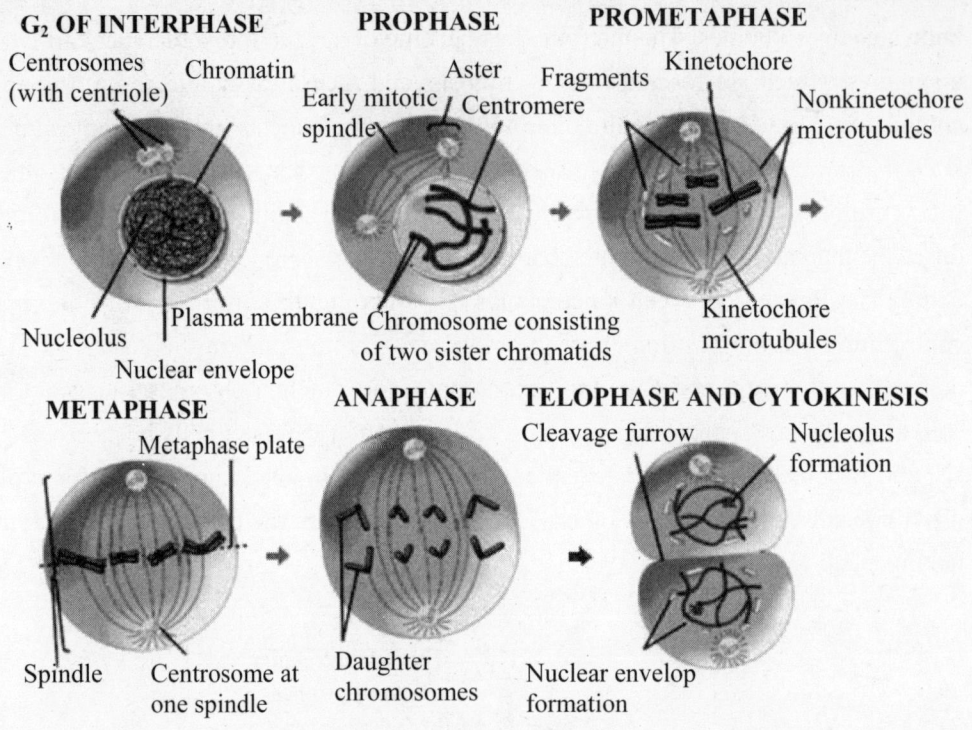

Figure 9.3: Stages of mitosis

9.2.2. Phases of Mitosis

The mitotic phase is a relatively short period of the cell cycle. It alternates with a much longer interphase, where the cell prepares itself for cell division. Interphase is therefore not considered to be part of mitosis. Interphase is divided into three phases, G_1 (first gap), S (synthesis), and G_2 (second gap). During all three phases, the cell grows synthesizing proteins and cytoplasmic organelles (Fig. 9.3). However, chromosomes are replicated only during the S phase. Thus, a cell growth (G_1), continues to grow as it duplicates its chromosomes (S), grows further and finally prepares itself for mitosis (G_2), where it divides (M).

Interphase: In this phase the cell performs the preparation for mitosis. Chromosomes are not clearly discerned in the nucleus, although a dark spot called the nucleolus may be visible. The cell may contain a pair of centrioles (or microtubule organizing centers in plants) both of which are organizational sites for microtubules.

Prophase: During prophase, the replicated chromosomes undergo extensive condensation (*i.e.,* coiling). The chromosomes are greatly thickened and shortened but are still contained within the nuclear envelope. Late in prophase, within about 6 min the nuclear envelope is breakdown, the mitotic spindle begins to grow, and two triangular 'clear zones' become visible, with one on each side of the nucleus. In three dimensions, the clear zones are actually conical and the nucleus appears spherical. Prophase ends with the sudden dispersion of the nuclear envelope, and the chromosomal mass is no longer occupying a discrete, spherically-shaped zone in the cell. Prophase in stamen hair cells can last for as long as several hours. In prophase, the chromatin condenses into chromosomes. Each chromosome has duplicated and now consists of two sister chromatids. At the end of prophase, the nuclear envelope breaks down into the vesicles.

Metaphase: Once the nuclear envelope is broken down, the spindle microtubules and the chromosomes are no longer separated by a (double) membrane boundary. The microtubules begin to interact with the chromosomes, and the chromosomes undergo congressional movement, where they ultimately end up with their centromeres all situated in middle of the spindle, at a site known as the metaphase plate. Each kinetochore of the replicated chromosome is pointed toward one side of the spindle; later, in anaphase, each kinetochore moves to one of the two spindle pole regions as the daughter chromosome. The arrangement of chromosomes and alignment of centromeres on the metaphase plate represent essential prerequisites for the orderly separation of the replicated genome into two equal parts with high fidelity.

The replicated chromosomes converge toward the center of the spindle, and once they reach there, further any significant movements cease. On either side of each centromere are the sites for microtubule attachment to the chromosome. Kinetochores are the specialized condensed region of each chromosome that appears during mitosis where the chromatids are held together to form an X shape. The kinetochores are not visible with the light microscope. At several points during metaphase, the chromatid arms may unwind from each other. This unwinding is especially apparent late in metaphase, just 1 or 2 minutes before the chromatids will split apart at their centromeres, with each replicated chromosome giving rise to two daughter chromosomes.

Anaphase: Anaphase commences with the initial splitting of sister chromatids at their respective centromeres. These daughter chromosomes then begin to separate from each other, each tends to move away from the metaphase plate towards one of the two spindle pole regions. The mechanisms that control chromosome separation clearly involve the interactions between microtubules and components in or near the kinetochore. The main events in anaphase are the divisions of centromeres, separation of sister chromatids and their movement towards the corresponding poles.

Telophase: In this stage the chromosomes have moved close to the spindle pole regions, and the spindle mid zone begins to clear. In the middle region of the spindle, a thin line of vesicles begins to accumulate. The vesicles aggregation event is the assembly of a new cell wall that will be formed midway along the length of the original cell. It forms the boundary between the newly separating daughter cells. Vesicles movement and aggregation in the spindle mid zone is facilitated by a microtubules network known as a phragmoplast and at this stage the vesicles begin to coalesce. Daughter chromosomes arrive at the poles and the microtubules disappear. The condensed chromatin expands and the nuclear envelope reappears. The cytoplasm divides; the cell membrane pinches inward ultimately producing two daughter cells.

Division of nucleus into two is often called karyokinesis and is followed by cytokinesis, in which the cytoplasm divides into two cells and can be brought about into two ways;

Cell furrow: In case of animals cells during cytokinesis a circular construction appears at the equator and it converges on all sides, finally separating into two daughter cells.

Cell plate: In plant cells a rigid cell plate is usually initiated at center and is completed towards periphery after the cell plate is formed the primary walls are deposited on either side as the result the thick secondary cell walls is formed.

9.3. Cell Cycle Regulation

Cell cycle research has primarily been performed on mutant strains of the fission yeast (Schizosaccharomyces pombe) and the budding yeast (Saccharomyces cerevisae) that have genetic lesions in some phase of the cell cycle. The cell division cycle (cdc) mutant strains have been quite useful in elucidating important steps. The cell cycle in yeast has two points where it is committed to proceed to the next stage in the cycle. The first point called start occurs near the end of the G1, and the cell becomes committed to DNA synthesis in the S phase of the cycle. The second commitment point is at the beginning of the M phase when the cell becomes committed to chromosomal condensation and the subsequent mitotic steps.

Cells like the skin which are constantly shed must renew themselves through the cell cycle on a regular basis. The cell cycle is also used during fetal development to allow a single fertilized egg to develop into an entire organism. Every process of the cell cycle is regulated by proteins which tell the cell what to do. These proteins are also used during interphase to confirm that conditions are appropriate for cell division. Sometimes the information is not copied exactly during interphase, and errors in a cell's genome are created. These errors can become harmful for the host organism, as in the case of an error which causes a cell to replicate and divide repeatedly, with no checks, forming a tumor as a cluster of cells grows out of control. Proper cell division requires a precisely ordered sequence of biochemical events that assures that every daughter cell contains a full complement of the molecules required for life. Protein kinase and protein phosphorylation are important to the timing mechanism that determines and controls entry into cell division and also ensures orderly passage through these events.

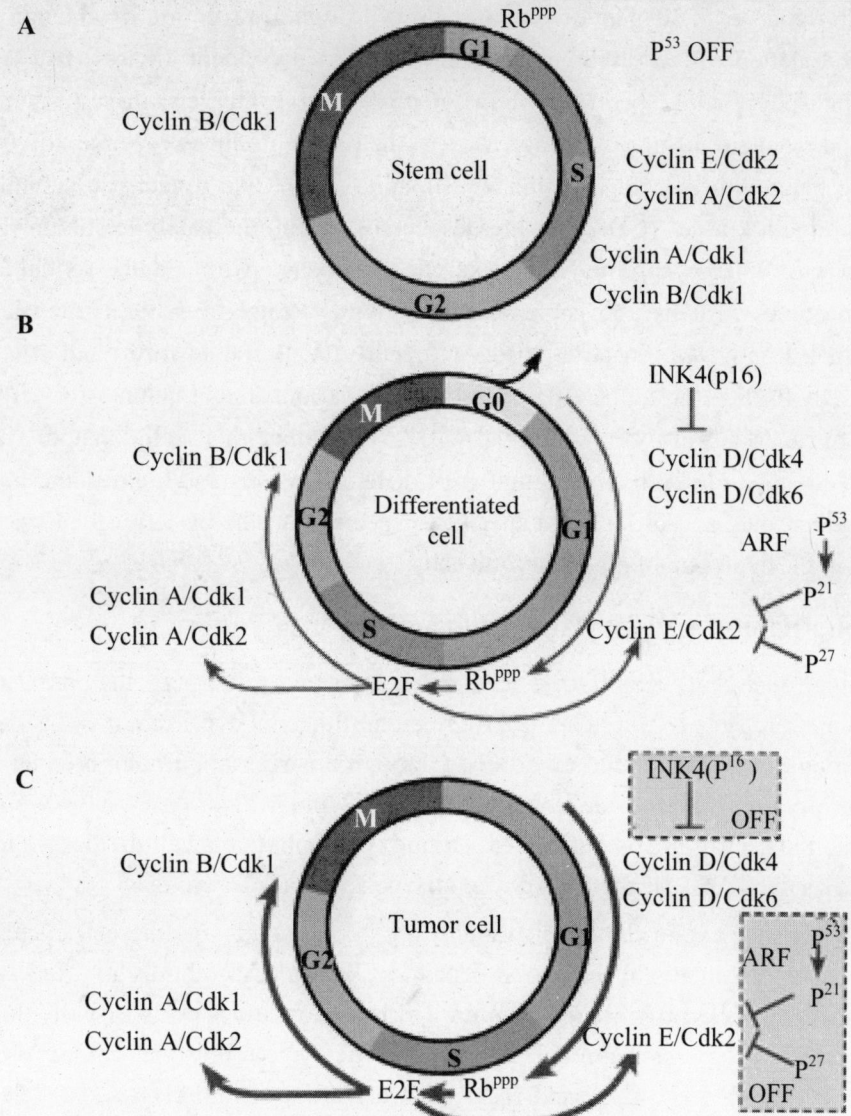

Figure 9.4: Pathways affecting proliferation in different cell types. The control of the cell cycle is essential to maintain a proper balance between proliferation and differentiation in most cells. Each cell type exhibits different proliferation characteristics and their response to the loss of Cdk activities varies. Embryonic stem cells proliferate very rapidly and are independent of D type cyclin activity (A). Moreover, they are not sensitive to the loss of other Cdks or cyclins (at least the ones that have been knockout), suggesting a high plasticity of the embryonic cell cycle. In contrast, differentiated cells (B) have acquired a G1/S checkpoint, do not proliferate indefinitely, and can enter quiescence (G0). It appears that tumor cells (C) are sometimes susceptible to Cdk inhibition, even if their proliferation features resemble the ones in stem cells (no G1/S checkpoint, no senescence, high telomerase activity, activation of proto-oncogenes, inactivation of tumor suppressor genes)

Regulation of the cell cycle involves processes crucial to the survival of a cell, including the detection and repair of genetic damage as well as the prevention of uncontrolled cell division. Regulation further involves the role of cyclin dependent kinases (Cdks) and cyclins. By phosphorylating specific proteins at precise time intervals, these protein kinases organize and maintain the metabolic activities of the cell to produce proper cell division. The kinases are heterodimers with a regulatory subunit, cyclin, and a catalytic subunit, cyclin dependent protein kinases (CDK). In the absence of cyclin, the catalytic subunits virtually remain inactive. When cyclin binds, the catalytic site opens up, a residue essential to catalysis which becomes virtually accessible, and the activity of catalytic subunit amplifies 10,000 folds. Animal cells have at least ten different cyclins (A, B and so forth) and at least eight different CDK (CDK1 through CDK8), which act in various combinations at specific points in the cell cycle. Plants also use a family of CDKs to regulate their cell division. The details of cell cycle regulation, such as the number of different cyclins and kinases and the combination in which they act, differ from species to species, but the basic mechanism has been conserved in the evolution of all eukaryotic cells.

9.4. Mechanism of Cyclin -Cdk Interaction

Non-dividing (quiescent) cells (Go) enter the cell division cycle at G1, the period when the cell grows and prepares for replication. Progression of the cell cycle requires that cell pass a restriction point in G1. Cells that do not pass through this restriction point re-enter Go. Cell cycles typically involve three additional phases, S, G2 and M. During S phase, DNA is synthesized and the centrosome is duplicated. During the M phase the cell divides (mitosis). G2 which follows the S phase is the period when the cell prepares for mitosis.

Members of the cyclin family of proteins are key regulators of the cell cycle. Cyclins bind and activate members of the cyclin-dependent kinase (Cdk) family to affect cell cycle progression. Cell cycle progression is controlled by the relative levels of individual cyclin family members. Progression through the G1-S-G2-M cycle follows successive oscillations in the levels of cyclins, D, E, A and B. Cyclins are grouped into classes that relate to the phase of the cell cycle they regulate. Cyclin D family members are G1 phase cyclins that regulate the entry of cells into G1 from Go. Cyclin D is up regulated by growth factor and external signals through the Ras GTPase signaling pathway. Cyclin D couples with Cdk4 and Cdk6. The cyclin-D-dependent kinases enforce commitment to enter S-phase. Cyclin D-Cdk4 hypophosphorylates retinoblastoma protein (pRB) and facilitates the expression of cyclin E. Cyclin E and Cyclin A are able to bind Cdk2 and promote the cell cycle progression through G1/S transition. Cyclin E-Cdk2 and Cyclin A-Cdk2 hyperphosphorylate and inactivate pRb. The inactivation of pRb leads to activation of E2F transcription factors. Cyclin E stimulates replication complex assembly through interaction with Cdc6.

Cyclin A activates DNA synthesis by the replication complex already assembled and inhibits assembly of new replication complex. Cyclin E reinitiates the replication complex that is blocked by cyclin A. Cyclins B1 and B2 are M-phase cyclins. Cyclin B1 and cyclin B2 and their catalytic partner, Cdk1 (cdc2, p34 kinase), are components of the M phase/maturation promoting (MPF) factor that regulates processes that lead to assembly of the mitotic spindle and sister-chromatid pair alignment on the spindle.

The G_1-cyclins bind to their Cdks and signal the cell to prepare the chromosomes for replication. A rising level of S-phase promoting factor (SPF) which includes cyclin A, that binds to Cdk2 enters the nucleus and prepares the cell to duplicate its DNA and centrosomes. Some cells shorten their cell cycle allowing repeated S phases without completing mitosis; this is called endoreplication for high copy number of the DNA.

9.5. Checkpoints

Cell cycle checkpoints are regulatory pathways that govern the order and timing of cell cycle transitions to ensure completion of one cellular event prior to commencement of another. The key regulators of the checkpoint pathways in the mammalian DNA damage response are the ATM (ataxia telangiectasia, mutated) and ATR (ATM and Rad3-related) protein kinases. Both of these proteins belong to a structurally unique family of serine-threonine kinases characterized by a C-terminal catalytic motif containing a phosphatidylinositol 3-kinase domain. Although ATM and ATR appear to phosphorylate many of the same cellular substrates, they generally respond to distinct types of DNA damage. ATM is the primary mediator of the response to DNA double strand breaks (DSBs) that can arise by exposure to ionizing radiation (IR). ATR, on the other hand, plays only a back-up role in the DSB response, but directs the principle response to UV damage and stalls in DNA replication.

(i) G1 Checkpoint

The G1 cell cycle checkpoint prevents damaged DNA from being replicated and is the best understood checkpoint in mammalian cells. Central to this checkpoint is the accumulation and activation of the p53 protein; two properties carefully controlled by the ATM and ATR kinases. In normally growing cells, p53 levels are low due to interaction with MDM2, which targets p53 for nuclear export and proteosome-mediated degradation in the cytoplasm. Following IR damage, ATM activates downstream kinase Chk2 (by phosphorylation at position T68), which in turn phosphorylates residue S20 of p53. The S20 phosphorylation of p53 blocks p53/MDM2 interaction, resulting in p53 accumulation. ATM exerts a second control measure on p53 stability by directly phosphorylating the p53 negative regulator, MDM2, on S395. This modification allows MDM2/p53 interaction, but prevents p53 nuclear export to the cytoplasm where degradation would normally occur. The role of ATR in p53 S20 phosphorylation (and subsequent stabilization) is less well established, but implied through *in vitro* evidence demonstrating S20 phosphorylation by the ATR-dependent kinase, Chk1.

While phosphorylation of S20 is important to p53 stability, it is the phosphorylation of S15 that appears crucial in enhancing p53 transcriptional transactivation activity. The S15 residue of p53 can be phosphorylated directly by ATM or ATR in response to IR (ATM and ATR), UV irradiation (ATR) and stalls of DNA replication forks (ATR). Activated p53 then up-regulates a number of target genes, several of which are also involved in the DNA damage response (MDM2, GADD45a, and p21/Cip). The accumulation of p21, a cyclin-dependent kinase inhibitor, suppresses Cyclin E/Cdk2 kinase activity thereby resulting in G1 arrest (Fig. 9.5).

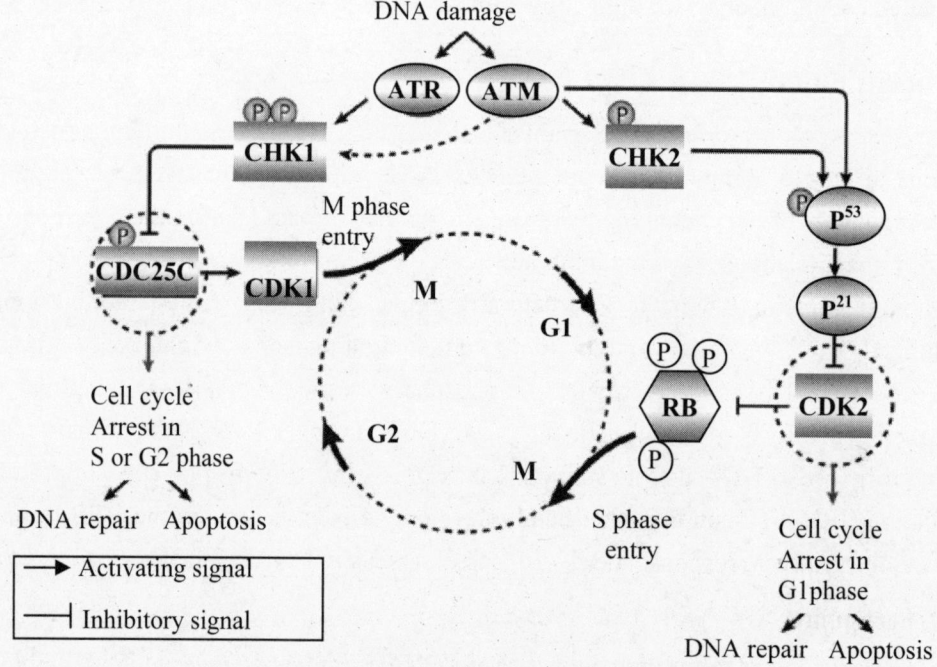

Figure 9.5: The ATM–ATR cascade

Induced or spontaneous DNA lesions are common events in the life of the cell. The ability of the cell to maintain homeostasis and protect itself from neoplastic transformation depends upon complex surveillance mechanisms and activation of repair pathways to preserve chromosomal integrity. The DNA damage checkpoint is a cardinal process. Genetic defects that perturb DNA repair mechanisms almost always cause severe diseases, including ataxia-telangiectasia and related syndromes, characterized by degeneration of the nervous and immune systems, sensitivity to ionizing radiation and DNA-damaging agents, and predisposition to cancer.

The serine–threonine protein kinases ataxia telangiectasia mutated (ATM; also known as serine protein kinase ATM) and ataxia telangiectasia and RAD3-related protein (ATR; also known as serine-threonine protein kinase ATR) are DNA damage sensor proteins that can induce cell cycle arrest, DNA damage repair or apoptosis, depending on the extent of the DNA lesions, whereas ATM responds primarily to DNA double-strand breaks, which are generally caused by ionizing radiation and radiomimetic drugs, ATR also responds to damage caused by ultraviolet light and stalled replication forks.

The ATM–ATR cascade is activated within minutes of a DNA damage alarm (Fig. 9.5). Both ATM and ATR can phosphorylate and activate the transcription factor p53, either directly or by means of prior activation of checkpoint kinase 2 (CHK2). Among the genes induced by p53 is the cyclin-dependent kinase 2 (CDK2) inhibitor *p21* (also known as *CDKN1A* and *CIP1*), the activity of which prevents damaged cells from entering the DNA synthesis (S) phase. Also, damaged cells that have already passed the transition from the first gap (G1) phase to S phase can be halted through the activation of another ATM–ATR effector, CHK1, which phosphorylates the dual-specificity phosphatase CDC25C, providing a signal that induces its sequestration in the cytoplasm. Because CDC25C is responsible for removing two inhibitory phosphates from CDK1, its inactivation prevents the cell from entry into the mitosis (M) phase. Cell cycle arrest in G1, S or G2 phase is maintained until DNA integrity is restored. If lesions are irreparable, programmed cell death is induced by the ATM–ATR signalling pathway. The ATM–CHK2 pathway predominantly regulates the G1 checkpoint, whereas the ATR–CHK1 pathway predominantly regulates the S and G2 checkpoints, although there is crosstalk between these pathways.

In most human cancers, however, the function of the DNA damage checkpoint in G1 is impaired owing to mutations in *p53* or the gene encoding the retinoblastoma protein (*RB1*). Treatment of these tumour cells with DNA-damaging agents, such as ionizing radiation and DNA-targeting drugs, results in S or G2 checkpoint-mediated arrest. Nonetheless, some of these cells might use this remaining checkpoint to protect themselves from radiation or cytotoxic agents. These cancer-favouring circumstances may be tackled by the combination of DNA-damaging drugs or ionizing radiation with inhibitors of the S or G2 checkpoints, or 'S or G2 checkpoint abrogators'. Such a combination should force cancer cells carrying DNA lesions into mitosis, a condition which prompts mitotic catastrophe and associated cell death. Abrogation of the DNA damage checkpoint in S or G2 is an attractive strategy for selectively targeting G1 checkpoint-defective cancer cells and is currently being explored in clinical trials.

p53: It is a tumor suppressor gene. The p53 protein senses DNA damage and halts progression of the cell cycle in G_1 by blocking the activity of cdk2. The p53 protein also plays a key role in apoptosis by forcing unfunctional or bad cells to commit suicide. p53 is a protein that functions to block the cell cycle if the DNA is damaged. If the damage is severe this protein can cause apoptosis (cell death).

1. p53 levels are increased in damaged cells. This allows time to repair DNA by blocking the cell cycle.

2. A p53 mutation is the most frequent mutation leading to cancer. An extreme case of this is Li Fraumeni syndrome, where a genetic defect in p53 leads to a high frequency of cancer in affected individuals.

One major function of the p53 protein, which is active as a homotetrameric transcription factor, is to serve as a component of the checkpoint that controls whether cells enter as well as progress through S-phase. The action of p53 is induced in response to DNA damage. Under normal circumstances p53 levels remain very low due to its interaction with a member of the ubiquitin ligase family called MDM2. MDM2 is so named since it was isolated as an amplified gene in the tumorigenic mouse cell line 3T3DM. In response to DNA damage, e.g. as a result of UV-irradiation or γ-irradiation, cells activate several kinases including checkpoint kinase 2 (ChK2) and ataxia telangiectasia mutated (ATM). One target of these kinases is p53. ATM also phosphorylates MDM2. When p53 is phosphorylated it is released from MDM2 and can carry out its transcriptional activation functions. One target of p53 is the cyclin inhibitor p21^{Cip1} gene. Activation of p21^{Cip1} leads to increased inhibition of the cyclin D1-CDK4 and cyclin E-CDK2 complexes thereby halting progression through the cell cycle either prior to S-phase entry or during S-phase. As a consequence of p53-induced synthesis of p21 expression, there is a convergence between the roles of p53 and pRB in regulation of cyclin-CDK complexes. In either case the aim is to allow the cell to repair its damaged DNA prior to replication or mitosis.

(ii) S-phase Checkpoint

The S-phase checkpoint monitors cell cycle progression and decreases the rate of DNA synthesis following DNA damage. Although, this pathway is the least understood of the mammalian checkpoints, recent studies on IR-induced S-phase checkpoint activation are beginning to provide important insight. Cells from cancer-prone individuals affected with ataxia telangiectasia (AT) or Nijmegen breakage syndrome (NBS) fail to slow their rate of DNA replication following IR exposure; a phenomenon known as radio-resistant DNA synthesis (RDS). This finding implicates the associated gene products (ATM and NBS1, respectively) in the S-phase checkpoint pathway. Experimental evidence indicates that IR damage activates the S-phase checkpoint via at least 2 parallel branches, both of which are regulated by ATM. In the first branch, IR damage induces the phosphorylation of the Chk2 kinase (at T68) by ATM. Chk2, once activated, targets the Cdc25A phosphatase for ubiquitin-dependent degradation by phosphorylating it on S123. The resultant destabilization of Cdc25A prevents it from performing its normal function of removing inhibitory phosphorylations (T14 and Y15) from Cdk2. The Cdk2/Cyclin E and Cdk2/Cyclin A complexes remain inactive thus preventing completion of DNA synthesis.

The second branch of the IR-induced S-phase checkpoint pathway is independent of Cdc25A, but requires the activities of both ATM and NBS1. Upon IR damage, ATM phosphorylates a number of downstream substrates including NBS1 (at multiple sites including S343), the product of the breast cancer susceptibility gene 1 (BRCA1; at multiple sites including S1387), and SMC1 (structural maintenance of chromosome protein 1; at S957 and S966). Loss of any of these proteins or mutation of the indicated phosphorylation sites results in attenuated S-phase checkpoint activation. The involvement of ATR in the S-phase checkpoint also remains relatively obscure. ATR has been shown to initiate a slow IR- induced S-phase checkpoint response by phosphorylating its effector kinase, Chk1 (on S317 and S345), which in turn phosphorylates Cdc25A targeting it for degradation. In addition, SMC1 undergoes S957 and S966 phosphorylation upon UV irradiation or hydroxyurea treatment in an ATM-independent manner.

(iii) G2 Checkpoint

The G2 cell cycle checkpoint is an important control measure that allows suspension of the cell cycle prior to chromosome segregation. Entry into mitosis is controlled by the activity of the cyclin dependent kinase Cdc2. Maintenance of the inhibitory phosphorylations on Cdc2 (on T14 andY15) is essential for G2 checkpoint activation. ATM and ATR indirectly modulate the phosphorylation status of these sites in response to DNA damage. Unlike other checkpoints, the response to IR is mediated primarily by ATR with ATM playing a back-up role; the response to UV damage and replication blocks is controlled by ATR. It should be noted that the stage of the cell cycle when the DNA damage occurs may influence whether the response is mediated through ATR or ATM. In any case, upon DNA damage, the downstream kinases Chk1 and Chk2 (activated by ATR- and ATM-dependent phosphorylation, respectively) phosphorylate the dual specificity phosphatase Cdc25C on position S216. Phosphorylation of this residue creates a binding site for the 14-3-3 proteins. The 14-3-3/Cdc25C protein complexes are sequestered in the cytoplasm, thereby preventing Cdc25C from activating Cdc2 through removal of the T14 and Y15 inhibitory phosphorylations. This results in the maintenance of the Cdc2/Cyclin B1 complex in its inactive state and blockage of entry into mitosis.

DNA damage checkpoints sense and detect DNA damage both before a cell enters S phase (a G_1 checkpoint) as well as after S phase (a G_2 checkpoint). Damage to DNA before the cell enters S phase inhibits the action of cdk2 thus stopping the progression of the cell cycle until the damage is repaired with the help of BRCA2. The BRCA2 gene (Breast Cancer Type 2 susceptibility protein) belongs to a class of genes known as tumor suppressor genes. Like many other tumor suppressors, the protein produced from the BRCA2 gene helps prevent cells from growing and dividing too rapidly or in an uncontrolled way. The BRCA2 gene provides instructions for making a protein that is directly involved in the repair of damaged DNA. In the nucleus of many types of normal cells, the BRCA2 protein interacts with several other proteins, including the proteins produced from the RAD51 and PALB2 genes, to prevent breaks in DNA. These breaks can be caused by natural and medical radiation or other environmental exposures, and also occur when chromosomes exchange genetic material in preparation for cell division. By helping repair DNA, BRCA2 plays a role in maintaining the stability of a cell's genetic information. If the damage is severe, while cannot be repaired, the cell undergoes destruction following apoptosis. Damage to DNA after S phase (the G_2 checkpoint), inhibits the action of cdk1 thus prevents the cell from proceeding from G_2 to mitosis.

In addition to intrinsic controls exerted by CDKs and checkpoints, many external controls affect cell division. Both normal and abnormal cell cycles can be triggered by such extrinsic controls. For example, the hormone estrogen affects the development of a wide variety of cell types in women. Estrogen exerts its effects on a receptive cell by binding to a specific receptor protein on the cell's nuclear membrane. By binding to an estrogen receptor, estrogen initiates a cascade of biochemical reactions that lead to changes in the cell-cycle program. Normally, estrogen moves cells out of a resting stage into an active cell cycle.

In a different context, however, even normal levels of estrogen encourage the growth of some forms of breast cancer. In these cases, estrogen increases the speed with which the cancerous cells complete their cell cycles, leading to more rapid growth of the tumor. The most effective current drug therapies for such breast cancers block the estrogen receptor's estrogen binding ability, making cells unresponsive to estrogen's proliferation signal. Thus, while estrogen itself does not cause breast cancer, it plays an important role in stimulating the growth of some cancers once they initiate by other mechanisms, such as by an unregulated CDK or a defect in a cell-cycle checkpoint.

Certain cyclins are present only during certain stages of the cell cycle. There are several cyclin-dependent kinases and several cyclins which control the G1 checkpoint (G1 Cdk's and G1 cyclins) and the G2 checkpoint (mitotic Cdk's and mitotic cyclins). Once bound to the cyclin, the mitotic cyclin-dependent kinase complex (or MPF) phosphorylates proteins involved in the early stages of mitosis. The active MPF stimulates the breakdown of the nuclear envelope, chromosome condensation, mitotic spindle formation and degradation of key proteins. The mitotic Cdk-cyclin complex (MPF) also controls the spindle assembly check-point by activating the anaphase promoting complex. The DNA damage checkpoint is regulated by p53, "the Guardian of the Genome". The G1 Cdk-cyclin complex controls the G1 checkpoint by the phosphorylation of a number of proteins. One main target is the retino-blastoma (Rb) protein. Phosphorylation of Rb prevents the binding and inactivation of the transcription factor E2F. When E2F is active it allows the transcription of a number of gene products that are essential to trigger S phase. During M phase, Rb is dephosphorylated and E2F is inhibited. In summary, the cell cycle is regulated by the control of checkpoints by cyclin-Cdk complexes (Fig. 9.6).

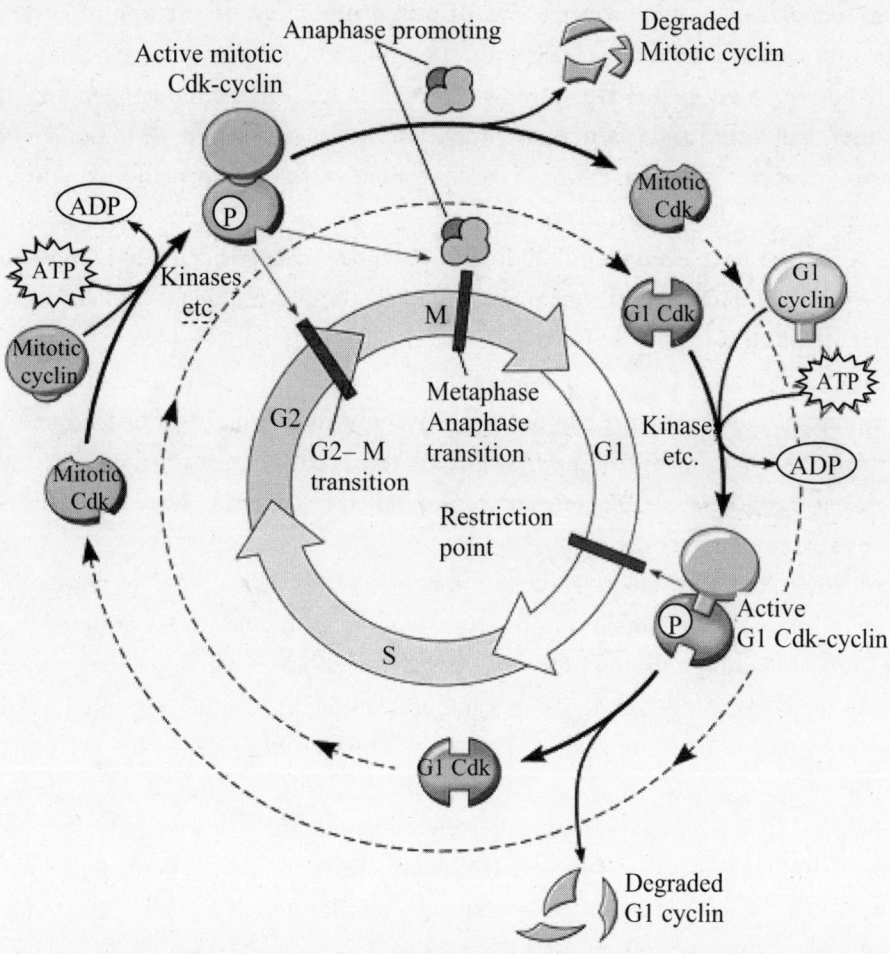

Figure 9.6: Control of checkpoints by cyclin-Cdk complexes

9.6. Cell Cycle and Cancer

Animals are multicellular organisms that require the normal function of all the organs of the body. These organs are developed from different tissues and each of the tissues is products of cell division. For the body to function normally, the organs and tissues must communicate to control the development of the cells and tissues. Otherwise, uncontrolled cell growth in one part of the body could infringe on the development of other cells or tissues. Then the normal functions of the individual would be seriously impaired. Oncogenes have been shown many times to be associated with cancer and uncontrolled cellular growth. This growth can lead to two types of tumors. Two types of tumors exist. Malignant tumors can induce secondary tumors by the release of cells that can lodge and begin growing in another location of the body. Benign tumors are cells that remain in the initial location.

The cell division process is dependent on a tightly controlled sequence of events. These events are dependent on the proper levels of transcription and translation of certain genes. When this process does not occur properly, unregulated cell growth may be the end result. Of the 30,000 or so genes that are currently thought to exist in the human genome, there is a small subset that seems to be particularly important in the prevention, development, and progression of cancer. These genes have been found to be either malfunctioning or nonfunctioning in many different kinds of cancer.

The genes that have been identified to date have been categorized into two broad categories, depending on their normal functions in the cell such as the genes, whose protein products stimulate or enhance the division and viability of cells. This first category also includes genes that contribute to tumor growth by inhibiting cell death. The second one are the genes whose protein products can directly or indirectly prevent cell division or lead to cell death. The normal versions of genes in the first group are called proto-oncogenes. The mutated or otherwise damaged versions of these genes are called oncogenes. The genes in the second group are called tumor suppressors.

The dis-regulation of the cell cycle components may lead to tumor formation. Some genes such as the cell cycle inhibitor p53 (tumor suppressor gene whose protein senses DNA damage and can halt progression of the cell cycle in G_1 phase), when mutates, may cause the cell to multiply uncontrollably, forming a tumor. Although, the duration of cell cycle in tumor cells is equal to that of normal cell cycle, the proportion of cells that are in active cell division versus quiescent cells in G_0 phase in tumors, is much higher than that in normal tissue because the cancerous cells rarely enter the resting phase. Thus there is a net increase in cell number and mass as the number of cells that die by apoptosis or senescence remains the same.

The proteins suppress the ability of cancer to develop are known as tumor suppressors because cancer ensues as a result of a loss of their normal function. It would seem obvious;

therefore, that one import function of tumor suppressors would be control of the progression of a cell through a round of the cell cycle. If cells are able to synthesize damaged DNA before it is repaired or to divide when the DNA is damaged then the resulting daughter cells can pass on the resultant DNA damage to their progeny. The result can be catastrophic resulting in cancer. For this reason, the two most important check points in the eukaryotic cell cycle are the G_1-S transition and the entry into mitosis. The former prevents DNA replication prior to repair of damaged DNA and the latter prevents damage that may have occurred to the DNA during replication to propagate into daughter cells during mitosis. Following the isolation and characterization of two tumor suppressor genes in particular it was found that they function to control the ability of cells to progress through these two important checkpoints. The protein encoded by the retinoblastoma susceptibility gene (pRB) and the p53 protein are both tumor suppressors. The function of pRB is to act as a brake preventing cells from exiting G_1 and that of p53 is to inhibit progression from S-phase to M-phase.

9.7. Apoptosis

Apoptosis is the term given when programmed cell death (PCD) occurs in multicellular organisms. Apoptosis is one of the main types of programmed cell death which involves a series of biochemical events leading to specific cell morphology characteristics and ultimately death of cells. The word apoptosis has ancient Greek origins, referring to the falling of leaves, or possibly "dropping of scabs" or "falling off of bones."Characteristic cell morphology of cells undergoing apoptosis include changes to the cell membrane such as loss of membrane asymmetry and attachment, cell shrinkage, nuclear fragmentation, chromatin condensation, and chromosomal DNA fragmentation. Apoptosis differentiates from necrosis as the processes associated with apoptosis in disposal of cellular debris do not damage the organism in apoptosis.

Cells die in response to a variety of stimuli and during apoptosis they do so in a controlled, regulated fashion. This makes apoptosis distinct from another form of cell death called necrosis in which uncontrolled cell death leads to lysis of cells, inflammatory responses and, potentially, to serious health problems. Apoptosis, by contrast, is a process in which cells play an active role in their own death (which is why apoptosis is often referred to as cell suicide).

This process of cell death has been termed also programmed cell death or active cell death because it requires controlled gene expression, which is activated in response to a variety of external or internal stimuli or their absence. Upon receiving specific signals instructing the cells to undergo apoptosis a number of distinctive changes occur in the cell. A family of proteins known as caspases is typically activated in the early stages of apoptosis. These proteins breakdown or cleave key cellular components that are required for normal cellular function including structural proteins in the cytoskeleton and nuclear proteins such as DNA repair enzymes. The caspases can also activate other degradative enzymes such as DNases, which begin to cleave the DNA in the nucleus.

Cell death can be triggered by a variety of stimuli, including gamma irradiation, cytotoxic lymphocytes, glucocorticoids, and various cytolytic cytokines, for example, TNF-alpha. In thymocytes apoptosis can be induced by treatment with glucocorticoids or irradiation. Many growth factors and cytokines act as cellular survival factors by preventing apoptosis. They are said to have anti-apoptotic activities. Apoptosis can also be initiated by cross-linking or engagement of one of several death receptor surface antigens. Some cell types such as neutrophils or eosinophils are constitutively programmed to undergo cell death by apoptosis.

In some cases the apoptotic stimuli comprise extrinsic signals such as the binding of death inducing ligands to cell surface receptors called death receptors. These ligands can either be soluble factors or can be expressed on the surface of cells such as cytotoxic T lymphocytes. The latter occurs when T-cells recognize damaged or virus infected cells and initiate apoptosis in order to prevent damaged cells from becoming neoplastic (cancerous) or virus-infected cells from spreading the infection. Apoptosis can also be induced by cytotoxic T-lymphocytes using the enzyme granzyme.

In other cases apoptosis can be initiated following intrinsic signals that are produced following cellular stress. Cellular stress may occur from exposure to radiation or chemicals or to viral infection. It might also be a consequence of growth factor deprivation or oxidative stress caused by free radicals. In general intrinsic signals initiate apoptosis via the involvement of the mitochondria. The relative ratios of the various bcl-2 proteins can often determine how much cellular stress is necessary to induce apoptosis.

Many physiological processes, including proper tissue development and homeostasis, require a balance between apoptosis and cell proliferation. All somatic cells proliferate via a mitotic process determined by progression through the cell cycle. Apoptosis (programmed cell death) occurs in a wide variety of physiological settings, where its role is to remove harmful, damaged or unwanted cells (Fig. 9.7). Apoptosis and cell proliferation are linked by cell-cycle regulators and apoptotic stimuli that affect both processes. As somatic cells proliferate, the cell-cycle progression is regulated by positive and negative signals. Apoptosis and mitosis share common morphological features such as cell shrinkage, chromatin condensation and membrane blebbing. Additionally, cell-cycle genes such as p53, RB and E2F have been shown to participate in both the cell cycle and in apoptosis. Thus, the balance between apoptosis and proliferation must be strictly maintained to sustain tissue homeostasis.

A damaged cell may undergo apoptosis if it is unable to repair genetic errors. There seem to be two major reasons for apoptosis. First, apoptosis is one means by which a developing organism shapes its tissues and organs. For instance, a human fetus has webbed hands and feet early on its development. Later, apoptosis removes skin cells, revealing individual fingers and toes. A fetus's eyelids form an opening by the process of apoptosis. During metamorphosis, tadpoles lose their tails through apoptosis. In young children, apoptosis is involved in the processes that literally shape the connections between brain cells, and in mature females, apoptosis of cells in the uterus causes the uterine lining to slough off at each menstrual cycle.

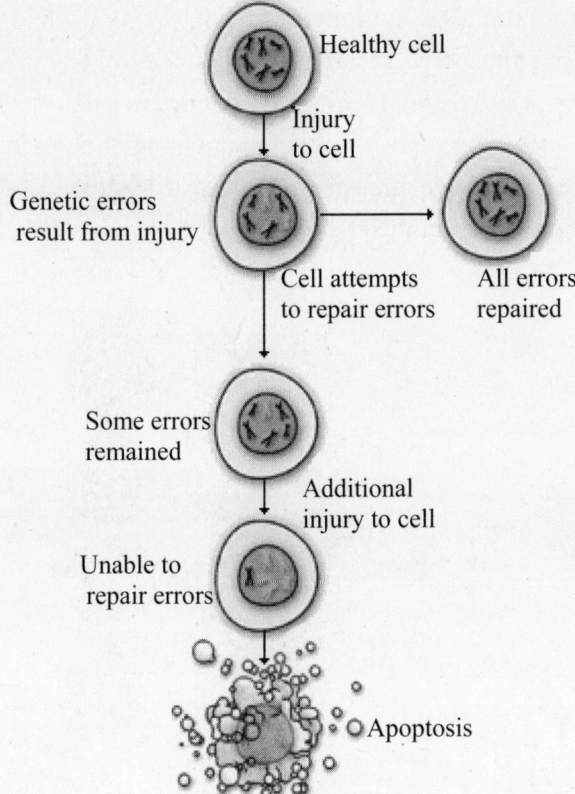

Figure 9.7: Steps involved in apoptosis

Cells may also commit suicide in times of distress, for the good of the organism as a whole. For example, in the case of a viral infection, certain cells of the immune system, called cytotoxic T lymphocytes, bind to infected cells and trigger them to undergo apoptosis. Also, cells that have suffered damage to their DNA, which can make them prone to becoming cancerous, are induced to commit apoptosis.

Malfunctions of apoptosis have been implicated in many forms of human diseases such as neurodegenerative diseases, AIDS and ischemic stroke. Reportedly, apoptosis is caused by various inducers such as chemical compounds, proteins or removal of NGF. The biochemical pathways of apoptosis are complex and depend on both the cells and the inducers.

9.8. Meiosis

Meiosis is a type of cell division that occurs only in eukaryotes, produces haploid (n) sex cells or gametes (which contain a single copy of each chromosome) from diploid (2n) cells (which contain two copies of each chromosome). In this process one DNA replication followed by two successive nuclear and cellular divisions (Meiosis I and Meiosis II). As in mitosis, meiosis is preceded by a process of DNA replication that converts each chromosome into two sister chromatids (Fig. 9.8). The resulting four gametes are haploid, meaning that they contain half the number of chromosomes. This is the reason as to why meiosis cell division is also referred to as reduction division. During fertilization, two gametes, one from the mother and another from the father, fuse, thus resulting in doubling of chromosome number. The fusion of gametes leads to the production of a zygote that has the same chromosome number of the parents. Variation occurs in the resulting zygote due to the process of meiosis and fertilization of gametes. Zygote after attaining maturity is capable of dividing into daughter cells.

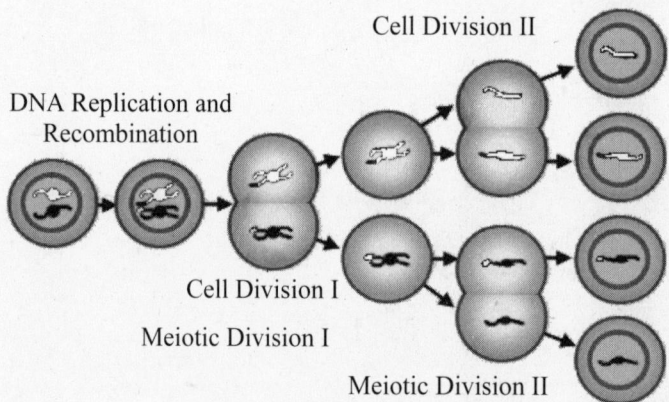

Figure 9.8: Meiotic Division

There are two different sex cells or gametes: sperm and eggs. Males produce sperm which females produce eggs because they are produced from germ cells, gametes are likewise haploid. In order to create a new individual via sexual reproduction, a sperm cell needs to activate an egg by joining it in a fertilization process. These two haploid cells can unite in to a diploid cell, which can then develop into a new individual. The sexual reproductive processes ensure the resulting offspring will have an equal maternal and paternal genetic contribution. Life cycles of all sexually-reproducing organisms follow this pattern of alternation of generations. The 2n adult produces 1n gametes by the process of meiosis. These unite in the process of syngamy to produce a new 2n generation. Thus, the life cycles alternate between 1n and 2n stages, and between the processes of meiosis and syngamy. Meiosis was discovered and described for the first time in sea urchin eggs in 1876, by a German biologist Oscar Hertwig (1849-1922). It was described again in 1883, at the level of chromosomes, by Belgian zoologist Edouard Van Beneden (1846-1910), in *Ascaris* worms' eggs. In animals meiosis helps in the production of the gametes: sperm and eggs, while in plants used to produce spores.

The process of meiosis is exhibited by higher forms of organisms, which reproduce sexually. In plants, meiosis is observed after spore production; whereas, in animals, meiosis takes place during gamete (sperm and egg) formation. Like other cell division, meiosis produces daughter cells. However, there is a significant difference between meiosis and other types of cell division like mitosis or binary fission. In meiosis, the parent cell divides and produces four gametes that are not capable of further division; whereas, in other types of cell division, the parent cell produces identical daughter cells, which can undergo division on their own.

9.8.1. Different Stages in the Process of Meiosis

The steps in meiosis are similar to mitosis and even known by having the same names. However, there is a significant difference in regions to the way the chromosomes line up initially. In mitosis, chromosomes line up individually, while in meiosis, the two chromosomes in each homologous pair line up next to each other as pairs. This pairing process is called synapsis, and the resulting homologous pair is called a bivalent in reference to the two chromosomes or a tetrad in reference to the four sister chromatids involved.

There are two stages of meiosis, namely, meiosis I and meiosis II. The parent cell or the dividing cell undergoes a preparatory phase, known as interphase, before entering the two stages of meiosis. In the interphase, the parent cell synthesizes more DNA (deoxyribonucleic acid) and proteins, increasing the overall size and mass of the cell. As a part of the preparatory phase, the dividing cell duplicates or doubles its chromosomes. With these major changes, the parent cell enters the first stage of meiosis.

Prior to meiosis, all chromosomes are duplicated in a process similar to chromosomes duplication prior to mitosis. Outside the nucleus of animal cells there are two centrosomes, each containing a pair of centrioles. The two centrosomes are produced by the duplication of a single centrosome during premeiotic interphase. The centrosomes serve as microtubule organizing centers (MTOCs). Microtubules extend radialy from centrosomes, forming an aster. Plant cells do not have centrosomes.

I. Meiosis I

(a) Prophase I

In beginning of prophase I, the chromosomes have already duplicated, and they coil and become shorter and thicker and visible under the light microscope (Fig. 9.9). The duplicated homologous chromosomes pair, and crossing-over (the physical exchange of chromosome parts) occurs. Crossing-over is the process that can give rise to genetic recombination. At this point, each homologous chromosome pair is visible as a bivalent (tetrad), a tight grouping of two chromosomes, each consisting of two sister chromatids. The sites of crossing-over are seen as crisscrossed non-sister chromatids and are called chiasmata (singular: chiasma). The homologous chromosomes pair and exchange DNA, to form recombinant chromosomes.

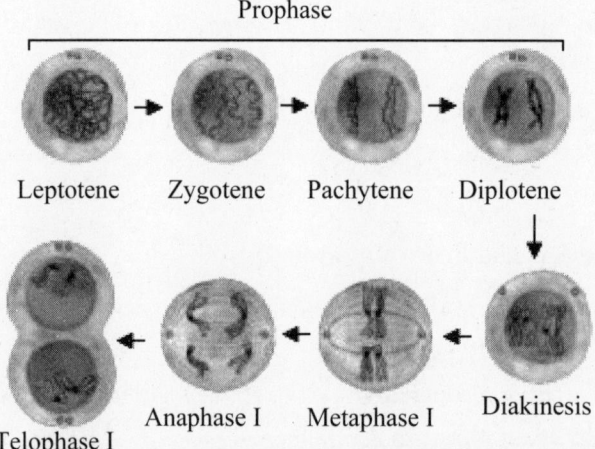

Prophase

Leptotene   Zygotene   Pachytene   Diplotene

Telophase I   Anaphase I   Metaphase I   Diakinesis

Figure 9.9: Stages of Meiosis I

Prophase I is divided into five phases:

(i) Leptotene: Chromosomes start to condense. Homologous dyads (pairs of sister chromatids) find each other and align themselves from end to end with the aid of an axial element (that contains cohesins). In budding yeast (and perhaps other eukaryotes) the process follows a period of trial-and-error. Any two dyads pair at their centromeres. If they are not homologs, they separate and try again. Double-stranded breaks (DSBs) often occur in the DNA of the chromatids, and these may be necessary for the homologs to recognize each other.

(ii) Zygotene: homologous chromosomes become closely associated (synapsis) to form pairs of chromosomes (bivalents) consisting of four chromatids (tetrads). The pairing of homologous chromosomes is known as synapsis (Gr. Synapsis= union). The synapsis begins at one or more points along the length of the homologues chromosomes. Three types of synapsis have been observed proterminal, procentric and localized on the basis of position of synapsis. The paired homologous chromosomes are joined by a roughly 0.2 μm thick protein containing synaptonemal complex (SC). Synaptonemal complex helps stabilize the pairing of homologous chromosomes and to facilitate the cytogenetical activity called crossing over or recombination.

(iii) Pachytene: Crossing over takes place between pairs of homologous chromosomes to form chiasmata (sing. chiasma). They are named for the idea that they represent points where DNA recombination is occurring. There must be at least one for each bivalent if meiosis is to succeed. There is often more, each one presumably representing the point of a crossover. They contain enzymes known to be needed for DNA recombination and repair. The steps in recombining DNA continue to the end of pachytene.

(iv) Diplotene: Homologous chromosomes start to separate but remain attached by chiasmata. DNA recombination is complete. The synaptonemal complex begins to break down. The chromatids begin to pull apart revealing chiasmata. At first the chiasmata are located at the sites of the recombination nodules, but later they migrate towards the ends of the chromatids.

(v) Diakinesis: Homologous chromosomes continue to separate, and chiasmata move to the ends of the chromosomes. In some organisms, the chromosomes decondense and begin to be transcribed for a time. This is followed by the chromosomes recondensing in preparation for metaphase I. In creatures where this does not occur, the chromosomes condense further in preparation for metaphase I.

(b) Metaphase I

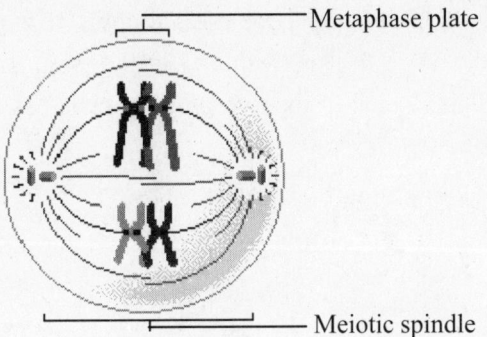

Metaphase plate

Meiotic spindle

Figure 9.10: The pairs of chromosomes (bivalents) become arranged on the metaphase plate and are attached to the now fully formed meiotic spindle

The centrioles are at opposite poles of the cell. The pairs of homologous chromosomes (the bivalents), now as tightly coiled and condensed as they will be in meiosis, become arranged on a plane equidistant from the poles called the metaphase plate. Spindle fibers from one pole of the cell attach to one chromosome of each pair (seen as sister-chromatids), and spindle fibers from the opposite pole attach to the homologous chromosome (again, seen as sister chromatids).

(c) Anaphase I

Anaphase I begin when the two chromosomes of each bivalent (tetrad) separate and start moving toward opposite poles of the cell as a result of the action of the spindle. In anaphase I the sister chromatids remain attached at their centromeres and move together toward the poles. A key difference between mitosis and meiosis is that sister chromatids remain joined after metaphase in meiosis I, whereas in mitosis they separate (Fig. 9.11).

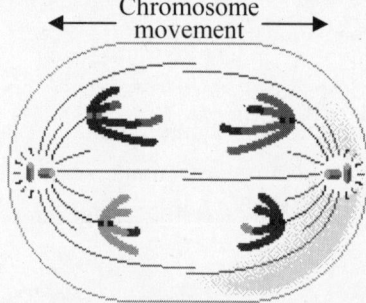

Figure 9.11: The two chromosomes in each bivalent separate and migrate toward opposite poles

(d) Telophase I

In Telophase I the homologous chromosome pairs complete their migration to the two poles as a result of the action of the spindle. Now a haploid set of chromosomes is at each pole, with each chromosome still having two chromatids. A nuclear envelope reforms around each chromosome set, the spindle disappears, and cytokinesis follows. In animal cells, cytokinesis involves the formation of a cleavage furrow, resulting in the pinching of the cell into two cells (Fig. 9.12). After cytokinesis, each of the two progeny cells has a nucleus with a haploid set of replicated chromosomes.

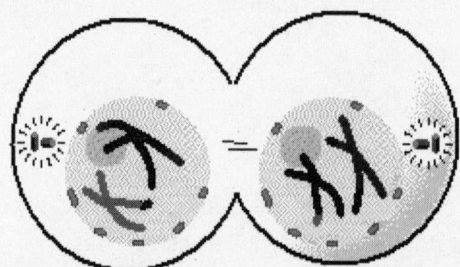

Figure 9.12: The homologous chromosome pairs reach the poles of the cell, nuclear envelopes form around them, and cytokinesis follows to produce two cells

II. Second division of meiosis: Gamete formation

(a) Prophase II

Meiosis II begins without any further replication of the chromosomes. In prophase II, the nuclear envelope breaks down and the spindle apparatus forms. Here, the centrioles duplicate. This occurs by separation of the two members of the pair, and then the formation of a daughter centriole perpendicular to each original centriole. The two pairs of centrioles separate into two centrosomes. The nuclear envelope breaks down, and the spindle apparatus forms.

(b) Metaphase II

The chromosomes become arranged on the metaphase plate, much as the chromosomes do in mitosis, and are attached to the now fully formed spindle (Fig. 9.13).

Metaphase plate

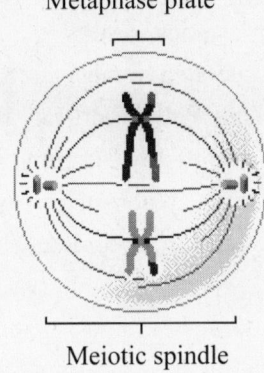

Meiotic spindle

Figure 9.13: Alignment of chromosome on metaphase plate

Each of the daughter cells completes the formation of a spindle apparatus. Single chromosomes align on the metaphase plate, much as chromosomes do in mitosis. This is in contrast to metaphase I, in which homologous pairs of chromosomes align on the metaphase plate. For each chromosome, the kinetochores of the sister chromatids face the opposite poles, and each is attached to a kinetochore microtubule coming from that pole.

(c) Anaphase II

The centromeres separate and the two chromatids of each chromosome move to opposite poles on the spindle. The separated chromatids are now called chromosomes.

d) Telophase II

In Telophase II a nuclear envelope forms around each set of chromosomes. Cytokinesis takes place, producing four daughter cells (gametes, in animals), each with a haploid set of chromosomes because of crossing-over, some chromosomes are seen to have recombined segments of the original parental chromosomes.

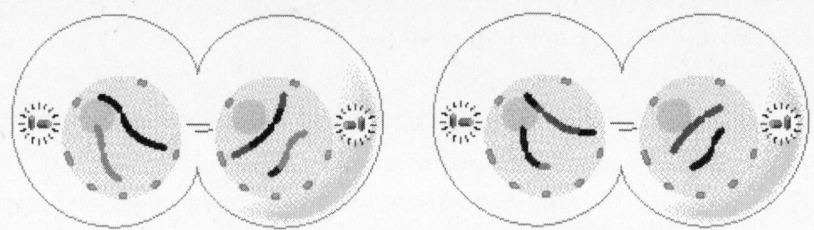

Figure 9.14: Cytokinesis: Four haploid daughter cells

9.9. The Significance of Meiosis

Meiosis facilitates stable sexual reproduction. Without the halving of ploidy, or chromosome count, fertilization would result in zygotes that have twice the number of chromosomes as the zygotes from the previous generation. Successive generations would have an exponential increase in chromosome count. In organisms that are normally diploid, polyploidy, the state of having three or more sets of chromosomes, results in extreme developmental abnormalities or lethality. Polyploidy is poorly tolerated in most animal species. Plants, however, regularly produce fertile, viable polyploids. Polyploidy has been implicated as an important mechanism in plant speciation. Most importantly, recombination and independent assortment of homologous chromosomes allow for a greater diversity of genotypes in the population. This produces genetic variation in gametes that promote genetic and phenotypic variation in a population of offspring.

The normal separation of chromosomes in meiosis I or sister chromatids in meiosis II is termed disjunction. When the separation is not normal, it is called nondisjunction. This results in the production of gametes which have either too or too a few of a particular chromosome, and is a common mechanism for trisomy or monosomy. Nondisjunction can occur in the meiosis I or meiosis II, phases of cellular reproduction, or during mitosis. This is a cause of several medical conditions in humans (such as):

- Down Syndrome - trisomy of chromosome 21
- Patau Syndrome - trisomy of chromosome 13
- Edward Syndrome - trisomy of chromosome 18
- Klinefelter Syndrome - extra X chromosomes in males – i.e. XXY, XXXY, XXXXY
- Turner Syndrome - lacking of one X chromosome in females - ie XO
- Triple X syndrome - and extra X chromosome in females

9.10. Gametogenesis

Gametogenesis is the process of forming gametes (haploid, n) from diploid cells of the germ line. Spermatogenesis is the process of forming sperm cells by meiosis (in animals, by mitosis in plants) in specialized organs known as gonads (in males these are termed testes). After division the cells undergo differentiation to become sperm cells. Oogenesis is the process of forming an ovum (egg) by meiosis (in animals, by mitosis in the gametophyte in plants) in specialized gonads known as ovaries, whereas in spermatogenesis all 4 meiotic products develop into gametes, oogenesis places most of the cytoplasm into the large egg. The other cells, the polar bodies, do not develop. Human males produce 200,000,000 sperm per day, while the female produces one egg (usually) each menstrual cycle.

- **Spermatogenesis**

Sperm production begins at puberty andat continues throughout life, with several hundred million sperm being produced each day. Once sperms form they move into the epididymis, where they are matured and stored (Fig. 9.15).

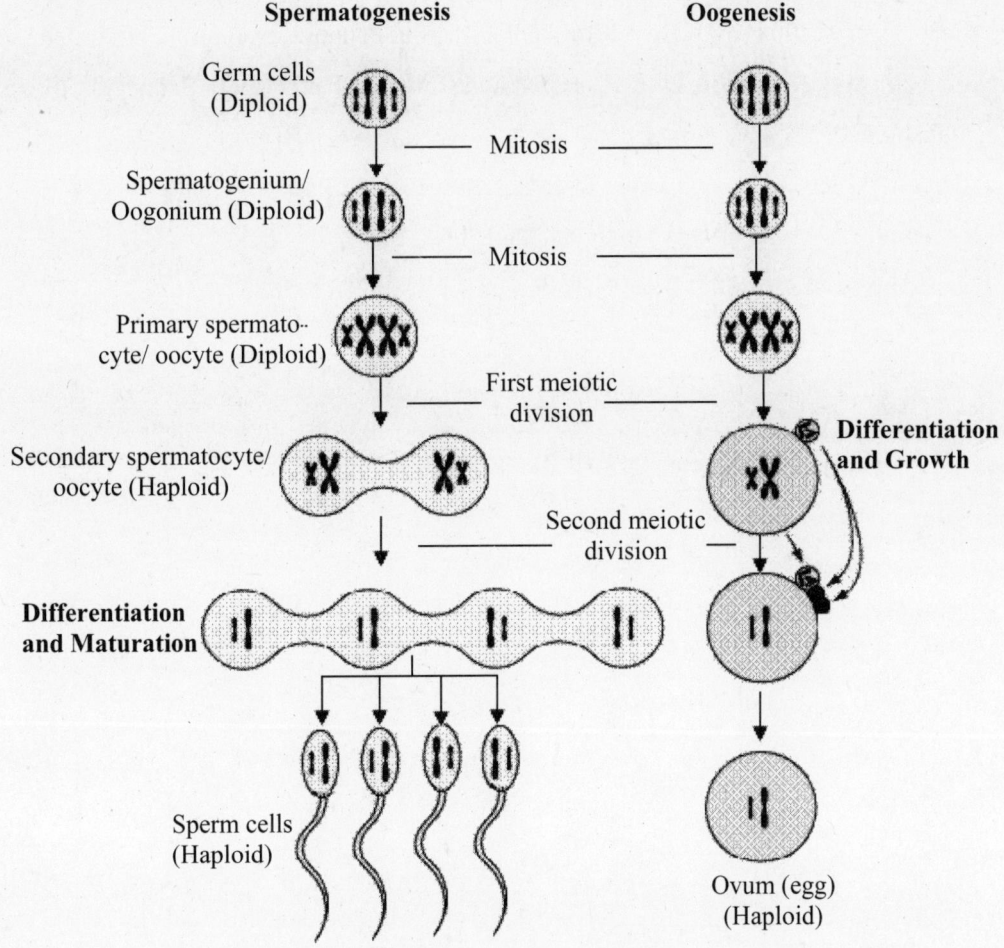

Figure 9.15: Gametogenesis

- **Oogenesis**

The ovary contains many follicles composed of a developing egg surrounded by an outer layer of follicle cells. Each egg begins oogenesis as a primary oocyte. At birth each female carries a lifetime supply of developing oocytes, each of which is in Prophase I. A developing egg (secondary oocyte) is released each month from puberty until menopause, a total of 400-500 eggs.

Suggested Readings

- Lodish, Harvey, et al. Molecular Cell Biology, 4th ed. New York: W. H. Freeman, 2000.

- Lehninger: Principles of Biochemistry, 4th edition, by David L. Nelson and M.M. Cox (2005) Maxmillan/ Worth publishers/ W.H. Freeman & Company.

- Biochemistry (2004) by J. David Rawn, Panima Publishing Corporation, New Delhi.

- Biochemistry, 2nd edition, by R H.Garrett and C.M. Grisham (1999). Saunders College Publishing, N.Y. Sons, NY.

- Alarcon-Vargas, D. & Z. Ronai (2002) Carcinogenesis **23**:541.

- Matsumoto, Y. *et al.* (1994) Mol. Cell. Biol. **14**:6187.

- Matsuoka, S. *et al.* (2000) Proc. Natl. Acad. Sci. USA **97**:10389.

CHAPTER 10

Genetic Engineering

- Molecular Tools in rDNA Technology
- Cutting and Joining DNA
- Restriction Endonuclease
- DNA Ligase
- Homopolymer Tailing
- Linker and Adaptor
- Problems with Ligation
- Vectors – The Cloning Vehicle
- Vectors for Cloning Large Pieces of DNA
- Hybrid Plasmid-Phage Vectors

- Artificial Chromosome Vectors
- Essential Steps of Genetic Engineering
- Methods of Gene Transfer
- Recombinant Selection
- Sources of DNA for Cloning
- Creation and Screening of DNA Libraries
- Expression Systems
- Purification of rDNA Products
- Transgenic Plants
- Edible Vaccines

The age of genetics has arrived. Society is in the midst of a genetic revolution that some futurists predict will have a greater impact on the culture than the industrial revolution. The future of genetics, like that of any other technology, offers great promise but also great peril. Nuclear technology has provided nuclear medicine, nuclear energy, and nuclear weapons. Genetic technology offers the promise of a diverse array of good, questionable, and bad technological applications.

Genetic engineering is relatively a **new discipline** of science which is used highly controllable laboratory conditions to alter the heredity apparatus of a living cell (i.e., the manipulation of genes under highly controllable laboratory conditions) so that the cell can produce different chemicals, or perform completely new functions. It is perhaps the finest of biologists who have been successful in tailoring and manipulating heredity to the best application to the mankind. The onset of this new revolutionary technology of genetic engineering took place at Massachusetts Institute of Technology (MIT), USA when H.G. Khorana, scientist of, Indian origin along with his colleagues in 1972 first reported total synthesis of an artificial gene, namely, tyrosine tRNA gene, with the potential for functioning within a living cell.

Research on genetic engineering is essentially involves *in vitro* joining or recombination of DNA fragments of different origins with the help of some highly specific enzymes to produce 'recombinant-DNA' which is subsequently introduced into appropriate hosts where it multiples (gene cloning). Thus the genetic engineering is also called "recombinant-DNA technology". Thus a multitude of possibilities prevails to bring about new gene combinations not occurring in nature. The science of recombinant-DNA technology or genetic engineering is still its infancy. Even then, its enormous potential impact both social and commercial, are clearly evident.

At present the microorganisms dominate in the sphere of this fascinating technology. Most of the basic information regarding this novel approach has been through microorganisms. Restriction enzymes, the enzymes that cleave DNA molecules to obtain desired genes, are obtained from microorganisms and so are the ligases that are used in joining the DNA fragments. Almost all the vectors, the vehicles that carry genes (DNA fragments) from donor DNA to recipient DNA, are microbial; for example, plasmids, cosmids and viral vectors. Not only these but, there are microorganisms which are predominantly cloned with new genes to produce products of choice.

Recombinant DNA works when the protein is expressed from the recombinant gene by host cell. A significant amount of recombinant protein will not be produced by the host unless expression factors are added. Protein expression depends upon the gene being influenced by a number of signals which provide instructions for the transcription and translation of the gene by the cell. These signals include the promoter, the ribosome binding site, and the terminator. Expression vectors, in which the foreign DNA is inserted, contain these signals. Signals are species specific. In the case of *E. coli*, these signals must be *E. coli* signals as *E. coli* is unlikely to follow the signals of human promoters and terminators.

The presence of introns or signals which act as terminators to a bacterial host in the gene of interest may results in premature termination, and the recombinant protein may expressed and processed improperly like folding, or even may suffer degradation. The preferential eukaryotic system for the production of recombinant proteins is yeast and filamentous fungi. Some proteins are too complex to be produced in bacterium, so eukaryotic cells must be used. Animal cells can also be used for this purpose but the main hindrances are its complex growth requirements such as solid support surface, unlike bacteria and other growth conditions.

10.1. Molecular Tools in rDNA Technology

10.1.1 Cutting and Joining DNA

Two major categories of enzymes represent the biological tools of importance critically used in the isolation of DNA and the preparation of recombinant DNA, restriction endonucleases and DNA ligases. Restriction endonucleases recognize a specific, rather short, nucleotide sequence on a double-stranded DNA molecule, called a restriction site, and cleave the DNA at this recognition site or elsewhere, depending on the type of enzyme. DNA ligase on the contrary joins two pieces of DNA by forming phosphodiester bonds.

10.1.2 Major Classes of Restriction Endonucleases- DNA Cutting Enzyme

Restriction enzymes protect bacteria from infections by viruses, and it is generally accepted that this is their role in nature. They function as microbial immune systems. When a strain of *E. coli* lacking a restriction enzyme is infected with a virus, most virus particles can initiate a successful infection. Restriction enzymes were discovered 40 years ago during investigations of the phenomenon of host-specific restriction and modification of bacterial viruses. Among the first restriction enzymes to be purified were EcoRI and EcoRII from *Escherichia coli*, and HindII and HindIII from *Haemophilus influenzae*. These enzymes were found to cleave DNA at specific sites, generating discrete, gene-size fragments that could be rejoined in the laboratory.

Restriction enzymes are generally classified into four types on the basis of their subunit composition, cleavage position, sequence specificity and cofactor requirements (Table 10.1).

Type I enzymes are complex, multisubunit, combination restriction-and-modification enzymes that cut DNA at random far from their recognition sequences. Originally, thought to be rare, we now know from the analysis of sequenced genomes that they are common. Type I enzymes are of considerable biochemical interest, but they have little practical value since they do not produce discrete restriction fragments or distinct gel-banding patterns.

Type II enzymes cut DNA at defined positions close to or within their recognition sequences. They produce discrete restriction fragments and accordingly distinct gel banding patterns. Thus they are used in the laboratory for DNA analysis and gene cloning. Rather than forming a single family of related proteins, Type II enzymes are a collection of unrelated proteins of many different sorts. Type II enzymes frequently differ in amino acid sequence from one another, and indeed from every other known protein, that they exemplify and represent for a class of rapidly evolving proteins that are often indicative of involvement in host-parasite interactions.

Type II restriction endonuclease is composed of two identical polypeptide subunits that join together to form a homodimer. These homodimers recognize short symmetric DNA sequences of 4–8 bp. six base pair cutters are the most commonly used in molecular biology research. Usually, the sequence read in the 5→3direction on one strand is the same as the sequence read in the 5→3direction on the complementary strand. Sequences that read the same in both directions are called palindromes (from the Greek word *palindromes* for "run back"). Some enzymes, such as *Eco*R1, generate a staggered cut, in which the single-stranded complementary tails are called "sticky" or cohesive ends because they can form hydrogen bond with the single-stranded complementary tails of other DNA fragments. If DNA molecules from different sources share the same palindromic recognition sites, both will contain complementary sticky ends (single-stranded tails) when digested with the same restriction endonuclease. Other type II enzymes, such as *Sm*aI, cut both strands of the DNA at the same position and generate blunt ends with no unpaired nucleotides when they cleave the DNA. Restriction endonucleases exhibit a much greater degree of sequence specificity in the enzymatic reaction than is exhibited in the binding of other regulatory proteins.

All structures of orthodox type II restriction endonucleases characterized by X-ray crystallography so far show a common structural core composed of four conserved β -strands and one α–helix. In the presence of the essential cofactor Mg^{2+}, the enzyme cleaves the DNA on both strands at the same time within or in close proximity to the recognition sequence (restriction site). The enzyme cuts the DNA duplex by breaking the covalent, phosphodiester bond between the phosphate of one nucleotide and the sugar of an adjacent nucleotide, to give free 5-phosphate and 3-OH ends. Type II restriction endonucleases do not require ATP hydrolysis for their nucleolytic activity.

Type III enzymes are also large combination of restriction-and-modification enzymes. They cleave outside of their recognition sequences and require two such sequences in opposite orientations within the same DNA molecule to accomplish cleavage; they rarely give complete digests.

Table 10.1: Major classes of restriction endonucleases

Class	Abundance	Recognition site	Composition	Use in recombinant DNA research
Type I	Less common than type II	Cut both strands at a nonspecific location > 1000 bp away from recognition site	Three-subunit complex: individual recognition, endonuclease, and methylase activities	Not useful
Type II	Most common	Cut both strands at a specific, usually palindromic, recognition site (4 –8 bp)	Endonuclease and methylase are separate, single-subunit enzyme	Very useful
Type III	Rare	Cleavage of one strand only, 24–26 bp downstream of the 3 recognition site	Endonuclease and methylase are separate two-subunit complexes with one subunit in common	Not useful

Type IV enzymes recognize modified, typically methylated DNA and are exemplified by the McrBC and Mrr systems of *E. coli*.

10.1.3. Patterns of DNA Cutting by Restriction Enzymes

Restriction enzymes hydrolyze the backbone of DNA between deoxyribose and phosphate groups. This leaves a phosphate group on the 5' ends and a hydroxyl on the 3' ends of both strands. A few restriction enzymes, however cleave single stranded DNA, although usually at low efficiency. Most of the restriction enzymes used in molecular biology labs cut within their recognition sites and generate one of three different types of ends.

- **5' overhangs:** The enzyme cuts asymmetrically within the recognition site such that a short single-stranded segment extends from the 5' ends. BamHI cuts in this manner.

```
5'                    3'              5'
  -A-T-G-G-A-T-C-C-A-A-      -A-T-G     G-A-T-C-C-A-A-
   | | | | | | | | | |    Bam-H1   | | |            | | |
  -T-A-C-C-T-A-G-G-T-T-      -T-A-C-C-T-A-G     G-T-T-
3'                    5'                    5'
```

- **3' overhangs:** Again, there is asymmetrical cutting within the recognition site, but the result is a single-stranded overhang from the two 3' ends. KpnI cuts in this manner.

```
5'                     3'              3'
  -G-A-G-G-T-A-C-C-C-T-      -G-A-G-G-T-A-C      C-C-T-
   | | | | | | | | | |   Kpn 1    | | |          | | |
3'-C-T-C-C-A-T-G-G-G-A-5'      -C-T-C     3'C-A-T-G-G-G-A-
```

- **Blunts:** Enzymes that cut at precisely opposite sites in the two strands of DNA generate blunt ends without overhangs. SmaI is an example of an enzyme that generates blunt ends. The 5' or 3' overhangs generated by enzymes that cut asymmetrically are called sticky ends or cohesive ends, because they readily stick or anneal with their partner by base pairing.

```
5'-T-A-C-C-C-G-G-G-T-C-3'              -T-A-C-C-C     G-G-G-T-C-
   | | | | | | | | | |   Sma 1     | | | | |    | | | | |
  -A-T-G-G-G-C-C-C-A-G-5'              -A-T-G-G-G     C-C-C-A-G-
3'
```

10.1.5. Restriction Endonclease Nomenclature

Restriction endonucleases are named by a standard procedure, with particular reference to the bacteria from which they are isolated. The first latter (in italics) of the enzyme indicates the genus name, followed by the first two letters (also in italics) of the species, then comes the strain of the organism and finally a Roman numeral indicating the order of discovery. For example, *Hin*dIII (pronounced "hindee-three") was discovered in *Haemophilus influenza* (strain d*)*. The *Hin* comes from the first letter of the genus name and the first two letters of the species name; d is for the strain type; and III is for the third enzyme of that type. *Sma*I is from *Serratia marcescens* and is pronounced "smah-one," *Eco*RI (pronounced "echo-r-one") was discovered in *Escherichia coli* (strain R), and *Ba*mHI is from *Bacillus amyloliquefaciens* (strain H). Over 3000 type II restriction endonucleases have been isolated and characterized to date. Approximately 240 are available commercially for use by molecular biologists (Table 10.2).

Table 10.2: Recognition sequences of some restriction endonucleases

Enzyme	Source	Recognition Sequence	Cutting pattern
EcoRI	*Escherichia coli*	5'GAATTC 3'CTTAAG	5'---G AATTC---3' 3'---CTTAA G---5'
BamHI	*Bacillus amyloliquefaciens*	5'GGATCC 3'CCTAGG	5'---G GATCC---3' 3'---CCTAG G---5'
HindIII	*Haemophilus influenzae*	5'AAGCTT 3'TTCGAA	5'---A AGCTT---3' 3'---TTCGA A---5'
TaqI	*Thermus aquaticus*	5'TCGA 3'AGCT	5'---T CGA---3' 3'---AGC T---5'
NotI	*Nocardia otitidis*	5'GCGGCCGC 3'CGCCGGCG	5'---GC GGCCGC---3' 3'---CGCCGG CG---5'
HinfI	*Haemophilus influenzae*	5'GANTC 3'CTNAG	5'---G ANTC---3' 3'---CTNA G---5'
Sau3A	*Staphylococcus aureus*	5'GATC 3'CTAG	5'--- GATC---3' 3'---CTAG ---5'
PstI	*Providencia stuartii*	5'CTGCAG 3'GACGTC	5'---CTGCA G---3' 3'---G ACGTC---5'
SmaI	*Serratia marcescens*	5'CCCGGG 3'GGGCCC	5'---CCC GGG---3' 3'---GGG CCC---5'
AluI	*Arthrobacter luteus*	5'AGCT 3'TCGA	5'---AG CT---3' 3'---TC GA---5'

10.1.6. DNA Ligase

The study of DNA replication and repair processes led to the discovery of the DNA-joining enzyme called DNA ligase. DNA ligases catalyze formation of a phosphodiester bond between the 5′-phosphate of a nucleotide on one fragment of DNA and the 3′-hydroxyl of another. This joining of linear DNA fragments together with covalent bonds is called ligation. Unlike the type II restriction endonucleases, DNA ligase requires ATP as a cofactor. As it can join two pieces of DNA, DNA ligase became a key enzyme in genetic engineering. If restriction-digested fragments of DNA are placed together under appropriate conditions, the DNA fragments from two sources can anneal to form recombinant molecules by hydrogen bonding between the complementary base pairs of the sticky ends. However, the two strands are not covalently bonded by phosphodiester bonds. DNA ligase is required to seal the gaps, covalently bonding the two strands and regenerating a circular molecule. The DNA ligase most widely used in the lab is derived from the bacteriophage T4. T4 DNA ligase will also ligate fragments with blunt ends, but the reaction is less efficient and higher concentrations of the enzyme are usually required *in vitro*. To increase the efficiency of the reaction, researchers often use the enyzme terminal deoxynucleotidyl transferase to modify the blunt ends by homopolymer tailing.

10.1.7. Homopolymer Tailing

This mechanism of homopolymer tailing is joining of complementary DNA stands by annealing. For example, if a single-stranded poly(dA) tail is added to DNA fragments from one source, and a single stranded poly(dT) tail is added to DNA from another source, the complementary tails can combine together through hydrogen bonds. Recombinant DNA molecules can then be created by ligation. The homopolymer extension (by adding 10-40 residues) can be synthesized by using terminal deoxy nucleotidyltransferase (of calf thymus).

10.1.8. Linker and Adaptor

Linker and adaptor are chemically synthesized, short, double stranded DNA possessing multiple cloning sites (also called the polylinker region) which have a number of unique target sites for restriction endonucleases. Cutting the circular plasmid vector with one of these enzymes results in a single cut, creating a linear plasmid. A foreign DNA molecule, referred to as the "insert," cut with the same enzyme, can then is joined to the vector in ligation reaction. They can be ligated to blunt ends of any DNA molecule and cut with specific restriction enzyme to produce DNA fragments with sticky ends. Adaptors are useful to be ligated to DNA fragments with blunt ends. The DNA fragments held to linker or adaptors are finally ligated to vector DNA molecule.

Ligations of the insert to vector are not 100% productive, because the two ends of a plasmid vector can be readily ligated together, which is called self-ligation. The degree of self-ligation can be reduced by treatment of the vector with the enzyme alkaline phosphatase. Alkaline phosphatase is an enzyme which removes the terminal 5′-phosphate. When the 5′-phosphate is removed from the plasmid it cannot be recircularized by ligase, since there is nothing with which to make a phosphodiester bond. But, if the vector is joined with a foreign insert, the 5′-phosphate is provided by the foreign DNA. Another strategy involves using two different restriction endonuclease cutting sites with noncomplementary sticky ends. This inhibits self-ligation and promotes annealing of the foreign DNA in the desired orientation within the vector.

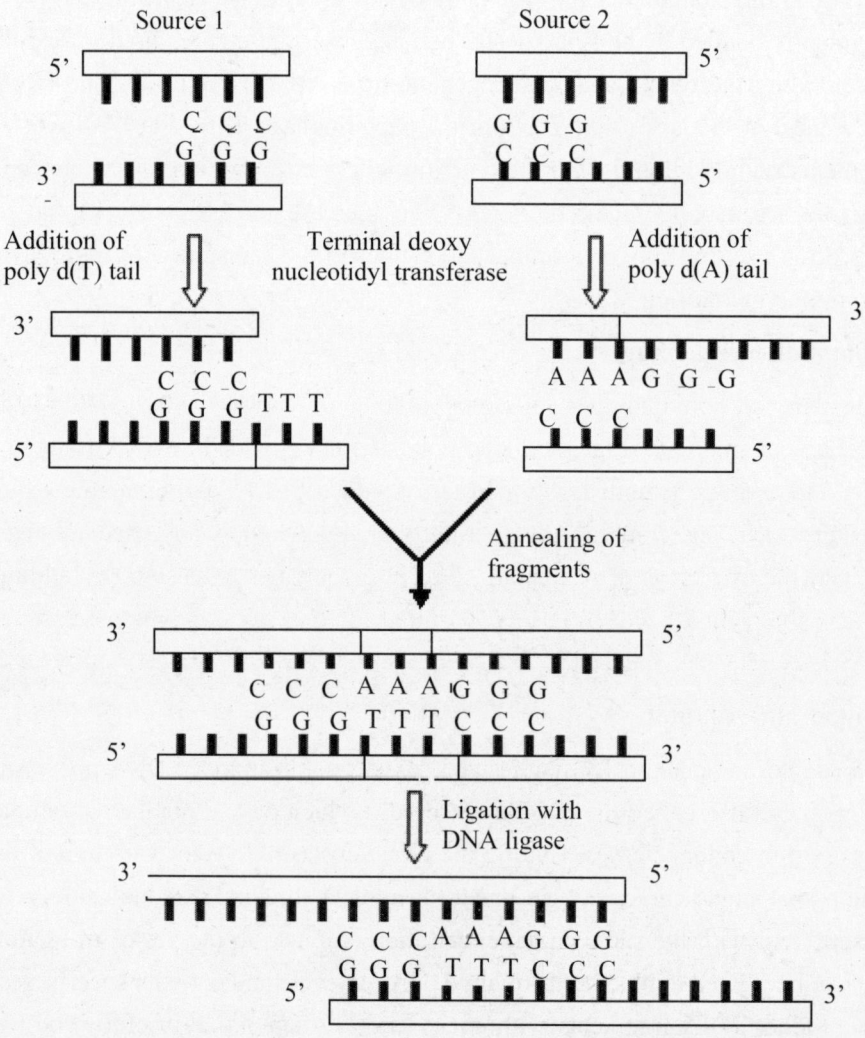

Figure 10.1: Modified blunt end ligation by homopolymer tailing

10.2. Vectors – The Cloning Vehicle

Vectors are the DNA molecules, which carry a foreign DNA fragment to be cloned. The ideal characteristics of a cloning vector are that they can independently replicate themselves as well as the foreign DNA segments they carry. They contain a number of unique restriction endonuclease cleavage sites that are present only once in the vector. They carry a selectable marker (usually in the form of antibiotic resistance genes or genes for enzymes missing in the host cell) to distinguish host cells that carry vectors from host cells that do not contain a vector and are relatively easy to recover from the host cell. The selection and choices of vector are depends on the purpose of cloning.

The classic cloning vectors are plasmids, phages, and cosmids, which are limited to the size insert they can accommodate, taking up to 10, 20, and 45 kb, respectively. A cosmid is a plasmid carrying a phage λ *cos* site, allowing it to be packaged into a phage head. Cosmids infect a host bacterium as do phages, but replicate like plasmids and the host cells are not lysed. Mammalian genes are often greater than 100 kb in size, so originally there were limitations in cloning complete gene sequences (Table 10.3). This new generation of artificial chromosome vectors includes bacterial artificial chromosomes (BACs), yeast artificial chromosomes (YACs), and mammalian artificial chromosomes (MACs).

Table 10.3: Principal features and applications of different cloning vector systems

Vector	Basis	Size limits of insert	Major application
Plasmid	Naturally occurring multicopy plasmids	≤ 10 kb	Subcloning and downstream manipulation, cDNA cloning and expression assays
Phage	Bacteriophage λ	5–20 kb	Genomic DNA cloning, cDNA cloning, and expression libraries
Cosmid	Plasmid containing a bacteriophage λ *cos* site	35–45 kb	Genomic library construction
BAC (bacterial artificial chromosome)	*Escherichia coli* F factor plasmid	75–300 kb	Analysis of large genomes
YAC (yeast artificial chromosome)	*Saccharomyces cerevisiae* centromere, telomere, and autonomously replicating sequence	100–1000 kb (1 Mb)	Analysis of large genomes, YAC transgenic mice
MAC (mammalian artificial chromosome)	Mammalian centromere, telomere, and origin of replication	100 kb to > 1 Mb	Under development for use in animal biotechnology and human gene therapy

10.2.1. Plasmid DNA as a vector

Plasmids are naturally occurring extra-chromosomal double-stranded circular DNA molecules that carry an origin of replication and replicate autonomously within bacterial cells. Almost all the bacteria have plasmids containing a low copy number (1-4 per cell) or a high copy number (10-100 per cell). The size of the plasmid varies from 1 to 500 kb. Usually plasmids contribute to about 0.5 to 5.0% of the total DNA of bacteria.

Plasmids are named with a system of uppercase letters and numbers, where the lowercase "p" stands for "plasmid." The plasmid vector *pBR322*, constructed in 1974, was one of the first genetically engineered plasmids to be used in recombinant DNA. In the case of *pBR322*, the BR identifies the original constructors of the vector (Bolivar and Rodriquez), and 322 is the identification number of the specific plasmid. Some plasmids are given names of the places where they are discovered e.g. pUC is the plasmid from University of California.

(a) *pBR322*- The most common plasmid vector

pBR322 has a DNA sequence of 4,361 bp. It carries ampicillin resistant and tetracycline resistant genes as markers for identification. The plasmid has unique recognition sites for the action of restriction endonucleases, namely *EcoRI, HindIII, BamHI* and *PstI*. These early vectors were often of low copy number, meaning that they replicate to yield only one or two copies in each cell. pUC18, is a derivative of *pBR322* (Fig. 10.2). This is a "high copy number" plasmid (500 copies per bacterial cell). Plasmid vectors are modified to contain a specific antibiotic resistance gene and a linker and adaptor.

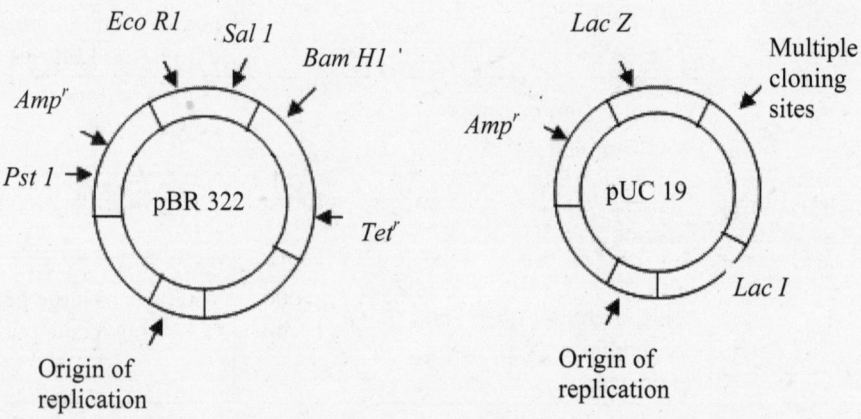

Figure 10.2: Genetic map of cloning vectors *pBR 322* and *pUC 19*

10.3. Vectors for Cloning Large Pieces of DNA

(a) Bacteriophage lambda (λ) as a vector

Bacteriophage lambda (λ) has been widely used in recombinant DNA since engineering of the first viral cloning vector in 1974. Phage λ vectors are particularly useful for preparing genomic libraries, because they can hold a larger piece of DNA than a plasmid vector. Today many variations of λ vectors exist. Insertion vectors have unique restriction endonuclease sites that allow the cloning of small DNA fragments in addition to the phage λ genome. These are often used for preparing cDNA expression libraries. Replacement vectors have paired cloning sites on either side of a central gene cluster. This central cluster contains genes for lysogeny and recombination, which are not essential for the lytic life cycle (Fig. 10.3).

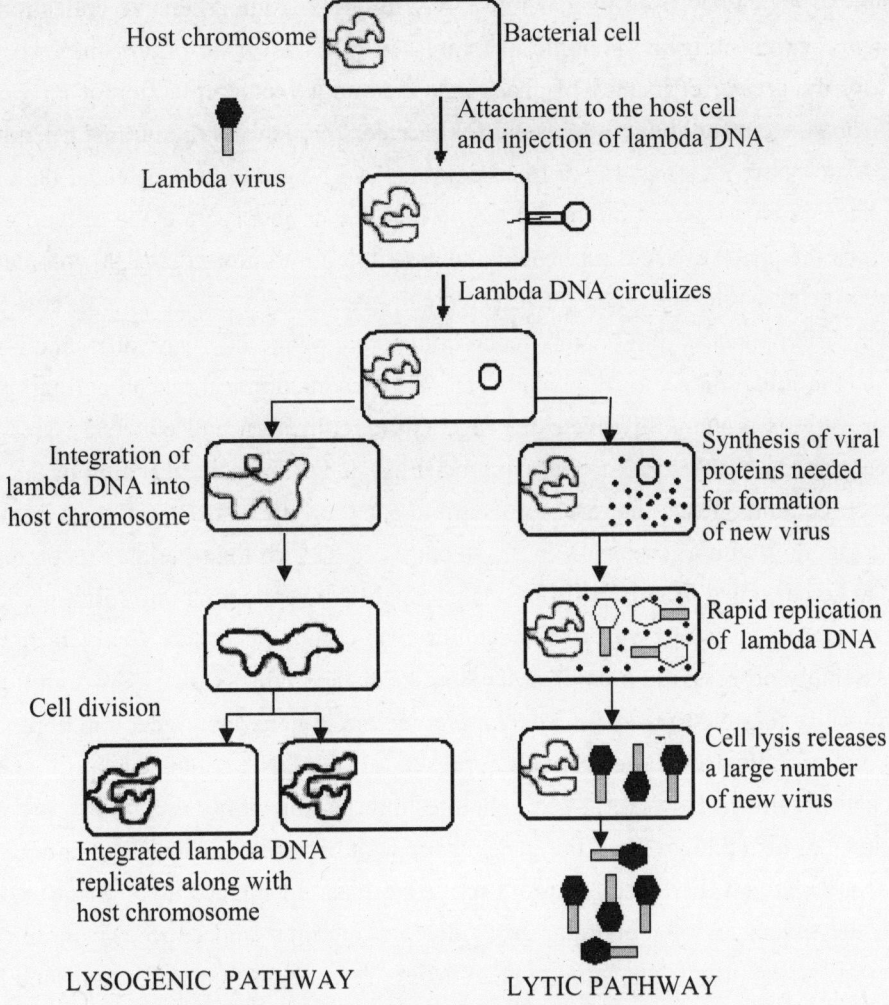

Figure 10.3: Life cycle of bacteriophage λ

The central gene cluster can be removed and foreign DNA inserted between the "arms." All phage vectors used as cloning vectors have been disarmed for safety and can only function in special laboratory conditions. The recombinant viral particle infects bacterial host cells, in a process called "transduction." The host cells lyse after phage reproduction, releasing progeny virus particles. The viral particles appear as a clear spot of lysed bacteria or "plaque" on an agar plate containing a lawn of bacteria. Each plaque represents progeny of a single recombinant phage and contains millions of recombinant phage particles. Most contemporary vectors carry a *lacZ′* gene allowing blue-white selection.

(b) Bacteriophage λ vectors permit efficient construction of large DNA libraries

Vectors constructed from bacteriophage λ are about a thousand times more efficient than plasmid vectors in cloning large numbers of DNA fragments. For this reason, phage λ vectors have been widely used to generate DNA libraries, comprehensive collections of DNA fragments representing the genome or expressed mRNAs of an organism. Two factors account for the greater efficiency of phage λ as a cloning vector. Infection of *E. coli* host cells by λ virions occurs at about a thousand fold greater frequencies than transformation by plasmids. Many more λ clones transformed colonies can be grown and detected on a single culture plate. When a λ virion infects an *E. coli* cell, it can undergo a cycle of lytic growth during which the phage DNA is replicated and assembled into more than 100 complete progeny phage, which are released when the infected cell lyses.

A λ virion consists of a head, which contains the phage DNA genome, and a tail, which functions in infecting *E. coli* host cells. The λ genes encoding the head and tail proteins, as well as various proteins involved in phage DNA replication and cell lysis, are grouped in discrete regions of the ≈50-kb viral genome (Fig. 10.4). The central region of the λ genome, however, contains genes that are not essential for the lytic pathway. Removing this region and replacing it with a foreign DNA fragment up to ≈25 kb long yields a recombinant DNA that can be packaged *in vitro* to form phage capable of replicating and forming plaques on a lawn of *E. coli* host cells. *In vitro* packaging of recombinant λ DNA, which mimics the *in vivo* assembly process, requires preassembled heads and tails as well as two viral proteins. It is technically feasible to use λ phage cloning vectors to generate a genomic library, that is, a collection of λ clones that collectively represent all the DNA sequences in the genome of a particular organism. However, such genomic libraries for higher eukaryotes present certain experimental difficulties. First, the genes from such organisms usually contain extensive intron sequences and therefore are too large to be inserted intact into λ phage vectors. As a result, the sequences of individual genes are broken apart and carried in more than one λ clone (this is also true for plasmid clones). Moreover, the presence of introns and long intergenic regions in genomic DNA often makes it difficult to identify the important parts of a gene that actually encode protein sequences. Thus for many studies, cellular mRNAs, which lack the noncoding regions present in genomic DNA, are a more useful starting material for generating a DNA library. In this approach, DNA copies of mRNAs, called complementary DNAs (cDNAs), are synthesized using reverse transcriptase and cloned in phage vectors. A large collection of the resulting cDNA clones, representing all the mRNAs expressed in a cell type is called a cDNA library.

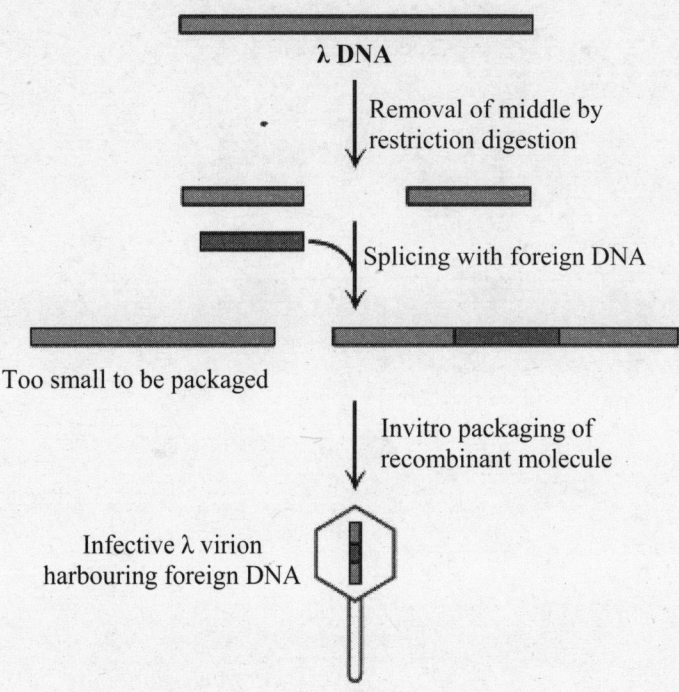

Figure 10.4: λ Phage as a cloning vector

10.4. Hybrid Plasmid-phage Vectors

Hybrid plasmid-phage vectors have been developed to overcome the inherent size limitation of the M13 cloning system and are now being widely used for applications such as DNA sequencing and the production of probes for use in hybridisation studies. One additional feature of phage vectors is that the technique of packaging *in vitro* is sequence independent, apart from the requirement of having the cos sites separated by DNA of packagable size (38-51 kb). This has been exploited in the construction of special vectors that contain plasmid sequences joined to the cos sites of phage λ. Such vectors are referred as cosmids (Fig. 10.5). They are relatively small (4-6 kb) and hence can accommodate cloned DNA fragments up to some 47 kb in size. As they lack phage genes, they behave as plasmids when introduced into

E. coli by the packaging/infection mechanism of λ. Cosmid vectors therefore offer an apparently ideal system as a highly efficient and specific tool for introducing the recombinant DNA into the host cell, with a cloning capacity nearly two fold greater than the best λ replacement vectors.

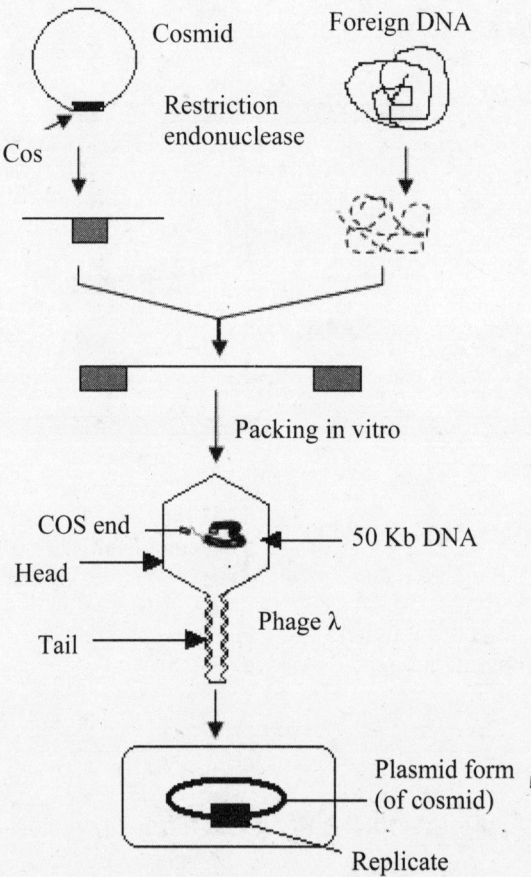

Figure 10.5: Cosmid vectors

However, they also suffer from disadvantages, as often the gains of using cosmids instead of phage vectors are offset by the losses in regard to the ease of use and further processing of cloned sequences. These vectors are essentially plasmids that contain the f1 (M13) phage origin of replication. When cells containing the plasmid are superinfected with phage, they produce single-stranded copies of the plasmid DNA and secrete them into the medium as M13-like particles. Vectors such as pEMBL9 or pBBR322 can accept DNA fragments of up to 10 kb.

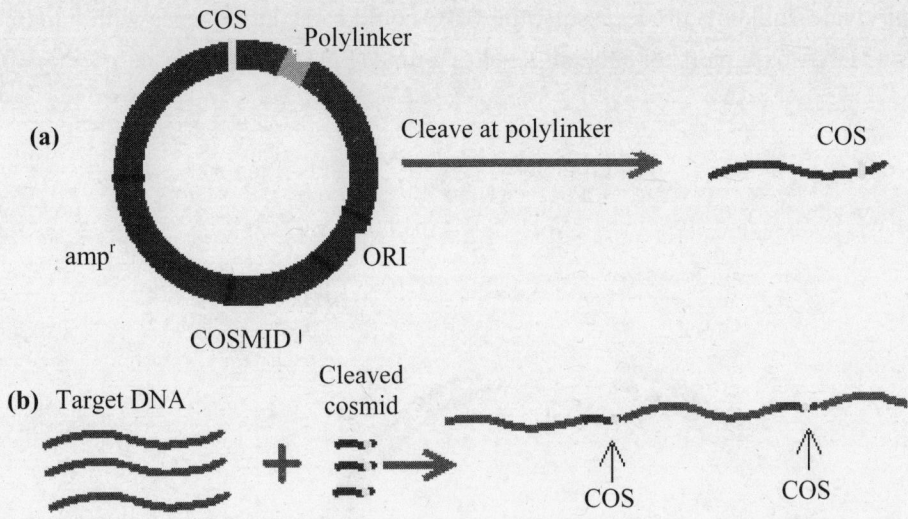

Figure 10.6: Cloning by using cosmid vectors. **(a)** In addition to *amp*^r, ORI, and polylinker as in the plasmid vector, the cosmid vector also contains a COS site. **(b)** After cosmid vectors are cleaved with restriction enzyme, they are ligated with DNA fragments. The subsequent assembly and transformation steps are the same as cloning with phages

10.5. Artificial Chromosome Vectors

Bacterial artificial chromosomes (BACs) and yeast artificial chromosomes (YACs) are important tools for mapping and analysis of complex eukaryotic genomes. Much of the work on the Human Genome Project and other genome sequencing projects depends on the use of BACs and YACs, because they can hold greater than 300 kb of foreign DNA. BACs are constructed using the fertility factor plasmid (F factor) of *E. coli* as a starting point.

(a) Bacterial Artificial Chromosome (BAC) Vectors

Over the years, scientists have developed a number of different kinds of vectors for modifying the genetic constitution of bacteria. The bacterial artificial chromosome is one of the plasmid-based vectors. Plasmids are the extra chromosomal DNA. A scientist can alter a strain of bacteria using a BAC, and then compare the altered bacteria to an unaltered strain to discover what role the inserted genes play in cell biology.

Plasmids like the bacterial artificial chromosome are inserted into bacteria using a process called electroporation. Electroporation involves disturbing the cell membrane with an electric shock, which creates temporary openings through which molecules may be inserted. Forerunners to the BAC included modified plasmids namely cosmid and the fosmid.

In 1992 the first bacterial artificial chromosome was created by Hiroaki Shizuya, a researcher at the California Institute of Technology, by modifying a plasmid called F-factor. F-factor plasmids are used naturally by bacteria to transfer DNA from one cell to another during periods of environmental stress, in order to increase genetic variability and the likelihood of survival. Unlike its predecessors, the BAC could carry large genes with hundreds of thousands of DNA base pairs, or several genes at a time (Fig. 10.7).

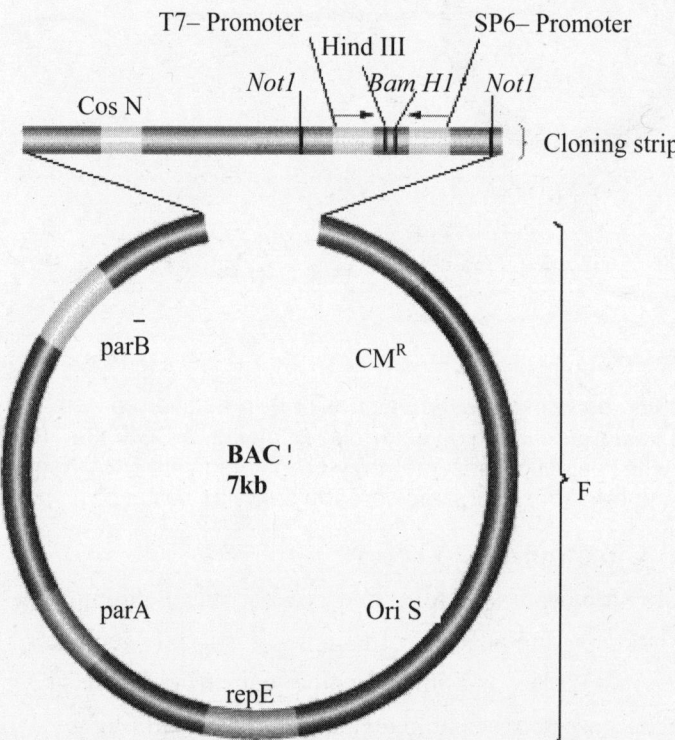

Figure 10.7: Structure of a bacterial artificial chromosome (BAC), used for cloning large fragments of donor DNA. CM^R is a selectable marker for chloramphenicol resistance. *oriS, repE, parA,* and *parB* are F genes for replication and regulation of copy number. *cosN* is the *cos* site from λ phage. *Hind*III and *Bam*HI are cloning sites at which foreign DNA is inserted. The two promoters are for transcribing the inserted fragment. The *Not*I sites are used for cutting out the inserted fragment

(b) Yeast artificial chromosome (YAC) vectors

Yeast is a single celled eukaryote that can be manipulated and grown in the lab much like bacteria. YAC vectors are designed to act like chromosomes. The yeast artificial chromosome (YAC) vector is capable of carrying a large DNA fragment (up to 2 Mb), however, its transformation efficiency is very low (Fig. 10.8). A YAC can be considered as a functional artificial chromosome (self replicating element), since it includes three specific DNA sequences that enable it to propagate from one cell to its offspring:

TEL: The **telomere** which is located at each chromosome end protects the linear DNA from degradation by nucleases.

CEN: The **centromere** which is the attachment site for mitotic spindle fibers "pulls" one copy of each duplicated chromosome into each new daughter cell.

ORI: Replication origin sequences which are specific DNA sequences that allows the DNA replication machinery to assemble on the DNA and move at the replication forks.

It also contains few other specific sequences like selectable markers that allow the easy isolation of yeast cells that have taken up the artificial chromosome recognition site for the restriction enzymes.

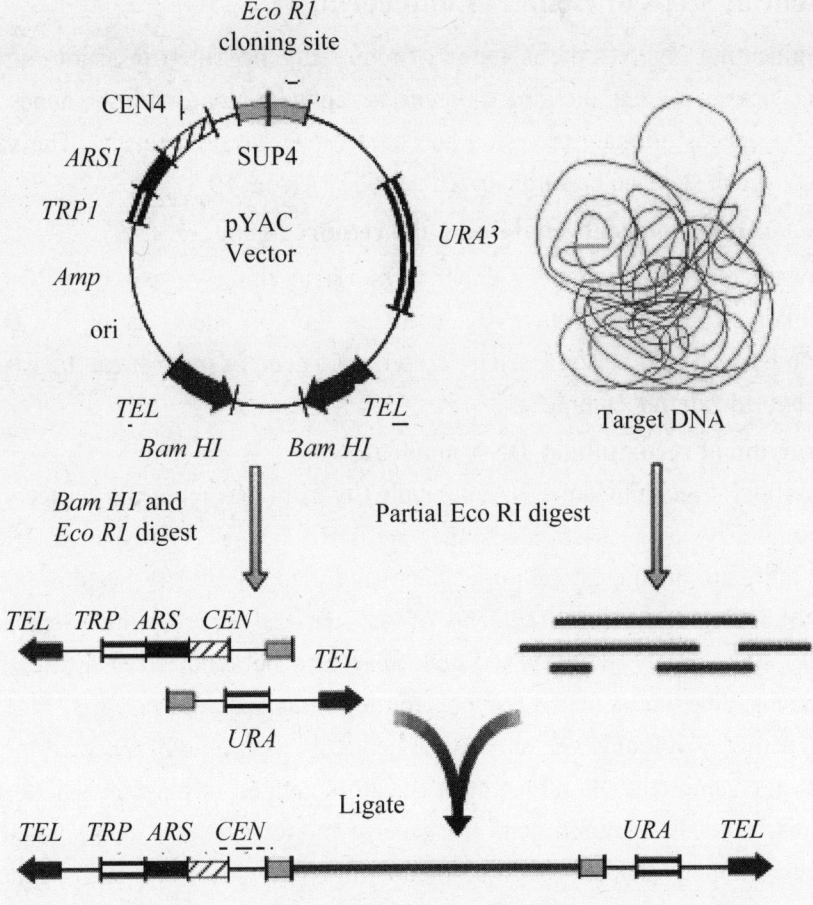

Figure 10.8: Yeast artificial chromosome (YAC) vectors

Table 10.4: Comparison between YAC and BAC Cloning Systems

Features	YAC	BAC
Configuration	Linear	Circular
Host	Yeast	Bacteria
Copy Number / Cell	1	1-2
Cloning Capacity	Unlimited	up-to 350 kb
Transformation	Spheroplast	Electroporation
Chimerism	up to 40%	None to low
DNA Isolation	Pulsed-field-gel-electrophoresis -Gel Isolation	Standard Plasmid Miniprep
Insert Stability	Unstable	Stable

10.6. Essential Steps of Genetic Engineering

Genetic engineering involves the isolation of required genes, their insertion into a bacterial cell (cloning organism) and allowing the gene to replicate along with the genes of bacterial cell. Each step needs ultimate precision and care for the desired results. The various techniques used in each step can be summarized as follows (Fig. 10.9).

(a) Isolation of DNA molecule containing the required gene

The gene of interest can be obtained either form a gene library or can be a PCR product. It can also obtain from natural sources by breaking the cell and isolating the DNA and its modification by restriction enzymes. The presence of gene of interest can be easily detected by various hybridization techniques.

(b) Construction of recombinant-DNA molecule

The construction of recombinant-DNA molecule (hybrid DNA molecule) is accomplished by the use of two enzymes: restriction enzymes and DNA ligases. The isolated DNA molecule containing the gene of interest (required gene) is treated with a restriction enzyme which cleaves DNA molecule to yield fragments of various sizes, one of which represents the required gene, alternatively, the required gene may also be synthesized artificially with the help of gene machine or automated polynucleotide synthesizer.

Simultaneously, a cloning vector (may be generally a plasmid or a bacteriophage) is also treated with the same restriction enzymes. A gap is created in plasmid where the required gene gets inserted. The required gene (or gene of interest) is now incorporated in the gap created in the cloning vector through co-incubating. The vector and target genes are combined by enzyme DNA ligase in a resulting-DNA molecule or hybrid DNA molecule.

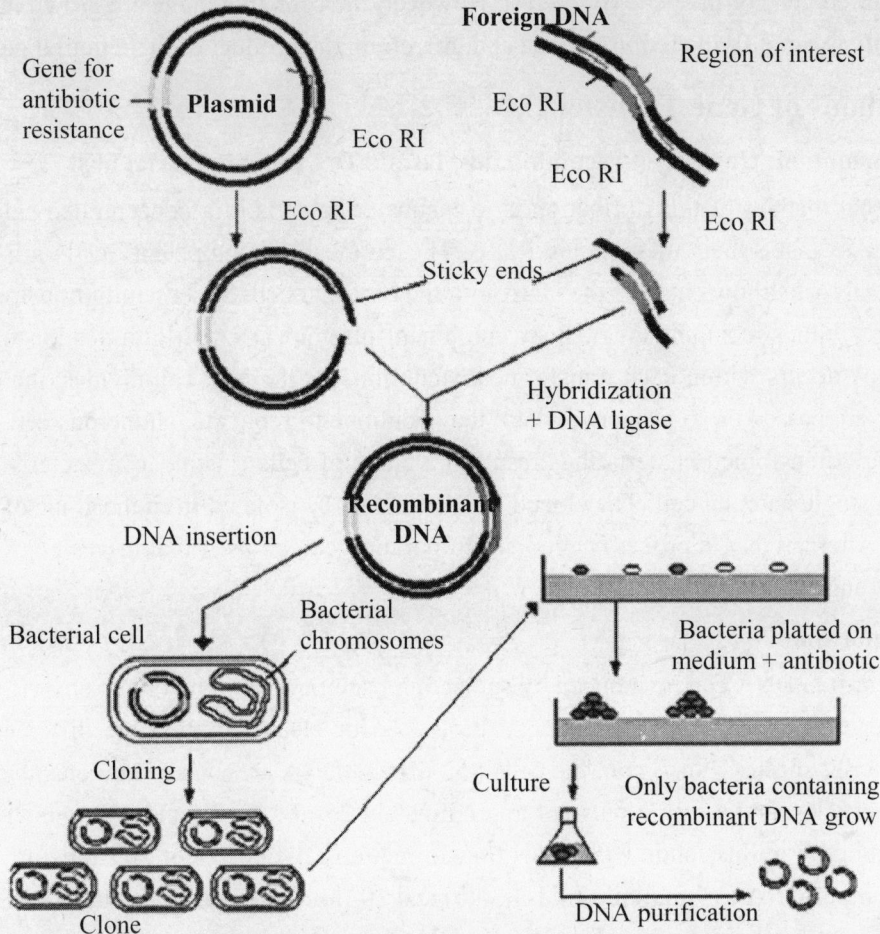

Figure 10.9: Steps involved in genetic engineering

(c) Insertion of recombinant DNA

The recombinant-DNA molecule is inserted into a competent host cell which is usually a bacterium. A competent host cell is one which accepts the recombinant-DNA molecule and allows it to replicate autonomously within it. The cell that accepts the recombinant-DNA molecule is called cloning organism which, finally, contains its own genes as well as the incorporated gene of interest.

(d) Production of clones

The final step in gene cloning is to allow the cloning organisms to multiply. The cloning organism is plated out on to agar medium where it divides. When it grows and divides, it yields a colony of identical cells possessing equivalent genetic, components and therefore physiological traits, such a colony is referred to as a clone as it has originated from a single cell and consisted of all identical cells. All cells of a clone, like the cloning organism, contain the required gene or the gene of interest. However, the cells of a clone are grown in limitless quantity to amplify the required gene and, therefore, the product of the required gene.

10.7. Methods of Gene Transfer

(a) Transformation: transfer of recombinant plasmid DNA to a bacterial host

The traditional method of transformation is to incubate the cells in a concentrated calcium salt solution to make their membranes leaky. The permeable "competent" cells are then mixed with DNA to allow entry of the DNA into the bacterial cell. Successfully transformed bacteria carry either recombinant or nonrecombinant plasmid DNA. Multiplication of the plasmid DNA occurs within each transformed bacterium. As the host cell divides, the plasmid vectors are passed on to progeny, where they continue to replicate. Numerous cell divisions of single transfomed bacteria thus result in a clone of cells (visible as a bacterial colony) from a single parental cell. The cloned DNA can then be isolated from the clone of bacterial cells. Alternatively, a process called electroporation can be used that drives DNA into cells by a strong electric current.

(b) Electroporation

The uptake of free DNA can be induced by subjecting bacteria to a high voltage electric field in the presence of DNA. The experimental protocols for electroporation are different for various bacterial species. For *E.coli*, the cells (-50 µl) and DNA are placed in a chamber fitted with electrodes, and a single pulse of approximately 25 µF, 2.5 kv and 200 ohms is applied for about 4.6 milliseconds will yields transformation efficiencies of 10^9 transforments per microgram of DNA for small plasmids (-3 kb) and 10^6 for large plasmids (-136 kb). Similar conditions are used to introduce BAC vector DNA into *E.coli*.

The supposed mechanism of DNA uptake during electroporation is of chemically induced transformation, that transient pores are formed in the cell wall as a result of the electroshock and that, after contact with the lipid bilayer of the cell membrane, the DNA is taken into the cell.

10.8. Recombinant Selection

(a) Selection by marker genes

The selection of transformed cell depends on the particular vector, for example in the case of *pUC*18, a selectable marker gene for resistance to the antibiotic ampicillin. Culturing of cells in a medium containing ampicillin will allow only those cells containing the marker gene. The ampicillin resistance genes carried by the recombinant plasmids produce an enzyme, β-lactamase that cleaves a specific bond in the four-membered ring (β -lactam ring) in the ampicillin molecule that is essential to its antibiotic action (Table 10.5). If the plasmid vector is introduced into a plasmid free antibiotic-sensitive bacterial cell, the cell becomes resistant to ampicillin. Nontransformed cells contain no pUC18 DNA, therefore they will not be antibiotic-resistant, and their growth will be inhibited on agar containing ampicillin. Transformed bacterial cells may contain either nonrecombinant pUC18 DNA (self ligated vector only) or recombinant pUC18 DNA (vector containing foreign DNA insert). Both types of transformed bacterial cells will be ampicillin-resistant (Fig. 10.10).

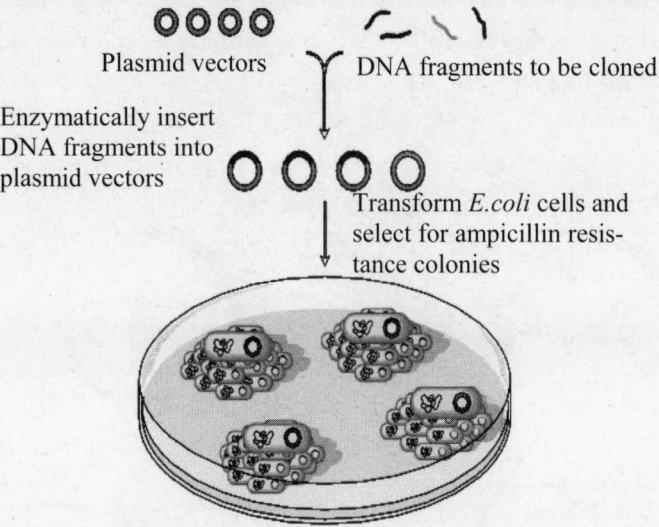

Figure 10.10: Selection by ampicillin resistance

Table: 10.5: Some commonly used antibiotics and antibiotic resistance genes

Antibiotic	Mode of action	Resistance
Ampicillin	Inhibits bacterial cell wall synthesis by disrupting peptidoglycan cross-linking	β-Lactamase (amp^r) gene product is secreted and hydrolyzes ampicillin
Tetracycline	Inhibits binding of aminoacyl tRNA to the 30S ribosomal subunit	tet^r gene product is membrane bound and prevents tetracycline accumulation by an efflux mechanism
Kanamycin	Inactivates translation by interfering with ribosome function	Neomycin or aminoglycoside phosphotransferase (neo^r) gene product inactivates kanamycin by phosphorylation

(b) Blue-white screening

To distinguish nonrecombinant from recombinant transformants, blue-white screening or "*lac* selection" (also called α-complementation) can be used with vector containing *lacZ* gene. Bacterial colonies are grown on selective medium containing ampicillin and a colorless chromogenic compound called X-gal (5-bromo-4-chloro-3-indolyl-β-d-galactoside). *pUC*18 carries a portion of the *lacZ* gene (called *lacZ* ') that encodes the first 146 amino acids for the enzyme β–galactosidase nonfunctional proteins. The multiple cloning sites reside in the coding region. If the *lacZ* 'region is not interrupted by inserted DNA, the aminoterminal portion of β-galactosidase is synthesized. However, by α-complementation the two partial proteins can associate and form a functional enzyme. When present the enzyme β -galactosidase, catalyzes hydrolysis of X-gal, converting the colorless substrate into a blue-colored product (Fig. 10.11).

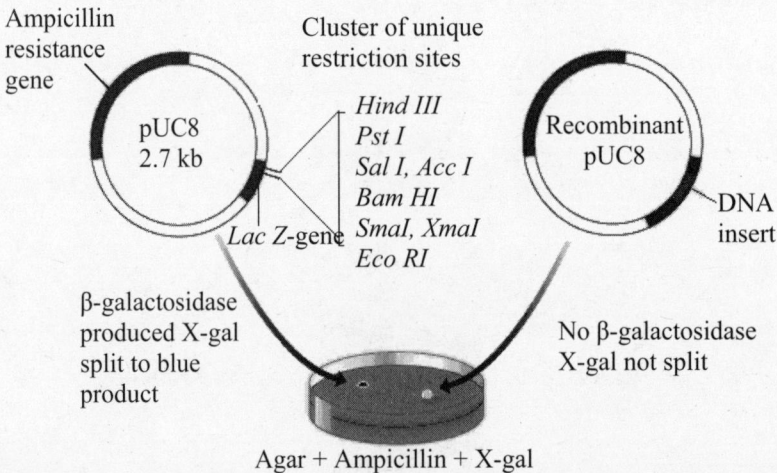

Figure 10.11: β-Galactosidase activity can be used as an indicator of the presence of a foreign DNA insert. Cleavage of X-gal produces a blue-colored product that can be visualized as a blue colony on agar plates. If a foreign insert has disrupted the *lacZ* 5′ coding sequence, then only the C-terminal polypeptide will be produced in the bacterial cell. Thus, X-gal is not cleaved and bacterial colonies remain white

Further screening of positive (white) colonies can be done by restriction endonuclease digest to confirm the presence and orientation of the insert. When a positive colony containing recombinant plasmid DNA is transferred aseptically to liquid growth medium, the cells continue to multiply exponentially. Within a day or two, a culture containing trillions of identical cells can be harvested. The final step in molecular cloning is the recovery of the cloned DNA. Plasmid DNA can be purified from crude cell lysates by chromatography using silica gel or anion exchange resins that preferentially bind nucleic acids under appropriate conditions and allow for the removal of proteins and polysaccharides. The purified plasmid DNA can then be eluted and recovered by ethanol precipitation in the presence of monovalent cations. Ethanol precipitation of plasmid DNA from aqueous solutions yields a clear pellet that can be easily dissolved in an appropriate buffered solution.

10.9. Sources of DNA for Cloning

Sources of DNA for cloning into vectors may be DNA fragments representing a specific gene or portion of a gene, or may be sequences of the entire genome of an organism. Typical "inserts" include genomic DNA, cDNA, polymerase chain reaction (PCR) products, and chemically synthesized oligonucleotides.

10.10. Creation and Screening of DNA Libraries

10.10.1 Gene Library

One of the fundamental objectives of molecular biology is the isolation of gene that encodes protein for industrial, agricultural and medical applications. In prokaryotic organisms the structural gene forms a continuous coding domain in the genomic DNA, whereas, in eukaryotes, the coding regions (exons) of structural genes are separated by noncoding regions (introns). Consequently, different cloning strategies have to be used for cloning prokaryotic and eukaryotic genes.

In a prokaryote, the desired sequence (target DNA, or gene of interest) is frequently a minuscule portion (about 0.02%) of the total chromosomal DNA. Vectors are used to compile a library of DNA fragments that have been isolated from the genomes of a variety of organisms. The collection of fragments of genomic DNA can then be used to isolate specific genes and other DNA sequences of interest. DNA fragments are generated by cutting the DNA with a specific restriction endonuclease. These fragments are ligated into vector molecules, and the collection of recombinant molecules is transferred into host cells, one molecule in each cell. The total number of all DNA molecules makes up the library. This library is searched, that is screened, with a molecular probe that specifically identifies the target DNA. Once prepared the library can be perpetuated indefinitely in the host cells and is readily retrieved whenever a new probe is available to seek out a particular fragment.

(a) Genomic library

A genomic library contains DNA fragments that represent the entire genome of an organism. The first step in creating a genomic library is to break the DNA into manageable size pieces (e.g. 15–20 kb for phage λ vectors), usually by partial restriction endonuclease digest. Under limiting conditions, any particular restriction site is cleaved only occasionally, so not all sites are cleaved in any particular DNA molecule. This generates a continuum of overlapping fragments. The second step is to purify fragments of optimal size by gel electrophoresis or centrifugation techniques. The final step is to insert the DNA fragments into a suitable vector. In humans, the genome size is approximately 3×10^9 bp. with an average insert size of 20 kb, the number of random fragments to ensure with high probability (95–99%) that every sequence represented is approximately 106 clones for humans. It actually works out to 1.5×10^5 (i.e. $(3 \times 10^9$ bp)/(2×10^4 bp)) but more clones are needed in practice, since insertion is random. Bacteriophage λ or cosmid vectors are typically used for genomic libraries. Since a larger insert size can be accommodated by these vectors compared with plasmids, there is a greater chance of cloning a gene sequence with both the coding sequence and the regulatory elements in a single clone.

(b) cDNA Library

The principle behind cDNA cloning is that a mRNA population isolated from a specific tissue, cell type, or developmental stage (e.g. embryo mRNA) should contain mRNAs specific for any protein expressed in that cell type or during that stage, along with "housekeeping" mRNAs that encode essential proteins such as the ribosomal-proteins, and other mRNAs common to many cell types or stages of development. Thus, if mRNA can be isolated, a small subset of all the genes in a genome can be studied. mRNA cannot be cloned directly, but a cDNA copy of the mRNA can be cloned. As cDNA library is derived from mRNA, the library contains the coding region of expressed genes only, with no introns or regulatory regions. This latter point becomes important for applications of recombinant DNA technology to the production of transgenic animals and for human gene therapy.

10.10.2. Screening by DNA Hybridization

The presence of a target nucleotide sequence in a DNA sample can be determined with a DNA probe. This procedure called hybridization depends on the formation of stable base pairs between the probe and the target sequence. DNA hybridization is feasible because double-stranded DNA can be converted into single-stranded DNA by heat or alkali treatment. Heating DNA breaks the hydrogen bonds that hold the base together (denaturation) but does not affect the phosphodiester bonds of the DNA backbone. If the heated solution is rapidly cooled, the strand remains single stranded. However, if the temperature of a heated DNA solution is lowered slowly, the double stranded, helical conformation of DNA can be reestablished because of the base pairing of complementary nucleotides (renaturation). The process of heating and slowly cooling double-stranded DNA is called annealing. When DNA from different sources with some shared (homologous) sequence are mixed, heated to 100°C, and slowly cooled, there will be some hybrid DNA molecules among the annealed products, that is, double stranded DNA in which the strands come from different sources.

In general, for a DNA hybridization assay, the target DNA is denatured and the single strands are irreversibly bound to a matrix, e.g., nitrocellulose or nylon. The binding process is often carried out at high temperature. Later, the single strands of a DNA probe, which are labeled with either a radioisotope or another tagging system, are incubated with the bound DNA sample. If the sequence of nucleotide in the DNA sample complements with the single stranded DNA probe, it will results in the base pairing, hybridization. The hybridization can be detected by autoradiography and other visualization procedures depending on the nature of the probe label. If the nucleotide sequence of the probe does not base pair with a DNA sequence in the sample, then no hybridization occurs and the assay gives a negative result. Generally, probe range in length from 100 to more than 1,000 bp, although both larger and smaller can be used. Depending on the condition of hybridization reaction, stable base requires a match of > 80% with a segment of 50 bases.

Genomic DNA libraries are often screened by plating out the transformed cells on the growth medium of a master plate and then transferring samples of each colony to a solid matrix such as nitrocellulose or nylon membrane, lysing breaking the cells, deproteinizing and denaturing the DNA, and binding the DNA to the matrix. At this stage, a labeled probe is added and, if hybridization occurs, the signals are detected on an auradiogaph. The colonies from the master plate that correspond to the samples containing hybridized DNA are then isolated and cultured. As most libraries are created by partial digestions, a number of colonies may give a positive response to the probe. The next task is to determine which clone, if any, contains the complete sequence of the target gene. Preliminary analysis, which use the results of gel electrophoresis and restriction endonuclease mapping reveal the length of each insert and identify those inserts that are same and those that share overlapping sequences. If an insert in any one of the clones is large enough to include the full gene, then the complete gene can be recognized by DNA sequencing because it will have start and stop codons and a contiguous set of nucleotides that code for the target protein. Alternatively, a gene can be assembled by using overlapping sequences from the different clones.

10.10.3. Screening by Immunological Assay

Alternative methods are used to screen a library when a DNA probe is not available. For example, when a cloned DNA sequence is transcribed and translated, the presence of the protein, or even part of it, can be determined by an immunological assay. Technically, this procedure has much in common with a DNA hybridization assay. All the clones of the library are grown separately on master plates. A sample of each colony is transferred to a known position on a matrix, where the cells are lysed and the released proteins are attached to the matrix. The matrix with the bound proteins is treated with a primary antibody that specifically binds with the target protein (antigen). Any unbound antibody is washed away, and the matrix is treated with a secondary antibody that is specific for the primary antibody. In many assay system, the secondary antibody has an enzyme, such as alkaline phosphatase, bound to the enzyme. After the matrix is washed, a colorless substrate is added. If the secondary antibody bound to the primary antibody, the colorless substrate is hydrolysed by the enzyme that produces a colored compound that accumulates at the site of the reaction. The colonies on master plate that corresponds to positive results (colored spots) on the matrix contain either an intact gene or a portion of the gene that is large enough to produce a protein product that is recognized by the primary antibody. After detection by immunoassay of genomic DNA libraries, the positive clones must be characterized to determine which, if any, carry a complete gene.

10.10.4. Screening by Protein Activity

DNA hybridization and immunological assays work well for many kinds of genes and gene products. If the target gene produces an enzyme that is not normally made by the host cell, a direct (*in situ*) plate assay can be devised to identify members of a library that carry the particular gene encoding that enzyme. The genes for α- amylase, endoglucanase, β-glucosidase and many other enzymes from various organisms have been isolated in this way. In some cases, the cells of a genomic library are plated onto the medium supplemented with a specific substrate; if the substrate is hydrolyzed, a colorimetric reaction identifies the colonies that carry the target gene. For example, to identify a cloned bacterial lipase gene, transformed cells are grown in the presence of trioleoglyceol and fluorescent dye rhodamine B. As a result of the hydrolysis of the substrate, positive colonies have orange fluorescent halos when viewed under ultraviolet light.

Functional (genetic) complementation is another useful means of isolating genes that encode enzymes. The procedure entails transforming host cells that have a particular genetic defect with plasmids of a DNA library constructed from a normal organism (wild-type) and selecting the transformed cells that function normally. The cloned gene may come from either the same or a different species, i.e., homologous or heterologous functional complementation, respectively. In practice, *E.coli* and yeast cells with mutations that affect various biochemical pathways have frequently been used as a host cells for functional complementation gene cloning. In many of these experiments, the protein derived from the cloned gene enables the host to grow on minimal medium; whereas gowth of the mutant cells requires the addition of a specific compound to the medium. As well, the genes that play a role in antibiotic biosynthesis, root nodulation, and other processes have been isolated in this way.

10.11. Expression Systems

Prokaryotic (bacteria) or eukaryotic (yeast, mammalian cell culture) systems are generally used as a host for the production of usable quantities of the desired rDNA product. Most of the rDNA products approved by FDA are being produced using these systems. Bacteria such as *Escherichia coli* are widely used for the expression of rDNA products. They offer several advantages due to high level of recombinant protein expression, rapid growth of cell and simple media requirement. However, there are some limitations such as intracellular accumulation of heterologous proteins, the potential for product degradation due to trace of protease impurities and production of endotoxin. Yeast such as *Saccharomyces cerevisiae*, *Hansenulla polymorpha* and *Pichia pastoris* are among the simplest eukaryotic organisms. They grow relatively quickly and are highly adaptable to large-scale production. These organisms do not produce endotoxin. They are capable of glycosylating proteins up to a certain extent like mammalian cells. Mammalian systems such as Chinese hamster ovary (CHO) cell and baby hamster kidney (BHK) cell systems are often the choice for production of human therapeutic proteins. The CHO and BHK cell systems are an ideal choice as these are capable of glycosylating the protein at the correct sites. However, cost of production of the products using these systems is high because of slow growth and expensive nutrient media. The choice of expression system can influence the character, quantity and cost of a final product. Recent advances have been made in producing therapeutic proteins by using transgenic animals. Transgenic milk production is currently most feasible. The advantages of this system are high expression levels and volume output, low capital investment, low operational costs and reproducible production facility, i.e. inbreeding could pass an animal's ability to produce transgenic protein to its offspring. Despite the attractiveness of this system, a number of issues remain to be solved before it is broadly accepted by the industries and regulatory authorities alike. These include variability of expression levels and characterization of the exact nature of the post-translational modification in the mammary systems. The use of genetically engineered plants to produce valuable proteins is increasing slowly. The system has potential advantages of economy and scalability. However, variation in product yield, contamination with agrochemical and fertilizer, impact of pest and disease, and variable cultivation conditions should also be considered. Plant cell culture system combines the advantages of whole plant system as well as animal cell culture. Although, no recombinant products have yet been produced commercially using plant cell culture, several companies are investigating the commercial feasibility of such a production system.

10.12. Production and Purification of rDNA Products

Recombinant DNA (rDNA) technology has made a revolutionary impact in the area of human healthcare by enabling mass production of safe, pure and effective rDNA expression products. As we have seen for the production of a desired rDNA product the gene of interest has to be identified and isolated. After isolation and characterization of the gene, it is inserted into a vector such as plasmid. The recombinant plasmid is then inserted into bacterial yeast or cultured animal cell. Clones of transformed host cell are isolated and those that produce the protein of interest in the desired quantities are preserved under suitable condition as a master cell bank. The cell banks are characterized and properly maintained for use in subsequent transformation procedures. The cell bank should be periodically tested for cell viability, genetic and phenotypic stability. When eukaryotic cells are used for production, distinguishing genetic, phenotypic and immunological markers of the cell are useful in establishing the identity of the cells. Likewise, when microbial cultures are used, specific phenotypic features which form a basis for identification should be described.

As manufacturing needs arise, cells from working cell can be scaled up to produce the product in roller bottles and/or fermentors. Traditional small-scale fermentors are generally used for expansion of cells in suspension culture such as the growth of *E. coli* or yeast. The presence, extent and nature of any microbial contamination in the culture vessels must be thoroughly examined at suitable stages during production. All the systems associated with fermentors must be validated before being routinely used.

Mammalian cells are often grown in roller bottles. Inoculation of host cells that contain an expression vector is added to defined volume of medium in either fermentors or roller bottles. The cells are allowed to grow until the nutrients in the medium are depleted or excreted by the products reaching inhibitory levels. By providing a balanced mixture of nutrients and/or chemicals to neutralize accumulating growth inhibitor, product yield in the medium or cell density can be improved. At the end of the run, the host cells are harvested and the recombinant product is isolated from culture medium or cells.

One of the main problems faced in industrial production of rDNA products is plasmid instability in continuous and large-scale fermentation, since these cultures go through many generations. The resulting effects are lower productivity and an increase in production cost, because of the build-up of non-productive plasmid free cells. Unintended variability in culture during production may lead to changes which cause alteration in the product. Such variations might result in differing yield of the products. Thus the steps in a production process should be validated to ensure that the process intermediates are within specifications. Any assay used during process validation must itself be standardized, before the process validation is commenced.

High level expression of rDNA products in different host systems can often result in aggregation and accumulation of inclusion bodies. Under appropriate conditions, the rDNA products may get deposited in inclusion bodies, approximately 50% or more of the total cell protein. The rDNA protein is highly pure, stable and compact and can be recovered from the inclusion bodies by proper techniques. The first step is the isolation of the inclusion body from disrupted cells by centrifugation. The inclusion body proteins were then solubilized by using a chaotrope (denaturant), a substance which disrupts the three dimensional structure in macromolecules such as proteins, DNA, or RNA and denatures them. Chaotropic agents such as urea and guanidinium chloride interfere with stabilizing inter-molecular interactions mediated by non-covalent forces such as hydrogen bonds, van der waals forces, and hydrophobic effects. The active protein will be then recovered by removal of denaturant under controlled conditions that allow the protein to adapt its native configuration.

The overall goal of purification is to bring as much product with as little loss as possible. In case the desired product is intracellular, fermentation is followed by harvesting of cells. This step is normally achieved by centrifugation or filtration. The cells are then disrupted or lysed and cell debris is removed by centrifugation, leaving behind a dilute solution of crude desired product.

If mammalian or yeast system is used, the desired product can be obtained directly from the medium. Nowadays, ultrafiltration has become the method of choice for concentration and chromatographic techniques for purification of rDNA products. Among the different chromatographic techniques generally employed in a typical downstream process, gel filtration and ion exchange chromatography are the most common. Affinity chromatography is employed wherever possible, as it has high biospecificity and one can achieve a high degree of purification.

Physico-chemical, biological and immunological characterizations of purified product should be ensured using a wide range of analytical tests. The purification process must be validated to ensure that it is effective and adequate to remove extraneous substances such as chemicals used in purification, column contaminations, endotoxin, residual cellular proteins and viruses. Analytical methods play a vital role in the determination of identity, purity and potency of rDNA products with respect to safe and efficacious medicine for human use. Characterization of products may include test for mainly amino acid composition, peptide mapping, electrophoretic assays (SDS–PAGE, Western blot, isoelectric focusing), HPLC, immunoassay, endotoxin test, potency determination test, etc.

Bicinchoninic acid and Bradford methods are generally used for the determination of protein concentration in rDNA product. Protein sequencing provides structure information. Amino acid analysis is used to identify rDNA products based on their amino acid composition. Peptide mapping is used to compare protein structure of the product with that of the reference standard and to confirm lot-to-lot consistency of primary structure. Electrophoretic assays (sodium dodecylsulphate polyacrylamide gel electrophoresis, Western blot and isoelectric focusing) are effectively used to evaluate rDNA product purity, identity, homogeneity and stability. More recently, capillary electrophoresis has generated considerable interest as a complementary technique in the analysis of rDNA products.

Chromatographic method, viz. reverse phase-HPLC, size exclusion chromatography and hydrophobic interaction chromatography are used in the determination of purity of the product as well as the level of known impurities or degradation of product. Immunoassay and DNA hybridization are used for determination of host cell impurities. Polymerase chain reaction, which involves DNA amplification, may prove useful in detection and identification of contaminant DNA. The limulus amebocyte lysate (LAL) test is the most sensitive and specific test used to detect and measure endotoxin. A comparative study demonstrated that LAL test is more sensitive than rabbit pyrogen test.

The potency of rDNA product is generally assessed by using specific techniques. The choice of assay is often determined by the nature of the product and its intended therapeutic application. Animal model assay, cell culture-based assay and *in vitro* (physico-chemical) assays used for determination of potency of rDNA product involves comparing the activity of the recovered product with that of reference standard (calibrated in international unit) and interpretation of the data with statistical support. Potency assays should have wide confidence limits and may include animal-based bioassay, *in vitro* cell culture assays or biochemical assay. All rDNA drugs undergo rigorous quality control testing in order to conform to predetermined specifications. The fundamental difference between quality control system for rDNA drugs and traditional pharmaceuticals lies in the types of method used to determine drug identity, purity and potency. The use of suitable reference standard from internationally recognized sources such as WHO, NIH, etc. is important for identification and purity of rDNA-derived drugs.

10.13. Transgenic Plants

For production of transgenic animals, DNA is usually microinjected into pronuclei of embryonic cells at a very early stage after fertilization, or alternatively gene targeting of embryo stem (ES) cells is employed. This is possible in animals due to the availability of specialized *in vitro* fertilization technology, which allows manipulation of ovule, zygote or early embryo. Such techniques are not available in plants. In contrast to this in higher plants, cells or protoplasts can be cultured and used for regeneration of whole plants. Therefore, these protoplasts can be used for gene transfer followed by regeneration leading to the production of transgenic plants. Besides cultured cells and protoplasts, other meristem cells (immature embryos or organs), pollen or zygotes can also be used for gene transfer in plants. To achieve genetic transformation in plants, we need the construction of a vector (genetic vehicle) which transports the genes of interest, flanked by the necessary controlling sequences i.e. promoter and terminator, and deliver the genes into the host plant. The two kinds of gene transfer methods in plants are:

(i) Vector-mediated or indirect gene transfer

Among the various vectors used in plant transformation, the Ti plasmid of *Agrobacterium tumefaciens* has been widely used. This bacteria is known as "natural genetic engineer" of plants because these bacteria have natural ability to transfer T-DNA of their plasmids into plant genome upon infection of cells at the wound site and cause an unorganized growth of a cell mass known as crown gall. Ti plasmids are used as gene vectors for delivering useful foreign genes into target plant cells and tissues (Fig. 10.12). The foreign gene is cloned in the T-DNA region of Ti-plasmid in place of unwanted sequences.

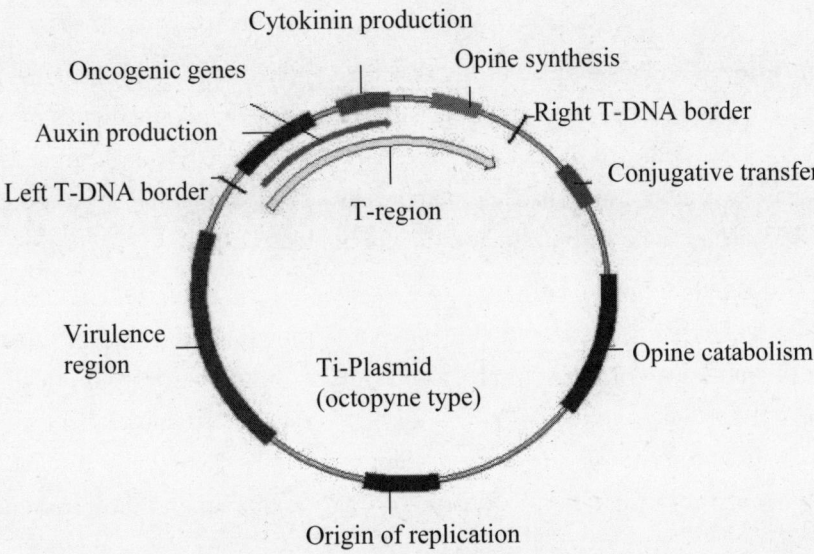

Figure 10.12: Ti plasmid

To transform plants, leaf discs (in case of dicots) or embryogenic callus (in case of monocots) are collected and infected with *Agrobacterium* carrying recombinant disarmed Ti-plasmid vector. The infected tissue is then cultured (co-cultivation) on shoot regeneration medium for 2-3 days during which time the transfer of T-DNA along with foreign genes takes place. After this, the transformed tissues (leaf discs/calli) are transferred onto selection cum plant regeneration medium supplemented with usually lethal concentration of an antibiotic to selectively eliminate non-transformed tissues. After 3-5 weeks, the regenerated shoots (from leaf discs) are transferred to root-inducing medium, and after another 3-4 weeks, the complete plants are transferred to soil following the hardening (acclimatization) of regenerated plants. The molecular techniques like PCR and southern hybridization are used to detect the presence of foreign genes in the transgenic plants.

(ii) Vectorless or direct gene transfer

In this method, the foreign gene of interest is delivered into the host plant cell without the help of a vector. The methods used for direct gene transfer in plants are:

- **Chemical mediated gene transfe**r e.g. chemicals like polyethylene glycol (PEG) and dextran sulphate induce DNA uptake into plant protoplasts. Calcium phosphate is also used to transfer DNA into cultured cells.

- **Microinjection,** where the DNA is directly injected into plant protoplasts or cell (specifically into the nucleus or cytoplasm) using fine tipped (0.5 - 1.0μm diameter) glassneedle or micropipette. This method of gene transfer is used to introduce DNA into large cells such as oocytes, eggs, and the cells of early embryo.

- **Electroporation,** involves a pulse of high voltage applied to protoplasts/cells/ tissues to make transient (temporary) pores in the plasma membrane which facilitates the uptake of foreign DNA. The cells are placed in a solution containing DNA and subjected to electrical shocks to cause holes in the membranes. The foreign DNA fragments enter through the holes into the cytoplasm and then to nucleus.

- **Particle gun/Particle bombardment** - In this method, the foreign DNA containing the genes to be transferred is coated onto the surface of minute gold or tungsten particles (1-3 μm) and bombarded onto the target tissue or cells using a particle gun (also called as gene gun/shot gun/microprojectile gun). The microprojectile bombardment method was initially named as biolistics by its inventor, Sanford (1988). Two types of plant tissue are commonly used for particle bombardment- Primary explants and the proliferating embryonic tissues.

- **Transformation** - This method is used for introducing foreign DNA into bacterial cells e.g. *E. coli*. The transformation frequency (the fraction of cell population that can be transferred) is very good in this method. e.g. the uptake of plasmid DNA by E. coli is carried out in ice cold $CaCl_2$ (0-5°C) followed by heat shock treatment at 37-45°C for about 90 sec. The transformation efficiency refers to the number of transformants per microgram of added DNA. The $CaCl_2$ breaks the cell wall at certain regions and binds the DNA to the cell surface.

- **Liposome mediated gene transfer or Lipofection** - Liposomes are circular lipid molecules with an aqueous interior that can carry nucleic acids. Liposomes encapsulate the DNA fragments and then adher to the cell membranes and fuse with them to transfer DNA fragments. Thus, the DNA enters the cell and then to the nucleus. Lipofection is very efficient technique used to transfer genes in bactcrial, animal and plant cells.

10.13.1. Selection of Tansformed Cells from Untransformed Cells

The selection of transformed plant cells from untransformed cells is an important step in the plant genetic engineering. For this, a marker gene (e.g. for antibiotic resistance) is introduced into the plant along with the transgene followed by the selection of an appropriate selection medium (containing the antibiotic). The segregation and stability of the transgene integration and expression in the subsequent generations can be studied by genetic and molecular analyses (Northern, Southern, Western blot, PCR).

10.13.2. Beneficial Traits of Transgenic Plants

During the last decades, a tremendous progress has been made in the development of transgenic plants using the various techniques of genetic engineering. The plants, in which a functional foreign gene has been incorporated by any biotechnological methods that generally not present in the plant, are called transgenic plants. Transgenic plants have many beneficial traits like insect resistance, herbicide tolerance, delayed fruit ripening, improved oil quality, weed control etc. Some of the traits introduced in these transgenic plants are as follows:

(a) Stress tolerance

Biotechnology strategies are being developed to overcome problems caused due to biotic stresses (viral, bacterial infections, pests and weeds) and abiotic stresses (physical factors such as temperature, humidity, salinity etc).

(b) Abiotic stress tolerance

The plants show their abiotic stress response reactions by the production of stress related osmolytes like sugars (e.g. trehalose and fructans), sugar alcohols (e.g. mannitol), amino acids (e.g. proline, glycine, betaine) and certain proteins (e.g. antifreeze proteins). Transgenic plants have been produced which over express the genes for one or more of the above mentioned compounds. Such plants show increased tolerance to environmental stresses. Resistance to abiotic stresses includes stress induced by herbicides, temperature (heat, chilling, freezing), drought, salinity, ozone and intense light. These environmental stresses result in the destruction, deterioration of crop plants which leads to low crop productivity. Several strategies have been used and developed to build resistance in the plants against these stresses.

(c) Herbicide tolerance

Several biotechnological strategies for weed control are being used e.g. the over-production of herbicide target enzyme (usually in the chloroplast) in the plant which makes the plant insensitive to the herbicide. This is done by the introduction of a modified gene that encodes for a resistant form of the enzyme targeted by the herbicide in weeds and crop plants. The biological manipulations using genetic engineering to develop herbicide resistant plants are: (a) over-expression of the target protein by integrating multiple copies of the gene or by using a strong promoter, (b) enhancing the plant detoxification system which helps in reducing the effect of herbicide, (c) detoxifying the herbicide by using a foreign gene, and (d) modification of the target protein by mutation. Some of the examples are:

(i) Glyphosate resistance - Glyphosate, a glycine derivative is a herbicide which is found to be effective against the 76 of the world's worst 78 weeds. It kills the plant by being the competitive inhibitor of the enzyme 5-enoyl-pyruvylshikimate 3- phosphate synthase (EPSPS) in the shikimic acid pathway. Due to it's structural similarity with the substrate phosphoenol pyruvate, glyphosate binds more tightly with EPSPS and thus blocks the shikimic acid pathway. Certain strategies were used to provide glyphosate resistance to plants. It was found that EPSPS gene was over-expressed in *Petunia* due to gene amplification. EPSPS gene was isolated from *Petunia* and introduced in to the other plants. These plants could tolerate glyphosate at a dose of 2–4 times higher than that required to kill wild type plants.

(ii) Phosphinothricin is a broad spectrum herbicide and is effective against broad-leafed weeds. It acts as a competitive inhibitor of the enzyme glutamine synthase which results in the inhibition of the enzyme glutamine synthase and accumulation of ammonia and finally the death of the plant. The disturbace in the glutamine synthesis also inhibits the photosynthetic activity. The enzyme phosphinothricin acetyl transferase (which was first observed in *Streptomyces* sp in natural detoxifying mechanism against phosphinothricin) acetylates phosphinothricin, and thus inactivates the herbicide. The gene encoding for phosphinothricin acetyl transferase (bar gene) was introduced in transgenic maize and oil seed rape to provide resistance against phosphinothricin.

(d) Other Abiotic Stresses

The abiotic stresses due to temperature, drought, and salinity are collectively also known as water deficit stresses. The plants produce osmolytes or osmoprotectants to overcome the osmotic stress. The attempts are on to use genetic engineering strategies to increase the production of osmoprotectants in the plants. The biosynthetic pathways for the production of many osmoprotectants have been established and genes coding the key enzymes have been isolated e.g. Glycine betaine is a cellular osmolyte which is produced by the participation of a number of key enzymes like choline dehydrogenase, choline monooxygenase etc. The choline oxidase gene from *Arthrobacter* sp. was used to produce transgenic rice with high levels of glycine betaine giving tolerance against water deficit stress. Scientists also developed cold-tolerant genes (around 20) in *Arabidopsis* when this plant was gradually exposed to slowly declining temperature. By introducing the coordinating gene (it encodes a protein which acts as transcription factor for regulating the expression of cold tolerant genes), expression of cold tolerant genes was triggered giving protection to the plants against the cold temperatures.

(i) Insect resistance

A variety of insects, mites and nematodes significantly reduce the yield and quality of the crop plants. The conventional method is to use synthetic pesticides, which also have severe effects on human health and environment. The transgenic technology uses an innovative and eco-friendly method to improve pest control management. About 40 genes obtained from microorganisms of higher plants and animals have been used to provide insect resistance in crop plants. The first genes available for genetic engineering of crop plants for pest resistance were Cry genes (popularly known as Bt genes) obtained from a bacterium *Bacillus thuringiensis*. These are specific to particular group of insect pests and are not harmful to other useful insects like butter flies and silk worms. Transgenic crops with Bt genes (e.g. cotton, rice, maize, potato, tomato, brinjal, cauliflower, cabbage, etc.) have been developed. This has proved to be an effective way of controlling the insect pests and has reduced the pesticide use. The most notable example is Bt cotton (which contains CrylAc gene) that is resistant to a notorious insect pest Bollworm *(Helicoperpa armigera)*. Certain genes from higher plants were also found to result in the synthesis of products possessing insecticidal activity. One of the examples is the Cowpea trypsin inhibitor gene (CpTi) which was introduced into tobacco, potato, and oilseed rape for develping transgenic plants. Cowpea trypsin inhibitor (CpTi) has no effect on mammalian trypsin, hence it is non-toxic to mammals.

(ii) Virus resistance

There are several strategies for engineering plants for viral resistance, and these utilizes the genes from virus itself (e.g. the viral coat protein gene). The virus-derived resistance has given promising results in a number of crop plants such as tobacco, tomato, potato, alfalfa, and papaya. The induction of virus resistance is done by employing virus-encoded genes-virus coat proteins, movement proteins, transmission proteins, satellite RNA, antisense RNAs, and ribozymes. The virus coat protein-mediated approach is the most successful one to provide virus resistance to plants. It was in 1986, transgenic tobacco plants expressing tobacco mosaic virus (TMV) coat protein gene were first developed. These plants exhibited high levels of resistance to TMV. The transgenic plant providing coat protein-mediated resistance to virus is rice, potato, peanut, sugar beet, alfalfa, etc.

(iii) Resistance Against Fungal and Bacterial Infections

As a defence strategy against the invading pathogens (fungi and bacteria) the plants accumulate low molecular weight proteins which are collectively known as pathogenesis-related (PR) proteins. Several transgenic crop plants with increased resistance to fungal pathogens are being raised with genes coding for the different compounds. One of the examples is the Glucanase enzyme that degrades the cell wall of many fungi. The most widely used glucanase is β-1,4-glucanase. The gene encoding for β-1,4 glucanase has been isolated from barley, introduced, and expressed in transgenic tobacco plants. This gene provided good protection against soil-borne fungal pathogen *Rhizoctonia solani*. Lysozyme degrades chitin and peptidoglycan of cell wall, and in this way fungal infection can be reduced. Transgenic potato plants with lysozyme gene providing resistance to *Erwinia carotovora* have been developed.

(e) Delayed Fruit Ripening

The ripening can be slowed down by blocking or reducing ethylene production since ethylene regulates the ripening of fruits. This can be achieved by introducing ethylene forming gene(s) in a way that will suppress its own expression in the crop plant. Such fruits ripen very slowly (however, they can be ripen by ethylene application) and this helps in exporting the fruits to longer distances without spoilage due to longer-shelf life. The main strategy used was the antisense RNA approach. In the normal tomato plant, the PG gene (for the enzyme polygalacturonase) encodes a normal mRNA that produces the enzyme polygalacturonase which is involved in the fruit ripening. The complimentary DNA of PG encodes for antisense mRNA, which is complimentary to normal (sense) mRNA. The hybridization between the sense and antisnse mRNAs renders the sense mRNA ineffective. Consequently, polygalacturonase is not produced causing delay in the fruit ripening. Similarly strategies have been developed to block the ethylene biosynthesis thereby reducing the fruit ripening.

(f) Male Sterility

The plants may inherit male sterility either from the nucleus or cytoplasm. It is possible to introduce male sterility through genetic manipulations while the female plants maintain fertility. In tobacco plants, these are created by introducing a gene coding for an enzyme (barnase, which is a RNA hydrolyzing enzyme) that inhibits pollen formation. This gene is expressed specifically in the tapetal cells of anther using tapetal specific promoter TA29 to restrict its activity only to the cells involved in pollen production. The restoration of male fertility is done by introducing another gene barstar that suppresses the activity of barnase at the onset of the breeding season. By using this approach, transgenic plants of tobacco, cauliflower, cotton, tomato, corn etc. with male sterility have been developed.

10.14. Edible Vaccines

Vaccines have been revolutionary for the prevention of infectious diseases. Edible vaccines hold great promise as a cost-effective, easy-to-administer, easy-to-store, fail-safe and socio-culturally readily acceptable vaccine delivery system, especially for the poor developing countries. It involves introduction of selected desired genes into plants and then inducing these altered plants to manufacture the encoded proteins. Crop plants offer cost-effective bioreactors to express antigens which can be used as edible vaccines. The approach is to isolate genes encoding antigenic proteins from the pathogens and then expressing them in plants. Such transgenic plants or their tissues producing antigens can be eaten for vaccination/immunization (edible vaccines). The expression of such antigenic proteins in crops like banana and tomato are useful for immunization of humans since banana and tomato fruits can be eaten raw.

Transgenic plants (tomato, potato) have been developed for expressing antigens derived from animal viruses e.g. rabies virus and herpes virus. In 1990, the first report of the production of edible vaccine (a surface protein from *Streptococcus*) in tobacco at 0.02% of total leaf protein level was published in the form of a patent application under the International Patent Cooperation Treaty (Mason and Arntzen, 1995).The first clinical trials in humans, using a plant derived vaccine were conducted in 1997 and were met with limited success. This involved the ingestion of transgenic potatoes with a toxin of *E. coli* causing diarrhea.

Creating edible vaccines involves introduction of selected desired genes into plants and then inducing these altered plants to manufacture the encoded proteins. This process is known as "transformation," and the altered plants are called "transgenic plants." The process of making of edible vaccines involves the incorporation of a plasmid carrying the antigen gene and an antibiotic resistance gene, into the bacterial cells, e.g. *Agrobacterium tumefaciens*. The small pieces of potato leaves are exposed to an antibiotic which can kill the cells that lack the new genes. The surviving cells with altered genes multiply and form a callus. This callus is allowed to grow and subsequently transferred to soil to form a complete plant. In about a few weeks, the plants bear potatoes with antigen vaccines.

Like conventional subunit vaccines, edible vaccines are composed of antigenic proteins and are devoid of pathogenic genes. Thus, they have no way of establishing infection, assuring its safety, especially in immunocompromised patients. The antigens in transgenic plants are delivered through bio-encapsulation, i.e, the tough outer wall of plant cells, which protects them from gastric secretions and finally break up in the intestines. The antigens are released, taken up by M cells in the intestinal lining that overlie Peyer's patches and gut-associated lymphoid tissue (GALT), passed on to macrophages, other antigen-presenting cells; and local lymphocyte populations, generating serum IgG, IgE responses, local IgA response and memory cells, which would promptly neutralize the attack by the real infectious agent.

Conventional subunit vaccines are expensive and technology-intensive, need purification, require refrigeration and produce poor mucosal response. In contrast, edible vaccines would enhance compliance, especially in children and because of oral administration, would eliminate the need for trained medical personnel. Their production is highly efficient and can be easily scaled up. The edible vaccines produced in transgenic plants will solve the storage problems, will ensure easy delivery system by feeding and will have low cost as compared to the recombinant vaccines produced by bacterial fermentation. The bacteria *E. coli, V. cholerae* cause acute watery diarrhea by colonizing the small intestine and by producing toxins. Another strategy adopted to produce a plant-based vaccine, is to infect the plants with recombinant virus carrying the desired antigen that is fused to viral coat protein. The infected plants are reported to produce the desired fusion protein in large amounts in a short duration. The technique involves either placing the gene downstream a subgenomic promoter, or fusing the gene with capsid protein that coats the virus.

10.15. Gene Therapy

Genes are specific sequences of bases that encode instructions on how to make proteins. Although genes get a lot of attention, it's the proteins that perform most life functions and even make up the majority of cellular structures. When genes are altered so that the encoded proteins are unable to carry out their normal functions, genetic disorders can result. Gene therapy is a technique for correcting defective genes responsible for disease development. Researchers may use one of several approaches for correcting faulty genes such as a normal gene may be inserted into a non-specific location within the genome to replace a nonfunctional gene. This approach is most common. An abnormal gene could be swapped for a normal gene through homologous recombination. The abnormal gene could be repaired through selective reverse mutation, which returns the gene to its normal function. The regulation (the degree to which a gene is turned on or off) of a particular gene could be altered.

In most gene therapy studies, a "normal" gene is inserted into the genome to replace an "abnormal," disease-causing gene. A carrier molecule called a vector must be used to deliver the therapeutic gene to the patient's target cells. Currently, the most common vector is a virus that has been genetically altered to carry normal human DNA. Viruses have evolved a way of encapsulating and delivering their genes to human cells in a pathogenic manner. Scientists have tried to take advantage of this capability and manipulate the virus genome to remove disease-causing genes (virulent) and insert therapeutic genes. Target cells such as the patient's liver or lung cells are infected with the viral vector. The vector then unloads its genetic material containing the therapeutic human gene into the target cell. The generation of a functional protein product from the therapeutic gene restores the target cell to a normal state. Some of the different types of viruses used as gene therapy vectors are:

- **Retroviruses:** They are the classes of viruses like Human immunodeficiency virus (HIV) that can create double-stranded DNA copies of their RNA genomes. These copies of its genome can be integrated into the chromosomes of host cells.

- **Adenoviruses:** A class of viruses with double-stranded DNA genomes that cause respiratory, intestinal, and eye infections in humans.

- **Adeno-associated viruses:** A class of small, single-stranded DNA viruses that can insert their genetic material at a specific site on chromosome 19.

- **Herpes simplex viruses:** A class of double-stranded DNA viruses that infect a particular cell type, neurons. Herpes simplex virus type 1 is a common human pathogen that causes cold sores.

Besides virus-mediated gene-delivery systems, there are several nonviral options for gene delivery. The simplest method is the direct introduction of therapeutic DNA into target cells. This approach is limited in its application because it can be used only with certain tissues and requires large amounts of DNA. It consists of approaches which involve the creation of an artificial lipid sphere with an aqueous core. This liposome, which carries the therapeutic DNA, is capable of passing the DNA through the target cell's membrane. Therapeutic DNA also can get inside target cells by chemically linking the DNA to a molecule that will bind to special cell receptors. Once bound to these receptors, the therapeutic DNA constructs are engulfed by the cell membrane and passed into the interior of the target cell. This delivery system tends to be less effective than other options.

The Food and Drug Administration (FDA) has not yet approved any human gene therapy product for sale. Current gene therapy is experimental and has not proven very successful in clinical trials. Little progress has been made since the first gene therapy clinical trial began in 1990. In 1999, gene therapy suffered a major setback with the death of 18-year-old Jesse Gelsinger. Jesse was participating in a gene therapy trial for ornithine transcarboxylase deficiency (OTCD). He died from multiple organ failures 4 days after starting the treatment. His death is believed to have been triggered by a severe immune response to the adenovirus carrier.

Suggested Readings

- Gene Cloning and DNA analysis (2006). An Introduction by T. A. Brown, Blackwell Science

- Molecular Biotechnology-Principles & applications of recombinant DNA (2009). Glick and Pasternak, ASM press.

- Principles of Gene Manipulation (2002). Old & Primose, Blackwell Scientific Publication

- Analysis of Genes and Genomes (2004). Richard Reese, John Wiley & Sons

- From Genes to Genomes- Concepts and applications of DNA Technology (2002). Dale & Von Schantz, John Wiley & Sons

- Culture of Animal Cells- A manual of Basic Technique, 5th Ed., (2005). R. Ian Freshney, John Wiley & Sons

- Plant Tissue Culture: Theory & Practice (2006). S.S. Bhojwani & M.K. Razdan, Elsevier Science

- Harrington, J.J., van Bokkelen, G., Mays, R.W., Gutashaw, K., Willard, H.F (1997). Formation of *de novo* centromeres and construction of first generation human artificial microchromosomes. Nature Genetics 125:345–355.

- Katoh, M., Ayabe, F., Norikane, S. (2004) Construction of a novel human artificial chromosome vector for gene delivery. Biochemical and Biophysical Research Communications 321:280–290.

- Kurpiewski, M.R., Engler, L.E., Wozniak, L.A., Kobylanska, A., Koziolkiewicz, M., Stec, W.J., Jen-Jacobsen, L. (2004) Mechanisms of coupling between DNA recognition and specificity and catalysis in *Eco*RI endonuclease. Structure 12:1775–1788.

- Morrow, J.F., Cohen, S.N., Chang, A.C.Y., Boyer, H.W., Goodman, H.M., Helling, R.B (1974). Replication and transcription of eukaryotic DNA in Escherichia coli. Proceedings of the National Academy of Science USA. 71:1743–1747.

CHAPTER 11

Tissue Culture

- Plant Tissue Culture
- Laboratory requirements
- Media components
- Media Preparation
- Techniques of Plant Tissue Culture
- Protoplast Culture
- Somatic hybridization
- Cytoplasmic Hybrids for Cybrids
- Selection of Hybrids and Cybrids
- Somaclonal Variation
- Advantages of somaclonal variation
- Isolation of somaclonal variation
- Culture Types
- Applications of Plant Tissue Culture
- Animal Tissue culture
- Development and maintenance
- Types of cell
- Laboratory facilities for tissue culture
- Growth Media
- Type of Cultures
- Hybridoma Technology
- Application of Animal cell culture

Tissue culture is the branch of biology in which tissues or cells of higher animals and plants are grown in an artificially controlled environment. Tissue cultures are used in the study of cell growth, multiplication and differentiation, as well as in cancer research, hereditary mechanisms, radiation biology, all hybridizations, and virus studies.

11.1 Plant Tissue Culture

Plant tissue culture is the method of culturing plant parts in an artificial medium to regenerate into a new plant. In horticulture, it is applied for the commercial production of disease and pest free plants on a commercial scale. It is a fascinating and useful tool which allows the rapid production of many genetically identical plants using relatively small amounts of space, supplies and time. Micro-propagation is the rapid vegetative propagation of plants via tissue culture techniques. It permits the manipulation of physical and chemical conditions in the production of large numbers of high quality plant material within a short period of time. Basically the technique consists of taking a piece of a plant (such as a stem tip, node, meristem, embryo, or even a seed) and placing it in a sterile, (usually gel-based) nutrient medium supplemented with growth hormones, where it multiplies. The formulation of the growth medium can be varied according to the need of culture like undifferentiated callus tissue, multiply the number of plantlets, rooting, or multiply embryos for "artificial seed".

The development of plant tissue began with the observation of French botanist George Morel (1965), while he was attempting to obtain a virus-free orchid plant and found that a millimetre-long shoot could be developed into complete plantlets by micropropagation. Thereafter, in the 1970s developed countries began commercial exploitation of this technology. It entered the developing world in the 1980s. It was earlier used to develop ornamental plants and flowering plants for export. The *in vitro* techniques were developed initially to demonstrate the totipotency of plant cells predicted by Haberlandt in 1902. Totipotency is the ability of a plant cell to perform all the functions of development, which are characteristic of zygote, *i.e.*, ability to develop into a complete plant. Haberlandt reported that culture of isolated single palisade cell from a leaf remained alive for up to 1 month, increased in size, accumulated starch but failed to divide in Knop's salt solution enriched with sucrose. Efforts to demonstrate totipotency led to the development of techniques for cultivation of plant cells under defined conditions. Most of the modern tissue culture media derive from the work of Skoog and coworkers during 1950s and 1960s.

A successful establishment of callus culture depended on the discovery during mid-thirties of IAA (idole-3-acetic acid), the endogenous *auxin*, and of the role of vitamins in plant growth and in root cultures. The first continuously growing callus cultures were established by Gautheret, White and Nobecourt in 1939 from cambium tissue. The subsequent discovery of kinetin by Miller and coworkers in 1955 enabled the initiation of callus cultures from differentiated tissues. Shoot bud differentiation from tobacco pith tissues cultured *in vitro* was reported by Skoog in 1944, and in 1957 Skoog and Miller proposed that root-shoot differentiation in this system, which was regulated by auxin-cytokinin ratio.

In 1972, Carlson and coworkers produced the first somatic hybrid plant by fusing the protoplasts of *Nicotiana glauca* and *N. langsdorfii*. Plant protoplasts are naked cells from which cell wall has been removed. In 1960, Cocking produced large quantities of protoplasts by using cell wall degrading enzymes. The techniques of protoplast production have now been considerably refined and are now possible to regenerate whole plants from protoplasts and also to fuse protoplasts of different plant species. Since then many divergent somatic hybrids have been produced. Details of all these techniques will be discussed later on.

The first embryo culture, although crude, was done by Hanning in 1904; he cultured nearly mature embryos of certain crucifers and grew them to maturity. Haploid plants from pollen grains were first produced by Maheshwari and Guha in 1964 by culturing anthers of *Datura*. This marked the beginning of anther culture or pollen culture for the production of haploid plants.

Tissue culture cells generally lack the distinctive features of most plant cells. They have a small vacuole, lack chloroplasts and photosynthetic pathways and the structural or chemical features that distinguish so many cell types, within the intact plant are found to be absent. They are most similar to the undifferentiated cells found in meristematic regions which become fated to develop into each cell type as the plant grows. Tissue cultured cells can also be induced to re-differentiate into whole plants by alterations to the growth media. Plant tissue cultures can be initiated from almost any part of a plant. The source, termed explant, must be healthy and free from obvious signs of disease or decay. Younger tissue contains a higher proportion of actively dividing cells (meristamatic) and is more responsive to a callus initiation programme. The exact conditions required to initiate and sustain plant cells in culture, or to regenerate intact plants from cultured cells, are different for each plant species.

11.1.1. Laboratory Requirements for Plant Tissue Culture

The essential requirements for proper tissue culture are analytical balance (for weighing nutrients for media), graduated cylinders and pipettes (for measuring stock solutions), pH meter (to regulate pH of media), microwave oven (to heat and dissolve gelling agent), glass containers (for heating and dissolving media), dispensing devices (to dispense equal quantities of media), de-ionizer (water needed for media), autoclave (for sterilizing instruments and media), transfer instruments (forceps, scalpels spatulas, blades), refrigerator (storage of chemicals and stock solutions), stereo-microscope (use for meristem culture) and laminar flow hood (provide a sterile area for transfers during initiation and sub-culturing).

11.1.2. Media Components

One of the most important factors governing the growth and morphogenesis of plant tissues in culture is the composition of the culture medium. The basic nutrient requirements of cultured plant cells are very similar to those of whole plants. Plant tissue and cell culture media are generally made up of some or all of the following components: macronutrients, micronutrients, vitamins, amino acids or other nitrogen supplements, sugar(s), other undefined organic supplements, solidifying agents or support systems, and growth regulators. Several media formulations are commonly used for the majority of all cell and tissue culture work. These media formulations include those described by many workers (White 1963; Murashige and Skoog 1962; Gamborg *et. al.*, 1968; Schenk and Hilderbrandt 1972). Murashige and Skoog's MS medium, Schenk and Hildebrand's SH medium, and Gamborg's B-5 medium are all high in macronutrients, while the other media formulations contain considerably less of the macronutrients. Composition of some of the general media are given in (Table 11.1).

Table 11.1: Different plant tissue cultures media and their compositions (mg/L DW)

Components	Murashige-Skoog (1962)	White (1963)	Gamborg (1968)	Heller (1953)	Schenk-Hildebrandt (1972)	Kohlenbach Schmidt (1975)
$(NH_4)_2SO_4$	-	-	134	-	-	-
$MgSO_{4\times}7H_2O$	370	720	500	250	400	185
Na_2SO_4	-	200	-	-	-	-
$KC1$	-	65	-	750	-	-
$CaC1_{2\times}2H_2O$	440	-	150	75	200	166
$NaNO_3$	-	-	-	600	-	-
KNO_3	1,900	80	3,000	-	2,500	950
$Ca(NO_3)_{2\times}4H_2O$	-	300	-	-	-	-
NH_4NO_3	1,650	-	-	-	-	720
$NaH_2PO_{4\times}H_2O$	-	16.5	150	125	-	-
$NH_4H_2PO_4$	-	-	-	-	300	-
KH_2PO_4	170	-	-	—	-	68
$FeSO_{4\times}7H_2)$	27.8	-	27.8	-	15	27.85
Na_2EDTA	37.3	-	37.3	-	20	37.25
$MnSO_{4\times}4H_2O$	22.3	7	10	0.1	10	25
$ZnSO_{4\times}7H_2O$	8.6	3	2	1	0.1	10
$CuSO_{4\times}5H_2O$	0.025	-	0.025	0.03	0.2	0.025
H_2SO_4	-	-	-	-	-	-
$Fe_2(SO_4)_3$	-	2.5	-	-	-	-
$NiC1_{2\times}6H_2O$	-	-	-	0.03	-	-
$CoC1_{2\times}6H_2O$	0.025	-	0.025	-	0.1	-
$A1C1_3$	-	-	-	0.03	-	-
$FeC1_{3\times}6H_2O$	-	-	-	1	-	-
$FeC_6O_5H_{7\times}5H_2O$	-	-	-	-	-	-
$K1$	0.83	0.75	0.75	0.01	1.0	-
H_3BO_3	6.2	1.5	3	1	5	10
$Na_2M_0O_{4\times}2H_2O$	0.25	-	0.25	-	0.1	0.25
Sucrose	30,000	20,000	20,000	20,000	30,000	10,000
Glucose	-	-	-	-	-	-
Myo-Inositol	100	-	100	-	1,000	100
Nicotinic Acid	0.5	0.5	1.0	-	0.5	5
Pyridoxine HC1	0.5	0.1	1.0	-	0.5	0.5
Thiamine HC1	0.1-1	0.1	10	1	5	0.5
Ca-Pantothenate	-	1	-	-	-	-
Biotin	-	-	-	-	-	0.05
Glycine	2	3	-	-	-	2
Cysteine HC1	-	1	-	-	-	-
Folic Acid	-	-	-	-	-	0.5
Glutamine	-	-	-	-	-	14.7

Plants grown *in vitro* require similar nutrients present in their natural environment. The basic components of any cultural medium are:

(a) Macronutrients

These elements are required in large amounts for plant growth and development. The macro-nutrients provide the six major elements-nitrogen (N), phosphorus (P), potassium (K), calcium (Ca), magnesium (Mg), and sulfur (S)-required for plant cell or tissue growth. The optimum concentration of each nutrient for achieving maximum growth rates varies considerably among species. Culture media should contain at least 25–60 mM of inorganic nitrogen for adequate plant cell growth. Plant cells may grow on nitrates alone, but considerably better results are obtained when the medium contains both a nitrate and ammonium nitrogen source. Certain species require ammonium or another source of reduced nitrogen for cell growth to occur. Nitrates are usually supplied in the range of 20–25 mM; typical ammonium concentrations range between 2 to 20 mM, however, excess of 8 mM may be deleterious to cell growth of certain species. Cells can grow on a culture medium containing ammonium as the sole nitrogen source if one or more of the TCA cycle acids (e.g., citrate, succinate, or malate) are also included in the culture medium at concentrations of approximately 10 mM. Potassium is required for cell growth of most plant species. Most media contain potassium, in the nitrate or chloride form, at concentrations of 20-30 mM. The optimum concentrations of P, Mg, S, and Ca range from 1–3 mM provide all other requirements.

(b) Micronutrients

These elements are required in trace amounts for plant growth and development. The essential micronutrients for plant cell and tissue growth include iron (Fe), manganese (Mn), zinc (Zn), boron (B), copper (Cu), and molybdenum (Mo). Chelated forms of iron and zinc are commonly used in preparing culture media. Iron may be the most critical of all the micronutrients. Iron citrate and tartrate may be used in culture media, but these compounds are difficult to dissolve and frequently precipitate after media are prepared. Murashige and Skoog used an ethylene diamine tetraacetic acid (EDTA)-iron chelate to bypass this problem. Cobalt (Co) and iodine (I) may also be added to certain media, but strict cell growth requirements for these elements have not been established. Sodium (Na) and chlorine (Cl) are also used in some media but are not essential for cell growth. Copper and Cobalt are normally added to culture media at concentrations of 0.1 µM, Fe and Mo at 1 µM, I at 5 µM, Zn at 5-30 µM, Mn at 20–90 µM, and B at 25-100 µM.

(c) Carbon and Energy Source

Sucrose is the most commonly used carbohydrate source in plant cell culture media, though glucose and fructose can be substituted in some cases. Other carbohydrates that have been tested include lactose, galactose, rafinose, maltose, and starch. Sucrose concentrations of culture media normally range between 2 to 3 percent. Carbohydrates must be supplied to the culture medium because few plant cell lines have been isolated that are fully autotropic, e.g., capable of supplying their own carbohydrate by CO_2 assimilation during photosynthesis.

(d) Vitamins

Normal plants synthesize the vitamins required for their growth and development. Vitamins are required by plants as catalysts in various metabolic processes. When plant cells and tissues are grown *in vitro*, some vitamins may become limiting factors for cell growth. The vitamins most frequently used in cell and tissue culture media include thiamin (B1), nicotinic acid, pyridoxine (B6), and *myo*-inositol. Thiamin is the one vitamin that is basically required by all cells for growth. Thiamin is normally used at concentrations ranging from 0.1 to 10.0 mg/liter. Nicotinic acid and pyridoxine are often added to culture media but are not essential for cell growth in many species. Nicotinic acid is normally used at concentrations of 0.1–5.0 mg/liter; pyridoxine is used at 0.1-10.0 mg/liter. *Myo*-inositol is commonly included in many vitamin stock solutions. Although it is a carbohydrate not a vitamin, it has been shown to stimulate growth in certain cell cultures. Its presence in the culture medium is not essential, but in small quantities *myo*-inositol stimulates cell growth in most species. It is generally used at concentrations of 50–5000 mg/liter.

Other vitamins such as biotin, folic acid, ascorbic acid, pantothenic acid, vitamin E (tocopherol), riboflavin, and p-aminobenzoic acid have been included in some cell culture media. The requirement for these vitamins by plant cell cultures is generally negligible, and they are not considered growth-limiting factors. These vitamins are generally added to the culture medium only when the concentration of thiamin is below the desired level or when it is desirable to grow cells at very low population densities.

(e) Amino Acids or other Nitrogen Supplements

Certain amino acids or amino acid mixtures are found to stimulate cell growth though cultured cells are normally capable of synthesizing all of the required amino acids. The use of amino acids is particularly important for establishing cell cultures and protoplast cultures. Amino acids provide plant cells with an immediately available source of nitrogen, which generally can be taken up by the cells more rapidly than inorganic nitrogen. The most common sources of organic nitrogen used in culture media are amino acid mixtures (e.g., casein hydrolysate), L-glutamine, L-asparagine, and adenine. Casein hydrolysate is generally used at concentrations between 0.05 and 0.1 percent. When amino acids are added alone, care must be taken, as they can be inhibitory to cell growth. Examples of amino acids included in culture media to enhance cell growth are glycine at 2 mg/liter, glutamine up to 8 mM, asparagine at 100 mg/liter, L-arginine and cysteine at 10 mg/liter, and L-tyrosine at 100 mg/liter. Tyrosine has been used to stimulate morphogenesis in cell cultures but should only be used in an agar medium. Supplementation of the culture medium with adenine sulfate can stimulate cell growth and greatly enhance shoot formation.

(f) Organic Supplements

Addition of a wide variety of organic extracts to culture media often results in favorable tissue responses. Supplements that have been tested include protein hydrolysates, coconut milk, yeast extracts, malt extracts, ground banana, orange juice and tomato juice. However, undefined organic supplements should only be used as a last resort, and only coconut milk and protein hydrolysates are used to any extent today. Protein (casein) hydrolysates are generally added to culture media at a concentration of 0.05-0.1%, while coconut milk is commonly used at 5-20% (v/v).

The addition of activated charcoal (AC) to culture media may have a beneficial effect. The effect of AC is generally attributed to one of three factors: absorption of inhibitory compounds, absorption of growth regulators from the culture medium, or darkening of the medium. The inhibition of growth in the presence of AC is generally attributed to the absorption of phytohormones to AC. 1-Napthaleneacetic acid (NAA), kinetin, 6-enzylamino-purine (BA), indole-3-acetic acid (IAA), and 6-α-α-dimethylallylaminopurine (2iP) all bind to AC, with the latter two growth regulators binding quite rapidly. The stimulation of cell growth by AC is generally attributed to its ability to bind to toxic phenolic compounds produced during culture. Activated charcoal is generally acid-washed prior to addition to the culture medium at a concentration of 0.5-3.0 percent.

(g) Solidifying Agents or Support Systems

Agar is the most commonly used gelling agent for preparing semisolid and solid plant tissue culture media. Agar has several advantages over other gelling agents. First, when agar is mixed with water, it forms a gel that melts at approximately 60-100 °C and solidifies at approximately 45°C; thus, agar gels are stable at all feasible incubation temperatures. Additionally, agar gels do not react with media constituents and are not digested by plant enzymes. The firmness of an agar gel is controlled by the concentration and brand of agar used in the culture medium and the pH of the medium. The agar concentrations commonly used in plant cell culture media range between 0.5 and 1.0%; these concentrations give a firm gel at the pH typical of plant cell culture media.

(h) Growth Regulators

Auxins, cytokinins, gibberellins, and abscisic acid are the four important classes of growth regulators in plant tissue culture. Skoog and Miller (1957) were the first to report that the ration of auxin to cytokinin determined the type and extent of organogenesis in plant cell cultures. Both, an auxin and cytokinin are usually added to culture media in order to obtain morphogenesis, although the ratio of hormones required for root and shoot induction is not universally the same. Considerable variability exists among genera, species, and even cultivars in the type and amount of auxin and cytokinin required for induction of morphogenesis. The auxins commonly used in plant tissue culture media are 1H-indole-3-acetic acid (IAA), 1H-indole-3-butyric acid (IBA), (2,4-dichlorophenoxy) acetic acid (2,4-D), and 1-napthaleneacetic acid (NAA). The only naturally occurring auxin found in plant tissues is IAA. Other synthetic auxins that have been used in plant cell culture include 4-chlorophenoxyacetic acid or p-chlorophenoxyacetic acid (4-CPA, PCPA), (2,4,5-trichlorophenoxy) acetic acid (2,4,5-T), 3,6- dichloro-2-methoxybenzoic acid and 4-amino-3,5,6-trichloropicolinic acid.

The cytokinins commonly used in the culture media include 6-benzylaminopurine or 6-benzyladenine (BAP, BA), N-(2-furanylmethyl)-1H-puring-6-amine (kinetin), and 6-(4-hydroxy-3-methyl-trans-2-butenylamino) purine (zeatin). Zeatin is considered to be naturally occurring cytokinin, while BAP and kinetin are synthetically derived cytokinins. The cytokinins are generally added to a culture medium to stimulate cell division, to induce shoot formation and axillary shoot proliferation, and to inhibit root formation. The type of morphogenesis that occurs in a plant tissue culture largely depends upon the ratio and concentrations of auxins and cytokinins present in the medium. Root initiation of plantlets, embryogenesis, and callus initiation all generally occur when the ratio of auxin to cytokinin is high, whereas adventitious and axillary shoot proliferation occurs when the ration is low. Gibberellins (GA3) and abscisic acid (ABA) are two other growth regulators occasionally used in culture media. Plant tissue cultures can usually be induced to grow without either GA3 or ABA, although, certain species may require these hormones for enhanced growth. Generally, GA3 is added to culture media to promote the growth of low-density cell cultures, to enhance callus growth, and to elongate dwarfed or stunted plantlets. Abscisic acid is generally added to culture media to either inhibit or stimulate callus growth (depending upon the species), to enhance, inhibit, or stimulate callus growth (depending upon the species), to enhance shoot or bud proliferation, and to inhibit latter stages of embryo development.

11.1.3. Media Preparation

Proper media preparation is apparent for successful results in plant tissue culture. The procedure involves the proper weighing of the individual media components according to the prescribed composition or requirement and dissolving it into approximately 90% of the required volume of de-ionized-distilled water by gentle heating. The pH of the medium is adjusted with NaOH or HCl and the final required volume will be made up with deionized-distilled water. Sterilize the medium by autoclaving at 15 psi (121°C) for appropriate time period. Higher temperature and duration may detrimental to the media. This medium will be then dispensed in to sterile culture vessels/tubes after the addition of thermo labile supplements.

11.1.4. Techniques of Plant Tissue Culture

In plant tissue culture, explants such as pieces of leave, steem or root is cultured in a specific plant medium, which contains essential plant nutrients and hormones. The explants are surface sterilized by using chemical solutions such as bleach or alcohol. Though, mercury chloride is an effective sterilizer, it is rarely used due to its potential toxicity. After sterilization, the explants are introduced into a plant medium, which can be either solid or liquid. Other plant growth factors like light and temperature are maintained and regulated by using artificial conditions. All the procedures of plant tissue culture are conducted under sterile (aseptic) conditions. Generally, these give rise to an unorganized mass of cells called callus (soft tissue that forms over a cut surface). The cells divide and differentiate into plant parts, thus giving rise to a complete plant (Fig. 11.1). The explants then develop stem, roots and leaves. The generated plantlets are hardened before planting in outdoor conditions. In addition to these ingredients, solid medium contains gelling agent (agar). Nutrient and plant hormones amount vary, depending on the objective of plant tissue culture. For example, in order to induce more roots, auxin amount should be high. Plant tissue culture techniques include the culture of protoplast (a cell without cell wall), meristem, node, anther, ovule, embryo and seed.

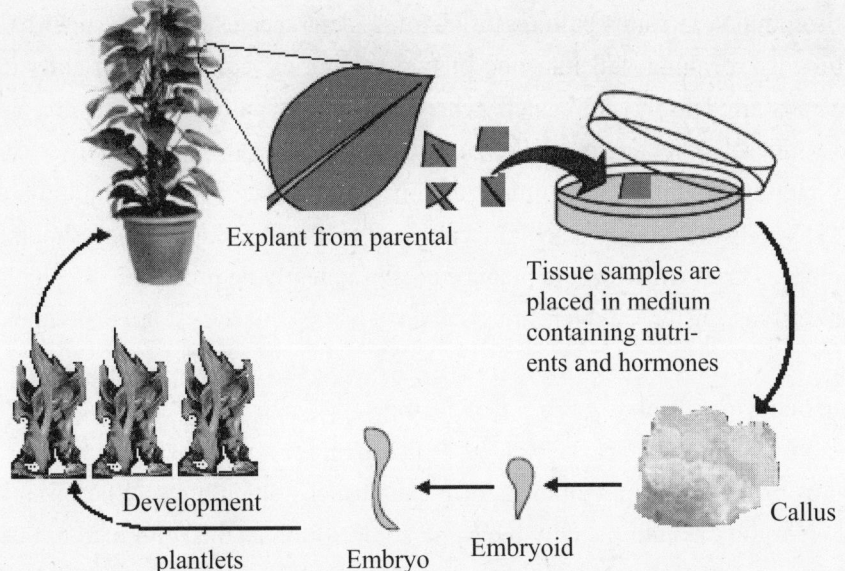

Figure 11.1: Diagrammatic representation of events in plant tissue culture

11.1.5. Culture Types

Cultures are generally initiated from sterile pieces of a whole plant, termed explants, and may consist of pieces of organs, such as leaves or roots, or may be specific cell types, such as pollen or endosperm. Many features of the explant are known to affect the efficiency of culture initiation. Generally, younger, more rapidly growing tissue (or tissue at an early stage of development) is most effective.

(1) Callus

Formation of callus, an unorganized, growing, and dividing mass of cells, can be induced on explants when they are cultured on an appropriate medium, usually with a supplementation of both auxin and cytokinin. In tissue culture, proliferation of callus can be maintained more or less indefinitely, provided that the callus is subcultured on to fresh medium periodically. During callus formation, there can be some degree of dedifferentiation (i.e. the changes that occur during development and specialization are, to some extent, reversed), both in morphology (a callus is usually composed of unspecialized parenchyma cells) and metabolism. One major consequence of this dedifferentiation is that most plant cultures lose the ability to photosynthesize. This has important consequences for the culture of callus tissue, as the metabolic profile will probably not match with that of the donor plant. This necessitates the addition of other components—such as vitamins and, most importantly, a carbon source—to the culture medium, in addition to the usual mineral nutrients.

Callus culture is often performed in the dark (the lack of photosynthetic capability being no drawback) as light can encourage differentiation of the callus. During long-term culture, the culture may lose the requirement for auxin and/or cytokinin. This process, known as habituation, is common in callus cultures from some plant species (such as sugar beet). Callus cultures, broadly speaking, fall into one of two categories: compact or friable. In compact callus, the cells are densely aggregated, whereas in friable callus, the cells are only loosely associated with each other and the callus becomes soft and breaks apart easily.

Callus cultures are extremely important in plant biotechnology. Manipulation of the auxin to cytokinin ratio in the medium can lead to the development of shoots, roots, or somatic embryos from which whole plants can subsequently be produced. It can also be used to initiate cell suspensions, which are used in a variety of ways in plant transformation studies.

(2) Cell-suspension cultures

In suspension culture, cells are suspended in the medium rather than adhering to a surface. Friable callus provides the inoculum to form cell-suspension cultures. When friable callus is placed into a liquid medium (usually the same composition as the solid medium used for the callus culture) and then agitated, single cells and/or small clumps of cells are released into the medium. Under the proper conditions, these released cells continue to grow and divide, eventually producing a cell-suspension culture. A relatively large inoculum should be used when initiating cell suspensions so that the released cell numbers build up quickly. The inoculum should not be too large though, as toxic products released from damaged or stressed cells can build up to lethal levels. Large cell clumps can be removed during subculture of the cell suspension.

Explants from some plant species or particular cell types tend not to form friable callus, making it difficult to initiate cell suspension. The friability of the callus can sometimes be improved by manipulating the medium components or by repeated subculturing. The friability of the callus can also sometimes be improved by culturing it on semi-solid medium (medium with a low concentration of gelling agent).

Cell suspensions can be maintained relatively simply as batch cultures in conical flasks. They are continually cultured by repeated subculturing into fresh medium. This results in dilution of the suspension and the initiation of another batch growth cycle. The degree of dilution during subculture should be determined empirically for each culture. A highdegree of dilution will result in a greatly extended lag period or, in extreme cases, death of the transferred cells. After subculture, the cells divide and the biomass of the culture increases in a characteristic fashion, until nutrients in the medium are exhausted and/or toxic by-products build up to inhibitory levels, called the stationary phase. If cells are left in the stationary phase for too long, they will die and the culture will be lost. Therefore, cells should be transferred as they enter the stationary phase. It is therefore important that the batch growth-cycle parameters are determined for each cell-suspension culture.

(3) Root cultures

Root cultures can be established *in vitro* from explants of the root tip of either primary or lateral roots and can be cultured on fairly simple media. The growth of roots *in vitro* is potentially unlimited, as roots are indeterminate organs. Although, the establishment of root cultures was one of the first achievements of modern plant tissue culture, they are not widely used in plant transformation studies.

(4) Anther culture

Anther culture is the process of using anthers to culture haploid plantlets. The technique was discovered in 1964 by Guha and Maheshwari. This technique can be used in over 200 species, including tomato, rice, tobacco, barley, and geranium. Some of the advantages which make this a valuable method for obtaining haploid plants. It is easy to induce cell division in the immature pollen cells in some species, high induction frequency and large number of haploids can be produced in a short period of time. For example in case of *Datura innoxia*, induction frequencies of almost 100% and a yield of more than one thousand plantlets or calluses have occurred under optimal conditions from one anther. Success can be determined within 24 hours as cells begin to divide (Fig. 11.2).

Some of the disadvantages of using anther culture to obtain haploids involves, when working with some species, the majority of plants produced have been non-haploid. Particularly in certain cases like cereals, very few green plants are obtained; many of the plants are albinos or green-albino chimeras. Generally, it is tedious to remove the anthers without causing damage and sometimes a particular orientation is necessary to achieve a desired response.

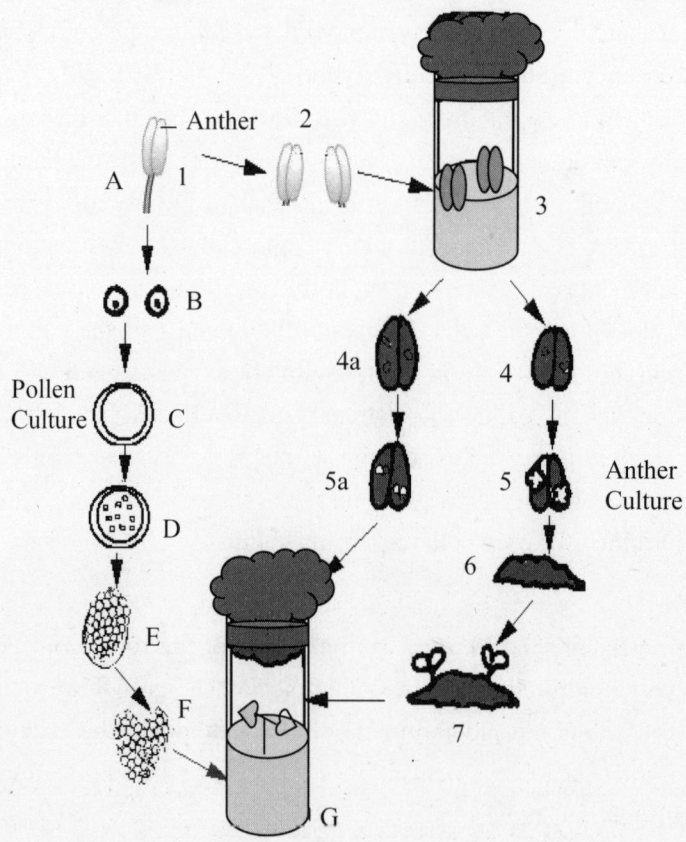

Figure 11.2: Diagram showing the various stages of anther and isolated pollen culture. The stages of anther culture from anther to haploid plantlet can be described as follows: 1) an unopened flower bud, 2) anthers, 3) the anthers in culture, 4) proliferating anther, 5) haploid callus, 6) differentiating callus, G) haploid plantlet. Isolated pollen culture is as follows: A) an unopened flower bud, B) isolated pollen from a cultured anther, C) pollen culture, D) multinucleate pollen, E) and F) pollen embryo. Homozygous plants can be obtained by treating the haploid plantlets with colchicine.

(5) Embryo culture

Embryos can be used as explants to generate callus cultures or somatic embryos. Both immature and mature embryos can be used as explants. Immature, embryo-derived embryogenic callus is the most popular method of monocotyledon plant regeneration.

(a) Somatic embryogenesis

In somatic (asexual) embryogenesis, embryo-like structures, which can develop into whole plants in a way analogous to zygotic embryos, are formed from somatic tissues. These somatic embryos can be produced either directly or indirectly. In direct somatic embryogenesis, the embryo is formed directly from a cell or small group of cells without the production of an intervening callus. Though, common from some tissues (usually reproductive tissues such as the nucellus, styles, or pollen), direct somatic embryogenesis is generally rare in comparison with indirect somatic embryogenesis.

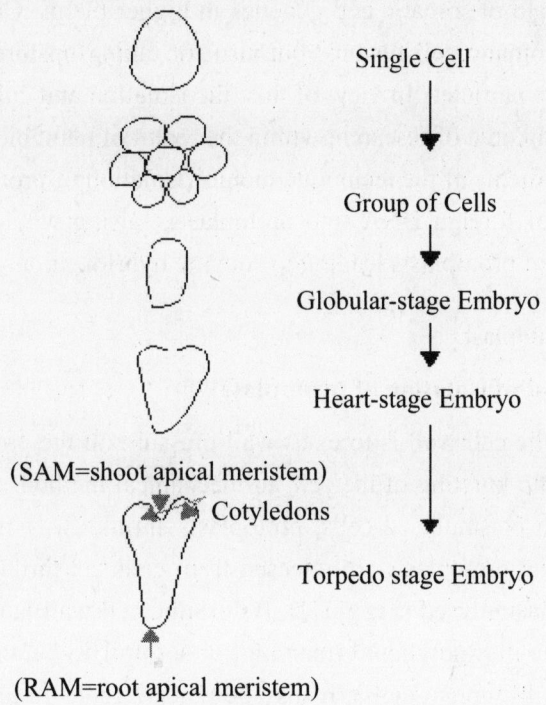

Figure 11.3: A schematic representation of the sequential stages of somatic embryo development

Somatic embryos may develop from single cells or from a small group of cells (Fig. 11.3). Repeated cell divisions lead to the production of a group of cells that develop into an organized structure known as a globular-stage embryo. Further development results in heart- and torpedo-stage embryos, from which plants can be regenerated. Zygotic embryos undergo a fundamentally similar development through the globular (which is formed after the 16-cell stage), heart and torpedo stages. Polarity is established early in embryo development. Signs of tissue differentiation become apparent at the globular stage and apical meristems are apparent in heart-stage embryos. Embryogenesis is particularly favored for transformation work.

11.1.6. Protoplast Culture

Protoplast is the living material of a plant or bacterial cell, including the protoplasm and plasma membrane after the cell wall has been removed. E.C. Cocking in 1960 at the University of Nottingham (U.K) demonstrated that naked cells called protoplasts can be obtained through enzymatic degradation of cell walls. Protoplast isolation, fusion and development of fused protoplast in to a complete plant are one of the most significant developments in the field of plant tissue culture, witnessed during the last few decades. This led to significant developments in the field of somatic cell genetics in higher plants. Cultured protoplasts can be used not only for somatic cell fusions, but also for taking up foreign DNA, cell organelles, bacteria and virus particles. In view of this, the isolation and culture of protoplasts has become a very important area of research, within the realm of plant biotechnology.

The essential ingredients of the technique include isolation of protoplasts, culture of protoplasts, introduction of foreign DNA into protoplasts, raising whole plants from cultured protoplasts and fusion of protoplasts leading to somatic hybridization.

11.1.6.1. Isolation of protoplast

(a) Mechanical method of isolation of protoplast

The chief function of the cell wall is to exert wall pressure on the protoplast preventing excessive water uptake and bursting of the cell. In mechanical method, cells are kept in a suitable plasmolyticum (in plasmolysed cells, protoplasts shrink away from cell wall) and cut with a fine knife, so that protoplasts are released from cells cut through the cell wall, when the tissue is again deplasmolysed (Fig. 11.4). Before the cell wall is removed, the cell must be placed in an isotonic plasmolyticum (mannitol or sorbitol 13 %, these sugar alcohols are less readily metabolised by plant cells). It may be advantageous to test a range of mannitol concentrations varying from 8 -15% (w/v). This method is suitable for isolation of protoplasts from vacuolated cells (e.g. onion bulbs, scales, radish roots). However, this method gives poor yield of protoplasts and is not suitable for isolating protoplst from meristematic and less vacuolated cells. The mechanical method, though, was used as early as 1892, is now only rarely used for isolation of protoplasts. One advantage, however, is that the deleterious effects of the wall-degrading enzymes on the metabolism of the protoplasts are eliminated.

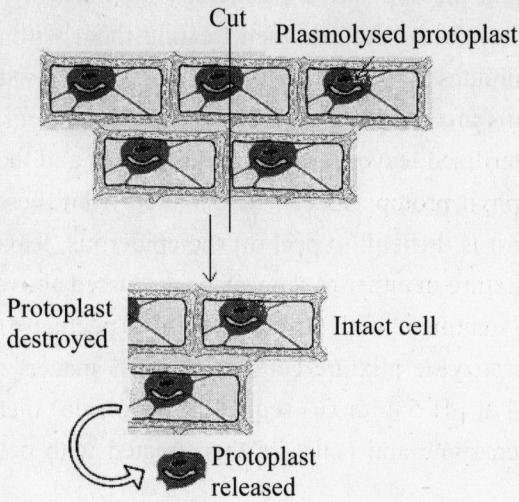

Figure 11.4: Mechanical method of isolation of protoplast

(b) Enzymatic method of isolation of protoplast

The enzymatic method has the advantage that it gives large quantities of protoplasts, where cells are not broken and osmotic shrinkage is minimum. But for better results sometimes mechanical and enzymatic methods are combined, where cells are first separated mechanically and later used for isolation of protoplasts through enzymatic treatment. The protoplasts can be isolated from a variety of tissues including leaves, roots, *in vitro* shoot cultures, callus, cell suspension and pollen. Young cell suspensions are particularly ideal for isolation of protoplasts in large quantities.

Protoplast isolation is achieved by using cellulase in combination with pectinase and hemicellulase. Commercial preparations of enzymes are derived from microorganisms, and may contain ribonucleases, proteases, and several other toxic enzymes. As a result of these deleterious enzymes, several purification procedures have been developed (one of the most often used procedures is column separation). There are two approaches to the use of wall-degrading enzymes.

- **Mixed-enzyme method:** pectinase and cellulase and/or hemicellulase are applied simultaneously.

- **Sequential method:** involves treatment with pectinase (loosen the cells), followed by cellulase and or hemicellulase.

The major steps employed for isolation of protoplasts involve (i) sterilization of leaves, (ii) peeling off the epidermis, (iii) enzymatic treatment and (iv) isolation and cleaning of protoplasts.

For protoplast isolation the explants are generally sterilized by first dipping them into 70% ethyl alcohol for about a minute and then treating them with 2% solution of sodium hypochlorite for 20-30 minutes. They are then rinsed three times with sterile distilled water and subsequent operations are carried out under aseptic conditions. In case of leaves the lower epidermis of the sterilized leaves is carefully peeled off and the stripped leaves are cut into small pieces. Mesophyll protoplasts can be obtained from these peeled leaf segments. In case of cereals, where it is difficult to peel off the epidermis, leaves are cut in long strips and used with enzyme mixture in either of the way as discussed above, such as (i) direct (one step) method, in which treatment with macerozyme (or pectinase) and cellulase is done simultaneously, here the enzyme mixture consists of 0.5% macerozyme + 2% cellulase in 13% sorbitol or mannitol at pH 5.4, or (ii) sequential (two step) method, in which cells are first isolated using macerozyme and cells are then treated with cellulase to isolate protoplasts.

11.1.6.2. Protoplast culture and regeneration of plants

The culture methods for isolated protoplasts are similar to those used for single cells. Both semi-solid and liquid medium can be used, although the liquid medium is preferred. Protoplasts can be suspended in a liquid medium in Erlenmeyer flasks without shaking and can be cultured in small quantities in 'hanging drops' or in 'microchambers'. Within 2-4 days, protoplasts start developing cell walls, which can be detected by staining with 0.1% calcofluor white (CPW) fluorescent stain, while the presence of a proper wall is essential for a regular division. The protoplasts, which are capable of dividing, undergo first division within 2–7 days and form multicellular colonies after 2– 3 weeks. After another two weeks, these colonies can be treated as standard tissue cultures. From these colonies or tissues in culture, plants can be regenerated. The regeneration technique involves transfer of callus to a medium capable of initiating differentiation and it behaves just like the callus derived from cells. Shooting and rooting can be induced by manipulating the hormone concentration. Subsequently, the generated plantlets may be transferred to pots or field after hardening.

11.1.6.3. Protoplast fusion and somatic hybridization

Protoplast fusion or somatic hybridization is one of the most important uses of protoplast culture. This is particularly significant for hybridization between species or genera, which can not be made to cross by conventional method of sexual hybridization. Although somatic hybridization was successfully achieved first in animals and later in plants, its significance has been realized fully in plants because the hybrid cells can be induced to regenerate into whole plants.

a. Spontaneous protoplast fusion: The spontaneous fusion of protoplast is found to be strictly intra-specific. However, spontaneous fusion of protoplasts can also be induced by bringing protoplasts into intimate contact through micromanipulators or micropipettes. There seems to be a correlation between the size of the leaf and the percentage of protoplasts undergoing spontaneous fusion; protoplasts from young leaves are more likely to undergo this fusion.

b. Induced protoplast fusion: Somatic hybridization is generally used for fusion of protoplasts either from two different species (interspecific fusion) or from two diverse sources belonging to the same species. In plants, however, the inducing agent (fusogen) first brings the protoplasts together and then causes them to adhere to one another for bringing about fusion. During the last two decades, a variety of treatments have been successfully utilized for fusion of plant protoplasts. It involves the treatments particularly with $NaNO_3$, high pH with high Ca^{++} ion concentration and polyehtylene glycol (PEG).

(i) $NaNO_3$ treatment

The method involves two steps such as isolated protoplasts are suspended in an aggregation mixture (5.5% sodium nitrate in 10% sucrose solution). This mixture works as a fusion inducing mixture and causes fusion on incubation at 35°C. In order to obtain a higher frequency of fused protoplasts, the mixture may be centrifuged and the pellet resuspended and incubated for one or more additional cycles. Finally the mixture is replaced by a liquid medium and the protoplasts in this mixture are incubated again; the cycle may be repeated once or twice before plating the protoplasts on a solid medium. The fusion of protoplasts can be monitored at different steps by examination under an inverted microscope.

This method was successfully utilized for fusion of protoplasts from root tips of oat and maize seedlings but is not preferred due to low frequency of fusion, particularly when highly vacuolated mesophyll protoplasts are used.

(ii) Treatment with calcium ions (Ca^{++}) at high pH

This method involves spinning (centrifugation) the protoplasts in a fusion inducing solution (0.05M $CaCl_2.2H_2O$ in 4M mannitol at pH 10 for 30 min at 50g, after which the tubes are placed in a water bath (37°) for 40–50 min. This leads to fusion of 20–50% of the protoplasts. A calcium solution buffered at high pH induces aggregation of the protoplasts and their fusion. The addition of Ca^{++} causes the potential of the surface negative charge on protoplasts to be reduced, facilitating protoplast adhesion. The high alkalinity (pH 9.5–10.4) induces the formation of intra-membranous lysophospholipids such as lysolecithin and lyso-phosphatidyl -ethanolamine that increase membrane fluidity, which results in fusion. This method has been successfully used in the production of numerous somatic hybrid plants.

(iii) Polyethylene glycol (PEG) treatment

PEG has been most widely used to fuse plant protoplasts. Both, the concentration and molecular weights of PEG are important in relation to fusion. PEG ($HOCH_2$-(CH_2-O-CH_2) - CH_2OH) is a water soluble compound whose linkages make the molecule slightly negative in charge. Thus, addition of Ca^{++} ($CaCl_2$ or Ca (NO_3)$_2$) links the compound with membrane surfaces. The high molecular weight of the polymer acts as a bridge connecting the protoplasts together. A strong affinity of PEG for water causes local membrane dehydration and increased fluidity. This in combination with the reduction of an exclusion volume between adjacent protoplasts causes diminishing mutual membrane electrostatic repulsion. The redistribution of glycoprotein and glycocalyx macromolecules causes fusion. Compounds structurally related to PEG, namely, polyvinyl alcohol, polyvinyl pyrrolidone and polyglycerol are known to induce fusion. Gelatin, and dextran sulphate also induce fusion to varying degrees.

The technique gives high frequency of fusion with reproducible results and involves low cytotoxicity. The technique can be used for fusion of protoplasts from unrelated plant taxa (e.g. soybean -tobacco, soybean, maize, and soybean - barley), from unrelated animal taxa and also between those from animal and plant cells. PEG has been used in combination with other treatments to enhance fusion frequency. An increase in the frequency of heterokaryon formation was observed when protoplasts were pre-incubated in lysozyme. Also, combination of PEG with high pH Ca^{++} solution, or the addition of DMSO or concanavalin A gave rise to higher fusion frequencies in comparison to treatments with PEG alone. After PEG treatment, protoplasts are gradually washed and during this process, most of the fusion is achieved. PEG is then replaced by culture medium to allow growth of fused protoplasts.

(iv) Electrical fusion

Protoplasts can be induced to fuse by placing them into a small culture cell containing electrodes and a potential difference is applied, then the protoplasts will line up between the electrodes. Application of an extremely short, square, wave of electric shock will now induce them to fuse.

After the fusion treatment the protoplast population consists of a mixture of parental types, homokaryons and heterokaryons of which heterokaryons (potential source of future hybrids) often make only 0. 5%–10%.

11.1.6.4. Somatic hybridization

Production of hybrid plants through the fusion of protoplasts of two different plant species/ varieties is called somatic hybridization and such hybrids are known as somatic hybrids. Protoplast technology, which includes the isolation, culture, and fusion of higher plant protoplasts leading to the production of whole plants, is considered one of the most exciting developments in experimental botany in recent years. Protoplast culture provides excellent opportunities for research on plant improvement, first by exploring genetic variations among the existing crops and then by attempting to transfer the available genetic information from one species to another through fusion of protoplasts isolated from somatic tissues of these crops. Somatic hybridization involves fusion of two distantly related, to closely related plant protoplasts at intraspecific, interspecific, intergeneric, and interfamily levels, with subsequent regeneration of hybrid cells into hybrid plants. Plastids and mitochondrial genomes (cytoplasmically encoded traits) are inherited maternally in sexual crossings. Through the fusion process, the nucleus and cytoplasm of both parents are mixed in the hybrid cell (heterokaryon). This results in various nucleocytoplasmic combinations. Sometimes interactions in the plastome and genome contribute to the formation of cybrids (cytoplasmid hybrids).

Conventional sexual crossing in higher plants is a highly regulated system of hybridization wherein sexual crosses are limited to phylogenetically related plant species. Also, the classical methods of breeding employed for transfer of beneficial traits from wild species to cultivated varieties are time consuming and require extensive backcrossing with the cultivated variety in order to eliminate most of the genome of the wild species while retaining the useful genes.

11.1.6.5. Cytoplasmic hybrids for cybrids

Cybrids, in contrast to conventional hybrids, possess a nuclear genome from only one parent but cytoplasmic genes, from both parents. The process of protoplast fusion resulting in the development of cybrids is known as cybridization. In cybridization, heterozygosity of extrachromosomal material can be obtained, which has direct application in plant breeding. The technique of cybrid production has been utilized for transfer of cytoplasmic male sterility as has been successfully done in *Nicotiana, Brassica* and *Petunia*. Other characters like streptomycin resistance have also been transferred from *N. tobacum* to *N. sylvestris*, using this technique. Ogura cytoplasmic-male sterility (CMS) lines with 'Ogura cytoplasm', an herbicide (atrazine) resistant line and lines with increased nectar production have also been obtained using cybrids in crop *Brassica*.

Cybrids can be obtained by methods such as fusion of normal protoplasts from one parent with enucleated protoplasts from the other parent; enucleated protoplasts can be obtained by high speed centrifugation (20,000 - 40,000g for 45-90 min) of protoplasts or by irradiation treatment, fusion of normal protoplasts from one parent and protoplasts containing non viable nuclei from the other, selective elimination of one of the nuclei from the heterokaryon or by selective elimination of chromosomes of one parent at a later stage after fusion of the nuclei.

11.1.6.6. Selection of somatic hybrids and cybrids

Proper selection of the hybrid cells or fusion products after fusion treatment is necessary since the protoplast populations consist of a heterogeneous mixture of unfused parental types, homokaryons, and heterokaryons. This is because the fusion induced by various methods is random and uncontrolled. The low number of true hybrid cells formed may get lost in the population of actively dividing homokaryotic fusion products and unfused parental protoplasts. Hence, selective recovery of the few hybrid cells formed from the mixed population of regenerating protoplasts is a key factor in successful somatic hybridization. The different selection procedures employed are:

(a) Biochemical selection of somatic hybrids

This selection procedure was based on a prior knowledge of the differential growth characteristics and nutritional requirements of unfused and hybrid protoplasts isolated from the genetically different species. Protoplasts of the hybrid are able to grow on a defined medium in culture to form calli, whereas parental types will fail to develop into calli. This selection system has an advantage in that the requirement of a mutant as one of the fusion partners is totally eliminated.

(b) Visual selection of somatic hybrids

In most of the somatic hybridization experiments selection procedures involve fusion of chlorophyll deficient (nongreen) protoplasts of one parent with the green protoplasts of the other parent (wild type), since this facilitates visual identification of heterokaryons at the light microscope level. Nongreen protoplasts are isolated from cultured cells, epidermal cells, or antibiotic induced albino plantlets. Even though the mechanical method of isolation of somatic fusion products is the most tedious procedure, it may be the most likely method for recovering osmotic hybrids in a variety of different plants, especially legumes, cereals, and tree species.

This approach suffers the draw back from the fact that it requires special culture media for each particular hybrid cell type to divide and form clusters. This is called the fishing method. Somatic hybrid callus has been similarly obtained in fusion between colorless protoplasts of *Glycine max* derived from cell cultures with the green mesophyll protoplasts of *Nicotiana glauca*.

(c) Morphological selection of somatic hybrids

Melchers *et al.* (1978) adopted the method of selection of somatic hybrids based on their abnormal morphology in regenerating intergeneric somatic hybrids such as "pomatoes" and 'topatoes' which are the fusion products of protoplasts of tomato and potato.

The regenerated plants showed abnormal morphology and proved to be somatic hybrids by analysis of chromosomal and fraction-1-protein, the ribulose1, 5-bisphosphate carboxylase. Intermediate morphology of the callus also determined the intergeneric somatic hybrids between *Vicia faba* and *Petunia hybrida*.

(d) Flow cytometry and sorting selection of somatic hybrids

Various laboratories are using techniques of flow cytometry and fluorescent activated cell sorting for analysis of plant protoplasts while maintaining their viability. These techniques have also been applied for sorting and selection of heterokaryons. The fused and unfused products are sorted in a "cell sorter" machine based on the presence or absence of fluorescence of both dyes in the fusion products. Galbraith *et al.* (1989) have described a universally applicable method for electronic sorting of heterokaryons formed by fusing the protoplasts of two parents labeled with different vital fluorescent dyes, such as rhodomine isothiocyanate and floreceine isothiocyanate.

11.1.6.7. Application of somatic hybridization and cybridization

- Somatic cell fusion appears to be the only means through which two different parental genomes can be recombined among plants that cannot reproduce sexually (asexual or sterile).
- Protoplasts of sexually sterile (haploid, triploid, and aneuploid) plants can be fused to produce fertile diploids and polyploids.
- Somatic cell fusion overcomes sexual incompatibility barriers. In some cases somatic hybrids between two incompatible plants have also found application in industry or agriculture.
- Somatic cell fusion is useful in the study of cytoplasmic genes and their activities and this information can be applied in plant-breeding experiments.

11.1.7. Somaclonal Variation

In plants genetic variation occurs at stages of development of the tissue culture process such as the variations occur as a part of mutation or as a part of clonal development have been termed as somaclonal variations. As these variations are not due to heredity, their transmissions to next generations are not possible. However, such variations combined with action of mutagens could result into ideal breeding material for crop improvement programme.

Somaclonal variations affect cytoplasmic genome as well as nuclear genome. These variations, when heritable are useful for improvement of crops such as resistance to insect pests and diseases, tolerance to environmental stress, male sterility etc.

Examples of somaclonal variations observed in crop species are:

- Rust resistance in wheat.
- Resistance for late blight in potato.
- Shortening of harvest duration in sugar cane.
- Increased shelf life in tomato.
- Tolerance to high temperature in wheat.
- Resistance for leaf hopper in rice.
- High protein content in potato.

11.1.7.1. Isolation of somoclonal variation

Mutants for several traits can be far more easily isolated from cell cultures than from whole plant populations. Mutants can be effectively selected for disease resistance, improvement of nutritional quality, adaptation of plants to stress conditions, e.g., saline soils, low temperature, toxic metals (e.g., aluminium), and resistance to herbicides and to increase the biosynthesis of plant products used for medicinal or industrial purposes. The various approaches for isolation of somaclonal variants can be categorized as screening and cell selection.

(i) Screening: It involves the observation of a large number of cells or regenerated plants for the detection of variant individuals. This approach is the only feasible technique for the isolation of mutants for yield and yield traits. Screening has been profitably and widely employed for the isolation of cell clones that produce higher quantities of certain biochemicals.

(ii) Cell Selection: In the cell selection approach, a suitable selection pressure is applied, which permits the preferential survival/growth of variant cells only. Some examples of cell selection are selection of cells resistant to various toxins, herbicides, high salt concentration, etc. When the selection pressure allows only the mutant cells to survive or divide, it is called positive selection. On the other hand, in the case of negative selection, the wild type cells divide normally and, therefore, are killed by a counter selection agent.

These cells are subsequently rescued by removal of the counter election agent. Negative selection approach is utilized for the isolation of auxotrophic mutants. The positive selection approach may be further subdivided into four categories: (i) direct selection, (ii) rescue method, (iii) stepwise selection and (iv) double selection. In direct selection, the cells resistant to the selection pressure survive and divide to form colonies; the wild type cells are killed by the selection agent. This is the most common selection method which it is used for the isolation of cells resistant to toxins (produced by pathogens), herbicides, elevated salt concentration, antibiotics, amino acid analogues, etc.

In the rescue method, the wild type cells are killed by the selection agent, while the variant cells remain alive but, usually, do not divide due to the unfavorable environment. The selection agent is then removed to recover the variant cells. This approach has been used to recover low temperature and aluminium resistant variant cells.

The selection pressure, e.g., salt concentration, may be gradually increased from a relatively low level to the cytotoxic level; the resistant clones isolated at each stage are subjected to the higher selection pressure. Such a selection approach is called stepwise selection.

Somaclonal variation has the advantages such as it occurs in rather high frequencies, which is a great advantage over conventional methods. Some 'new' alleles or even 'new' mutations may be isolated, which were not available in the germplasm or through mutagenesis. The use of somaclonal variation may reduce the time required for the release of new variety as compared to mutation breeding. This is the only approach for the isolation of biochemical mutants, especially auxotrophic mutants, in plants. A very effective selection can be practiced at the cell level for several traits, e.g., disease resistance.

One major advantage of plant tissue culture is the production of disease and/or pest resistant varieties, thus indirectly increasing the crop yield. Commercially, it is used directly for the propagation of plants that are hard to propagate in natural conditions. Horticultural plants such as orchids, roses, banana, strawberries, potatoes, apples, etc. are successfully cultured in *in-vitro* conditions. Plants with valuable secondary products are grown in the controlled conditions by using plant tissue culture technique. It is also used for the propagation of medicinal herbs on a large scale. With plant tissue culture, it is possible to generate virus-free plantlet of vegetatively propagated plants.

In experimental biology such as plant breeding, cell biology, biotechnology and genetics, plant tissue culture is applied in order to solve plant related problems. It allows screening of cells for the desirable characters such as early fruit bearing, disease resistance and drought resistance. Another important application is generation of a novel hybrid by crossing two distantly related species having advantageous traits. *In-vitro* fertilization and/or pollination of plants is possible, irrespective of the hindrances in natural conditions. In short plant tissue culture is one of the methods for conservation of germplasm.

> *HeLa cells are a human epithelial cervical cancer, and the first human cells, from which a permanent cell line was established. On 9 February 1951, surgeon Lawrence Wharton Jr. removed the tissue from the patient Henrietta Lacks, a 31-year-old African American woman from Baltimore, in the Women's Clinic of the Johns Hopkins Hospital.*

11.2. Animal Tissue Culture

Tissue Culture is the general term for the removal of cells, tissues, or organs from an animal or plant and their subsequent placement into an artificial environment favorable to growth. This environment usually consists of a suitable glass or plastic culture vessel containing a liquid or semisolid medium that supplies the nutrients essential for survival and growth. The culture of whole organs or intact organ fragments with the intent of studying their continued function or development is called organ culture. When the cells are removed from the organ fragments prior to, or during cultivation, thus disrupting their normal relationships with neighboring cells, it is called cell culture. Cell culture is the process by which cells are grown under controlled conditions. Cell culture has become one of the major tools used in the life sciences today.

In the beginning of 19th century, Sydney Ringer, English physiologist developed salt solutions containing the chlorides of sodium, potassium, calcium and magnesium suitable for maintaining the beating of an isolated animal heart outside of the body. In 1885, Wilhelm Roux removed a portion of the medullary plate of an embryonic chicken and maintained it in a warm saline solution for several days, establishing the principle of tissue culture. Rose Harrison (1907) developed a reproducible technique for tissue culture and later Alexis Carrel (1912) used tissue and embryo extracts as culture media. They successfully demonstrated that animal cells can be grown indefinitely *in vitro*, just like protozoa and microorganisms. Although animal cell culture was first successfully undertaken by Ross Harrison in 1907, it was not until the late 1940s to early 1950s that several developments occurred that made cell culture widely available as a tool for scientists. First, there was the development of antibiotics that made it easier to avoid many of the contamination problems that plagued earlier cell culture attempts. Second, was the development of the techniques, such as the use of trypsin to remove cells from culture vessels, necessary to obtain continuously growing cell lines (such as HeLa cells). Third, using these cell lines, scientists were able to develop standardized, chemically defined culture media that made it far easier to grow cells. These three areas combined to allow many more scientists to use cell, tissue and organ culture in their research.

11.2.1. Development and Maintenance of Cell Culture

Tissue culture is often a generic term that refers to both organ culture and cell culture and the terms are often used interchangeably. Cell cultures are derived from either primary tissue explants or cell suspensions. Primary cell cultures typically will have a finite life span in culture whereas continuous cell lines are, by definition, abnormal and are often transformed cell lines.

When cells are surgically removed from an organism and placed into a suitable culture environment, they will attach, divide and grow. This is called a primary culture. There are two basic methods for doing this. First, for explant cultures, small pieces of tissue are attached to a glass or treated plastic culture vessel containing suitable culture medium. After a few days, individual cells will move from the tissue explant out onto the culture vessel surface or substrate, where they will begin to divide and grow. The second, more widely used method speeds up this process by adding digesting (proteolytic) enzymes, such as trypsin or collagenase, to the tissue fragments to dissolve the cement holding the cells together. This creates a suspension of single cells that are then placed into culture vessels containing culture medium and allowed to grow and divide. This method is called subculturing.

When the cells in the primary culture vessel have grown and filled up all of the available culture substrate, they must be subcultured to give them room for continued growth. This is usually done by removing them as gently as possible from the substrate with enzymes. These are similar to the enzymes used in obtaining the primary culture and are used to break the protein bonds attaching the cells to the substrate. Once released, the cell suspension can then be subdivided and placed into new culture vessels. Once a surplus of cells is available, they can be treated with suitable cryoprotective agents, such as dimethylsulfoxide (DMSO) or glycerol, carefully frozen and then stored at cryogenic temperatures (below -130°C) until they are needed. Organizations such as American Type Culture Collection (ATCC) also provide high quality cell lines that are carefully tested to ensure the authenticity of the cells.

The basic culture systems can be of two types, based on the ability of the cells to either grow attached to a glass or treated plastic substrate (Monolayer culture sytems) or floating free in the culture medium (suspension culture systems). Monolayer cultures are usually grown in tissue culture treated dishes, T-flasks, roller bottles, or multiple well plates, the choice being based on the number of cells needed, the nature of the culture environment, cost and personal preference. Suspension cultures are usually grown either in magnetically rotated spinner flasks or shaken Erlenmeyer flasks where the cells are kept actively suspended in the medium. Many cell lines, especially those derived from normal tissues, are considered to be anchorage-dependent, that is, they can only grow when attached to a suitable substrate. Some cell lines that are no longer considered normal (transformed cells) are frequently able to grow either attached to a substrate or floating free in suspension; they are anchorage-independent. In addition, some normal cells, such as those found in the blood, do not normally attach to substrates and always grow in suspension.

Once in culture, cells exhibit a wide range of behaviors, characteristics and shapes. Cultured cells are usually described based on their morphology or their functional characteristics. The culture conditions play an important role in determining shape and that many cell cultures are capable of exhibiting multiple morphologies. The three basic types of cells based on the morphologies are epithelial-like cells, which consists of cells that are attached to a substrate and appear flattened and polygonal in shape, the lymphoblast-like cells, here the cells that do not attach normally to a substrate but remain in suspension with a spherical shape and third type fibroblast like cells that are attached to a substrate and appear elongated and bipolar, frequently forming swirls in heavy cultures.

The characteristics of cultured cells result from both their origin (liver, heart, etc.) and how well they adapt to the culture conditions. Biochemical markers can be used to determine if cells are still carrying on specialized functions that they performed *in vivo* (e.g., liver cells secreting albumin). Some cell lines will eventually stop dividing and show signs of aging. These lines are called finite. Other lines are, or become immortal; these can continue to divide indefinitely and are called continuous cell lines. When a "normal" finite cell line becomes immortal, it undergoes a fundamental irreversible change or "transformation". This can occur spontaneously or be brought about intentionally using drugs, radiation or viruses. Transformed cells are usually easier and fast growing, may often have extra or abnormal chromosomes such as aneuploidy and frequently can be grown in suspension.

11.2.3. Laboratory Facilities for Tissue Culture

The laboratory facilities for animal culture should include facilities for sterile handling, incubation of cultured cells, glassware needed for preparation and handling of media and tissue, sterilization and storage. Tissue culture facilities required in any laboratory can be divided into essential and beneficial requirements on the basis of priority (Table 11.2).

11.2.4. Growth Media

For growing cells in vitro, the environment should be as close as that expected *in vivo*. The nutrient media used for animal cell and tissue culture must be able to support their survival as well as growth, i.e., must provide nutritional, hormonal and stromal factors. Nine amino acids, referred to as the essential amino acids, cannot be synthesized by adult vertebrate animals and thus must be obtained from their diet. Animal cells grown in culture also must be supplied with these nine amino acids, namely, histidine, isoleucine, leucine, lysine, methionine, phenylalanine, threonine, tryptophan, and valine. In addition, most cultured cells require cysteine, glutamine and tyrosine. In the intact animal, these three amino acids are synthesized by specialized cells; for example, liver cells make tyrosine from phenylalanine, and both liver and kidney cells can make glutamine. Animal cells both within the organism and in culture can synthesize the 8 remaining amino acids; thus these amino acids need not be present in the diet or culture medium.

Table 11.2: Tissue culture facilities required in laboratory

Minimum require-ments (essential)	Desirable features (beneficial)	Useful additions
Laminar flow hood(s)	Cell counter	Glassware washing machine
Incubator	Vacuum pump	-70°C freezer
5%CO_2 cylinder (for gassing cultures)	Pipetter(s)	Closed-circuit TV for inverted microscope (s)
Liquid CO_2 (for incubator)	pH meter	Colony counter
Balance (coarse & fine)	Osmometer	High –capacity centrifuge (6× 1 litre)
Sterilizer (autoclave, pressure cooker, oven)	Drying oven	Cell sizer (e.g., Coulter ZB series
Freezer (for - 20°C storage)	Phase-contrast and fluorescence microscope (s)	Interference-contrast microscope
Inverted microscope	Portable temperature recorder	Polythene bag sealer (for packaging sterile items of long-term storage)
Soaking bath or sink	Permanent temperature recorders on sterilizing oven and autoclave	Controlled-rate cooler (for cell freezing)
Deep washing sink	Roller racks for roller bottle culture	Filing for freeze records and catalogue
Pipette cylinder (s)	Magnetic stirrer racks for suspension cultures	Centrifugal elutriator centrifuge and rotor
Pipette washer	Pipette drier	Fluorescence-activated cell sorter
Water purifier	Pipette plugger	Densitometer
Bench centrifuge	Trolleys for collecting soiled glassware and redistributing fresh supplies	Density meter (for density) gradient cell separation
liquid N_2 freezer (35I, 500-3,000 ampules)	Pipette aid	Conductivity meter
Liquid N_2 storage flask (~251)	Autopipette or other form of automatic dispenser, diluter	Computer for records and database
	Separate sterilizing oven and drying oven	Confocal microscope

The other essential components of a medium for culturing animal cells are vitamins, which the cells cannot make at all or in adequate amounts; various salts, glucose, and serum, the noncellular part of the blood. Serum, a mixture of hundreds of proteins, contains various factors needed for proliferation of cells in culture. For example, it contains insulin, a hormone required for growth of many cultured vertebrate cells, and transferrin, an iron-transporting protein essential for incorporation of iron by cells in culture. Although, many animal cells can grow in a serum-containing medium, such as Eagle's medium, certain cell types require specific protein growth factors, which are not present in serum. For instance, precursors of red blood cells require the hormone erythropoietin, and T lymphocytes of the immune system require interleukin 2 (IL-2). These factors bind to receptor proteins that span the plasma membrane, signaling the cells to increase in size and mass and undergo cell division. The medium is an important factor in this. The various types of media used for tissue culture may be grouped into two broad categories:

1. Natural media

Natural media is the most preferred medium, since it is the cheapest and most convenient. The natural media, which promotes cell growth, falls into the following three categories.

(a) Coagula such as plasma clots

Plasma clots have been in use and plasma can be collected from male fowl, where efforts are made to prevent coagulation of blood by adding heparin as an anticoagulant.

(b) Biological fluids such as serum

The most commonly used biological fluid is serum, which is obtained from human adult blood, placental cord blood, horse blood or calf blood. Out of these, human placental cord serum and foetal calf serum satisfactory. The serum can be obtained as exuded liquid from blood undergoing coagulation and is filtered using millipore filters. The serum should be tested for sterility and toxicity before using and stored at low temperature. The toxicity of sera can be reduced by heat inactivation. Besides serum, other biological fluids used as natural media includes amniotic fluid, ascitic fluid and pleural fluid, aqueous humour (from eye), serum ultrafiltrate and insect haemolymph

2. Artificial media

The various artificial media developed for cell culture may be grouped into 4 classes: (a) Serum-containing media (b) Serum-free media (c) Chemically defined media and (d) Protein-free media.

(a) Serum-containing media

The various defined media, such as Eagle's minimum essential media, when supplemented with 5–20% serum are good nutrient media for culture of most types of cells. The serum provides various plasma proteins, peptides, lipids, carbohydrates, minerals, and some enzymes. Serum serves several major functions like providing basic nutrients for cells, hormones, binding proteins and several minerals. It contains several growth factors and protease inhibitors. A major role of serum is to supply proteins and also act as a buffer. However, there are few disadvantages like it may inhibit growth of some cell types, like epidermal keratinocytes. Also the serum may contain cytotoxic constituents. Sometimes serum may interfere with downstream processing.

(b) Serum-free media

Considering the disadvantages due to serum, extensive investigations have been made to develop serum-free formulations of culture media. These efforts were mainly based on analytical approach based on the analysis of serum constituents, synthetic approach to supplement basal media by various combinations of growth factors and the limiting-factor approach consisting of lowering the serum level in the medium till growth stops and then supplementing the medium with vitamins, amino acids, hormones, etc., till growth resumes.

Serum-free media has the advantages such as improved reproducibility of results over time from different laboratories since variation due to batch change of serum is avoided. It made easier downstream processing of products from cultured cells. Bioassays are free from interference due to serum proteins. There is no danger of degradation of sensitive proteins by serum proteases. They permit selective culture of differentiated and reproducing cell types from the heterogeneous cultures. It also has some disadvantages like most of them are specific to one cell type and the growth rate and the maximum cell density attained are lower than those with serum-containing media.

(c) Chemically defined media
These media contain contamination-free ultra-pure inorganic and organic constituents, and may contain pure protein additives like insulin, epidermal growth factors, etc., that have been produced in bacteria or yeast by genetic engineering.

(d) Protein-free media
In contrast to the above, protein-free media do not contain any protein; they only contain non-protein constituents necessary for culture of the cells.

In addition to the basic nutritional requirement of the cells, the medium should also control the pH range of the culture and buffers from abrupt changes. Usually a CO_2-bicarbonate based buffer or an organic buffer, such as HEPES (4-(2-hydroxyethyl)-1-piperazine-ethanesulfonic acid) is a zwitterionic organic chemical buffering agent and is used to help, keep the medium pH in a range from 7.0 to 7.4 depending on the type of cell being cultured. When using a CO_2-bicarbonate buffer, it is necessary to regulate the amount of CO_2 dissolved in the medium. This is usually done using an incubator with CO_2 controls set to provide an atmosphere with between 2% and 10% CO_2 (for Earle's salts-based buffers). However, some media use a CO_2-bicarbonate buffer (for Hanks' salts-based buffers) that requires no additional CO_2, but it must be used in a sealed vessel (not dishes or plates). Finally, the osmolality (osmotic pressure) of the culture medium is important since it helps to regulate the flow of substances in and out of the cell. It is controlled by the addition or subtraction of salt in the culture medium. Evaporation of culture media from open culture vessels will rapidly increase the osmolality of the medium which affects the cell attachment. Appropriate medium and incubator that maintains the correct pH and osmolality is necessary to maintain proper growth rate.

The viability of cells can be observed visually using an inverted phase contrast microscope. Live cells are phase bright; suspension cells are typically rounded and somewhat symmetrical; adherent cells will form projections when they attach to the growth surface. Viability can also be assessed using the vital dye, trypan blue, which is excluded by live cells but accumulates in dead cells. Cell numbers are determined using a hemocytometer.

Table 11.3: Different commonly used media (with serum), for animal cell and tissue culture and their constituents (mg/l)

Components	Eagle's MEM	Dulbecco's modification	Ham's F12	CMRL 1066	RPMI 1640	199	L15	Fischer'	Waymouth MB 752
Amino acids									
L- alanine	-	-	8.90	25.0	-	25.0	225	-	-
L-Arginine (free base)	-	-	-	-	200	-	550	-	-
L-Arginine-HCL	126	84.0	211	70.0	-	70.0	-	15.0	75.0
L-Asparagine	-	-	-	-	50.0	-	-	-	-
L-Asparagine-H20	-	15.0	-	-	-	260	11.4	-	
L- aspartic acid	-	13.3	30.0	20.0	30.0	-	-	60.0	
L-Cysteine (free base)	-	-	-	-	-	-	120	-	61.0
L-Cysteine	24	48.0	-	20.0	50.0	-	-	-	15.0
L-Cysteine.2Na	-	-	-	-	-	23.7	-	23.7	-
L-Cysteine. HCL. H_2O	-	-	35.1	260	-	0.09	-	-	-

Pyridoxal. HCL	1.00	4.00	0.062	0.025	-	0.02	-	0.50	-
Riboflavin	0.10	0.40	0.038	0.010	0.20	0.01	-	0.50	1.00
Thiamin. HCL	1.00	4.00	0.34	0.010	1.00	0.100	-	1.00	10.0
Vitamin B12	-	-	1.36	-	0.005	-	-	-	0.20
Pyridoxine HCL	-	-	0.062	0.025	1.00	0.02	-	-	1.00
Cholesterol	-	-	-	0.200	-	-	-	-	-
Para-amino ben-zoic acid	-	-	-	0.050	1.00	0.50	-	-	-
Nicotinic acid	-	-	-	-	-	0.025	-	-	-
Menaphthone sodium bissul-phite 3 H20	-	-	-	-	-	0.019	-	-	-
DI-A tocopherol PO4. 2Na	-	-	-	-	-	0.10	-	-	-
Vitamin A ace-tate	-	-	-	-	-	0.115	-	-	-
Riboflavin	-	-	-	-	-	-	0.10	-	-
PO4.2Na Thiamin mono PO4, 2H20	-	-	-	-	-	-	1.00	-	-
Inorganic salts									
CaCl2 (anhyd.)	200	200	-	200	-	-	-	-	-
CaCl2. 2H20	-	-	44.0	-	-	186	186	91.0	120
Fe (NO3)3. 9H20	-	0.10	-	-	-	0.10	-	-	-
KCL	400	400	224	400	400	400	400	400	150
KH2PO4	-	-	-	-	-	60.0	60.0	-	80.0
MgCl2. 6H20	-	-	122	-	-	-	-	-	240
MgSO4. 7H20	200	200	-	200	100	200	400	121	200
NaCL	6,800	6,400	7,599	6, 799	6,000	8.000	8,000	8,000	6,000

L- Hydroxyproline	-	-	-	10.0	20.0	10.0	-	-	-
L- isoleucine	52.0	105	3.94	20.0	50.0	20.0	125	75.0	25.0
L- leucine	52.0	105	13.1	60.0	50.0	60.0	125	30.0	50.0
L- lysine.HCL	73.1	146	36.5	70.0	40.0	70.0	93	50.0	240
L- methionine	15.0	30.0	4.48	15.0	15.0	15.0	75.0	100	50.0
L- phenylalanine	33.0	66.0	4.96	25.0	15.0	25.0	125	67.0	50.0
L- proline	-	-	34.5	40.0	20.0	40.0	-	-	50.0
L- serine	-	42.0	10.5	25.0	30.0	25.0	200	15.0	-
L-threonine	48.0	95.0	11.9	30.0	20.0	30.0	300	40.0	75.0
L-tryptophan	10.0	16.0	2.04	10.0	5.0	10.0	20.0	10.0	40.0
L-tyrosine	36.0	72.0	5.40	40.0	20.0	-	-	-	40.0
L-tyrosine. 2Na	-	-	-	-	-	49.7	373	74.6	-
L-valine	47.0	94.0	11.7	25.0	20.0	25.0	100	70.0	65.0
Vitamins									
L-ascorbic acid	-	-	-	50.0	-	0.05	-	-	17.5
Biotin	-	-	0.0073	0.010	0.200	0.01	-	0.010	0.02
D-Ca-pantothenate Calciferol	1.00	4.00	0.480	0.010	0.250	0.10	1.00	0.500	1.00
Calciferol	-	-	-	-	-	0.10	-	-	-
Choline chloride	1.00	4.00	14.0	0.500	3.00	0.50	1.00	1.50	250
Folic acid	1.00	4.00	1.30	0.010	1.00	0.01	1.00	10.0	0.40
i-inositol	2.00	7.20	18.0	0.050	35.0	0.05	2.00	1.50	1.00
Nicotinamide	1.00	4.00	0.04	0.025	1.00	0.02	1.00	0.50	1.00

NaHCO3	2.200	3,700	1,176	2,200	2,200	350	-	1,125	2,240
Na2H2PO4.H20	140	125	-	140	-	-	-	78.0	-
Na2HPO4 (anhyd)	-	-	-	-	-	47.5	190	60.0	-
Na2HPO4. 7H20	-	-	268	-	1,512	-	-	-	566
CuSO4. 5H20	-	-	0,0024	-	-	-	-	-	-
FeSO4. 7H20	-	-	0.834	-	-	-	-	-	-
ZnSO4. 7H20	-	-	0.836	-	-	-	-	-	-
CaNO3. 4H20	-	-	-	-	100	-	-	-	-
Other compounds									
D-glucose	1,000	4,500	1,802	1,000	2,000	1,000	-	1,000	5,000
D-galactose	-	-	-	-	-	-	9,000	-	-
Lipoic acid	-	-	0.21	-	-	-	-	-	-
Phenol red									
Sodium pyru-vate	-	110	110	-	-	-	550	-	-
Hypoxanthine	-	-	4.10	-	-	0.30	-	-	-
Linoleic acid	-	0.084	-	-	-	-	-	-	25.0
Putrescine 2HCL	-	-	0.161	-	-	-	-	-	-
Thymidine	-	-	0.73	10.0	-	-	-	-	-
Cocarboxylase	-	-	-	1.00	-	-	-	-	-
Coenzyme A	-	-	-	2.50	-	-	-	-	-
Dexyadenosine	-	-	-	10.0	-	-	-	-	-
Deoxycytidine. HCL	-	-	-	10.0	-	-	-	-	-
Deoxyguanosine	-	-	-	10.0	-	-	-	-	-
Diphosphopyri-dine nucleotide	-	-	-	10.0	-	-	-	-	-

11.2.5. Type of Cultures

Cell culture is defined as the technique in which tissue or outgrowth from an explant is dispersed, most enzymatically, into a cell suspension, which may then be cultured as a monolayer or suspension culture. Some normal functions may be maintained but the original organization of tissue is lost. Cell cultures may contain the following three types of cells.

1. Stem cells

2. Precursor cells

3. Differentiated cells

Stem cells are undifferentiated cells, which can differentiate under correct inducing conditions into one of sever kinds of cells. Different kinds of stem cells differ markedly in terms of the kinds of cells they will differentiate into. Precursor cells are derived from stem cells and are committed to differentiation. These cells retain the capacity for proliferation. In contrast, differentiated cells usually do not have the capacity to divide. Some cell cultures like epidermal keratinocyte cultures contain all the three types of cells. In such cell cultures, stem cells constantly provide new cells, which develop into precursors; the precursor cells proliferate and mature into the differentiated cell types. Thus stem cells are necessary for the maintenance of such cultures, which by nature are heterogeneous. On the other hand fibroblast cultures contain a more or less uniform population of dividing cells at low cell densities ($<10^4$ cells/cm^2), but at high cell densities (10^5 cells/cm^2) are uniformly composed of non-proliferating differentiated cells. The cells begin to proliferate once the cell density is approximately reduced.

Differentiation and cell proliferation are affected not only by cell density but also by factors like serum, Ca^{2+} ions, hormones, cell-to-cell and cell-to-matrix interactions, etc. Generally cell proliferation is promoted by low cell density, low Ca^{2+} (100–600µm), and high growth factor levels, while differentiation is promoted by the exact opposite conditions and by the presence of differentiation-inducing factors, e.g. cortisone nerve growth factor, etc. The proportion of stem, precursor and differentiated cells are markedly affected by the source tissue used for obtaining the cultures. For example, cultures derived from embryos and those derived from even adult tissues where continuous cell renewal occurs naturally (intestinal epithelium, haemopoietic cells, etc.), stem cells are likely to be more frequent than in other cell cultures. In contrast, cell cultures from tissues where renewal occurs only under stress, e.g. fibroblasts, muscle, etc., may contain only precursor cells.

Cell cultures can be grown as monolayers (adherent cell lines) or as suspension cultures (non-adherent cell lines). Propagation in suspension cultures is limited to haemopoietic cell lines, ascites, tumours and transformed cells (those cells that have become phenotypically modified during *in vitro* culture to become anchorage-independent and are able to grow in layers of several cells thick, as against monolayer growth of non-transformed cells). Therefore cells in culture need a surface or substrate to adhere to so that they are able to proliferate. Cells that are unable to adhere to a substrate are unable to divide, i.e., their growth is anchorage-dependent.

Cells of both adherent and non-adherent types may be i) primary cell lines, ii) immortal cell lines or iii) transformed cell lines. Primary cell cultures are established by inoculating growth medium with cells taken from animal tissue. The excised tissue is fragmented into small pieces with forceps and scissors. Then it is placed in sterile medium in a petri dish. The excised fragment is then treated with proteolytic enzymes such as trypsin to desegregate the tissue into individual cells. Such a culture may contain variety of differentiated cell types. In case of connective tissue, fibroblasts start growing within 7 days. Fibroblasts outgrow other cell types. Careful control of medium composition allows selective growth of certain cell types. Subculture of primary culture leads to secondary and tertiary cultures. Primary cell lines have limited lifespan and are also called finite cell cultures. Cells from primary cultures multiply at a constant rate over successive transfers and such cells comprise a cell strain. Human cells generally divide only 50-100 times before dying. The natural aging of cells can be arrested by storage in liquid nitrogen. Immortal cell lines are capable of unlimited growth in culture and they do not die. They are altered to produce a continuous cell line from cells of primary culture. They are not necessarily malignant cells.

To be able to clone individual cells, modify cell behavior, or select mutants, biologists often want to maintain cell cultures for many more than 100 doublings. This is possible with cells derived from some tumors and with rare cells that arise spontaneously because they have undergone genetic changes that endow them with the ability to grow indefinitely. The genetic changes that allow these cells to grow indefinitely are collectively called oncogenic transformation, and the cells are said to be oncogenically transformed, or simply transformed. A culture of cells with an indefinite life span is considered immortal; such a culture is called a cell line to distinguish it from an impermanent cell strain.

The ability of cultured cells to grow indefinitely or their tendency to be transformed varies depending on the animal species from which the cells originate. Normal chicken cells rarely are transformed and die out after only a few doublings; even tumor cells from chickens almost never exhibit immortality. Among human cells, only tumor cells grow indefinitely. The HeLa cell, the first human cell type to be grown in culture, was originally obtained in 1952 from a malignant tumor (carcinoma) of the uterine cervix. This cell line has been invaluable for research on human cells. During repeated serial transfer, cell lines can undergo extensive changes in their cultural properties; such cells may grow in clumps rather than in a monolayer, and cells may also be irregularly oriented with respect to each other.

Such cells are said to be transformed and are generally neoplastic. Transformed cell lines are either cells derived from tumour cells or cells manipulated by transfection with oncogenes, or obtained by treatment with carcinogens to produce cells with novel phenotype. These cell lines are quite robust. They have low doubling time and low requirement for growth factors. Although transformed cells are much easier to grow in culture, there is some reluctance to use them for large-scale production of biologicals. The concern is due to fear of contamination of products with tumorigenic agents.

11.2.6. Hybridoma Technology

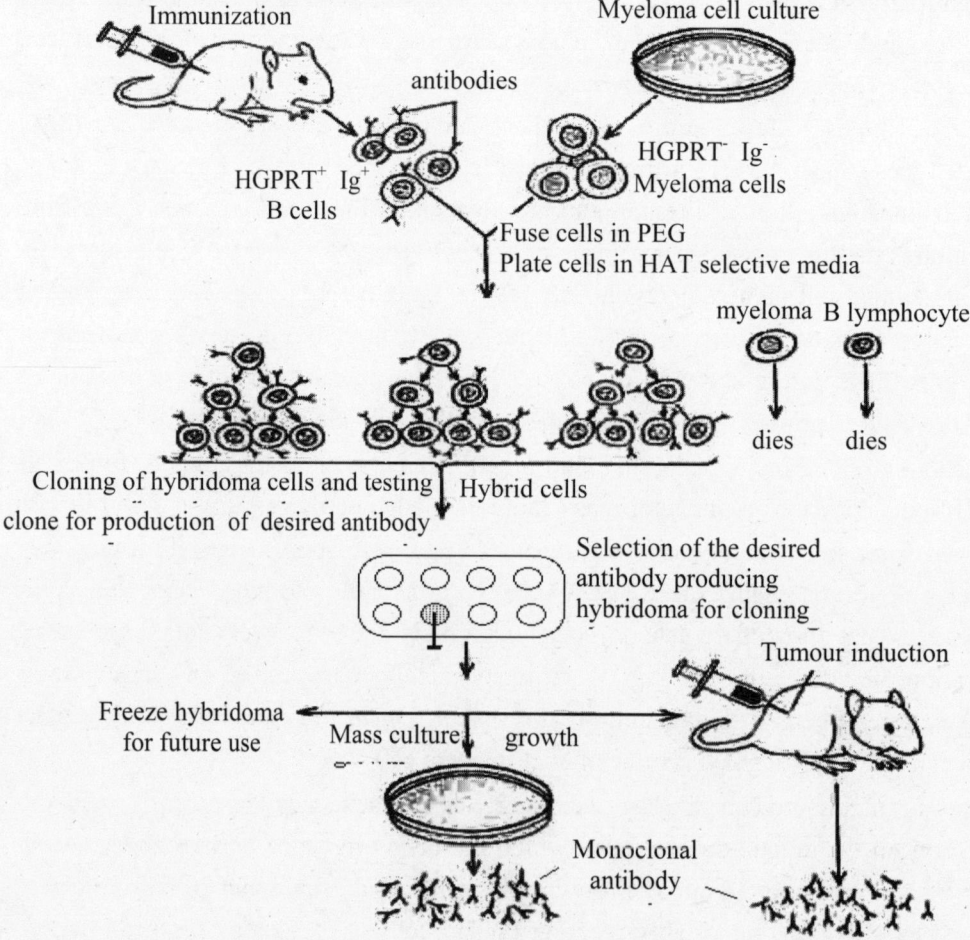

Figure 11.5: Hybridoma technology: production of monoclonal antibodies

Antibodies are proteins produced by the B lymphocytes of the immune system in response to foreign proteins, called antigens. Antibodies function as markers, binding to the antigen so that the antigen molecules can be recognized and destroyed by phagocytes. The part of the antigen that the antibody binds to is called the epitope. The epitope is thus a short amino acid sequence that enable the antibody to recognize. Two features of the antibody-epitope relationship of monoclonal antibodies such as specificity, the antibody binds only to its particular epitope and sufficiency, the epitope can bind to the antibody on its own, i.e. the presence of the whole antigen molecule is not necessary make it as a molecular tool.

In 1975 Cesar Milstein, Georges Kohler and Niels Jeme developed monoclonal antibody technology by fusing immortal tumor cells (myeloma cells) with antibody-producing B lymphocyte cells to produce "hybridomas," that continuously synthesize identical (or "monoclonal") antibodies. Milstein, Kohler and Jeme were awarded the 1984 Nobel Prize in Medicine.

For isolation of B lymphocyte producing a certain antibody, we first have to induce the production of such a B cell in an organism. This is typically done in two doses, an initial "priming" dose and a second "booster" dose, 10 days later. Since the protein is of foreign origin, the mouse immune system recognizes it as such and soon some of the B cells in the mouse would begin production of the antibody against antigen. A sample of B cells is extracted from the spleen of the mouse and added to a culture of myeloma cells (cancer cells). The intended result is the formation of hybridomas, cells formed by the fusion of a B cell and a myeloma cell. The fusion is done by using polyethylene glycol, a virus or by electroporation.

The next step is to select for the hybridomas. The myeloma cells are HGPRT- and the B cells are HGPRT+. HGPRT is hypoxanthine-guanine phosphoribosyl transferase, an enzyme involved in the synthesis of nucleotides from hypoxanthine, an amino acid. The culture is grown in HAT (hypoxanthine-aminopterin-thymine) medium, which can sustain only HGPRT+ cells. The myeloma cells that fuse with another myeloma cell or do not fuse at all die in the HAT medium since they are HGPRT-. The B cells that fuse with another B cell or do not fuse at all die because they do not have the capacity to divide indefinitely. Only hybridomas between B cells and myeloma cells survive, being both HGPRT+ and cancerous. The initial collection of B cells used is heterogenous, i.e. they do not all produce the same antibody. Therefore the hybridoma population too does not produce a single antibody. There is also another complication. A hybridoma cell is initially tetraploid, having been formed by the fusion of two diploid cells. However the extra chromosomes are somehow lost in subsequent divisions in a random manner. This means that we cannot be certain that the hybridomas will all produce the desired antibody or even any antibody at all. Screening is required to decide which hybridoma cells are actually producing the desired antibody (Fig. 11.5).

Each hybridoma is cultured and screened after doing SDS-PAGE (sodium dodecyl sulfate - polyacrylamide gel electrophoresis) and Western blots. The probe used is the epitope of the antibody that is desired, which may be labeled by radioactivity or immunofluorescence. Once it is sure that a certain hybridoma is producing the right antibody, it can be indefinitely cultured and monoclonal antibodies can be harvested from it. The resulting hybridomas can produce large quantities of the desired antibody. These antibodies, called monoclonal antibodies due to their purity, have many important clinical, diagnostic, and industrial applications with a yearly value of well over a billion dollars.

11.2.7. Application of Animal Cell Culture

Cell culture has become one of the major tools used in cell and molecular biology. Some of the important areas where cell culture is currently playing a major role for studying basic cell biology and biochemistry, the interactions between disease-causing agents and cells, the effects of drugs on cells, the process and triggers for aging, and nutritional studies. A variety of areas of research in biotechnology depend largely on tissue culture and, therefore, these areas have given the desired impetus to the development of tissue culture methods in animals. These areas include the following: (i) production of antiviral vaccines, which required the standardization of cell lines for the multiplication and assay of viruses; (ii) cancer research, which required the study of uncontrolled cell division in cultures; (iii) cell fusion techniques; (iv) genetic manipulation, which is possible in cells or organs in culture; (v) monoclonal antibodies whose production, requires cell lines in culture; (vi) production of pharmaceutical drugs using cell lines; (vii) chromosome analysis of cells derived from womb; (viii) study of the effects of toxins and pollutants using cell lines; (ix) use of artificial skin; (x) study of the function of nerve cells (even though neurons can not be propagated *in vitro,* without resorting to the use of transformed cells). The major research fields in which cell lines find applications include

(a) Toxicity Testing: Cultured cells are widely used alone or in conjunction with animal tests to study the effects of new drugs, cosmetics and chemicals on survival and growth in a wide variety of cell types. Especially important are liver- and kidney-derived cell cultures.

(b) Cancer Research: Since both normal cells and cancer cells can be grown in culture, the basic differences between them can be closely studied. In addition, it is possible, by the use of chemicals, viruses and radiation, to convert normal cultured cells to cancer causing cells. Thus, the mechanisms that cause the change can be studied.

(c) Virology: One of the earliest and major uses of cell culture is the replication of viruses in cell cultures (in place of animals) for use in vaccine production. Cell cultures are also widely used in the clinical detection and isolation of viruses, as well as basic research into how they grow and infect organisms.

(d) Cell-Based Manufacturing: While cultured cells can be used to produce many important products, three areas are generating the most interest. The first is the large-scale production of viruses for use in vaccine production. These include vaccines for polio, rabies, chicken pox, hepatitis B and measles, the large-scale production of cells that have been genetically engineered to produce proteins that have medicinal or commercial value. These include monoclonal antibodies, insulin, hormones, etc. and the use of cells as replacement tissues and organs. Artificial skin for use in treating burns and ulcers is the first commercially available product. A potential supply of replacement cells and tissues may come out of work currently being done with both embryonic and adult stem cells. These are cells that have the potential to differentiate into a variety of different cell types and it may offer new treatment approaches for a wide variety of medical conditions.

(e) Genetic Counseling: Amniocentesis, a diagnostic technique that enables doctors to remove and culture fetal cells from pregnant women, an important tool for the early diagnosis of fetal disorders. These cells can then be examined for abnormalities in their chromosomes and genes using karyotyping, chromosome painting and other molecular techniques.

(f) Genetic Engineering: The ability to transfect or reprogram cultured cells with new genetic material (DNA and genes) has provided a major tool to molecular biologists wishing to study the cellular effects of the expression of theses genes (new proteins). These techniques can also be used to produce these new proteins in large quantity in cultured cells for further study.

(g) Gene Therapy: The ability to genetically engineer cells has also led to their use for gene therapy. Cells can be removed from a patient lacking a functional gene and the missing or damaged gene can then be replaced. The cells can be grown for a while in culture and then replaced into the patient. An alternative approach is to place the missing gene into a viral vector and then "infect" the patient with the virus in the hope that the missing gene will then be expressed in the patient's cells.

(h) Drug Screening and Development: Cell-based assays have become increasingly important for the pharmaceutical industry, not just for cytotoxicity testing but also for high throughput screening of compounds that may have potential use as drugs.

Suggested Readings

- Gene Cloning and DNA analysis- an Introduction by T. A. Brown (2006). Blackwell Science
- Molecular Biotechnology-Principles & applications of recombinant DNA by Glick and Pasternak (2009), ASM press.
- Principles of Gene Manipulation by Old & Primose. (2002). Blackwell Scientific Publication

- Culture of Animal Cells- A manual of Basic Technique, 5th Ed., 2005, R. Ian Freshney, John Wiley & Sons
- Plant Tissue Culture: Theory & Practice by S.S. Bhojwani & M.K. Razdan (1996), Elsevier Science
- Culture of Animal Cells, A Manual of Basic Technique (1994) R. Ian Freshney, 3rd edition, Alan R. Liss, Inc., New York.
- Methods in Enzymology: Cell Culture, Vol. 58, (1979) W. B. Jacoby and I. H. Pasten, eds. Academic Press, New York.
- Cell and Tissue Culture (1975) John Paul, 5th edition, Churchill Livingstone, Edinburgh.

CHAPTER 12

Basic Immunology

- The Organs of the Immune System
- Bone marrow
- Thymus
- Spleen
- Lymph Nodes
- Fluid Systems of the Body
- The Blood System
- The Lymph Systems
- The Cells of the Immune System
- The Immune Response
- Immunoglobulin Classes
- Acute Phase Reactants

- Cytokines
- Regulation of Humoral Response
- Passive Immunity
- Complement system
- Major Histocompatibility Complex
- Structure of the T cell Receptor (TCR)
- Toll like Receptors and innate immunity
- Antigens
- Mitogens
- Immunomodulating Substances
- Vaccines

The immune system is a highly sensitive, responsive and adaptive versatile defence system that has evolved to protect animals from invading pathogenic microorganisms and cancer. It is able to generate an enormous variety of cells and molecules capable of specifically recognizing and eliminating an apparently limitless variety of foreign invaders. It protects us against billions of bacteria, viruses, and other parasites. Functionally, an immune response can be divided into two related activities—recognition and response. Immune recognition is remarkable for its specificity. It is able to recognize subtle chemical differences that distinguish one foreign pathogen from another and even discriminate between foreign molecules and the body's own cells and proteins. Once a foreign organism has been recognized, the immune system recruits a variety of cells and molecules to mount an appropriate response, called as an effector response, that eliminates or neutralizes the foreign organism. Thus system becomes able to convert the initial recognition event into a variety of effector responses, each uniquely suited for eliminating a particular type of pathogen. Subsequent exposure to the same foreign organism induces a memory response, characterized by a more rapid and heightened immune reaction that serves to eliminate the pathogen and prevents the disease.

The immune system is composed of many interdependent cell types that interplay to protect the body from bacterial, parasitic, fungal, viral infections and from the growth of tumor cells (Fig. 12.1). Many of these cell types have specialized functions. The cells of the immune system can engulf bacteria, kill parasites or tumor cells, or kill viral-infected cells. Often, these cells depend on the T helper subset for activation signals in the form of secretions formally known as cytokines, lymphokines, or more specifically interleukins.

12.1 The Organs of the Immune System

The thymus and bone marrow are the primary (or central) lymphoid organs, where maturation of lymphocytes takes place. The lymph nodes, spleen, and various mucosal associated lymphoid tissues (MALT) such as gut-associated lymphoid tissue (GALT) are the secondary (or peripheral) lymphoid organs, which trap antigen and provide sites for mature lymphocytes to interact with that antigen. In addition, tertiary lymphoid tissues, which normally contain fewer lymphoid cells than secondary lymphoid organs, can import lymphoid cells during an inflammatory response (Fig. 12.1).

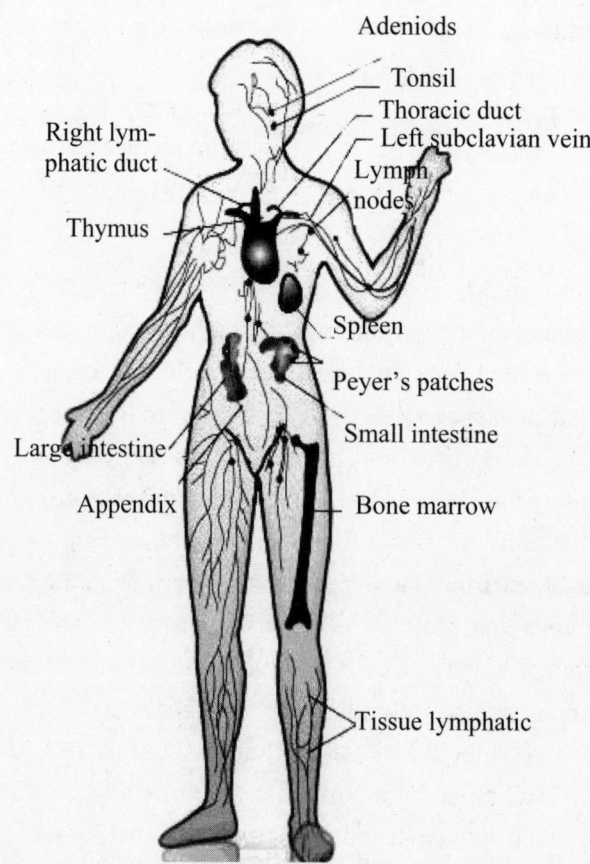

Figure 12.1: Anatomy of the Immunological System: The major components of the immunological system are lymph nodes connected by lymph ducts, Peyer's patches (masses of lymphocytes in the lower gastrointestinal tract), thymus, spleen, and bone marrow

12.1.1 Bone Marrow

The cells of the immune system are basically derived from the bone marrow through a process called hematopoiesis. During this process, the bone marrow-derived stem cells differentiate into either mature cells of the immune system or into precursor cells that migrate out of the bone marrow to continue their maturation elsewhere like thymus, spleen or lymphatic tissues. The bone marrow produces B cells, natural killer cells, granulocytes and immature thymocytes, in addition to red blood cells and platelets.

12.1.2. Thymus

Thymus is the site of maturation of T cells. Immature thymocytes (prothymocytes) leave the bone marrow and migrate into the thymus, there they under go remarkable maturation process, referred to as thymic education and are then released into the bloodstream. It is a flat, bilobed organ situated above the heart. Each lobe is surrounded by a capsule and is divided into lobules, which are separated from each other by strands of connective tissue called trabeculae. Each lobule is organized into two compartments: the outer compartment, or cortex, is densely packed with immature T cells, called thymocytes, whereas the inner compartment, or medulla, is sparsely populated with thymocytes (Fig. 12.2). The function of the thymus is to generate and select a repertoire of T cells that will protect the body from infection. As thymocytes develop, an enormous diversity of T-cell receptors is generated by a random process that produces some T cells with receptors capable of recognizing antigen-MHC complexes.

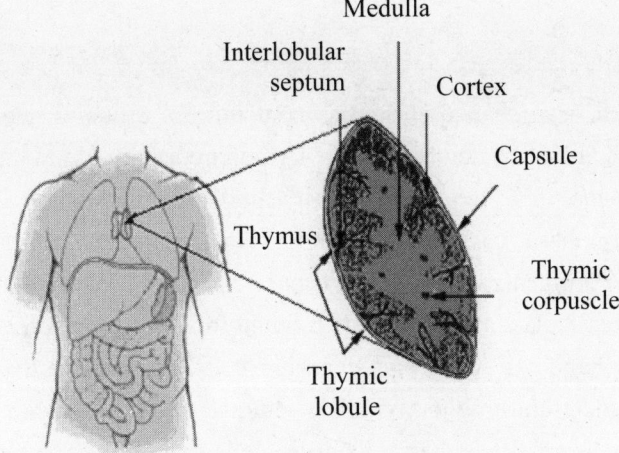

Figure 12.2: Thymus

12.1.3. Spleen

The spleen is an immunologic filter of the blood. It is a reserve of B cells, T cells, macrophages, dendritic cells, natural killer cells and red blood cells. It is a large, ovoid secondary lymphoid organ situated high in the left abdominal cavity. While lymph nodes are specialized for trapping antigen from local tissues, the spleen specializes in filtering blood and trapping blood-borne antigens; thus, it can respond to systemic infections. Unlike the lymph nodes, the spleen is not supplied by lymphatic vessels. Instead, blood borne antigens and lymphocytes are carried into the spleen through the splenic artery. In addition to capturing foreign materials (antigens) from the blood that passes through the spleen, migratory macrophages and dendritic cells bring antigens to the spleen via the bloodstream. An immune response is initiated when the macrophage or dendritic cells present the antigen to the appropriate B or T cells. In the spleen, B cells become activated and produce large amounts of antibody. Also, old red blood cells are destroyed in the spleen (Fig. 12.3).

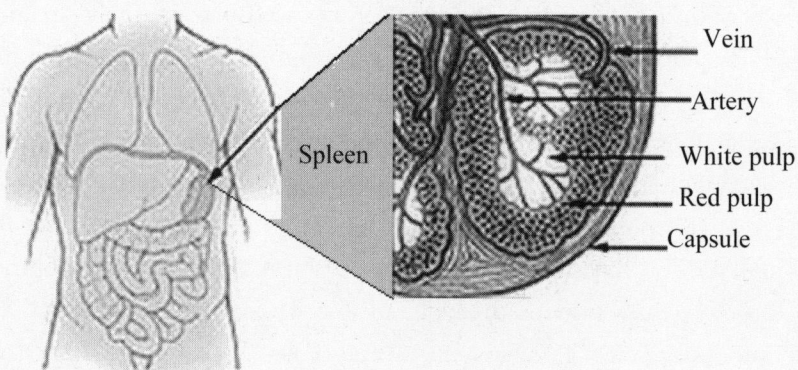

Figure 12.3: Spleen

12.1.4. Lymph Nodes

They are encapsulated bean shaped structures containing a reticular network packed with lymphocytes, macrophages, and dendritic cells. Lymph nodes are found throughout the body and serves as an immunologic filter for the bodily fluid known as lymph. They are clustered at junctions of the lymphatic vessels; lymph nodes are the first organized lymphoid structures which encounter antigens that enter the tissue spaces (Fig. 12.4). As lymph percolates through a node, any particulate antigen that is brought in with the lymph gets trapped by the cellular network of phagocytic cells and dendritic cells. Antigens are filtered out of the lymph in the lymph node returning the lymph is returned to the circulation in a similar fashion as the spleen, the macrophages and dendritic cells that capture antigens present these foreign materials to T and B cells, consequently initiating an immune response. As antigen is carried to a regional node by the lymph, it is trapped, processed, and presented together with class II MHC molecules by interdigitating dendritic cells in the paracortex, resulting in the activation of T_H cells.

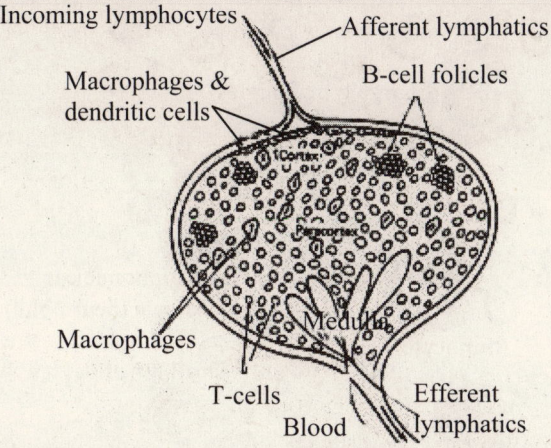

Figure 12.4: A lymph node. Afferent lymph ducts bring lymph-containing antigens into the lymph node. Macrophages, dendritic cells and B-cells in the cortical region make contact with the antigen and process it for presentation to immunocompetent B-cells and T- cells, thereby initiating an immune response

12.2. Fluid Systems of the Body

There are two main dynamic fluid systems exist in the body namely blood and lymph. The blood and lymph systems are intertwined throughout the body and they are mainly responsible for transporting the agents of the immune system.

12.2.1. The Blood System

Blood is the major transporter of the body, which flows from the heart into arteries, then to capillaries, and returns to the heart through veins. On an average the body of 70 kg person contains 5 liters of blood, which constitutes about 7% of the total body weight. Blood is composed of 52–62% liquid plasma and 38–48% cells. The plasma is mostly water (91.5%) and acts as a vehicle for transporting other materials (7% protein [consisting of albumins (54%), globulins (38%), fibrinogen (7%), and assorted other remaining stuffs]). Blood is slightly alkaline (pH = 7.40 ± .05) and heavier than water (density = 1.057 ± .009).

Blood cells are derived from hematopoietic stem cells, which are mainly found in the bone marrow, via a process called hematopoiesis. The stem cells produce hemocytoblasts that differentiate into the precursors for all the different types of blood cells (Fig. 12.5). Hemocytoblasts mature into three types of blood cells: erythrocytes (red blood cells or RBCs), leukocytes (white blood cells) and platelets.

The leukocytes are further subdivided into granulocytes (containing large granules in the cytoplasm) and agranulocytes (without granules). The granulocytes are consisted of neutrophils (55–70%), eosinophils (1–3%), and basophils (0.5–1.0%). The agranulocytes are lymphocytes (consisting of B cells and T cells) and monocytes. Lymphocytes circulate in the blood and lymph systems, and make their home in the lymphoid organs.

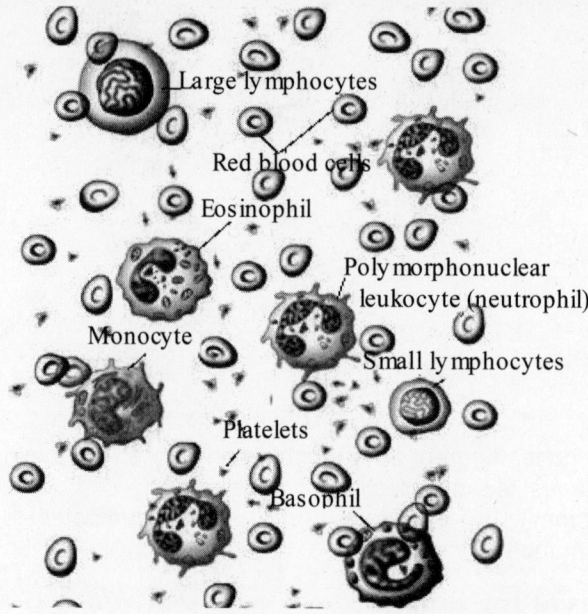

Large lymphocytes

Red blood cells

Eosinophil

Polymorphonuclear
leukocyte (neutrophil)

Monocyte

Small lymphocytes

Platelets

Basophil

Figure 12.5: Major cells in the blood system

There are 5000–10,000 WBCs per mm^3 and biological life is 5–9 days. About 2,400,000 RBCs are produced each second and each of them of them lives for about 120 days (They migrate to the spleen to die. Once there, that organ scavenges usable proteins from their carcasses). A healthy male has about 5 million RBCs per mm^3, whereas females have a bit fewer than 5 million.

12.2.2. The Lymph System

Lymph is an alkaline (pH > 7.0) fluid that is usually clear, transparent, and colorless. It flows in the lymphatic vessels and bathes tissues and organs in its protective covering. There are no RBCs in lymph and it has relatively lower protein content than blood. Like blood, it is slightly heavier than water (density = 1.019 ± .003).

The lymph flows from the interstitial fluid through lymphatic vessels up to either the thoracic duct or right lymph duct, which terminates in the subclavian veins, where lymph is mixed with the blood. (The right lymph duct drains the right sides of the thorax, neck, and head, whereas the thoracic duct drains the rest of the body.) Lymph carries lipids and lipid-soluble vitamins absorbed from the gastrointestinal (GI) tract. Since there is no active pump in the lymph system, there is no back-pressure produced. The lymphatic vessels, like veins, have one-way valves that prevent backflow. Additionally, along these vessels there are small bean-shaped lymph nodes which serve as filters of the lymphatic fluid. It is in the lymph nodes where antigen is usually presented to the immune system.

The human lymphoid system consists of the followings:

- Primary organs: bone marrow (in the hollow center of bones) and the thymus gland (located behind the breastbone above the heart), and

- Secondary organs at or near possible portals of entry for pathogens: adenoids, tonsils, spleen (located at the upper left of the abdomen), lymph nodes (along the lymphatic vessels with concentrations in the neck, armpits, abdomen, and groin), Peyer's patches (within the intestines), and the appendix.

Lymphocytes originate in the bone marrow but migrate to the parts of the lymphatic system such as the lymph nodes, spleen, and thymus. There are two main types of lymphatic cells, T cells and B cells. The lymphatic system also involves a transportation system - lymph vessels - for transportation and storage of lymphocyte cells within the body. The lymphatic system feeds cells into the body while filters out dead cells and invading organisms such as bacteria.

12.3. The Cells of the Immune System

T cell–dependent acquired immune responses typically require antigen-presenting cells (APCs) to present Ag-derived peptides within major histocompatibility complex (MHC) molecules though some antigens can stimulate the immune response directly. Intracellular Ag (e.g., viruses) can be processed and presented to $CD8^+$ cytotoxic T cells by any nucleated cell because all nucleated cells express class I MHC molecules. However, extracellular antigen must be processed into peptides and complexed with surface class II MHC molecules present on professional APCs to be recognized by $CD4^+$ helper T (T_H) cells.

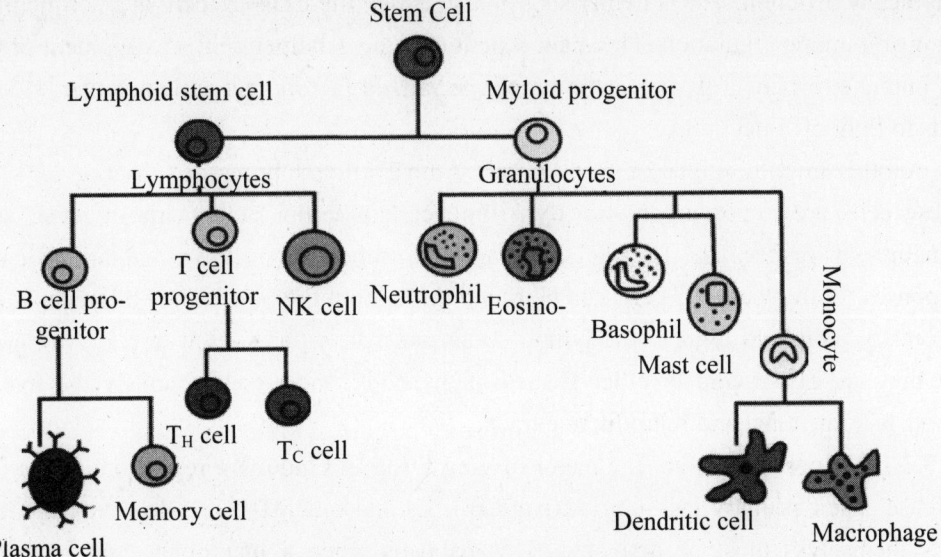

Figure 12.6: Cell of the immune system

12.3.1. Monocytes in the circulation are precursors to tissue macrophages. During hemato-poiesis in the bone marrow, granulocyte-monocyte progenitor cells differentiate into promonocytes, which leave the bone marrow and enter the blood, where they further differ-entiate into mature monocytes. Monocytes migrate into tissues, where over about 8 h, they develop into macrophages under the influence of macrophage colony-stimulating factor (M-CSF), secreted by various cell types (e.g., endothelial cells, fibroblasts). At infection sites, activated T cells secrete cytokines (e.g., interferon-γ [IFN-γ]) that induce production of macrophage migration inhibitory factor, preventing macrophages migration (Fig. 12.7).

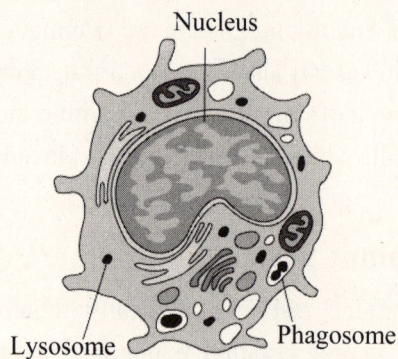

Figure 12.7: Monocyte

12.3.2. T-Cells

T cells got the name from its organ of maturation thymus, an organ situated under the breast bone. T cells are produced in the bone marrow and later move to the thymus where they ma-ture. T lymphocytes are usually divided into two major subsets that are functionally and phe-notypically different. The T helper subset, also called the CD4+ T cell, is a pertinent coordi-nator of immune regulation. The main function of the T helper cell is to augment or potenti-ate immune responses by the secretion of specialized factors that activate other white blood cells to fight off infection.

Another important type of T cell is called the T killer/suppressor subset or CD8+ T cell. These cells are important in directly killing certain tumor cells, viral-infected cells and sometimes parasites. The CD8+ T cells are also important in down-regulation of immune responses. Both types of T cells can be found throughout the body. They often depend on the secondary lymphoid organs (the lymph nodes and spleen) as sites where activation occurs, but they are also found in other tissues of the body, most conspicuously the liver, lung, blood, and intestinal and reproductive tracts.

12.3.2.1. Helper T cells are the major driving force and the main regulators of the immune defense. Their primary task is to activate B cells and killer T cells. However, the helper T cells themselves must be activated. This happens when a macrophage or dendritic cell, which has uptaken an invader, travels to the nearest lymph node to present information about the captured pathogen. The phagocyte displays an antigen fragment from the invader on its own surface, a process called antigen presentation. When the receptor of a helper T cell recognizes the antigen, the T cell is activated. Once activated, helper T cells start to divide and to produce proteins that activate B and T cells as well as other immune cells.

12.3.2.2. The killer T cell is specialized in attacking cells of the body infected by viruses and sometimes also by bacteria. It can also attack cancer cells. The killer T cell has receptors that are used to search each cell that it meets. If a cell is infected, it is swiftly killed. Infected cells are recognized because tiny traces of the intruder, antigen, can be found on their surface.

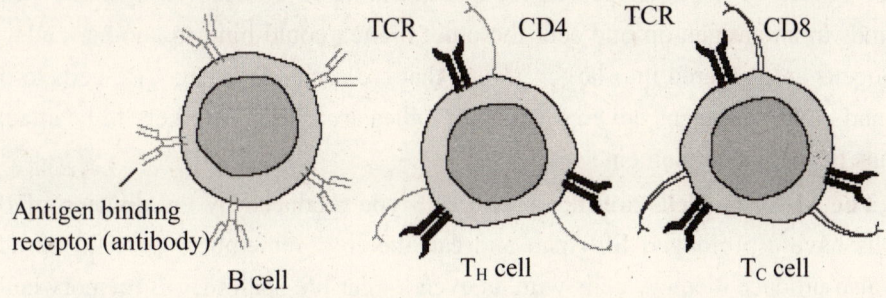

Figure 12.8: Different lymphocytic cells. (a) B cells have about 105 molecules of membrane-bound antibody per cell. (b) T cells bearing CD4 (CD4+ cells) recognize only antigen bound to class II MHC molecules. (c) T cells bearing CD8 (CD8+ cells) recognize only antigen associated with class I MHC molecules

12.3.2.3. Natural Killer Cells

Natural killer cells, often referred to as NK cells, are similar to the killer T cell subset (CD8+ T cells). They function as effector cells that directly kill certain tumors such as melanomas, lymphomas and viral-infected cells, most notably herpes and cytomegalovirus-infected cells. NK cells, unlike the CD8+ (killer) T cells, kill their targets without a prior "conference" in the lymphoid organs. However, NK cells that have been activated by secretions from CD4+ T cells will kill their tumor or viral-infected targets more effectively.

12.3.3. B Cells

The major function of B lymphocytes is the production of antibodies in response to foreign proteins of bacteria, viruses, and tumor cells. Antibodies are specialized proteins that specifically recognize and bind to antigen. Antibody production and binding to a foreign substance or antigen, often is critical as a means of signaling other cells to engulf, kill or remove that substance from the body. The B lymphocyte cell searches for antigen matching its receptors. If it finds such antigen it connects to it, and inside the B cell a triggering signal is set off.

The B cell now needs proteins produced by helper T cells to become fully activated. When this happens, the B cell starts to divide to produce clones of it. During this process, two new cell types are created, plasma cells and B memory cells.

12.3.3.1. The plasma cell is specialized in producing a specific protein, called an antibody that will respond to the same antigen that matched the B cell receptor. Antibodies are released from the plasma cell so that they can seek out intruders and help destroy them. Plasma cells produce antibodies at an amazing rate and can release tens of thousands of antibodies per second. When the Y-shaped antibody finds a matching antigen, it attaches to it. The attached antibodies serve as an appetizing coating for eater cells such as the macrophage. Antibodies also neutralize toxins and incapacitate viruses, preventing them from infecting new cells. Each branch of the Y-shaped antibody can bind to a different antigen, so while one branch binds to an antigen on one cell, the other branch could bind to another cell - in this way pathogens are gathered into larger groups that are easier for phagocyte cells to devour. Bacteria and other pathogens covered with antibodies are also more likely to be attacked by the proteins from the complement system.

12.3.3.2. The Memory Cells are the second cell type produced by the division of B cells. These cells have a prolonged life span and can thereby "remember" specific intruders. T cells can also produce memory cells with an even longer life span than B memory cells. The second time an intruder tries to invade the body, B and T memory cells help the immune system to activate much faster. The invaders are wiped out before the infected human feels any symptoms. The body has achieved immunity against the invader.

12.3.4. Granulocytes or Polymorphonuclear (PMN) Leukocytes

Another group of white blood cells is collectively referred to as granulocytes or polymorphonuclear leukocytes (PMNs). Granulocytes are composed of three cell types identified as neutrophils, eosinophils and basophils, based on their staining characteristics with certain dyes. These cells are predominantly important in the removal of bacteria and parasites from the body. They engulf these foreign bodies and degrade them using their powerful enzymes.

12.3.5. Macrophages

Macrophages are important in the regulation of immune responses. They are often referred to as scavengers or antigen-presenting cells (APC) because they pick up and ingest foreign materials and present these antigens to other cells of the immune system such as T cells and B cells. This is one of the important first steps in the initiation of an immune response. Stimulated macrophages exhibit increased levels of phagocytosis and are also secretory.

12.3.6. Dendritic Cells

Another cell type, addressed only recently, is the dendritic cell. Dendritic cells, which also originate in the bone marrow, function as antigen presenting cells (APC). In fact, the dendritic cells are more efficient APCs than macrophages. These cells are usually found in the structural compartment of the lymphoid organs such as the thymus, lymph nodes and spleen. However, they are also found in the bloodstream and other tissues of the body. It is believed that they capture antigen or bring it to the lymphoid organs where an immune response is initiated.

12.3.7. Mast cells are found in different tissues of the body. Mucosal mast cell granules contain tryptase and chondroitin sulfate; connective tissue mast cell granules contain tryptase, chymase, and heparin. By releasing these mediators, mast cells play a key role in generating protective acute inflammatory responses; basophils and mast cells are the source of type I hypersensitivity reactions associated with atopic allergy. Degranulation can be triggered by cross-linking of IgE receptors or by the anaphylatoxin complement fragments C3a and C5a.

Table 12.1: Cells of the immune system

Leukocytes	White blood cells. These are the cells which provide immunity, and they can be subdivided into three classes: lymphocytes, granulocytes and monocytes
Lymphocytes	Small white blood cells which are responsible for much of the work of the immune system. Lymphocytes can be divided into three classes: B cells, T cells and null cells.
Granulocytes	Leukocytes (white blood cells) containing granules in the cytoplasm. Also known as a granular leukocyte. They seem to act as a first line of defense, as they rush towards an infected area and engulf the offending microbes. Granulocytes kill microbes by digesting them with killer enzymes contained in small units called lysosomes.
Antigen-presenting cells	Cells which do not have antigen-specific receptors. Instead, they capture and process antigens, present them to T cell receptors. These cells include macrophages, dentritic cells and B cells.
B cells	Also known as B cell lymphocytes. B cells spend their entire early life in the bone marrow. Upon maturity, they is to travel throughout the blood and lymph looking for antigens with which they can interlock Once a B cell has identified an antigen, it starts replicating itself. These cloned cells mature into antibody-manufacturing plasma cells.
Plasma cells	Specialized B cells which churn out antibodies—more than two thousand per second. Most of these die after four to five days; however, a few survive to become memory cells.
Memory cells	Specialized B cells which confer the body the ability to manufacture more of a particular antibody as needed, in case a particular antigen is ever encountered again.

T cells	Also known as T cell lymphocytes. Unlike B cells, these cells leave the marrow at an early age and travel to the thymus, where they mature. Here they are imprinted with critical information for recognizing "self" and "non-self" substances. Among the sub-classes of T cells are helper T cells and cytotoxic (or killer) T cells.
Helper T cells	These cells travel through the blood and lymph, looking for antigens (such as those captured by antigen-presenting cells). Upon locating an antigen, they notify other cells to assist in combating the invader. This is sometimes done through the use of cytokines (or specifically, lymphokines) which help destroy target cells and stimulate the production of healthy new tissue. Interferon is an example of such a cytokine.
Cytotoxic T cells	Also called cytotoxic T lymphocytes or CTLs.
Dendritic cells	Mostly found in the skin and mucosal epithelium, where they are referred to as Langerhan's cells. Unlike macrophages, dendritic cells can also recognize viral particles as non-self. In addition, they can present antigens via both MHC I and MHC II, and can thus activate both CD8 and CD4 T cells, directly.
Basophils	Similar to mast cells, but distributed throughout the body. Like mast cells, basophils release histamine upon encountering certain antigens, thereby triggering an allergic reaction.
Macrophages	Literally, "large eaters." These are large, long-lived phagocytes which capture foreign cells, digest them and present protein fragments (peptides) from these cells and manifest them on their exterior. In this manner, they present the antigens to the T cells. Macrophages are strategically located in lymphoid tissues, connective tissues and body cavities, where they are likely to encounter antigens. They also act as effector cells in cell-mediated immunity.
Mast cells	Cells concentrated within the respiratory and gastrointestinal tracts, and within the deep layers of the skin. These cells release histamine upon encountering certain antigens, thereby triggering an allergic reaction.
Monocytes	Large, agranular leukocytes with relatively small, eccentric, oval or kidney-shaped nuclei.

12.3.8. Antigen Presenting Cells (APCs)

Induction of the humoral immune response begins with the recognition of antigen. Through a process of clonal selection, specific B-cells are stimulated to proliferate and differentiate. However, this process requires the intervention of specific T-cells that are themselves stimulated to produce lymphokines that are responsible for activation of the antigen-induced B-cells. In other words, B cells recognize antigen via immunoglobulin receptors on their surface but are unable to proliferate and differentiate unless prompted by the action of T-cell lymphokines. In order for the T-cells to become stimulated to release lymphokines, they must also recognize specific antigen. However, while T-cells recognize antigen via their T-cell receptors, they can only do so in the context of the MHC molecules. This "antigen-presentation" is the responsibility of the antigen-presenting cells (APCs).

Several types of cells may serve the APC function. Perhaps the best APC is, in fact, the B-cell itself. When B-cells bind antigen, the antigen becomes internalized, processed and expressed on the surface of the B-cell. Expression occurs within the class II MHC molecule, which can then be recognized by T-helper cells (CD4$^+$).

Other types of antigen-presenting cells include the macrophage and dendritic cells. These cells either actively phagocytose or pinocytose foreign antigens. The antigens are then processed in a manner similar to that observed for the B-cells. Next, specific antigen epitopes are expressed on the macrophage or dendritic cell surface. Again, this expression occurs within the class II MHC molecule, where T-cell recognition occurs. The stimulated T-cells then release lymphokines that act upon "primed" B-cells (B-cells that have already encountered antigen), inducing B-cell proliferation and differentiation.

12.4. The Immune Response

The immune system protects the body from potentially harmful substances by recognizing and responding to antigens. Antigens are molecules (usually proteins) on the surface of cells, viruses, fungi, or bacteria. Non-living substances such as toxins, chemicals, drugs, and foreign particles (such as a splinter) can be antigens. The immune system recognizes and destroys substances that contain these antigens.

An immune response to foreign antigen requires the presence of an antigen-presenting cell (APC), (usually either a macrophage or dendritic cell) in combination with a B cell or T cell. When an APC presents an antigen on its cell surface to a B cell, the B cell is signaled to proliferate and produce antibodies that specifically bind to that antigen. If the antibodies bind to antigens on bacteria or parasites it acts as a signal for pmns or macrophages to engulf (phagocytose) and kill them. Another important function of antibodies is to initiate the "complement destruction cascade." When antibodies bind to cells or bacteria, serum proteins called complement bind to the immobilized antibodies and destroy the bacteria by creating holes in them. Antibodies can also signal natural killer cells and macrophages to kill viral or bacterial-infected cells.

If the APC presents the antigen to T cells, the T cells become activated. Activated T cells proliferate and become secretory in the case of CD4+ T cells, or, if they are CD8+ T cells, they become activated to kill target cells that specifically express the antigen presented by the APC. The production of antibodies and the activity of CD8+ killer T cells are highly regulated by the CD4+ helper T cell subset. The CD4+ T cells provide growth factors or signals to these cells that signal them to proliferate and function more efficiently. This multitude of interleukins or cytokines that are produced and secreted by CD4+ T cells are often crucial to ensure the activation of natural killer cells, macrophages, CD8+ T cells, and PMNs.

12.4.1. Innate Immunity

The term, innate immunity, refers to the basic resistance to disease that a species possesses - the first line of defense against infection. The characteristics of the innate immune response include the following:

- Responses are Broad-Spectrum (non-specific)
- There is no memory or lasting protective immunity
- There is a limited repertoire of recognition molecules
- The responses are phylogenetically ancient

Potential pathogens are encountered routinely, but only rarely cause disease. The vast majority of microorganisms are destroyed within minutes or hours by innate defenses. The acquired specific immune response comes into play only if these innate defenses are breached.

The elements of the innate immune response involves

Anatomic Barriers

1. Skin

- **Epidermis** - thin outer layer containing tightly packed epidermal cells and keratin (water -proofing) completely renewed every 15-30 days. **Dermis** - thicker inner layer contains sebaceous glands associated with hair follicles - produce sebum which consists of lactic and fatty acids maintaining a pH 3–5.
- **Mucous membranes** (ciliated epithelial cells; saliva, tears and mucous secretions) - GI, urogenital, respiratory tracts - collectively represents a huge surface area.
- **Physiologic Barriers**
- **Temperature** - normal body temperature inhibits growth of most microorganisms.

- **Elevated body temperature** (fever) can have a direct effect on pathogenic microorganisms.
- **pH** - low pH of stomach, skin, & vagina (inhibits microbial growth)

2. Chemical factors

- Fatty acids, lactic acid
- Pepsin (digestive enzyme which hydrolyzes proteins)
- Lysozyme -hydrolytic enzyme found in mucous secretions - able to cleave the petidoglycan layer of the bacterial cell wall
- Anti-microbial substances which directly destroy microorganims: cryptidins and a-defensins (produced in base of crypts of small intestine - damage cell membranes) b-defensins (produced within skin, respiratory tract - also damages cell membranes) surfactant proteins A & D (present in lungs - function as opsonins which enhance the efficiency of phagocytosis)
- Interferons - group of proteins produced by cells following viral infection. Secreted by the cells, and then binds to nearby cells and induces mechanisms which inhibit viral replication.
- Complement - a group of serum proteins that circulate in an inactive proenzyme state. These proteins can be activated by a variety of specific and nonspecific immunologic mechanisms that convert the inactive proenzymes into active enzymes. The activated complement components participate in a controlled enzymatic cascade that results in membrane-damaging reactions which destroy pathogenic organisms by formation of a membrane attack comples (MAC).

3. Endocytic and Phagocytic Barriers

Endocytosis is the process by which macromolecules contained within the extracellular tissue fluid are internalized by cells. Internalization occurs as small regions of the plasma membrane invaginate, or fold inward, forming small endocytic vesicles known as endosomes. Occurs through pinocytosis or receptor-mediated endocytosis:

- **Pinocytosis** - nonspecific membrane invagination
- **Receptor-mediated endocytosis** - specific, macromolecules are selectively internalized after binding to specific membrane receptors.

Following internalization, the endosomes fuse with primary lysosmes. Lysosomes contain large numbers of degradative enzymes (> 20 different hydrolytic enzymes including proteases, nucleases, lipases, etc). The ingested macromolecules are subsequently digested into small breakdown products. Products not utilized by the cell are released through the process known as exocytosis.

Phagocytosis involves the ingestion of particulate material including whole pathogenic microorganisms. The plasma membrane expands around the particulate material to form large vesicles called phagosomes (10-20times larger than endosome). Only specialized cells are capable of phagocytosis, whereas endocytosis is carried out by virtually all cells. Once particulate matter is ingested into phagosomes, the phagosomes fuse with lysosomes and the ingested material is then digested by a process similar to that seen in endocytosis. The so-called "professional phagocytes" include: monocytes & macrophages, neutrophils, and dendritic cells.

Phagocytic cells distinguish between self/ and non-self by the recognition of common molecular pattern of the invading microorganisms. These microbial patterns involves,

- LPS- lipopolysaccharide (associated with the outer membrane of Gram - bacteria)
- Mannose, fucose, and other sugar residues (not just absence/presence but also factors like spacing between sugars on the cell surface)
- Teichoic acid (associated with the peptidoglycan cell wall of Gram+ bacteria)
- N-formyl peptides (recall that all prokaryotic protein sequences begin with a formyl-methionine)

These common microbial patterns are recognized by host proteins which have been termed as Pattern Recognition Molecules (PRMs) or Pattern Recognition Receptors (PRRs), which includes

- f-Met-Leu-Phe receptor (binds to N-formyl peptides, and when present attracts neutrophils)
- Complement receptors- designated CRs - (binds to complement components such as C3b and C4b which opsonize microorganims as a consequence of the activation of the complement cascade)
- Macrophage Mannose receptor (binds to mannose residues commonly present on surface of microorganisms)
- Scavenger Receptors - at least 6 different scavenger receptors with different specificities have been described (recognize certain anionic polymers and acetylated low-density lipoproteins)
- CD14 (receptor on the surface of phagocytes which allows for the recognition of LPS)

The interaction between a PRM and its microbial pattern leads to a rapid cascade of events. Toll like receptors (TLR) were first identified in the fruitfly, Drosophila, and were shown to play a very important role in the development of the insect. More recently, toll receptors have been shown to also be involved in the innate immune response of fruit flies and other insects and even in vertebrate organisms including humans reported to possess several similar proteins. TLR-4 plays an important role in signal transduction (transfer of the signal received at the cell membrane eventually to DNA sequences located in the nucleus of the cell). Importantly, TLR-4 is now known to activate a transcription factor known as NFkB. NFkB activation eventually leads to transcriptional activation resulting in the synthesis of:

- ROIs (Reactive oxygen intermediates) and RNIs (Reactive nitrogen intermediates) - highly toxic to microorganisms anti-microbial peptides (such as the defensins)
- Cytokines (the small proteins which function as the chemical messengers of the immune response facilitating cell-cell communication)
- Chemokines (small proteins which function in the chemotaxis of leucocytes) adhesion molecules (proteins which regulate the adhesive properties of leucocytes leading to alterations in leucocyte migration and trafficking)
- Acute phase proteins (proteins synthesized largely in the liver and secreted rapidly following infection or tissue injury)

12.4.2. Adaptive or Acquired Immunity

Natural immunity alone cannot protect the body from invading pathogens. Hence, immunity is provided by either stimulating an individual's antibody production or by introducing antibodies acquired from other sources. Adaptive immunity involves the lymphocytes and develops as people are exposed to diseases or immunized against diseases through vaccination. The adaptive (or active) immunity, which develops throughout our lives and particularly, develops when a person is exposed to natural infection by pathogens or to some antigens in day-to-day life. Following exposure, the immune system responds by producing specialized lymphocytes and special proteins called antibodies. Immunity of this kind lasts long in most cases. Immunity developed following clinical and sub-clinical infections also falls under this category. Artificially acquired active immunity arises from the stimulation of antibody production following the administration of specially prepared antigens called vaccines into the body by safe means. This is termed as vaccination or active immunization. Vaccines are composed of inactivated bacterial toxins (toxoids), killed micro-organisms or living but attenuated (weakened) micro-organisms that are subjected to treatment wherein they lose their toxicity or the ability to cause a disease but are still capable of stimulating the immune system. There are two fundamental adaptive mechanisms: cell-mediated immunity and humoral immunity.

12.4.2.1. Cell-mediated Immunity

In 1883 Elie Metchnikoff observed that blood cells also contribute to the immune system. He noted that some white blood cells were able to engulf invading micro-organisms, and he named these white blood cells as phagocytes. Macrophages engulf antigens, process them internally and then display parts of them on their surface together with some of their own proteins. This sensitizes the T cells to recognize these antigens. All cells are coated with various substances. CD stands for cluster of differentiation and there are more than one hundred and sixty clusters, each of which is a different chemical molecule that coats the surface. CD8+ is read "CD8 positive." Every T and B cell has about $10^5 = 100,000$ molecules on its surface. B cells are coated with CD21, CD35, CD40, and CD45 in addition to other non-CD molecules. T cells have CD2, CD3, CD4, CD28, CD45R, and other non-CD molecules on their surfaces.

The large number of molecules on the surfaces of lymphocytes allow a huge variability in the forms of the receptors. They are produced with random configurations on their surfaces. There are some 10^{18} different structurally different receptors. Essentially, an antigen may find a near-perfect fit with a very small number of lymphocytes, perhaps as few as one.

T cells are primed in the thymus, where they undergo two selection processes. The first positive selection process weeds out only those T cells with the correct set of receptors that can recognize the MHC molecules responsible for self-recognition. Then a negative selection process begins whereby T cells that can recognize MHC molecules complexed with foreign peptides are allowed to pass out of the thymus.

Cytotoxic or killer T cells (CD8+) do their work by releasing lymphotoxins, which cause cell lysis. Helper T cells (CD4+) serve as managers, directing the immune response. They secrete chemicals called lymphokines that stimulate cytotoxic T cells and B cells to grow and divide, attract neutrophils, and enhance the ability of macrophages to engulf and destroy microbes. Suppressor T cells inhibit the production of cytotoxic T cells once they are not needed, lest they cause more damage than necessary. Memory T cells are programmed to recognize and respond to a pathogen once it has invaded and has been thus repelled and neutralized.

T cells, like B cells, have specificity for a single antigen indicating the presence of T cell receptors, which recognize the antigen. However, the response is not on the same line because being soluble antigens are unable to stimulate T cells as they cannot bind to T cells. A T cell responds only to those antigens processed by an antigen-presenting cell (APC). The major difference between T cell response and B cell response is that the T cell recognizes an antigen only when it is in close association with a major histocompatibility complex (MHC). This type of recognition is known as associative recognition. Various cells involved in cell mediated immunity are summarized in Table 12.2.

Once the APC is stimulated by an antigen, the cell secretes a substance called interleukin -l (IL-I), a monokine secreted by macrophages, activates the T cell, which in turn begins to synthesize interleukin-2 (IL-2). The T cell also synthesizes surface receptors for IL-2. When the receptors bind to the IL-2, the T cells proliferate and differentiate into different effector cells, IL-2 receptors on T cells appear only if the T cell has been stimulated by an antigen.

Table 12.2: Different cells involved in cell-mediated immunity and their functions

Cell	Function
Helper T Cell (TH)	Required for B cells activation by T -dependent antigens
Suppressor T cells (Ts)	Regulates immune response and helps In maintaining immune tolerance
Delayed hypersensitivity T cell (TD)	Protects against infectious agents; causes inflammation in association to tissue transplant rejection
Cytotoxic T cell (Tc)	Destroys target cells on contact
Killer Cell (K)	Attacks antibody-coated target cells
Natural Killer cell (NK)	Attacks and destroys target cells

12.4.2.2. Humoral Immunity

Emil von Behring and Shibasaburo Kitasato in 1890 demonstrated that serum from previously immunized animals, when administered to non-immunized animals, they got immunized. Since the immunity was mediated by antibodies contained in body fluids (in early days it was known as humors), this kind of immunity was named humoral immunity.

Humoral immunity or response is carried out by B cells, which produce antibodies. Humoral response is involved in the elimination of extracellular pathogens. It produces a large number of antibody molecules. B cells produced in the bone marrow mature and migrate into the lymphoidal organs, where they encounter antigens. When an appropriate antigen contacts the antigen receptor antibodies on a B cell, the latter proliferates into a large clone of cells. This phenomenon is known as clonal selection. Sometimes, the production of antibodies by a B cell depends on other cells, thus production of antibodies against T-dependent antigens requires the help of certain macrophages and T cells. The humoral immune system operates through antibodies found in blood plasma and lymph.

An immunocompetent but yet immature B-lymphocyte is stimulated to maturity when an antigen binds to its surface receptors and there is a T helper cell nearby (to release a cytokine). This sensitizes or primes the B cell and it undergoes clonal selection, and most of the family of clones becomes plasma cells. These cells, after an initial lag, produce highly specific antibodies at a rate of as many as 2000 molecules per second for four to five days. The other B cells become long-lived memory cells.

Antibodies, also called immunoglobulins or Igs (with molecular weights of 150–900 Md), constitute the gamma globulin part of the blood proteins. They are soluble proteins secreted by the plasma offspring clones of primed B cells. The antibodies inactivate antigens by, (a) complement fixation (proteins attach to antigen surface and cause holes to form, i.e., cell lysis), (b) neutralization (binding to specific sites to prevent attachment (c) agglutination (clumping), (d) precipitation (forcing insolubility and settling out of solution), and other more arcane methods.

Constituents of gamma globulin are: IgG-76%, IgA-15%, IgM-8%, IgD-1%, and IgE-0.002% (responsible for autoimmune responses, such as allergies and diseases like arthritis, multiple sclerosis, and systemic lupus erythematosus). IgG is the only antibody that can cross the placental barrier to the fetus and it is responsible for the 3 to 6 month immune protection of newborns that is conferred by the mother. IgM is the dominant antibody produced in primary immune responses, while IgG dominates in secondary immune responses. IgM is physically much larger than the other immunoglobulins.

The upper part or Fab (antigen binding) portion of the antibody molecule (physically and not necessarily chemically) attaches to specific proteins (called epitopes) on the antigen. Thus antibody recognizes the epitope and not the entire antigen. The Fc region is crystallizable and is responsible for effector functions, i.e., the end to which immune cells can attach. In addition to these antibody produced, it has been found that the B cells can produce as many as 10^{14} conformationally different forms.

All of these mechanisms hinge on the attachment of antigen and cell receptors. Since there are many receptor shapes available, WBCs seek to optimize the degree of confluence between the two receptors. The number of these "best fit" receptors may be quite small, even as few as a single cell. This attests he specificity of the interaction. Nevertheless, cells can bind to receptors whose fit is less than optimal when required. This is referred to as cross-reactivity.

12.5. Immunoglobulin Classes

12.5.1. Immunoglobulin G (IgG)

70-75% of the total human serum immunoglobulin consists of Immunoglobulin G. IgG is a monomeric protein with two γ heavy chains and two k or l light chains. It has a molecular weight of 1,46,000 with a sedimentation coefficient of 7S. The IgG class is distributed evenly between the intra and extra-vascular pools. It is the major antibody of secondary immune responses and the exclusive-toxin class. There are four IgG subclasses namely IgG 1, IgG2, IgG3 and IgG4 numbered in accordance with their order of occurrence in the serum. One important thing to be noted is that no two subclasses are identical. This may be either with reference to the number or the distribution of inter-chain disulfide linkages. The four subclasses are encoded by different germ-line CH genes whose DNA sequences are 90–95% homologous. The differences in amino acid sequence in IgG subclasses are directly related to biological activity. While IgG1, IgG3 and IgG4 cross the placenta and play an important role in protecting the fetus, IgG2 crosses only partially in some cases. Complement activation efficiency also differs; IgG3 is the most effective, followed by IgG 1, IgG2 and IgG4. The opsonin activity of IgG is attributed to its binding to Fc receptors on phagocytic cells. Again, the different subclasses have different affinity. IgG1 and IgG3 have a higher affinity to Fc receptors while IgG4 has an intermediate affinity, IgG2 shows an extremely low affinity.

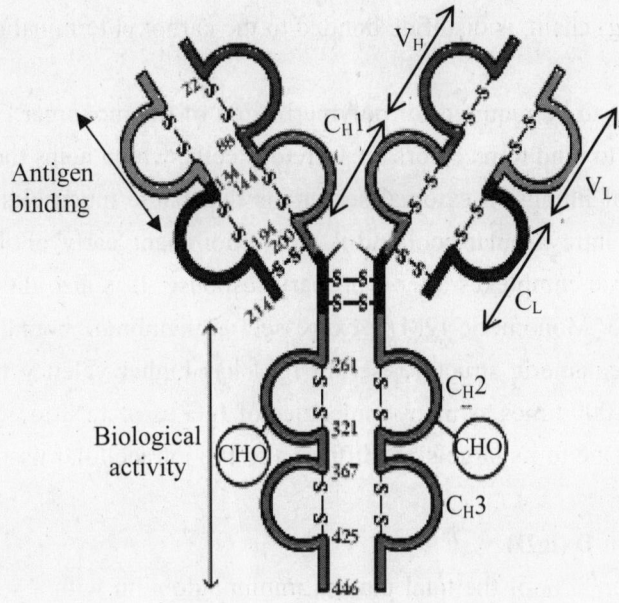

Figure 12.9: Structure of IgG

12.5.2. Immunoglobulin A (IgA)

Immunoglobulin A (IgA), the predominant immunoglobulin in seromucous secretions, constitutes 15-20% of the normal human serum immunoglobulin pool. It is protected from proteolysis by combination with another protein; the secretory component IgA is predominantly seen in external secretions such as breast milk, saliva, tears and mucus of the bronchial, genitourinary and digestive tracts. Hence, they are frequently known as secretory IgA (sIgA). In serum, IgA exists as a monomer; however, in most cases it is polymeric, i.e. dimers, trimers, etc. The sIgA consists of a dimer or tetramer, a J chain polypeptide and a polypeptide chain called secretory component. The secretory component is a polypeptide with a molecular weight of 70,000 and is produced by epithelial cells of mucous membranes. It has five immunoglobulin like domains that bind to the Fc regions of the IgA dimmer (Fig. 12.10)

12.5.3. Immunoglobulin M (IgM)

IgM accounts for about 10% of the total serum immunoglobulin with an average serum concentration of 1.5% mg/ml. Unlike IgG or IgA, IgM has a pentameric structure in which individual heavy chains have a molecular weight of approximately 65,000 while the total molecular weight amounts to 9,70,000. The monomeric units consist of two m heavy chains and two light chains. The subunits are held together by disulfide bonds between their carboxyl terminal (Cm 4/Cm4) domains and Cm3/Cm3. The subunits are so arranged that their Fc region lies in the center of the pentamer. It is believed that IgM has 10 antigen binding sites but they are unable to combine with the antigen with similar efficiency; this makes it difficult to demonstrate the presence of 10 sites. In addition to the above, a Fc linked polypeptide called J (joining) chain, is disulfide bonded to the carboxyl terminal cysteine residue of two of the 10m chains.

The J chain appears to be required for polymerization of the monomer. The presence of the J chain allows IgM to bind to receptors on secretory cells, which helps them in transporting across the epithelial linings to external secretions that bathe mucosal surfaces. IgM is largely confined to the intravascular pool and is the predominant 'early' antibody frequently directed against antigenic complexes after a primary response. It is also the first to be synthesized by the neonate. Monomeric IgM is expressed as membrane bound antibody on B cells. Because of its pentameric structure, serum IgM has higher valency than others. For example, it takes 100-1000 times as many molecules of IgG as of IgM to achieve the same level of agglutination. Due to its large size, diffusion to the intracellular tissue fluids is very low (fig. 12.10).

12.5.4 Immunoglobulin D (IgD)

IgD constitutes less than 1 % of the total plasma immunoglobulin with a serum concentration of 30mg/ml. IgD, together with IgM, is the major membrane bound immunoglobulin expressed by mature B cells. Though their exact biological function is not clear they are thought to function in the activation of B cells by an antigen. IgD is more susceptible to proteolysis than any other immunoglobulin class. IgD has a simple disulfide bond between the d chains and a high content of carbohydrate distributed in multiple oligosaccharide units. One of these units is rich in N-acetyl galactosamine (Fig. 12.10).

12.5.5. Immunoglobulin E (IgE)

IgE is present in low levels in serum and in respiratory and gastro-intestinal mucous secretions. IgE binds with high affinity to receptors present in high levels on mast cells and basophils and to a lesser extent on several other hematopoietic cells, including dendritic cells. If Ag bridges 2 IgE molecules bound to the mast cell or basophil surface, the cells degranulate, releasing chemical mediators that cause an inflammatory response. IgE levels are elevated in atopic disorders (e.g., allergic or extrinsic asthma, hay fever, atopic dermatitis) and parasitic infections (Fig. 12.10).

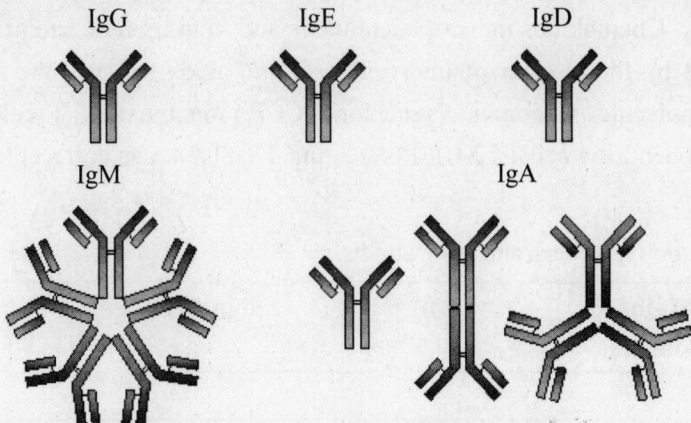

Figure 12.10: Structure of immunoglobulins

12.6. Acute Phase Reactants

Acute phase reactants are plasma proteins whose levels dramatically increase if infection or tissue damage occurs. Most dramatically increased are C-reactive protein and mannose-binding lectin (which fix complement and act as opsonins), the transport protein α_1-acid glycoprotein, and serum amyloid P component. Many acute phase reactants are synthesized in the liver. Collectively, they may help limit tissue injury, enhance host resistance to infection, and promote tissue repair and resolution of inflammation.

12.7. Cytokines

Cytokines are polypeptides secreted by immune and other cells when the cell interacts with a specific Ag, endotoxin, or other cytokines. Main categories include

- IFNs (IFN-α, IFN-β, IFN-γ)
- TNFs (TNF-α, lymphotoxin-α, lymphotoxin-β)
- ILs
- Chemokines
- TGFs
- Hematopoietic colony-stimulating factors (CSFs)

Although lymphocytes interaction with a specific Ag triggers cytokine secretion, cytokines themselves are not Ag-specific; thus, they bridge innate and acquired immunity and generally influence the magnitude of inflammatory or immune responses. They act sequentially, synergistically, or antagonistically and may act in an autocrine or paracrine manner.

Cytokines deliver their signals via cell surface receptors. For example, the IL-2 receptor consists of 3 chains: α, β, and γ. The receptor's affinity for IL-2 is high if all 3 chains are expressed, intermediate if only the β and γ chains are expressed, or low if only the α chain is expressed. Mutations or deletion of the γ chain is the basis for X-linked severe combined immunodeficiency. Chemokines induces chemotaxis and migration of leukocytes. There are 4 subsets, defined by the number of intervening amino acids between the first 2 cysteine residues in the molecule. Chemokine receptors (CCR5 on memory T cells, monocytes/macrophages, and dendritic cells; CXCR4 on resting T cells) act as co-receptors for entry of HIV into cells.

Table 12.3: Selected Cytokines and their effects

Cytokine	Major Sources	Significance
Interleukins (IL)		
IL-1α IL-1β	B cells, dendritic cells, endothelium, macrophages, monocytes, NK cells	• Co-stimulates T-cell activation by enhancing production of cytokines (e.g., IL-2 and its receptor) • Enhances B-cell proliferation and maturation • Enhances NK-cell cytotoxicity • Induces IL-1, IL-6, IL-8, TNF, GM-CSF, and prostaglandin E_2 production by macrophages • Is pro-inflammatory by inducing chemokines, ICAM-1, and VCAM-1 (intercellular adhesion molecule and vascular adhesion molecule), on endothelium • Induces sleep, anorexia, release of tissue factor, acute phase reactants, and bone resorption by osteoclasts • Is an endogenous pyrogen
IL-2	T_H1 cells	• Induces proliferation of activated T and B cells • Enhances NK-cell cytotoxicity and killing of tumor cells and bacteria by monocytes and macrophages
IL-3	Mast cells, NK cells, T cells	• Induces growth and differentiation of hematopoietic precursors and growth of mast cells
IL-4	Mast cells, NK cells, NK-T cells, γ δ T cells, T_C2 cells, T_H2 cells	• Induces T_H2 cells • Stimulates proliferation of activated B, T, and mast cells • Up-regulates class II MHC molecules on B cells and on macrophages and CD23 on B cells • Down regulates IL-12 production and thereby inhibits T_H1 cell-differentiation • Increases macrophage phagocytosis • Induces switch to IgG1 and IgE

IL-6	Dendritic cells, fibroblasts, macrophages, monocytes, T_H2 cells	• Induces differentiation of myeloid stem cells and B cells into plasma cells • Induces acute phase reactants • Enhances T-cell proliferation • Induces T_C-cell differentiation • Is a pyrogen
IL-7	Bone marrow and thymus stromal cells	• Induces differentiation of lymphoid stem cells into T- and B-cell precursors • Activates mature T cells
IL-8 (chemokine)	Endothelial cells, macrophages, monocytes	• Mediates chemotaxis and activation of neutrophils
IL-9	T_H cells	• Induces proliferation of thymocytes • Enhances mast cell growth • Acts synergistically with IL-4 to induce switch to IgG1 and IgE
IL-10	B cells, macrophages, monocytes, T_C cells, T_H2 cells	• Inhibits IL-2 secretion by human T_H1 cells • Downregulates production of class II MHC molecules and cytokines (eg, IL-12) by monocytes, macrophages, and dendritic cells and thereby inhibits T_H1-cell differentiation • Inhibits T-cell proliferation • Enhances B-cell differentiation
IL-11	Bone marrow stromal cells	• Promotes differentiation of pro-B cells and megakaryocytes • Induces acute phase reactants • Stimulates macrophage precursors
IL-12	B cells, dendritic cells, macrophages, monocytes	• Critical for T_H1 differentiation • Induces proliferation of T_H1 cells, CD8 T cells, γ δ T cells, and NK cells and their production of IFN-γ • Enhances NK and CD8 T-cell cytotoxicity
IL-13	Mast cells, T_H2 cells	• Inhibits activation and cytokine secretion by macrophages • Coactivates B-cell proliferation • Upregulates class II MHC molecules and CD23 on B cells and monocytes • Induces switch to IgG1 and IgE • Induces VCAM-1 on endothelium
IL-14	—	• Originally thought to stimulate B cells, but gene and protein sequence have not been confirmed • IL-14 may not exist

IL-15	B cells, dendritic cells, macrophages, monocytes, NK cells, T cells	• Induces proliferation of T, NK, and activated B cells • Induces cytokine production and cytotoxicity of NK cells and CD8 T cells • Is chemotactic for T cells • Stimulates growth of intestinal epithelium
IL-16	T_C cells, T_H cells	• chemo-attractant for CD4 T cells, monocytes, and eosinophils • Induces class II MHC molecules
IL-17	T cells	• Is pro-inflammatory • Stimulates production of cytokines (eg, TNF, IL-1β, IL-6, IL-8, G-CSF)
IL-18	Monocytes, dendritic cells	• Induces IFN-γ production by T cells • Enhances NK-cell cytotoxicity
IL-19	B cells, monocytes, macrophages	• Induces proliferation and proinflammatory activities in keratinocytes • Promotes T_H2-cell responses • Induces apoptosis in monocytes
IL-20	Keratinocytes, macrophages	• Induces proliferation and proinflammatory activities in keratinocytes
IL-21	NK cells, T_H cells	• Stimulates B-cell proliferation after CD40 cross-linking • Stimulates proliferation of bone marrow precursor cells
IL-22	Mast cells, NK cells, T cells	• Is pro-inflammatory • Induces synthesis of acute phase reactants
IL-23	Dendritic cells, macrophages	• Induces proliferation of T_H cells
IL-24	B cells, macrophages, monocytes, T cells	• Suppresses tumor cell growth • Induces apoptosis in tumor cells
IL-25	Bone marrow stromal cells	• Induces production of cytokines that promote eosinophilia
IL-26	T cells	• Is proinflammatory • Induces IL-8 and IL-10 production and ICAM-1 expression in epithelial cells
IL-27	Dendritic cells, macrophages	• Induces T_H1 cells • Is a heterodimer consisting of IL-30 and Epstein-Barr virus–induced gene 3

IL-28	Mononuclear cells in response to viral infection	• Is antiviral
IL-29	Mononuclear cells in response to viral infection	• Is antiviral
IL-30	Dendritic cells, macrophages	• Induces T_H1 cells • Is a subunit of IL-27

Interferons (IFN)

IFN-α	Leukocytes	• Inhibits viral replication • Increases class I MHC expression
IFN-β	Fibroblasts	• Inhibits viral replication • Increases class I MHC expression
IFN-γ	NK cells, T_C1 cells, T_H1 cells	• Inhibits viral replication • Increases class I and II MHC expression • Activates macrophages • Antagonizes several actions of IL-4 • Inhibits proliferation of T_H2 cells

Tumour necrosis factors (TNF)

TNF-α (cachectin)	B cells, dendritic cells, macrophages, mast cells, monocytes, NK cells, T_H cells	• Is cytotoxic to tumor cells • Induces secretion of several cytokines (eg, IL-1, GM-CSF, IFN-γ) • Induces E-selectin on endothelium • Activates macrophages • Is antiviral
TNF-β (lymphotoxin)	T_C cells, T_H1 cells	• Is cytotoxic to tumor cells and antiviral • Enhances phagocytosis by neutrophils and macrophages • Is involved in lymphoid organ development

Colony-stimulating factors (CSF)

G-CSF	Endothelial cells, fibroblasts	• Stimulates growth of neutrophil precursors
GM-CSF	Endothelial cells, fibroblasts, macrophages, mast cells, T_H cells	• Stimulates growth of precursors of monocytes, neutrophils, eosinophils, and basophils • Activates macrophages
M-CSF	Endothelial cells, epithelial cells, fibroblasts	• Stimulates growth of monocyte precursors
SCF	Bone marrow stromal cells	• Stimulates stem cell division

Transforming growth factors (TGF)		
TGF-α	Monocytes, solid tumors (carcinoma more so than sarcomas)	Induces angiogenesis, keratinocyte proliferation, bone resorption, and tumor growth
TGF-β	B cells, macrophages, mast cells, T_H3 cells	Is proinflammatory (eg, by chemoattraction of monocytes and macrophages) but also anti-inflammatory (eg, by inhibiting lymphocyte proliferation) Induces switch to IgA Promotes tissue repair

NK = natural killer; TNF = tumor necrosis factor; GM-CSF = granulocyte-macrophage colony-stimulating factor; ICAM-1 = intercellular adhesion molecule 1; VCAM-1 = vascular cell adhesion molecule 1; T_H cell = helper T cell; T_C cell = cytotoxic T cell; MHC = major histocompatibility complex; CD = cluster of differentiation; G-CSF = granulocyte colony-stimulating factor; SCF = stem cell factor.

12.8. Regulation of the Humoral response

Immune responses are tightly regulated complex interaction of cells and mediators and operates through a mechanism that prevents anti self reactivity. Regulation of the immune response is possibly mediated in several ways. First, a specific group of T-cells, suppressor T-cells, are thought to be involved in turning down the immune response. Like helper T-cells, suppressor T-cells are stimulated by antigen but instead of releasing lymphokines that activate B-cells (and other cells), suppressor T-cells release factors that suppress the B-cell response. While immunosuppression is not completely understood, it appears to be more complicated than the activation pathway, possibly involves additional cells in the overall process.

Other means of regulation involve interactions between antibody and B-cells. One mechanism, "antigen blocking", occurs when high doses of antibody interact with all of the antigenic epitopes, thereby inhibiting interactions with B-cell receptors. A second mechanism, "receptor cross linking", results when antibody, bound to a B-cell via its Fc receptor and the B-cell receptor both combine with antigen. This "cross-linking" inhibits the B-cell from producing further antibody. Another means of regulation that has been proposed is the idiotypic network hypothesis. This theory suggests that the idiotypic determinants of antibody molecules are so unique that they appear foreign to the immune system and are, therefore, antigenic. Thus, production of antibody in response to antigen leads to the production of anti-antibody in response, and anti-anti-antibody and so on. Eventually, however, the level of [anti]$_n$-antibody is not sufficient to induce another round and the cascade thus ends.

12.9. Passive Immunity

Passive immunity is the immunity acquired by the transfer of antibodies from another individual, as through injection or placental transfer to a fetus. Protection from passive immunity diminishes in a relatively short time, usually a few weeks or months. Infants have passive immunity because they are born with antibodies that are transferred to them through the placenta from the mother. These antibodies disappear between 6 and 12 months of age. Here, the fetus is immune to those diseases to which the mother is immune, but only for a short period. For example, if the mother is immune to diphtheria, chicken pox, and polio, the newborn is also immune to the same diseases but only for a period not exceeding six months. Similarly, certain amount of immunity is provided through breast-feeding. Certain antibodies can pass from the mother to the infant via the breast milk.

Passive immunization involves injection of antiserum, which contains antibodies that are formed by another person or animal. It provides immediate protection against an antigen, but does not provide long-lasting protection. Gamma globulin (given for hepatitis exposure) and tetanus antitoxin are examples of passive immunization. These antibodies are produced either in animals or humans and then administered to the subject.

Table 12.4: Comparison between active and passive immunity

Active	Passive
Developed immunity	Produced immunity
Develops slowly and last long	Relatively fast and short lived
If required, a booster dose can be given to provide life long immunity	A booster dose also doesn't help in maintaining it for long
It is mainly to prevent a disease and is administered before infection Given in long term prophylaxis	Generally develops after the subject has been exposed to an infection. Given in short term prophylaxis and therapeutically
Antigens are administered	Antibodies are administered

12.10. Complement System

The complement system is believed to play important functions in the innate immune response to infections, the generation of adaptive immune responses and the initiation of some autoimmune disorders. It is one of the oldest families of pattern recognition molecules and is involved in promoting opsonophagocytosis of bacterial and fungal pathogens, attraction and activation of phagocytes, clearance of immune complexes and apoptotic cells, and inducing inflammation and anaphylatoxins. The system consists of more than 30 soluble and cell-surface associated molecules responsible for initiation, effector functions, and regulation of three different enzyme cascades, termed the alternative-, classical- and mannose-binding lectin (MBL) pathways.

Historically, the term complement (C) was used to refer a heat-labile serum component that was able to lyse bacteria (activity is destroyed (inactivated) by heating serum at 56° C for 30 min). However, complement is now known to contribute to host defenses in other ways as well. Complement can opsonize bacteria for enhanced phagocytosis; it can recruit and activate various cells including polymorphonuclear cells (PMNs) and macrophages; it can participate in regulation of antibody responses and it can aid in the clearance of immune complexes and apoptotic cells. Complement can also have detrimental effects for the host; it contributes to inflammation and tissue damage and can trigger anaphylaxis.

Complement comprises over 20 different serum proteins that are produced by a variety of cells including, hepatocytes, macrophages and gut epithelial cells. Some complement proteins bind to immunoglobulins or to membrane components of cells. Others are proenzymes that, when activated, cleave one or more other complement proteins. Upon cleavage some of the complement proteins yield fragments that activate cells, increase vascular permeability or opsonize bacteria.

12.10.1. Complement Activation

The complement system is an enzyme cascade that helps defend against infection. Many complement proteins occur in serum as inactive enzyme precursors (zymogens); others reside on cell surfaces. The complement system bridges innate and acquired immunity by augmenting antibody (Ab) responses and immunologic memory, lysing foreign cells and clearing immune complexes and apoptotic cells. They have many biologic functions such as stimulation of chemotaxis and triggering of mast cell de-granulation independent of IgE). There are 3 pathways of complement activation

- Classical
- Lectin
- Alternative

Classical pathway components are labeled with a C and a number (e.g., C1, C3), based on the order in which they were identified. Alternative pathway components are often lettered (e.g., factor B, factor D) or named (e.g., properdin). Classical pathway activation is Ab-dependent, occurring when C1 interacts with Ag-IgM or aggregated Ag-IgG complexes, or Ab-independent, occurring when polyanions (e.g., heparin, protamine, DNA and RNA from apoptotic cells), gram-negative bacteria, or bound C-reactive protein reacts directly with C1. This pathway is regulated by C1 inhibitor (C1-INH).

The three pathways all generate homologous variants of the protease, C3-convertase. C3-convertase cleaves and activates C3, creating C3a and C3b and causing a cascade of further cleavage and activation events. C3b binds to the surface of pathogens leading to greater internalization by phagocytic cells. C5a is an important chemokine, which leads to the recruitment of inflammatory cells. C5b is initiates the membrane attack pathway which results in the membrane attack complex (MAC), consisting of C5b, C6, C7, C8, and polymeric C9. MAC is the cytolytic end product of the complement cascade; it forms a transmembrane channel which causes osmotic lysis of the target cell.

(a) Classical Pathway

IgM or IgG antibody molecules, bound to the surface of micro-organisms, activate the complement system. The complement proteins actually recognize and bind the antibody on the surface of the pathogen. In this scenario the complement system could be considered as specific, but the antibody brings about the specificity so it merely complements the specific function of antibody. A series of proteins bind to the immune complex (C1, C2, C4), resulting in the formation of C3 convertase activity.

The classical pathway is triggered by activation of the C1-complex (which consist of one molecule C1q and two molecules C1r and C1s respectively), either by C1q binding to antibodies from classes M and G, complexed with antigens, or by binding C1q to the surface of the pathogen (Fig. 12.11). This binding leads to conformational changes in C1q molecule, which leads to the activation of two C1r (serine protease) molecules. Then they cleave C1s (another serine protease). The C1-complex now binds to and splits C2 and C4, producing C2a and C4b. The inhibition of C1r and C1s is controlled by C1-inhibitor. C4b and C2a bind to form C3-convertase (C4b2a complex). Production of C3-convertase signals the end of the classical pathway, but cleavage of C3 by this enzyme brings to the start of the alternative pathway.

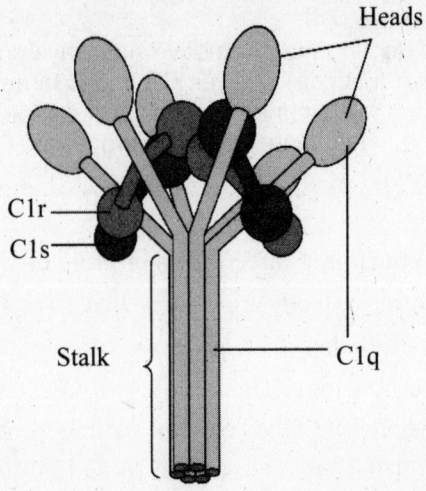

Figure 12.11: Proteins of the classical pathway: C1complex

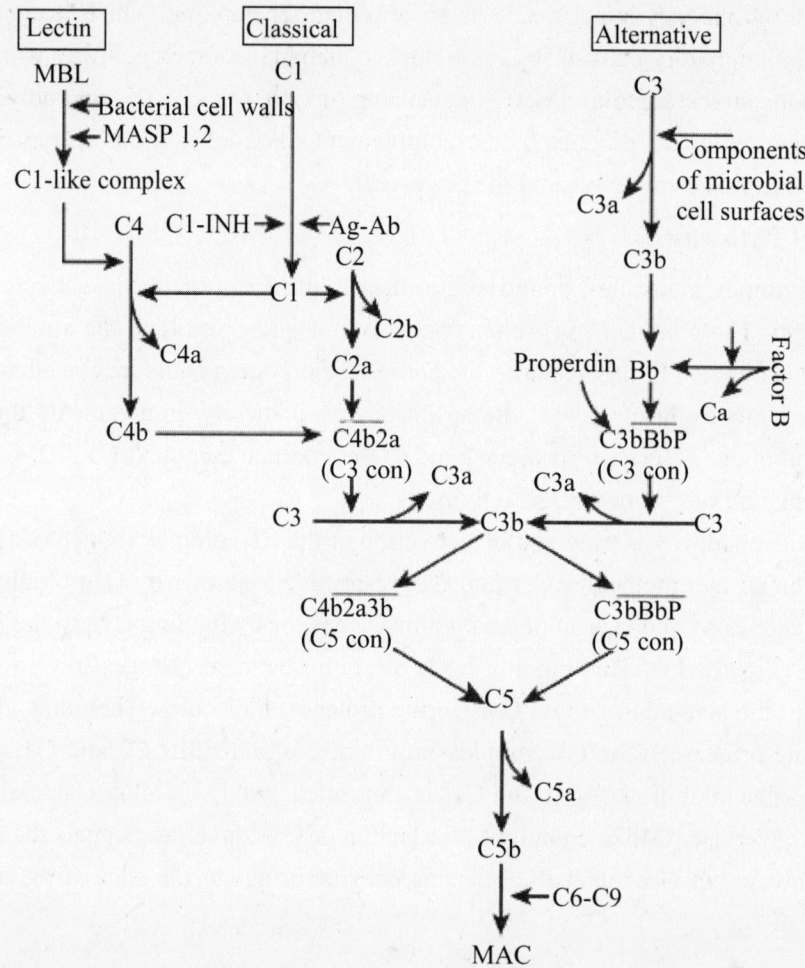

Figure 12.12: The classical, lectin, and alternative pathways converge into a final common pathway when C3 convertase (C3 con) cleaves C3 into C3a and C3b. Ab = antibody; Ag = antigen; C1-INH = C1 inhibitor; MAC = membrane attack complex; MASP = MBL-associated serine protease; MBL = mannose-binding lectin; P = properdin. Overbar indicates activation

(i) C1 activation

C1, a multi-subunit protein containing three different proteins (C1q, C1r and C1s), binds to the Fc region of IgG and IgM antibody molecules that have interacted with antigen. C1 binding does not occur to antibodies that have not complexed with antigen and binding requires calcium and magnesium ions. (In some cases C1 can bind to aggregated immunoglobulin (e.g. aggregated IgG) or to certain pathogen surfaces in the absence of antibody). The binding of C1 to antibody is via C1q and C1q must cross link at least two antibody molecules before it is firmly fixed. The binding of C1q results in the activation of

C1r which in turn activates C1s. The result is the formation of an activated "C1qrs", which is an enzyme that cleaves C4 into two fragments C4a and C4b.

(ii) C4 and C2 activation (generation of C3 convertase)

The C4b fragment binds to the membrane and the C4a fragment is released into the microenvironment. Activated "C1qrs" also cleaves C2 into C2a and C2b. C2a binds to the membrane in association with C4b, and C2b is released into the microenvironment. The resulting C4bC2a complex is a C3 convertase, which cleaves C3 into C3a and C3b.

Table12.5: Proteins of the Complement system

Classical Pathway	Lectin Pathway	Alternative Pathway	Lytic Pathway
Activation Proteins: C1qrs, C2, C3, C4 Control Proteins: C1-INH, C4-BP	Mannan binding protein (MBP), mannan-asociated serine protease (MASP, MASP2)	C3, Factors <u>B</u> & D*, Properdin (P) Factors I* & H, decay accelerating factor (DAF), Complement receptor 1(CR1), *etc.*	C5, C6, C7, C8, C9 Protein S
Components underlined acquire enzymatic activity when activated. Components marked with an asterisk have enzymatic activity in their native form.			

(iii) C3 activation (generation of C5 convertase)

C3b binds to the membrane in association with C4b and C2a, and C3a is released into the microenvironment. The resulting C4bC2aC3b is a C5 convertase. The generation of C5 convertase is the end of the classical pathway. Several of the products of the classical pathway have potent biological activities that contribute to host defenses. Some of these products may also have detrimental effects if produced in an unregulated manner (Fig. 12.13).

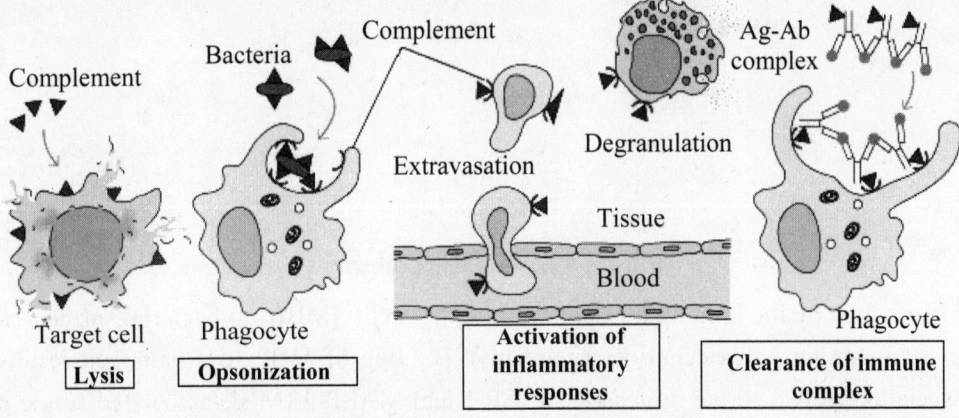

Figure 12.13: Immune responses

If the classical pathway were not regulated there would be continued production of C2b, C3a, and C4a. Thus, there must be some way to regulate the activity of the classical pathway. Table 3 summarizes the ways in which the classical pathway is regulated (Table 12.6).

Table 12.6: Regulation of the Classical Pathway

Component	Regulation
All	**C1-INH**; dissociates C1r and C1s from C1q
C3a	**C3a inactivator (C3a-INA;Carboxypeptidase B)**; inactivates C3a
C3b	**Factors H and I**; Factor H facilitates the degradation of C3b by Factor I
C4a	**C3-INA**
C4b	**C4 binding protein(C4-BP) and Factor I**; C4-BP facilitates degradation of C4b by Factor I; C4-BP also prevents association of C2a with C4b thus blocking the formation of C3 convertase

(b) Lectin Pathway

Lectin pathway activation is Ab-independent; it occurs when mannose-binding lectin (MBL), a serum protein, binds to mannose or fructose groups on bacterial cell walls, yeast walls, or viruses. This pathway otherwise resembles the classical pathway structurally and functionally.

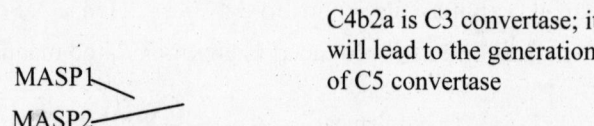

MASP1

MASP2

C4b2a is C3 convertase; it will lead to the generation of C5 convertase

Figure 12.14: Lectin pathway

It is initiated by the binding of mannose-binding lectin (MBL) to bacterial surfaces with mannose-containing polysaccharides (mannans). Binding of MBL to a pathogen results in the association of two serine proteases, MASP-1 and MASP-2 (MBL-associated serine proteases). MASP-1 and MASP-2 are similar to C1r and C1s, respectively and MBL is similar to C1q. Formation of the MBL/MASP-1/MASP-2 tri-molecular complex results in the activation of the MASPs and subsequent cleavage of C4 into C4a and C4b. The C4b fragment binds to the membrane and the C4a fragment is released into the microenvironment. Activated MASPs also cleave C2 into C2a and C2b. C2a binds to the membrane in association with C4b and C2b is released into the microenvironment. The resulting C4bC2a complex is a C3 convertase, which cleaves C3 into C3a and C3b. C3b binds to the membrane in association with C4b and C2a and C3a is released into the microenvironment. The resulting C4bC2aC3b is a C5 convertase. The generation of C5 convertase is the end of the lectin pathway.

(c) Alternate Pathway

Alternate pathway activation occurs when components of microbial cell surfaces (e.g., yeast walls, bacterial cell wall lipopolysaccharide (endotoxin) or Ig (e.g., nephritic factor, aggregated IgA) cleave small amounts of C3. This pathway is regulated by properdin, factor H, and decay-accelerating factor. The alternative pathway begins with the activation of C3 and requires Factors B and D and Mg^{++} cation, all present in normal serum.

Amplification loop of C3b formation

In serum there is low level spontaneous hydrolysis of C3 to produce C3i. Factor B binds to C3i and becomes susceptible to Factor D, which cleaves Factor B into Bb. The C3iBb complex acts as a C3 convertase and cleaves C3 into C3a and C3b. Once C3b is formed, Factor B will bind to it and becomes susceptible to cleavage by Factor D. The resulting C3bBb complex is a C3 convertase that will continue to generate more C3b, thus amplifying C3b production. If this process continues unchecked, the result would be the consumption of all C3 in the serum. Thus, the spontaneous production of C3b is tightly controlled.

(ii) Control of the amplification loop

As spontaneously produced C3b binds to autologous host membranes, it interacts with DAF (decay accelerating factor), which blocks the association of Factor B with C3b thereby preventing the formation of additional C3 convertase. In addition, DAF accelerates the dissociation of Bb from C3b in C3 convertase that has already formed, thereby stopping the production of additional C3b. Some cells possess complement receptor 1 (CR1). Binding of C3b to CR1 facilitates the enzymatic degradation of C3b by Factor I. In addition, binding of C3 convertase (C3bBb) to CR1 also dissociates Bb from the complex. Thus, in cells possessing complement receptors, CR1 also plays a role in controlling the amplification loop. Finally, Factor H can bind to C3b bound to a cell or in the in the fluid phase and facilitate the enzymatic degradation of C3b by Factor I. Thus, the amplification loop is controlled by either blocking the formation of C3 convertase, dissociating C3 convertase, or by enzymatically digesting C3b. The importance of controlling this amplification loop is illustrated in patients with genetic deficiencies of Factor H or I. These patients have a C3 deficiency and increased susceptibility to certain infections.

(iii) Stabilization of C convertase by activator (protector) surfaces

C3b when bound to an appropriate activator of the alternative pathway, it will bind Factor B, which is enzymatically cleaved by Factor D to produce C3 convertase (C3bBb). However, C3b is resistant to degradation by Factor I and the C3 convertase is not rapidly degraded, since it is stabilized by the activator surface. The complex is further stabilized by properdin binding to C3bBb. Activators of the alternate pathway are components on the surface of pathogens and include LPS of Gram-negative bacteria and the cell walls of some bacteria and yeasts. Thus, when C3b binds to an activator surface, the C3 convertase formed will be stable and continue to generate additional C3a and C3b by cleavage of C3.

12.10.5. Generation of C5 Convertase

Some of the C3b is generated by the stabilized C3 convertase on the activator surface associates with the C3bBb complex to form a C3bBbC3b complex. This is the C5 convertase of the alternative pathway. The generation of C5 convertase is the end of the alternative pathway. The alternative pathway can be activated by many Gram-negative (most significantly, *Neisseria meningitidis* and *N. gonorrhoea*), some Gram-positive bacteria and certain viruses and parasites, and results in the lysis of these organisms. Thus, the alternative pathway of C activation provides another means of protection against certain pathogens before an antibody response is mounted. A deficiency of C3 results in an increased susceptibility to these organisms. The alternate pathway may be the more primitive pathway and the classical and lectin pathways probably developed from it.

12.10.6. Membrane Attack (Lytic) Pathway

C5 convertase from the classical (C4b2a3b), lectin (C4b2a3b) or alternative (C3bBb3b) pathway cleaves C5 into C5a and C5b. C5a remains in the fluid phase and the C5b rapidly associates with C6 and C7 and inserts into the membrane. Subsequently C8 binds, followed by several molecules of C9. The C9 molecules form a pore in the membrane through which the cellular contents leak and lysis occurs. Lysis is not an enzymatic process; it is thought to be due to physical damage to the membrane. The complex consisting of C5bC6C7C8C9 is referred to as the membrane attack complex (MAC).

C5a generated in the lytic pathway has several potent biological activities. It is the most potent anaphylotoxin. In addition, it is a chemotactic factor for neutrophils and stimulates the respiratory burst in them and it stimulates inflammatory cytokine production by macrophages. Its activities are controlled by inactivation by carboxypeptidase B (C3-INA).

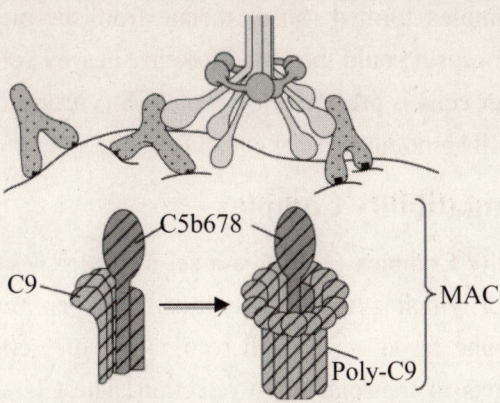

Figure 12.15: MAC and lysis (C5b6789$_n$)

Table 12.7: Complement components and their effects

Fragment	Activity	Effect	Control Factor (s)
C2a	Prokinin, accumulation of fluids	Edema	C1-INH
C3a	Basophil and mast cells degranulation; enhanced vascular permeability, smooth muscle contraction	Anaphylaxis	C3a-INA
C3b	Opsonin, phagocyte activation	Phagocytosis	Factors H and I
C4a	Basophil and mast cells degranulation; enhanced vascular permeability, smooth muscle contraction	Anaphylaxis (least potent)	C3a-INA
C4b	Opsonin	Phagocytosis	C4-BP and Factor I
C5a	Basophil and mast cells degranulation; enhanced vascular permeability, smooth muscle contraction	Anaphylaxis (most potent)	C3a-INA
	Chemotaxis, stimulation of respiratory burst, activation of phagocytes, stimulation of inflammatory cytokines	Inflammation	
C5bC6C7	Chemotaxis	Inflammation	Protein S (vitronectin)
	Attaches to other membranes	Tissue damage	

Some of the C5b67 complex formed can dissociate from the membrane and enter the fluid phase. If this were to occur it could then bind to other nearby cells and lead to their lysis. The damage to bystander cells is prevented by Protein S (vitronectin). Protein S binds to soluble C5b67 and prevents its binding to other cells (Table 12.7).

12.11. Major Histocompatibility Complex

The Major Histocompatibility Complex (MHC) is a set of molecules displayed on cell surfaces that are responsible for lymphocyte recognition and "antigen presentation". The MHC molecules control the immune response through recognition of "self" and "non-self" and, consequently, serve as targets in transplantation rejection. The Class I and Class II MHC molecules belong to a group of molecules known as the Immunoglobulin Supergene Family (Fig. 12.16), which includes immunoglobulins, T-cell receptors, CD4, CD8, and others.

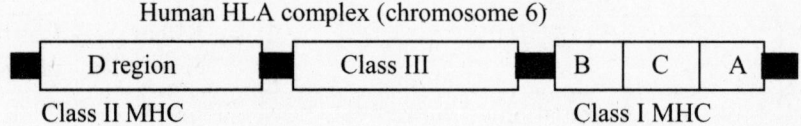

Figure 12.16: Genetic organization of Human HLA complex gene

The major histocompatibility complex is encoded by several genes located on human chromosome 6: Class I molecules are encoded by the BCA region while class II molecules are encoded by the D region. A region between these two on chromosome 6 encodes class III molecules, including some complement components.

Gene products encoded in the Major Histocompatibility Complex (MHC) were first identified as being important in rejection of transplanted tissues. Furthermore, genes in the MHC were found to be highly polymorphic (i.e. in the population there were many different allelic forms of the genes). Studies with inbred strains of mice showed that genes in the MHC were also involved in controlling both humoral and cell-mediated immune responses. For example, some strains of mice could respond to a particular antigen but other strains could not and these strains differed only in one or more of the genes in the MHC. Subsequent studies showed that there were two kinds of molecules encoded by the MHC – Class I molecules and class II molecules. Class I molecules were found on all nucleated cells whereas class II molecules were found only on antigen presenting cells, (APCs) which included dendritic cells, macrophages, B cells and a few other types.

It was not until the discovery of how the T cell receptor (TCR) recognizes antigen that the role of MHC genes in immune responses was understood. The TCR was shown to recognize antigenic peptides in association with MHC molecules. T cells recognize portions of protein antigens that are bound non-covalently to MHC gene products. Cytotoxic T cells (Tc) recognize peptides bound to class I MHC molecules and helper T cells (Th) recognize peptides bound to class II MHC molecules. The mechanism by which the TCR, MHC gene products and antigen interact has been elucidated by the three dimensional structures of MHC molecules and the TCR determined by X-ray crystallography.

12.11.1. Structure of Class I MHC Molecules

Class I molecules are composed of two polypeptide chains; one encoded by the BCA region and another (β2-microglobulin) that is encoded elsewhere. The MHC-encoded polypeptide is about 350 amino acids long and glycosylated, giving a total molecular weight of about 45 kDa. This polypeptide folds into three separate domains called alpha-1, alpha-2 and alpha-3. β2-microglobulin is a 12 kDa polypeptide that is non-covalently associated with the alpha-3 domain. Between the alpha-1 and alpha-2 domains lies a region bounded by a beta-pleated sheet on the bottom and two alpha helices on the sides. This region is capable of binding (via non-covalent interactions) a small peptide of about 10 amino acids. This small peptide is "presented" to a T-cell and defines the antigen "epitope" that the T-cell recognizes.

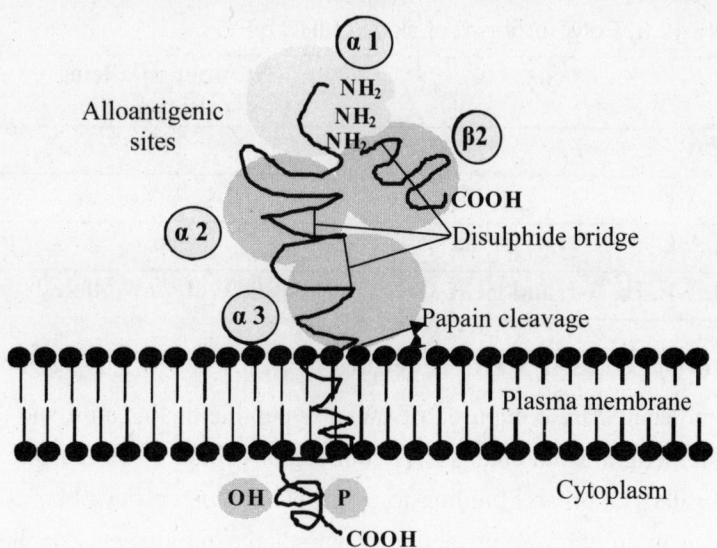

Figure 12.17: The MHC class 1 molecule

Class I MHC molecules are composed of two polypeptide chains, a long α chain and a short β chain called β2-microglobulin. The α chain has four regions. First, a cytoplasmic region, containing sites for phosphoylation and binding to cytoskeletal elements. Second, a transmembrane region containing hydrophic amino acids by which the molecule is anchored in the cell membrane. Third, a highly conserved α3 immunoglubilin-like domain to which CD8 binds. Fourth, a highly polymorphic peptide binding region formed from the α1 and α2 domains. The β2- microglobulin associates with the α chain and helps maintain the proper conformation of the molecule (Fig. 12.17).

The α1 and α2 domains of the class I MHC molecules, which comprise the peptide binding region is found to be the most variable region. The structure of the peptide binding groove, revealed by X-ray crystallography, shows that the groove is composed of two α helices forming a wall on each side and eight β-pleated sheets forming a floor. The peptide is bound in the groove and the residues that line the groove make contact with the peptide. These are the residues that are most polymorphic. The groove will accommodate peptides of approximately 8-10 amino acids long. Whether a particular peptide will bind to the groove will depend on the amino acids that line the groove. Because class I molecules are polymorphic, different class I molecules will bind different peptides. Each class I molecule will bind only certain peptides and will have a set of criteria that a peptide must have in order to bind to the groove. Within the MHC there are 6 genes that encode class I molecules HLA-A, HLA –B, HLA-C, HLA-E, HLA-F and HLA-G. Among these HLA-A, HLA –B, and HLA-C are the most important and also most polymorphic. Table 12.8 shows the degree of polymorphism at each of these loci.

Table 12.8: Polymorphism of class I MHC genes

Locus	Number of alleles (allotypes)
HLA-A	218
HLA-B	439
HLA-C	96
HLA-E, HLA-F and HLA-G	Relatively few alleles

12.11.2. Structure of Class II MHC Molecules

Class II MHC molecules are composed of two polypeptide chains an α and a β chain of approximately equal length. Both chains have four regions: first, a cytoplasmic region containing sites for phosphoylation and binding to cytoskeletal elements; second, a transmembrane region containing hydrophic amino acids by which the molecule is anchored in the cell membrane, third, a highly conserved α2 domain and a highly conserved β2 domain to which CD4 binds and fourth, a highly polymorphic peptide binding region formed from the α1 and β1 domains.

The α1 and β2 domains of the class II MHC molecules, which comprise the peptide binding region are found to be the most variable regions. The structure of the peptide binding groove, revealed by X-ray crystallography, shows that, like class I MHC molecules, the groove is composed of two α helices forming a wall on each side and eight β-pleated sheets forming a floor. Both the α1 and β1 chain contribute to the peptide binding groove. The peptide is bound in the groove and the residues that line the groove make contact with the peptide. These are the residues that are the most polymorphic. The groove of Class II molecules is open at one end so that the groove can accommodate longer peptides of approximately 13-25 amino acids long with some of the amino acids located outside of the groove. Whether a particular peptide will bind to the groove will depend on the amino acids that line the groove. Because class II molecules are polymorphic, different class II molecules will bind different peptides. Like class I molecules, each class II molecule will bind only certain peptides and will have a set of criteria that a peptide must have in order to bind to the groove.

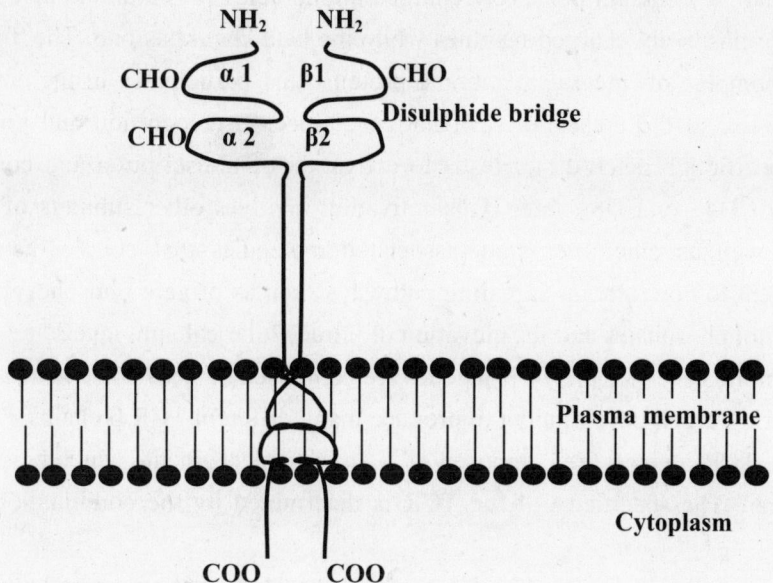

Figure 12.18: MHC class II molecules comprise two non-identical peptides (alpha and beta) which are non-covalently associated and traverse the plasma membrane with the N terminus to the outside of the cell

Within the MHC there are 5 loci that encode class II molecules, each of which contains a gene for an α chain and at least one gene for a β chain. The loci are designated as HLA-DP, HLA-DQ, HLA-DR, HLA-DM, and HLA-DO. Among these, HLA-DP, HLA –DQ, and HLA-DR are the most important and polymorphic in nature.

12.12. Structure of the T cell Receptor (TCR)

The TCR is a heterodimer composed of one α and one β chain of approximately equal length. Each chain has a short cytoplasmic tail but it is too small to be able to transduce an activation signal to the cell. Both chains have a transmembrane region comprised of hydrophobic amino acids by which the molecule is anchored in the cell membrane. Both chains have a constant region and a variable region similar to the immunoglobulin chains. The variable region of both the chains contains hypervariable regions that determine the specificity for antigen. Each T cell bears a TCR of only one specificity (*i.e.* there is allelic exclusion). The T cell receptor heterodimer comprises of two transmembrane glycoproteins, the alpha and beta chains. There are two domains in the external part of each chain and these resemble immunoglobulin variable and constant regions. There are sugar chains on each domain. There is a short sequence similar to the immunoglobulin hinge region that connects the immunoglobulin-like domains to the transmembrane sequence. This contains cysteines that form a disulfide bridge. The hydrophobic transmembrane helical structures are unusual in that they contain positively charged amino acids (basic amino acids). The alpha chain has two positively charged residues while the beta chain has one. The T cell receptor (TCR) is a complex of integral membrane proteins that participates in the activation of T cells in response to the presentation of antigen. Specific recognition and binding by the clonotype-specific a/b heterodimer leads to activation of transcription and commitment of the T cell to CD4+ or CD8+ fate. This activation involves other subunits of the receptor complex as well as other membrane-associated molecules that couple the extracellular liganding event to downstream signaling pathways such as protein phosphorylation, the release of inositol phosphates and the elevation of intracellular calcium levels.

The germline genes for the TCR β genes are composed of V, D and J gene segments that rearrange during T cell development to produce many different TCR β chains. The germline genes for the TCR α genes are composed of V and J gene segments which rearrange to produce α chains. The specificity of the TCR is determined by the combination of α and β chains.

There is a small population of T cells that express TCRs that have γ and δ chains instead of α and β chains. These gamma/delta T cells predominate in the mucosal epithelium and have a repertoire biased toward certain bacterial and viral antigens. The genes for the δ chains have V, D and J gene segments whereas the genes for the γ chains have only V and J gene segments but the repertoire is considerably smaller than that of the alpha/beta T cells. The γ/δ T cells recognize antigen in an MHC-independent manner unlike the α/β T cells.

GENES		
Properties	**Ig**	**TCR**
Many VDJs, Few C's	Yes	Yes
VDJ Rearrangement	Yes	Yes
V pairs form antigen-recognition site	Yes	Yes
Somatic hypermutation	Yes	No

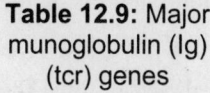

Table 12.9: Major munoglobulin (Ig) (tcr) genes

properties of im- and t-cell receptor

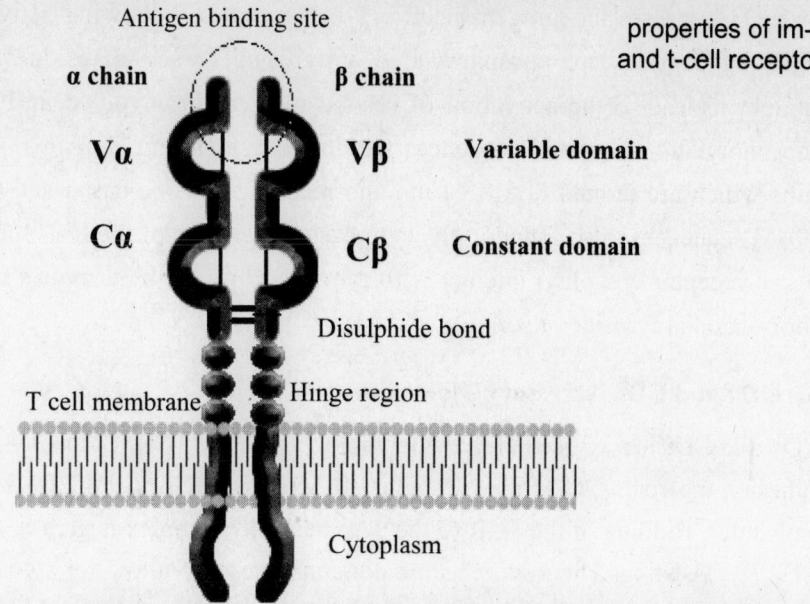

Figure 12.19: Structure of T-Cell receptor

(i) TCR and CD3 Complex

The TCR is closely associated with a group of 5 proteins collectively called CD3 complex. The CD3 complex is composed of one γ, one δ, two ε and 2 ξ chains. The CD3 is actually a complex of 5 polypeptides. Gamma, delta, and epsilon occur as 2 dimers [gamma-epsilon and delta-epsilon] complexed with either a homodimer of two zeta chains or a heterodimer of zeta and eta chains. Zeta and eta are encoded by the same gene and only differ in their carboxyl terminus. The two forms are generated by differential RNA splicing of the primary transcript. All of the proteins of the CD3 complex are invariant and they do not contribute to the specificity in any way. The CD 3 complex is necessary for cell surface expression of the TCR during T cell development. In addition, the CD3 complex transduces activation signals to the cell following antigen interaction with the TCR.

Short length of the cytoplasmic tail of the alpha & beta chains suggests that they are unsuitable for signal transduction. CD3 functions in this regard. The TcR exists on the membrane as a molecular complex with CD3. Mutation in either the CD3 or the TcR results in loss of the entire complex from the membrane. The transmembrane domain of all CD3 polypeptides contains a –ve charged aspartic acid. Correspondingly, there are either 1 or 2 + charged amino acids in the transmembrane domain of each TcR chain. The alpha chain contains a lysine and an arginine while the beta chain contains a single lysine. Once the TcR recognizes an antigen-MHC complex, the associated CD3 complex is thought to transmit a signal to the cell interior that contributes to cellular activation. Monoclonal antibody specific for CD3 bypasses the antigen-specific T cell receptor. Following activation, several of the CD3 polypeptides are phosphorylated at tyrosine or serine residues. Phosphorylation is thought to lead to the activation of second messengers involved in T cell activation. The phosphorylation occurs at sequences within the cytoplasmic domains of the CD3 glycoproteins which are termed ITAMS (immuno-receptor tyrosine-based activation motifs). These ITAM sequences (also found in the cytoplasmic domains of the Iga / Igb heterodimers of the B cell receptor complex) interact with tyrosine kinases (the enzymes which catalyze phosphorylation at tyrosine or serine).

(ii) CD4 and CD8 Accessory Molecules

CD4 and CD8 are associated in the membrane with the TCR. Both CD4 and CD8 function as adhesion molecules; CD4 binds to Class II MHC molecules and CD8 binds to Class I MHC molecules. Binding of the TCR to the peptide/MHC complex is greatly augmented if CD4 or CD8 are assisting. Their cytoplasmic domains may also allow for signal transduction to occur. The signal-transduction property of CD4 and CD8 is mediated through their cytoplasmic domains. Both CD4 and CD8 are noncovalently associated with the protein kinase Lck.

Variety of other membrane molecules plays an important accessory role in antigen recognition and T cell activation. In addition to CD4 and CD8, T cells possess several other accessory molecules including LFA-1 and CD28. LFA-1 is an adhesion molecule which strengthens the interaction of the T cell with an APC or target cell. LFA-1 is an integrin which binds to ICAM-1 (inter-cell adhesion molecule on the APC or target cell. CD28 on Th cell binds to B7 on an APC or target cell. This interaction functions as a co-stimulatory signal leading to activation of the T lymphocyte. Without this co-stimulatory signal, the T lymphocyte experiences anergy (non-responsive, basically the opposite of activation).

The interactions between the TCR and MHC molecules are not very strong. Accessory molecules are necessary to help stabilize the interaction. These include: 1) CD4 binding to Class II MCH, ensures that Th cells only interact with APCs; 2) CD8 binding to class I MHC, which ensures that Tc cells can interact with target cells; 3) CD2binding to LFA-3 and 4) LFA-1 binding to ICAM-1. The accessory molecules are invariant and do not contribute to the specificity of the interaction, which is solely determined by the TCR. The expression of accessory molecules can be increased in response to cytokine, which is one way that cytokines can modulate immune responses. In addition to accessory molecules which help stabilize the interaction between the TCR and antigen in association with MHC molecules, other molecules are also needed for T cell activation. Two signals are required for T cell activation; one is the engagement of the TCR with Ag/MHC and the other signal comes from the engagement of co-stimulatory molecules with their ligands. One of the most important (but not the only) co-stimulatory molecule is CD28 on T cells which must interact with B7-1 (CD80) or B7-2 (CD81) on APCs. Like accessory molecules the co-stimulatory molecules are invariant and do not contribute to the specificity of the interaction. The multiple interactions of TCR with Ag/MHC and the accessory and co-stimulatory molecules with their ligands have been termed the "immunological synapse."

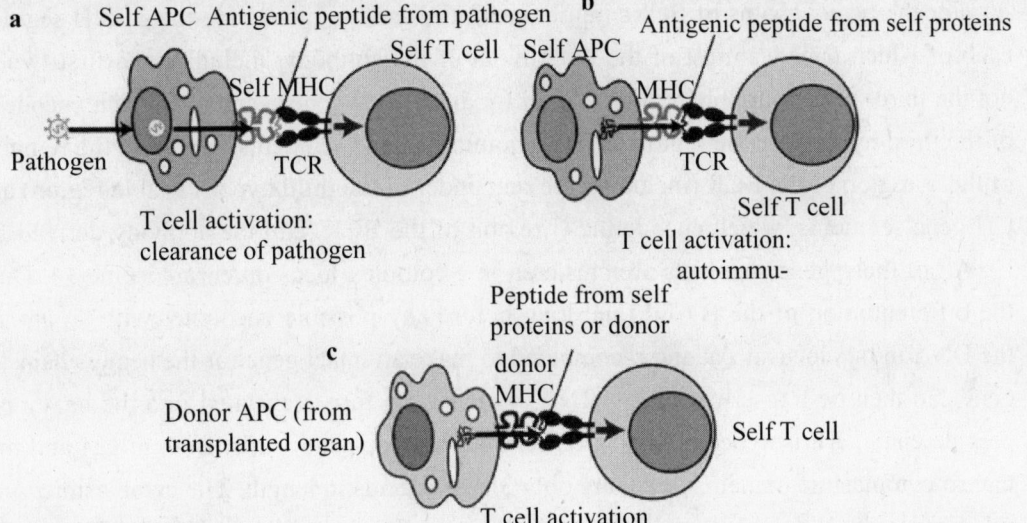

Figure 12.20: Three consequences of T cells recognizing antigenic peptides presented by major histocompatibility complex

There are three consequences of T cells recognizing antigenic peptides presented by major histocompatibility complex (MHC) molecules on antigen-presenting cells (a) During an infection, T cells recognize antigenic peptide fragments of the pathogen that are presented on the surface of MHC molecules. This recognition is mediated by the T-cell receptor (TCR) and stabilized by additional cell-surface molecules (b) The nature of T-cell development means that potentially self-reactive T cells are produced that can respond to self MHC molecules, even in the absence of infection. (c) In transplantation, T-cell activation in response to foreign (allogeneic) MHC molecules on the surface of donor antigen-presenting cells (APCs) induces destructive immune responses (Fig. 12.20).

12.13. B- Cell Receptor

B-Lymphocytes and T-Lymphocytes are the most abundant lymphocytes. B-Cells are produced and mature in the bone marrow and are specific for a particular antigen. The specificity of binding resides in the BCR (B-Cell receptor) for antigen. They are integral membrane proteins. They are present in thousands of identical copies exposed at the cell surface. They are made before the cell ever encounters an antigen. B-Cell receptor complex usually consist of an antigen-binding subunit (the membrane immunoglobulin or MIg), which is composed of two IgHs (Immunoglobulin Heavy Chains) and two IgLs (Immunoglobulin Light Chains), and a signaling subunit, which is a disulfide-linked heterodimer of Ig-Alpha (CD79A) and Ig -Beta (CD79B) proteins.

For the heavy chains of BCRs (antibodies), the gene segments are the 51 VH segments, each of which encodes most of the N-terminal of the antibody, including the first two (but not the third) hyper variable region, 25 DH (="diversity") gene segments, which encode part of the third hyper variable region, 6 JH (="joining") gene segments, encoding the remainder of the V region of the BCR (including the remainder of the third hyper variable region) and 9 CH gene segments, which encode the C region of the BCR (and the antibody derived from it). All of these gene segments are clustered in a complex locus on chromosome 14. During the differentiation of the B-Cell (and long before any possible encounter with an antigen), the DNA in this locus is cut and recombined to make an intact gene for the heavy chain. This gene can then be transcribed into mRNA, which is, in turn, translated into the heavy poly-peptide chain. All isotypes of mIg have very short cytoplasmic tails. Both mIgM and mIgD have a cytoplasmic domain, which are only 3 amino acids in length. The cytoplasmic tails of mIg are too short to be able to associate with intracellular signaling molecules. Since mIg is always associated with the Ig-alpha/Ig-beta heterodimer collectively forming B-Cell receptor complex (BCR), two molecules of this heterodimer associate with one mIg to form a single BCR. The Ig-alpha/Ig-beta heterodimer carries out the signal transducing function of the complex. The Ig-alpha chain has a long cytoplasmic domain containing 61 amino acids while the Ig-beta chain has a long cytoplasmic domain containing 48 amino acids.

BCR have a unique binding site. This site binds to a portion of the antigen called an anti-genic determinant or epitope. The binding depends on complementarity of the surface of the receptor and the surface of the epitope. The binding occurs by non-covalent forces. In the absence of specific antigen, mature B-Cells survive in the peripheral circulation for only a few days. Cells which do not encounter antigen within this period of time undergo apoptosis. This is necessary in order to maintain an optimal circulation of B-lymphocytes in the periph-eral circulation. The receptor on the cell surface of B-lymphocytes functions to transmit in-tracellular signals that regulate cell growth and differentiation and it binds to antigen for the generation of the immune response.

Most B-Cell antigens are T dependent. In other words, the B-Cell requires direct contact by T$_H$ lymphocytes as well as exposure to T$_H$ lymphocyte cytokines in order to be fully acti-vated. There are a few T independent antigens. One of the best-known examples of a T independent antigen is LPS (Lipopolysaccharide). At low concentrations, LPS stimulates the production of specific antibodies (LPS-specific) but at high concentrations it can cause the polyclonal activation of B-Cells. The polyclonal activation of B-Cells leads to the proliferation and differentiation of large numbers of B-Cells, regardless of their antigen specificity.

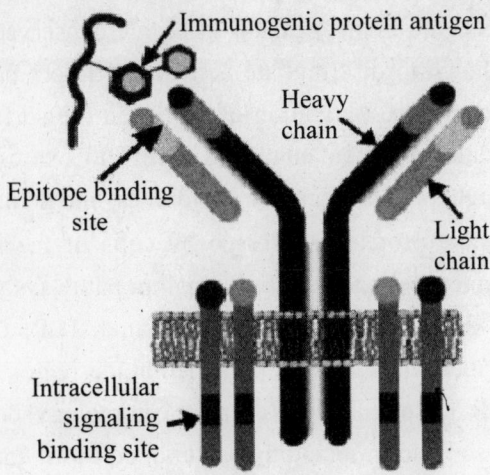

Figure 12.21: B cell receptor

12.14. Toll-Like Receptors and Innate Immunity

The ability of the host organism to discriminate between infectious nonself and self is essential for identification and for the fight against invading pathogens, thus allowing it to survive in an environment heavily populated with infectious agents. In response to this challenge, multicellular organisms have evolved several distinct immune-recognition systems. In vertebrate animals, these systems can be broadly categorized as 'innate' and 'adaptive'. Both components of immunity recognize invading microorganisms as non-self, which triggers immune responses to eliminate them. To date, both components have been characterized independently, and the main research interest in the immunology field has been confined to the acquired immunity. In acquired immunity, B and T lymphocytes utilize antigen receptors such as immunoglobulins and T cell receptors to recognize non-self. The mechanisms by which these antigen receptors recognize foreign antigens have been intensively analyzed, and the major mechanisms, such as diversity, clonality and memory, have been well characterized.

The adaptive immune response depends on B and T lymphocytes which are specific for particular antigens. This system involves clonal selection of antibody producing B cells to respond to foreign antigens, and works well, but has a major limitation in that it takes from 4 to 7 days to ramp up. In that time period, pathogens could overwhelm the organism. In contrast, the innate immune system is immediately available to combat threats. There is no memory to responds to the same threat upon the second or third exposure. Instead, the innate immune system responds to common structures shared by a vast majority of threats. These common structures are called pathogen associated molecular patterns, or PAMPs, and are recognized by the toll-like receptors. In addition to the cellular TLRs, an important part of the innate immune system is the humoral complement system that opsonizes and kills pathogens through the PAMP recognition mechanism. TLRs are conserved molecules, cloned initially in *Drosophila* and shown to discriminate between different pathogens and induce an appropriate antimicrobial response. Activation of TLRs on the surface of the immune and epithelial cells is accompanied by their enhanced ability to express co-stimulatory molecules, present antigens, secrete pro-inflammatory cytokines, and mediate microbial killing.

TLRs are transmembrane proteins expressed by cells of the innate immune system, which recognize invading microbes and activate signaling pathways that launch immune and inflammatory responses to destroy the invaders. Mammalian TLRs consist of an extracellular portion containing leucine-rich repeats, a transmembrane region and a cytoplasmic tail, called the TIR (Toll-IL-1R (Interleukin-1-Receptor)) homology domain. Different TLRs serve as receptors for diverse ligands, including bacterial cell wall components, viral double-stranded RNA and small-molecule such as anti-viral or immunomodulatory compounds. Activation of TLRs occurs after binding of a cognate ligand to the extracellular leucine-rich repeats portion of the TLR. In humans, TLR1, 2,4,5 and 6 are outer membrane associated, and respond primarily to bacterial surface associated PAMPs. The second group, TLR3,7,8 and 9 are found on the surface of endosomes, where they respond primarily to nucleic acid based PAMPs from viruses and bacteria. Upon binding with their cognates, TLRs activate two major signaling pathways. The core pathway utilized by most TLRs leads to activation of the transcription factor NF-κ B (Nuclear Factor-κ B) and the MAPKs (Mitogen-Activated Protein Kinases) p38 and JNK (c-Jun N-termal Kinase). The second pathway involves TLR3 and TLR4 and leads to the activation of both NF-κB and another transcription factor IRF3 (Interferon Regulatory Factor-3), allowing for an additional set of genes to be induced, including anti-viral genes such as IFN-β (Interferon-Beta) and others. The innate immune response is a complex set of interactions that have evolved to optimize the response to pathogens. While the structure of the TLRs has been highly conserved, the innate immune response for each organism has selectively been driven to protect against the pathogens found in the host's environment.

12.14.1. TLRs and Ligands

TLRs recognize the specific microbial patterns. Since the last decade there has been a steady increase in the number of TLR family members and their ligands (Table 12.10). Most of the ligand studies are based on the knockout mice. Different TLRs seem to play crucial roles in the activation of the immune response to PAMPs.

TLR1

TLR1, the first member of the TLR family, was identified by the presence of a domain homology found in both *Drosophila* Toll and human IL-1 receptors. TLR1 is expressed at higher levels in the spleen and peripheral blood cells. No direct ligands have been identified so far for TLR1, and its function remains unclear. TLR1 seems to act as a co-receptor. TLR1 was shown to associate with TLR2 in response to triacylated lipopeptides, but not diacylated lipopeptides. These observations indicate that TLR1 is able to discriminate among lipoproteins by recognizing the lipid configuration.

TLR2 and TLR 6

TLR2 has been shown to be involved in the recognition of a broad range of microbial products, including: peptidoglycan from Gram-positive bacteria, bacterial lipoproteins, mycobacterial cell-wall lipoarabinomannan, glycosylphosphatidylinositol lipid from *Trypanosoma Cruzi*, a phenol-soluble modulin produced by *Staphylococcus epidermidis*, and yeast cell walls. This unusually broad range of ligands recognized by TLR2 is explained, in part, by cooperation between TLR2 and at least two other TLRs: TLR1 and TLR6. So, the formation of heterodimers between TLR2 and either TLR1 or TLR6 dictates the specificity of ligand recognition. Thus, TLR2 recognizes a wide range of microbial products through functional cooperation with several proteins that are either structurally related or unrelated. For example, TLR2 cooperates with TLR6 for the recognition of mycoplasmal macrophage-activating lipopeptide 2 kDa (MALP-2). Interestingly, it is TLR6 that discriminates between bacterial lipoproteins, which are triacylated at the amino-terminal cysteine residue, and the diacylated mycoplasmal lipoprotein MALP-2.

TLR 3

TLR3 recognizes double-stranded RNA (dsRNA), a molecular pattern associated with viral infection. Expression of human TLR3 in the double-stranded RNA (dsRNA)-non-responsive cell line 293 confers enhanced activation of NF-κB in response to dsRNA. In addition, TLR3 -deficient mice are impaired in their response to dsRNA. dsRNA is produced by most viruses during their replication and induces the synthesis of type I interferons (IFN-/αß), which exert anti-viral and immunostimulatory activities. Thus, TLR3 is implicated in the recognition of dsRNA and viruses.

TLR4

TLR4 is the principal LPS receptor. LPS, a major component of the outer membrane of Gram-negative bacteria is composed of polysaccharides extending outward from the bacterial cell surface and a lipid portion, lipid A, which is embedded in the cell surface. LPS can provoke a variety of immunostimulatory responses; for example, production of proinflammatory cytokines such as IL-12 and inflammatory effector substances such as nitric oxide. Lipid A portion of LPS is mainly responsible for its biological activities. LPS can cause a clinically life-threatening condition called endotoxin shock. In addition to TLR4, a glycosylphosphatidylinositol anchoring protein, CD14, has been identified that facilitates LPS action by binding and retaining LPS on the cell surface.

Table 12.10: Receptors and ligands of TCR

Receptor	Ligand(s)	Ligand location
TLR 1	multiple triacyl lipopeptides	Bacteria
TLR 2	multiple glycolipids	Bacteria
	multiple lipopeptides	
	multiple lipoproteins	
	lipoteichoic acid	
	HSP70	Host cells
	zymosan (Beta-glucan)	Fungi
TLR 3	double-stranded RNA, poly I:C	viruses
TLR 4	lipopolysaccharide	Gram-negative bacteria
	several heat shock proteins	Bacteria and host cells
	fibrinogen	host cells
	heparan sulfate fragments	host cells
	hyaluronic acid fragments	host cells
TLR 5	flagellin	Bacteria
TLR 6	multiple diacyl lipopeptides	Mycoplasma
TLR 7	imidazoquinoline	small synthetic compounds
	loxoribine (a guanosine analogue)	
	bropirimine	
	single-stranded RNA	
TLR 8	small synthetic compounds; single-stranded RNA	
TLR 9	unmethylated CpG Oligodeoxynucleotide DNA	Bacteria

TLR 5

TLR5 recognizes flagellin from both Gram-positive and Gram-negative bacteria. Flagellin is the monomeric subunit of bacterial flagella. Flagellin shows potent pro-inflammatory activity by inducing expression of IL-8. TLR5 was identified by the presence of the TIR domain and is expressed in the spleen, peripheral blood leukocytes and epithelial cells. Enforced expression of human TLR5 in CHO cells confers response to flagellin, a monomeric constituent of bacterial flagella. TLR5 has further been shown to recognize an evolutionarily conserved domain of flagellin through close physical interaction between TLR5 and flagellin. TLR5 is expressed on the basolateral, but not the apical side of intestinal epithelial cells. TLR5 expression is also observed in the intestinal endothelial cells of the subepithelial compartment.

TLR7 and TLR8

TLR7 and TLR8 are structurally highly conserved proteins, and recognize the same ligand in some cases. Analysis of TLR7-deficient mice revealed that murine TLR7 recognize synthetic compounds, imidazoquinolines, which are clinically used for treatment of genital warts associated with viral infection. Human TLR7 and TLR8, but not murine TLR8, recognizes imidazoquinoline compounds. Murine TLR7 has also been shown to recognize another synthetic compound, loxoribine, which has anti-viral and anti-tumor activities. Both imidazoquinoline and loxoribine are structurally related to guanosine nucleoside.

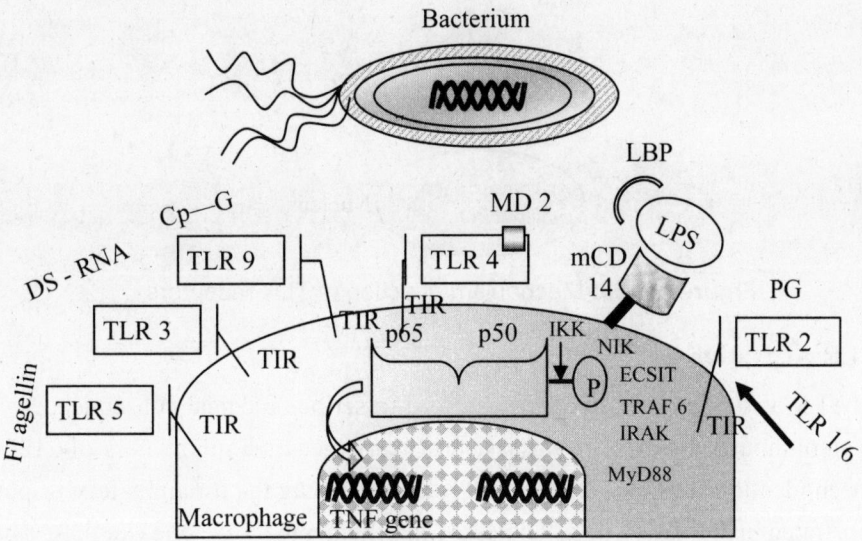

Figure 12.22: The human Toll-like receptors and their known ligands. CpG, cytosine-phosphoryl-quanine; ECSIT, evolutionarily conserved signaling intermediate of Toll; IκB, inhibitory kappaB; IKK, IκB inducing kinase; IRAK, IL-1 receptor associated kinase; LBP-lipopolysaccharide-binding protein; LPS, lipopolysaccharide; MyD88, myeloid differentiation factor 88; NF-κB, nuclear factor-κ for B cells; NIK, NF-κB inducing kinase; PG, peptidoglycan; TIR, Toll IL-1 receptor domain; TRAF6, Tumor necrosis factor receptor associated factor-6

TLR9

TLR9, which is localized intracellularly, is involved in the recognition of specific unmethylated CpG-ODN sequences that distinguishes bacterial DNA from mammalian DNA. CpG oligodeoxynucleotides (or CpG ODN) are short single stranded synthetic DNA molecules that contain a cytosine "C" followed by a guanine "G". The "p" refers to the phosphodiester backbone of DNA, however some ODN have a modified phosphorothioate (PS) backbone. Bacterial DNA can stimulate immune cells. This activity is mainly because of the unmethylated CpG motifs, which are rarely detected in vertebrate DNA and, if present, are highly methylated. This stimulation leads to the production of Th1 (T helper 1) cytokines and co-stimulatory molecule upregulation.

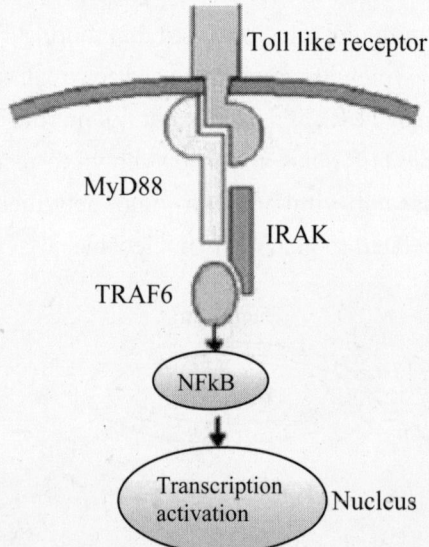

Figure 12. 23: Mechanism of action of TLR receptors

12.14.2: TLR Activation

Unchecked TLR activation by pathogens can lead to serious medical consequences, such as sepsis and autoimmune diseases. In the last few years, negative modulators of TLR activation have been identified, and their important role in reducing the inflammatory response has been demonstrated in animal models. The TAM family members are one example. The TAM (Tyro3/Axl/Mer) family has been found to be central to the fine tuning of the TLR response. Loss of function of the three members of this family (Tyro3/Axl/Mer) in a triple knockout mouse results in a profound disregulation of the immune response. This includes massive splenomegaly and lymphadenopathy, lymphocyte infiltration into all tissues, and high levels of autoimmunity. Even a single knockout of just Mcr is sufficient to elevate susceptibility to

LPS induced shock via the TLR4 signaling. These mice have elevated levels of dendritic cells, and the cells express elevated levels of activation markers, including MHC class II antigens. This effect was not restricted to TLR4, as hypersensitivity to the TLR3 activator polyIC was also observed.

Figure 12.23 shows how TLR receptor works. Recognition of an appropriate ligand (for example, lipopolysaccharide) triggers the Toll-like receptor to recruit MyD88. MyD88 interacts with the Toll-like receptor through its own Toll/IL-1 receptor domain and in turn engages the serine-threonine kinase IRAK though a death domain. Signal transduction factors such as TRAF6 carry the signal through a series of phosphorylations until NFκB is ultimately released to the nucleus where it can activate the transcription of appropriate genes.

12.15. Antigens

Antigen could be any substance that when introduced into the body stimulates the production of an antibody. Antigens include toxins, bacteria, foreign blood cells, and the cells of transplanted organs. Based on the immunological properties, antigens can be categorized as immunogenic, antigenic, allergenic and tolerogenic. Immunogenic substances are those which can induce a humoral or cell-mediated immune response.

$$B \text{ cells} + \text{antigen} \rightarrow \text{plasma cells} + \text{memory cells}$$

$$T \text{ cells} + \text{antigen} \rightarrow T \text{ effector cells} + \text{memory cells}$$

In contrast, some small molecules referred to as haptens are not capable by themselves of inducing a specific immune response. In simple terms, they lack immunogenicity. In order to induce immune response, the hapten requires to be attached to a carrier molecule (usually a serum protein such as albumin). The hapten molecule then acts as a determinant of antigenic specificity and is referred to as an antigenic determinant. Classical haptens include di- and trinitrophenol (DNP and TNP), dimethyl aminonaphthalene sulfonate (dansyl), and a number of toxins, including urushiol, which is the toxin found in poison ivy. Carriers are macromolecules that bind haptens and enable them to induce an immune response. Most carriers are secretory proteins or proteins on the cell surface, where cells of the immune system can reach them. First, step in the induction of immune response by a hapten is binding to its carrier. The carrier, normally ignored by the immune system now has a different surface structure that can act as an antigen (the hapten on its own is too small). Depending on the type of immune cell that recognizes the antigen, two pathways can be distinguished: a) The B-cell mediated pathway. It leads to the production of immunoglobulins against the hapten-carrier compound. A great variety of haptens and carriers have been shown to act this way. b) The T-cell mediated pathway. It leads to cytotoxic T-cell activity and to the recruitment of inflammatory cells. Usually, the carrier is a MHC molecule recognized by the T-cell receptor. In contact dermatitis, a well-resolved subgroup of this pathway, the haptens travel a long way with Langerhans cells before being checked by T cells in the lymphatic system.

Allergenic substances are those which have the ability to induce various types of allergic responses. Allergens are immunogens that tend to activate specific types of humoral or cell-mediated responses. Tolerogenic substances are those which can induce specific immunologic non-responsiveness in either the humoral or cell-mediated branch.

12.16. Mitogens

Mitogens are agents that can induce cell division in a high percentage of T or B cells. Unlike immunogens, which activate only lymphocytes bearing specific receptors, mitogens activate many clones of T or B cells regardless of their antigen specificity. Because of this ability, mitogens are known as polyclonal activators. Various diverse agents function as mitogens. Many common mitogens are proteins (called lectins) that are derived from plants and bind sugars. Lectins recognize different glycoproteins on the surface of various cells, including lymphocytes. Their binding often leads to agglutination, or clustering of the cells, followed by cellular activation. Some mitogens preferentially activate B cells, others activate T cells, and some activate both. Three commonly used lectins with mitogenic activity are concanavalin A (Con A), phyto-hemagglutinin (PHA) and pokeweed mitogen. Each of these binds to carbohydrate residues in glycoproteins and is able to crosslink glycoproteins on the surface of cells. The lipopolysaccharide (LPS) component of the gram-negative bacterial cell wall functions as a B-cell mitogen, Con A and PHA are T-cell mitogens, while pokeweed mitogen acts as both. Among the group of T cell mitogens, an unusual group of substances, known as superantigens, is found to be most potent.

12.17. Immunomodulating Substances

A variety of substances, when used as adjuvants, in combination with specific vaccines, enhance immunity levels above those which the vaccine elicits by itself, Agar, tapioca, lecithin, and some other substances show this potentiating effect. Certain peptides of animal origin are potent stimulants (or adjuvants) of the immune system whereas others act as inhibitors and in some cases the same peptide stimulates under certain conditions and on the contrary inhibits under other conditions the immune response. These peptides with dual function are called immunomodulators. Good examples of immunomodulator peptides include interferon, interleukin, muramyl peptides of microbial origin (e.g., murabutide and lipopeptides which attack phagocytic cells and T-lymphocytes), several peptides of animal origin, including thymic hormones (e.g., thymulin promotes many T-cell functions and inhibits the generation of cytotoxic T-lymphocytes), tuftsin (stimulates phagocytic cells, pinocytosis, phagocytosis, motility, and antigen processing), peptides derived from fibrinogen, and certain peptides from colostrums and from milk. Furthermore, some neuropeptides (neuroendocrine hormones) are thought to play an essential role as chemo signals from the central nervous system to the immune system. Somatostatin is a tetradecapeptide, isolated from the hypothalamus that inhibit the secretion of growth hormone. It is present in neural and gastrointestinal tissues and can also inhibit secretion from several endocrine and exocrine glands. Specific functional receptors for a variety of neuropeptides have been demonstrated in diverse cell populations of the immune system.

12.18. Vaccines

Recent advances in immunology have led to the development of new and promising vaccine strategies. Knowledge of differences in epitopes recognized by T cells and B cells has enabled immunologists to design vaccines to maximize activation of the humoral or cell-mediated branch of the immune system. Genetic engineering techniques facilitate development of vaccines which maximize the immune response to selected epitopes. Table 12.11 indicates some currently used vaccines.

Vaccines work by priming the immune system to swiftly destroy the disease causing agents before they can multiply enough to cause symptoms. To date, this priming has been achieved by presenting the immune system with whole viruses or bacteria that have been killed or attenuated (made too weak to proliferate much). The immune system responds to this vaccine as if it was under attack by a fully potent antagonist and mobilizes its forces to destroy the foreign body. Memory cells are then left behind on alert, ready to unleash whole armies of defenders if the real pathogen ever finds its way into the body.

Classical vaccines pose a small risk in that the killed or attenuated microorganism may sometimes spring back to life, causing the disease the vaccine was meant to prevent. For this reason, 'subunit' vaccines (which contain no genes, just proteins derived from them) are now favored since they reduce this risk. They are, however, often not as effective as live vaccines. Subunit vaccines are also expensive, because they are produced in cultures of bacteria or animal cells and have to be purified and refrigerated.

Many researchers hope to develop edible vaccines which are similar to subunit preparations, containing only the genes coding for certain antigens, not the whole virus or bacterium. One main hurdle to be overcome here is that the antigens could be degraded in the stomach before having time to act. Typical subunit vaccines have to be delivered by injection precisely because of this. Researchers working on an edible hepatitis B vaccine suggest that oral doses may need to be 10-100 times higher than an injectable dose to elicit a comparable immune response.

One of the aims of the edible vaccine proponents is to reduce immunization costs. They feel that edible vaccines would be far cheaper than current injectable vaccines since they would not have to undergo the expensive purification and refrigeration of traditional vaccines, and shipping costs may be less. However, shipping costs may not necessarily be significantly reduced, and edible vaccines may still require refrigeration. Even if edible vaccines are cheaper, it does not follow that this will lead to increased vaccination coverage, since the cost of the vaccine is only a small part of the whole package.

Table 12.11: Classification of commonly used vaccines

Disease	Type of vaccine
Whole organism	
Bacterial cells	
Tuberculosis	Attenuated
Cholera	Inactivated
Viral particles	
Polio (Sabin)	Attenuated
Influenza	Inactivated
Mumps	Attenuated
Purified Macromolecules	
Toxoids	
Diphtheria	Inactivated exotoxin
Tetanus	Inactivated exotoxin
Capsular polysaccharide	
H. influenza type b	Polysaccharide + protein
S. pneumoniae	23 distinct capsular polysaccharides
N. meningitis	Polysaccharide

Producing stable and reliable amounts of vaccines in plants is complicated by the fact that tomatoes and bananas do not come in standard sizes. In many developing countries, stringent quality control for standard drugs do not exist. People could ingest too much of the vaccine, which could be toxic, or too little — which could lead to disease outbreaks among populations believed to be immune. Oral vaccines are also more difficult to formulate than injectables (for example, the oral polio vaccine is more convenient but less effective than the injectable one). The vaccines are likely to need cofactors (adjuvants) such as cholera toxin to enhance their uptake and increase their effectiveness; in addition, new vaccines have to be tested worldwide, since their effectiveness is not uniform in different contexts.

12.19. The Ideal Vaccine

An ideal vaccine should be safe, efficacious, cheap, easily administrable (e.g. orally), and thermally stable. It should confer long-term immunity. A single vaccine should preferably protect against several locally important infectious diseases, i.e. should be multivalent. Some of the currently available viral vaccines meet many of these requirements. The efficacy of a vaccine depends primarily upon the nature and persistence of the induced immune response. Some understanding has come from the study of model viral-host systems, such as the *murine influenza* model. Four stages are readily identified and include (1) prevention of infection, (2) limitation of viral replication, (3) recovery from infection, and (4) generation of memory cells.

Vaccines function by stimulating adaptive immune response. They are usually administered before exposure to the wild-type agent has occurred. The time interval may be weeks, months or years. The vaccine should stimulate B-cells, T-helper (Th) cells, and Tc cells. In the case of an antigenically stable infectious agent, neutralizing antibody is the immune parameter of most importance.

The four requirements of an ideal vaccine are: (1) activation of antigen-presenting cells to initiate antigen processing and production of interleukins; (2) activation of both T- and B-cells to give a high yield of memory cells; (3) due generation of antibody to two or three B-cell epitopes and of Th and Tc cells to several epitopes; and (4) persistence of antigen, probably mainly on follicular dendritic cells in lymphoid tissue resulting in the continuing presence of antibody.

Suggested Readings

- Roitt I, Brostoff J and Male D (1989). Immunology. J.B. Lippincott Co.

- Thomas J. Kindt, Richard A. Goldsby, Barbara Anne Osborne, Janis Kuby (2007). Kuby Immunology

- Nandini Shetty (2007). Immunology. New age international publications

- Mosmann TR and Coffman RL (1989). TH1 and TH2 cells: Different patterns of lymphokine secretion lead to different functional properties. Annual Review of Immunology 7; 145-173

- Yarchoan R, Mitsuya H and Broder S (1993). Challenges in the therapy of HIV infection. Immunology Today 14: 303-309.

Immunology - Pioneers

Ehrlich had hit upon the key concept that the body produces substances, which we today call antibodies, to help in the destruction of invaders, while Mechnikov had discovered that certain body cells could destroy pathogens by simply engulfing or "eating" them. We now know that the incredibly complex immune system mounts attacks in both of these ways. It's entirely fitting, therefore, that Ilya Mechnikov and Paul Ehrlich shared the 1908 Nobel Prize in Physiology or Medicine in recognition of their work on immunity.

Ilya Mechnikov and the Phagocyte Cells

In 1882, the Russian scientist Ilya Mechnikov was working in Messina, Italy, studying the larvae of the sea star. When he inserted a thorn into a larva, something weird happened. Mechnikov noticed strange cells gathering at the point of insertion. The cells surrounded the thorn, eating any foreign substances that entered through the ruptured skin. Mechnikov was thrilled. He decided to name these new cells phagocytes from the Greek words meaning "devouring cells."

The discovery of the phagocyte cells was very important since it helped scientists understand the concept of immunity and how the body defends itself against disease. If the phagocyte cells come upon anything alien, they absorb it and destroy it. The phagocytes also play an important role in activating the rest of the immune system

Paul Ehrlich and the Side-chain Theory

At the end of the nineteenth century, the German scientist Paul Ehrlich proposed the "side-chain theory" to explain immunity and how antibodies were formed. Although we now know that some of his ideas were incorrect, this theory allowed him to accomplish important work and provided the groundwork for later researchers in this field.

Ehrlich argued that all cells have a wide variety of special receptors that he called side-chains. He thought that these receptors worked like gatekeepers or locks for the cell. Each receptor/side-chain had a unique structure, and only substances matching this structure were allowed to enter the cell.

The side-chain receptors' primary function was to absorb nutrients for the cell. Unfortunately, the receptors also allowed many toxic substances to enter. According to Ehrlich, the body defended itself against these toxins in the following way: When a cell was attacked by a toxin, it started to produce excess side-chains matching the toxin. These excess side-chains then were released, flooding the body and neutralizing free toxins by attaching to them. The toxin was wiped out and remaining healthy cells protected.

CHAPTER 13

Instrumentation in Cell Biology

- Microscopy
- History of Microscope
- Light Microscopy
- Brightfeild Microscopy
- Darkfield Microscopy
- Phase Contrast Microscopy
- The Fluorescence Microscope
- Electron Microscope
  - TEM
  - SEM
- Centrifugation
- Cell Fractionation
- Chromatography

- Spectroscopy
  - UV-Visible Spectroscopy
  - IR Spectroscopy
- NMR Spectroscopy
- Mass Spectroscopy
- Electrophoresis
- Blotting Techniques
  - Western Blotting
  - Southern blotting
  - Northern Blotting
- ELISA
- Polymerase Chain Reaction (PCR)
- Flow Cytometry

Biophysics is that branch of knowledge that applies the principles of physics and chemistry and the methods of mathematical analysis and computer modeling to understand how biological systems work. A technique is a procedure used to accomplish a specific activity or task. In the present chapter the general techniques which are used to unravel the cellular world, are described.

13.1. Microscopy

The term microscopic means minute or very small, not visible with an unaided eye. Modern biologists work with fairly small components of living organisms, tissues, cells and biomolecules. To actually see them, one needs optical instruments which can magnify these components. The invention of the light microscope is one of the remarkable events in the development of science. It made visible the fascinating details of worlds within worlds.

There were no suitable means of magnifying invisible organisms prior to the 17th century. Anton van Leeuwenhoek is honored for providing the first accurate report of the occurrence of bacteria with the help of his single-lens microscopes of simplest possible design. He could make lenses and used them to build magnifying glasses to provide a magnification of about 200 times. It is true that Robert Hooke had used a compound microscope in

18th century, but these were incapable of good performance, due to defects such as chromatic and spherical aberration inherent in their basic design.

13.1.1. History of Microscope

It is believed that in unrecorded past, someone picked up a piece of transparent crystal thicker in the middle than at the edges, looked through it, and discovered that it made things look larger and such a crystal would focus the sun's rays and set fire to a piece of parchment or cloth. Magnifiers and "burning glasses" or "magnifying glasses" are mentioned in the writings of Seneca and Pliny the Elder, Roman philosophers during the first century AD They were named lenses because they shaped like the seeds of a lentil. The major milestones in the history of microscopy are the following events

Circa 1000AD: The first vision aid was invented (inventor unknown) called a reading stone. It was a glass sphere that magnified when laid on top of reading materials.

Circa 1284: Italian, Salvino D'Armate is credited with inventing the first wearable eye glasses.

1590: Two Dutch eye glass makers, Zaccharias Janssen and son Hans Janssen experimented with multiple lenses placed in a tube. The Janssens observed that viewed objects in front of the tube appeared greatly enlarged, predecessor of the compound microscope and the telescope.

1665: English physicist, Robert Hooke looked at a cork through a microscope lens and noticed some "pores" or "cells" in it.

1674: Anton van Leeuwenhoek built a simple microscope with only one lens to examine blood, yeast, insects and many other tiny objects. Leeuwenhoek was the first person to describe bacteria, and he invented new methods for grinding and polishing microscope lenses.

18th century: Technical innovations improved microscopes, leading to microscopy becoming popular among scientists. Lenses combining two types of glass reduced the "chromatic effect" the disturbing halos resulting from differences in refraction of light.

1830: Joseph Jackson Lister reduces spherical aberration or the "chromatic effect" by showing that several weak lenses used together at certain distances gave good magnification without blurring the image. This was the prototype for the compound microscope.

1872: Ernst Abbe, then research director of the Zeiss Optical Works, wrote a mathematical formula called the "Abbe Sine Condition". His formula provided calculations that allowed for the maximum resolution in microscopes possible.

1903: Richard Zsigmondy developed the ultra-microscope that could study objects below the wavelength of light. He won the Nobel Prize in Chemistry in 1925.

1931: Ernst Ruska co-invented the electron microscope for which he won the Nobel Prize in Physics in 1986. An electron microscope depends on electrons rather than light to view an object, electrons are speeded up in a vacuum until their wavelength is extremely short, only one hundred-thousandth that of white light. Electron microscopes make it possible to view objects as small as the diameter of an atom.

1932: Frits Zernike invented the phase-contrast microscope that allowed for the study of colorless and transparent biological materials for which he won the Nobel Prize in Physics in 1953.

1981: Gerd Binnig and Heinrich Rohrer invented the scanning tunneling microscope that gives three-dimensional images of objects down to the atomic level. Binnig and Rohrer won the Nobel Prize in Physics in 1986. The powerful scanning tunneling microscope is the strongest microscope to date.

13.1.2. Birth of the Light Microscope

Dutch spectacle makers, Zaccharias Janssen and his son Hans (1590), while experimenting with several lenses in a tube, discovered that nearby objects appeared greatly enlarged. That was the forerunner of the compound microscope and of the telescope. In 1609, Galileo, father of modern physics and astronomy, heard of these early experiments, worked out the principles of lenses, and made a much better instrument with a focusing device.

Anton van Leeuwenhoek, the father of microscopy, started his career as an apprentice in a dry goods store where magnifying glasses were used to count the threads in cloth. He made tiny lenses of great curvature which gave magnifications up to 270 diameters, the finest known at that time by grinding and polishing. He was the first to see and describe bacteria, yeast plants, the teeming life in a drop of water, and the circulation of blood corpuscles in capillaries. During a long life he used his lenses to make pioneer studies on an extraordinary variety of things, both living and non living, and reported his findings in over a hundred letters to the Royal Society of England and the French Academy.

Robert Hooke, re-confirmed Anton van Leeuwenhoek's discoveries of the existence of tiny living organisms in a drop of water. Hooke made a copy of Leeuwenhoek's light microscope and then improved upon his design.

13.1.3. General Terms used in Microscopy

Amplitude, frequency, wave length, interference, diffraction and phase are the most important parameters to describe a wave. The wavelength of visible light is between 400 and 800 nm. Interference is the mutual influence of two waves on each other, whereby the resulting crests may be either enhanced or flattened (enhancement of amplitude/reduction of amplitude).

- **Resolving power** is the ability of a lens to enable the observer to see fine details in a specimen. The better the resolving power, the closer two small objects can and still be distinguished as two objects. Thus, a lens system with a resolving power of 2.5 m has poorer resolving power than a lens with a resolving power of 1.0 m. The practical resolving power of the microscope is limited by that of the human eye. From a distance of 25 cm, which is approximately the distance of the optical tube in a microscope, the human eye can distinguish two small objects that are 0.1 mm apart. Therefore, the practical limit of resolving power for optical microscopes that use visible light is about 0.2 m.

The resolving power of a microscope depends upon the wavelength of light and numerical aperture (NA). The minimum resolvable distance between two lumi-nous points (v) is given by the following formula

$$v = \frac{0.61 \times \lambda}{NA}$$

where λ = Wavelength of light and N.A. = Numerical aperture.

Thus, the shorter the wavelength of light used and lowers the N.A., greater is the resolving power. That's why, with electron beam as the source of illumination has more resolution than with visible light. The above equation specifies the minimum distance between two minute structures that allows them to be seen as two structures. According to the equation, resolving power is better in blue light than in red light:

400 nm---------490 nm----------560 nm---------590 nm---------630 nm---------700 nm
    blue   green   yellow   orange   red

While blue light will theoretically provide better resolving power, the visual acuity of the human eye is higher in green light. Thus, green filters are generally used.

- **Numerical Aperture**

When light strikes a specimen on a microscope stage, some light passes straight through while some is bent by the specimen and goes off at an angle. Numerical aperture is an expression of the ability of an objective to collect these angled, image-forming rays of light. Theoretically it is the sine of the vertex angle of the largest cone of meridional rays that can enter or leave an optical system or element, multiplied by the refractive index of the medium in which the vertex of the cone is located. NA= n sin θ, where *n* is the refractive index of the medium in which the lens is working and θ is the half-angle of the maximum cone of light that can enter or exit the lens. Refractive index (n) of a medium is the ratio of the velocity of propagation of an electromagnetic wave in vacuum to its velocity in the medium.

In microscopy, NA is important because it indicates the resolving power of a lens. The size of the finest detail that can be resolved is proportional to λ/NA, where λ is the wavelength of the light. A lens with a larger numerical aperture will be able to visualize finer details than a lens with a smaller numerical aperture. Lenses with larger numerical apertures also collect more light and will generally provide a brighter image. The larger the N.A., the greater the ability of the objective to collect the rays and hence, the better its resolving power. The theoretical maximum N.A. possible for dry objectives is 1.0. The actual highest numerical aperture for a dry objective is about 0.95. The only way to have an objective of N.A. equal to or greater than 1.0 is to place a liquid medium of higher refractive index between the lens and the specimen slide. Air has a refractive index of 1.0, oil has 1.51, while water has 1.333. When immersion oil is used, image-forming rays of light are bent less than they would be in air and thus more of them enter the objective; hence, resolution is increased. Some image-forming rays of light are lost due to reflection where air meets the surface of the glass cover slip. Immersion oil used has a refractive index equal to that of the glass used in cover slips.

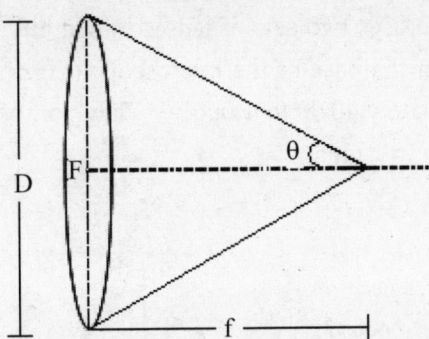

Figure 13.1: Half-angle of the maximum cone of light that can enter or exit the lens

Magnification: Magnification is how much bigger a sample appears to be under the microscope than it is in real life. In a microscope where more than one lenses are present, the resultant magnification will be the product of magnifications of individual lenses.

13.2. Light Microscopy

The light microscope, so called because it employs visible light to detect small objects, is probably the most well-known and well-used research tool in biology. Microscope must gather light from a tiny area of a thin, well-illuminated specimen that is close-by. So the lens of a microscope is small and spherical, which means that it has a much shorter focal length on either side. It brings the image of the object into focus at a short distance within the microscope's tube. The image is then magnified by a second lens, called an ocular lens or eyepiece, as it is brought to your eye. Microscope has a light source and a condenser. The condenser is a lens system that focuses the light from the source on to a tiny, bright spot of the specimen, which is the same area that the objective lens examines.

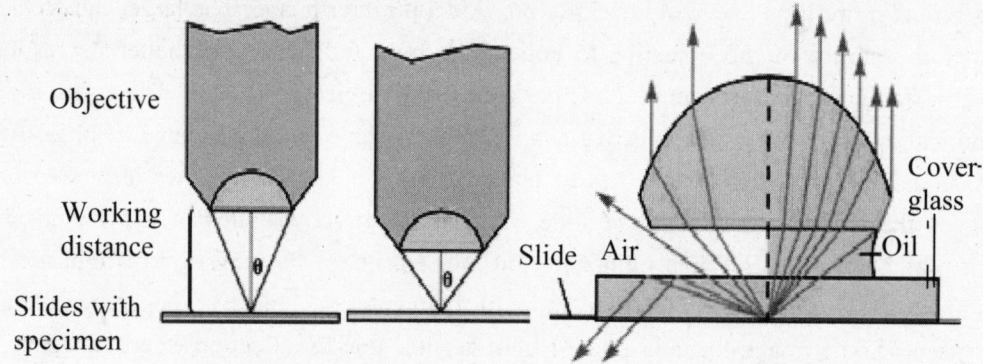

Figure 13.2: Working distance of oil immersion and dry lenses

13.2.1. Compound Light Microscope

The compound light microscope uses two sets of lenses to magnify the object. Illumination is provided by a light source on the base of the microscope (Fig. 13.3). The magnification typically ranges from approximately 40 X to 1,000 X. They can be used with objects that range in size from about 100 nm to 2 mm.

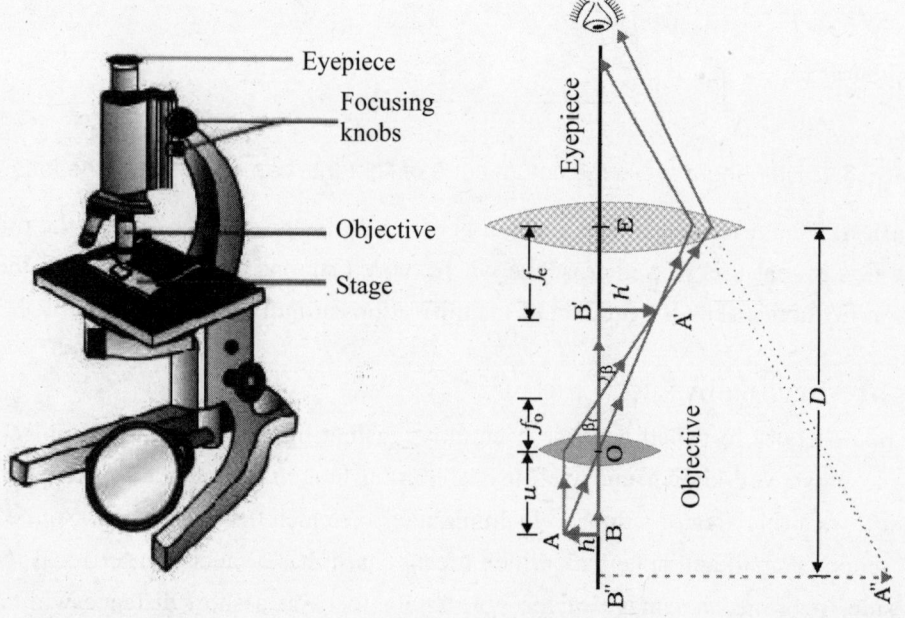

Figure 13.3: Compound light microscope, showing the parts and the light path

13.2.2. Parts of the Light Microscope

The stage is a platform that holds the slide containing the specimen to be viewed. A mechanical stage has a mechanism for moving the slide. A light microscope must have a light source. This is usually a light bulb located beneath the stage. An adjustable diaphragm located beneath the stage is used to regulate the amount of light that passes through. A condenser contains two sets of lenses that concentrate light. It is located directly underneath the stage. Light from the light source passes through the diaphragm and condenser before continuing up through the specimen to be viewed. The body tube contains an ocular lens (eyepiece) and a nosepiece with several objective lenses. Each objective lens is used for a different magnification and is moved into place by rotating the nosepiece. The image is brought into focus by adjusting the coarse and fine focus knobs.

13.2.3. Types of Light Microscopy

(a) Bright Field Microscopy

In conventional bright field microscope, light from a source is aimed towards a lens beneath the stage called the condenser, that passes through the specimen, followed by an objective lens and finally reaches to the eye through a second magnifying lens, referred to as ocular or eyepiece. The bright field condenser usually contains an aperture diaphragm, a device that controls the diameter of the light beam coming up through the condenser, so that when the diaphragm is stopped down (nearly closed) the light comes straight up through the center of the condenser lens and contrast is high. When the diaphragm is wide open the image tend to be brighter, while contrast turns to be low.

Basic dyes, used to stain, have a positively charged chromophore (color-bearing ion) that is attracted to the slightly negatively charged cells. The specimen will appear as a colored shape in a bright background. Bright field microscopy is best suited to viewing stained or naturally pigmented specimens such as stained prepared slides of tissue sections or living photosynthetic organisms. It is useless for living specimens of bacteria, and inferior for non-photosynthetic protists or metazoans, or unstained cell suspensions or tissue sections.

(b) Darkfield Microscopy

Dark field microscopy is a method which also creates contrast between the object and the surrounding field. As the name implies, the background is dark and the object is bright. An annular stop is also used for dark field. Only light coming from the outside of the beam passes through the object and it cannot be seen directly. The following diagram shows the setup of the dark field light path (Fig. 13.4).

To view a specimen in dark field, an opaque disc is placed underneath the condenser lens, so that only light that is scattered by objects on the slide can reach the eye. Instead of coming up through the specimen, the light is reflected by particles on the slide. Everything is visible regardless of color, usually bright white against a dark background. Pigmented objects are often seen in "false colors," that is, the reflected light is of a color different than the color of the object. Better resolution can be obtained using dark field as opposed to bright field viewing.

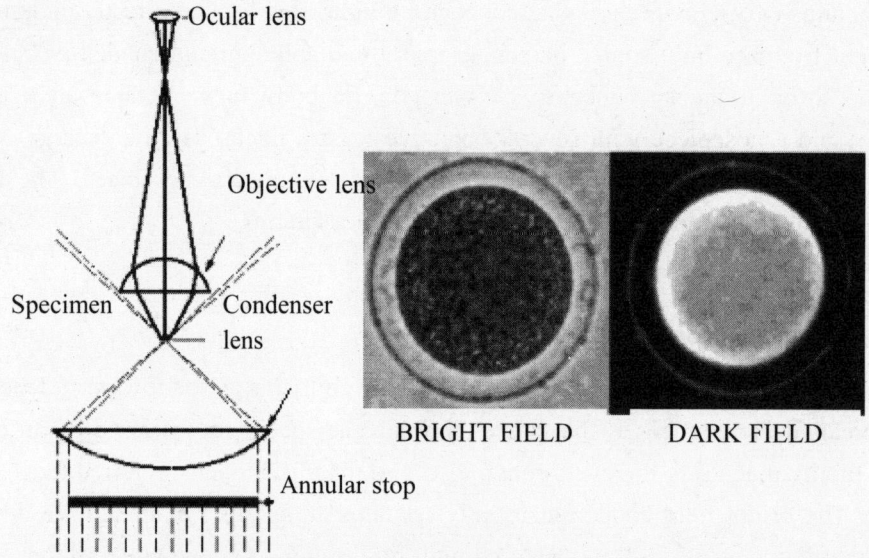

Figure 13.4: Schematic representation of dark field microscope

(c) Phase Contrast Microscopy

Phase contrast microscopy, first described in 1934 by Dutch physicist Frits Zernike, is a contrast-enhancing optical technique that can be utilized to produce high-contrast images of transparent specimens, such as living cells (usually in culture), microorganisms, thin tissue slices, and subcellular particles (including nuclei and other organelles).

Most of the detail of living cells is undetectable in bright field microscopy because there is too little contrast between structures with similar transparency and there is insufficient natural pigmentation. However, the various organelles show wide variation in refractive index, that is, the tendency of the materials to bend light, providing an opportunity to distinguish them. Highly refractive structures bend light to a much greater angle than do structures of low refractive index. The same properties that cause the light to bend also delay the passage of light by a quarter of a wavelength or so. In a light microscope in bright field mode, light from highly refractive structures bends farther away from the center of the lens than light from less refractive structures and arrives about a quarter of a wavelength out of phase.

Light from most objects passes through the center of the lens as well as to the periphery. Now, if the light from an object to the edges of the objective lens is retarded a half wavelength and the light to the center is not retarded at all, then the light rays are out of phase by a half wavelength. They cancel each other when the objective lens brings the image into focus. A reduction in brightness of the object is observed. The degree of reduction in brightness depends on the refractive index of the object.

Phase contrast is preferable to bright field microscopy when high magnifications (400x, 1000x) are needed and the specimen is colorless or the details so fine that color does not show up well. Cilia and flagella, for example, are nearly invisible in bright field but show up in sharp contrast in phase contrast. Amoebae look like vague outlines in bright field, but show a great deal of detail in phase. Most living microscopic organisms are much more obvious in phase contrast (Fig. 13.5).

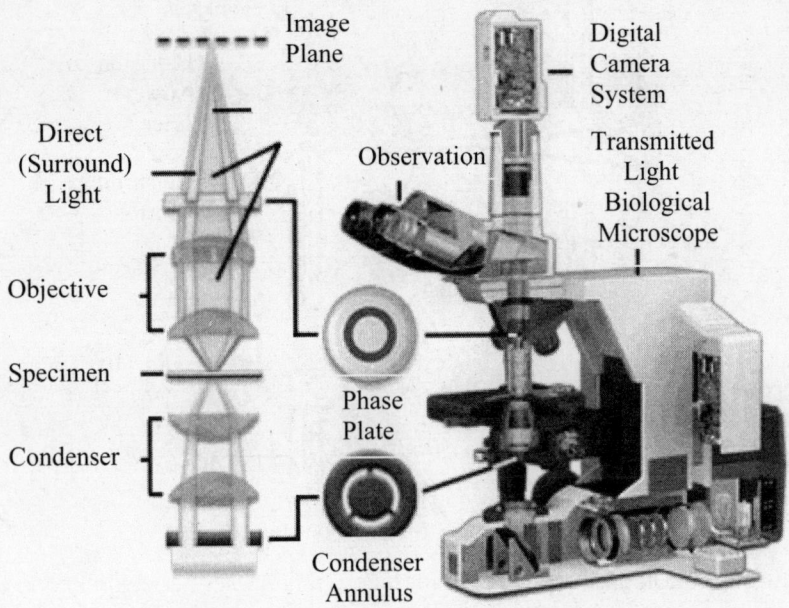

Figure 13.5: Phase contrast microscope

(d) The Fluorescence Microscope

Fluorescence microscopy works on the principle of fluorescence. Energy is absorbed by the atom which becomes excited. The electron jumps to a higher energy level. Soon, the electron drops back to the ground state, emitting a photon (or a packet of light) - the atom is fluorescing. The technique is used to study specimens, which can be made to fluoresce. The fluorescence microscope is based on the phenomenon that certain material emits energy detectable as visible light when irradiated with the light of a specific wavelength. The sample can either be fluorescing in its natural form like chlorophyll and some minerals, or treated with fluorescing chemicals (Fig. 13.6).

The basic task of the fluorescence microscope is to let excitation light radiate the specimen and then sort out the much weaker emitted light to make up the image. First, the microscope has a filter that only lets through radiation with the desired wavelength that matches fluorescing material. The radiation collides with the atoms in the specimen and electrons are excited to a higher energy level. When they relax to a lower level, they emit light. To become visible, the emitted light is separated from the much brighter excitation light in a second filter. Here, the fact that the emitted light is of lower energy and has a longer wavelength is used. The fluorescing areas can be observed in the microscope and shine out against a dark background with high contrast.

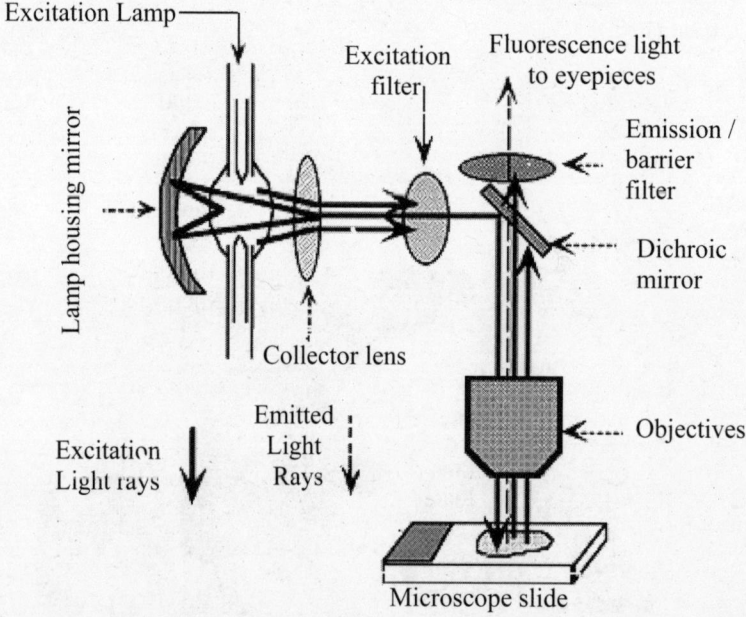

Figure 13.6: Diagrammatic representation of fluorescence microscope

13.3. Electron Microscope

Electron Microscopes were developed due to the limitations of light microscopes which are limited to 500x or 1000x magnification and a resolution of 0.2 micrometers. Simple light microscopy cannot be used to distinguish objects that are smaller than half the wavelength of light. White light has an average wavelength of 0.55 micrometers, half of which is 0.275 micrometers. Any two lines that are closer together than 0.275 micrometers will be seen as a single line, and any object with a diameter smaller than 0.275 micrometers will be invisible or, at best, show up as a blur. By using blue/violet light (400 nm) by decreasing the wavelength. It can approximately double the resolution that can be obtained using red (600 nm) or white (mean 500 nm) light, but a doubling of the resolution is hardly a great improvement. .

Max Knoll and Ernst Ruska in 1931 introduced the electron microscope. Ernst Ruska was awarded the Nobel Prize for Physics in 1986 for his invention. A stream of electrons is formed (by the electron source) and accelerated toward the specimen using a positive electrical potential. This stream is confined and focused using metal apertures and magnetic lenses (condenser) into a thin, focused, monochromatic beam. This beam is focused onto the sample using a magnetic lens. Interactions occur inside the irradiated sample, affecting the electron beam. These interactions and effects are detected and transformed into an image, which contains information such as structure and composition (Fig. 13.7).

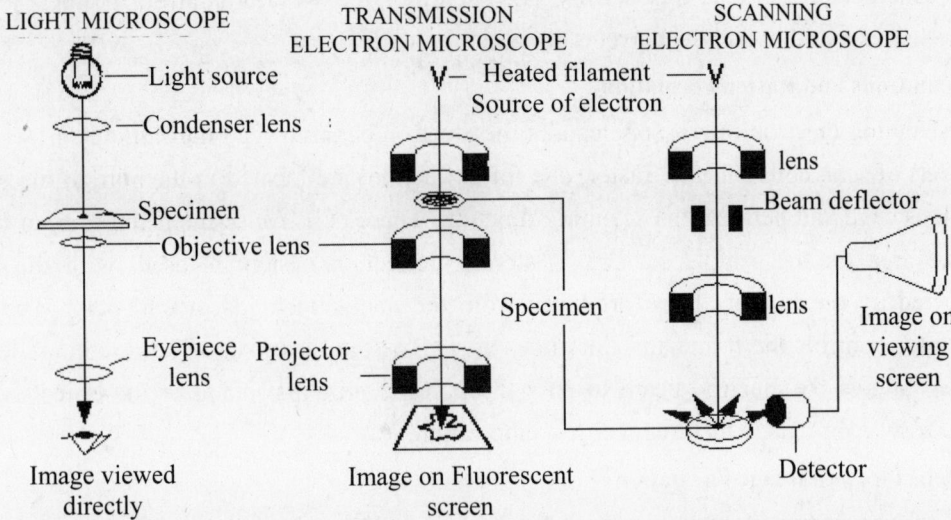

Figure 13. 7: Comparative instrumentation of light microscope with electron microscope

13.3.1. Components of Electron Microscope

The various components of the microscope can be categorized as (1) the electron column, (2) the specimen chamber, (3) the vacuum pumping system and (4) the electron control and imaging system.

(a) The Electron Gun

The electron gun produces a narrowly divergent beam of electrons directed down the centerline of the column. The electrons are produced by thermionic emission at filament and are attracted to the anode. The anode is maintained at a positive voltage relative to the filament, ranging from 5 to 30 kV in scanning electron microscopes. This voltage, controlled by the operator, is generally held at 20 kV, but variations can be useful for structure and X-ray analysis.

(b) Lenses

Electron microscopes have magnetic lenses that are similar to simple solenoids. A coil of copper wire produces a magnetic field that is shaped by the surrounding iron fixture into an optimum geometry. As an electron moves through the magnetic field, it experiences a radial force inward, which is proportional to the Lorenz force; v x B, where v is the electron velocity and B is the magnetic flux density. The lensing action is similar to that of an optical lens, in which a ray parallel to the axis of the lens is bent to the lens axis at the focal length f, of the lens. In an optical lens, the focal length is fixed by the curvature of the lens surfaces and cannot be changed. In the electromagnetic lens, the focal length depends on two factors: the gun voltage (which determines the electron velocity v and the amount of current through the coil (which determines the flux density, B). Therefore, the operator controls the focal lengths of the lenses by adjusting the currents supplied to them.

(c) Scan Coils and Raster Formation

The scanning electron microscope causes the electron beam to scan the sample surface. The two sets of scan coils (one for raster, one for deflection) are located in the bore of the objective lens cage and perform the scanning function. These coils cause the beam to scan over a square area on the sample surface. A double-deflection system is used, with the beam deflected by the Lorentz force produced from the magnetic fields of coil pairs. The scan generator controls the frame and line times as well as the raster size. The double-deflection system allows the electron beam to pass through the principal plane of the objective lens very close to on-axis, which reduces lens aberration.

(d) Detectors and Image Formation

Detector use specimen current, secondary electron, backscattered electron and x-ray signals. The secondary electron detector is generally used for image formation with the scanning electron microscope. The secondary electron detector has a screen on its outer surface that is bias at about 200 V. Electrons that pass through the screen are accelerated by a high voltage into a quartz light pipe coated with a scintillation material. The photons generated by the scintillator pass down the light pipe to a photomultiplier tube outside the vacuum system. A significant amplification is achieved, having high signal to noise characteristics. The secondary electron energies are low (approximately 5eV); consequently, the 200 V on the screen will pull many of the electrons to the screen even though that is not their initial direction.

13.3.2. Transmission Electron Microscopy

In Transmission electron microscopy, the ray of electrons is produced by a pin-shaped cathode heated up by current. The electrons are collected by the anode. The acceleration voltage is between 50 and 150 kV. The higher it is, the shorter are the electron waves and the higher is the power of resolution. But this factor is hardly ever limiting. The power of resolution of electron microscopy is usually restrained by the quality of the lens-systems and especially by the technique with which the preparation has been achieved. Modern gadgets have powers of resolution that range from 0.5 - 10 nm. The useful magnification is therefore more than 1,000,000X. In transmission electron microscopy the two dimensional image of a thin section of a specimen is obtained (Fig. 13.8).

Preparation in TEM

Transmission Electron Microscopy (TEM) allows visualization of fine cellular structures of nanometer-size.

Fixation: The specimen, a piece of biological tissue of a few millimeters or single cell, is fixed with chemical products (e.g. glutaraldehyde) or cold (liquid propane at - 90°C, for physical fixation). Fixation is done to preserve the fine structure in the cells in a state as close as possible to the living state and to make the cells permeable for the components required in the next steps of preparation.

Rinsing and staining: After fixation the next step is rinsing away of the fixative. The material is treated with heavy metal compounds (osmiumtetroxide, uranylacetate or potassium permanganate) that bind preferably to certain regions like lipid-rich membranes of organelles, DNA-clusters in the cell nucleus, and protein-rich structures like cytoskeletal elements. Such metal-compounds have the property to reflect electrons so that labeled structures appear as dark areas in the electron microscopic view.

Dehydration: To be able to cut extremely thin sections (60–90 nm) that keep their consistency and yet allow electrons to pass the stained samples are imbedded in resins (plastics). As most of these resins are hydrophobic, it is necessary to remove all water from the sample through wash steps of increasing ethanol or acetone concentration, followed by final washes in another non-polar substance like propylene oxide.

Imbedding in resin: Later the material is gradually infiltrated with the still unpolymerized resin (e.g. methacrylates, polyester and epoxy-resins, acryls, polyethyleneglycol and others) desolved in the non-polar and volatile transition medium that evaporates.

Trimming of the block of resin and ultra-thin sectioning: Sections with a thickness of about 70 nm can only be cut with special knifes of cleaved glass of high purity made with a glass-knife maker (which breaks glass in triangles with extremely sharp edges) or with a diamond knife. The cutting is done with an ultra-microtome (a precision cutting instrument) with numerous setting possibilities.

Picking up sections on a grid: Water in a tiny container behind the knife contributes to lubrification of the cut edge. Sections float on that surface (in air they would easily become electrostatic and jump aside or be blown away). The thickness of the section can be estimated with quite high accuracy from the reflection color of the floating section. These very fragile rows of trapezoid-shaped sections can be lift up like with a spoon from the water surface onto a so-called grid. Grids are later inserted into the electron microscope with help of a rod-shaped holder.

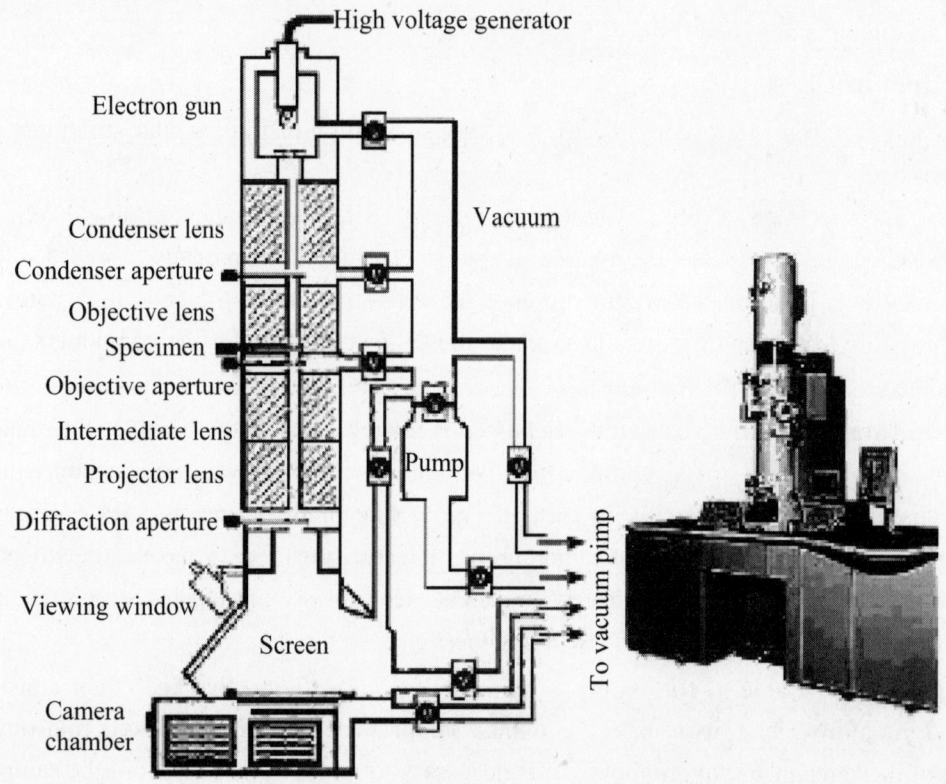

Figure 13.8: Transmission electron microscope

13.3.3. Scanning Electron Microscopy (SEM)

The SEM is a microscope that uses electrons instead of light to form an image, in the early 1950s. It uses a focused beam of high-energy electrons to generate a variety of signals at the surface of solid specimens. The signals that derive from electron-sample interactions reveal information about the sample including external morphology (texture), chemical composition, crystalline structure and orientation of materials making up the sample. Areas ranging from approximately 1 μm to 5 microns in width can be imaged in a scanning mode using conventional SEM techniques (magnification ranging from 20X to approximately 30,000X, spatial resolution of 50 to 100 nm).

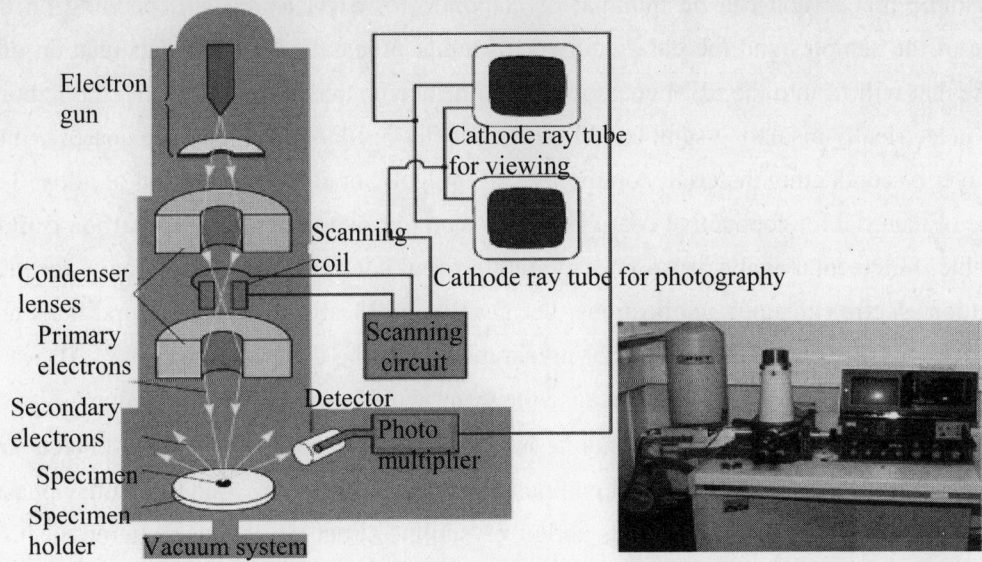

Figure 13.9: Scanning electron micrograph

The SEM has allowed researchers to examine a much bigger variety of specimens. The scanning electron microscope has many advantages over traditional microscopes. The SEM has a large depth of field, which allows more of a specimen to be in focus at one time. The SEM also has much higher resolution, so closely spaced specimens can be magnified at much higher levels. As the SEM uses electromagnets rather than lenses,; it has much more control on the degree of magnification. All of these advantages, as well as the actual strikingly clear images make the scanning electron microscope one of the most useful instruments in research today.

A beam of electrons is produced at the top of the microscope by an electron gun. The electron beam follows a vertical path through the microscope, which is held within a vacuum. The beam travels through electromagnetic fields and lenses, which focus the beam down toward the sample. Once the beam hits the sample, electrons and X-rays are ejected from the sample. In SEM the image is formed from secondary electrons that have been dislocated at the surface of the scanned sample by bombarding primary electrons from the electron gun. Those ejected electrons are captured by a detector and the information is converted into an electric signal, amplified and digitalized. The result is a topographical image of the surface of the object. Besides secondary electrons, radiation in particular X-rays and cathodoluminescence are produced upon interaction of atoms in the surface layer of the sample with the primary electron beam. These emission signals, which contain information among others on the element composition of the upper layer, can be received by selected detectors and convert them into signal that is sent to a screen similar to television screen (Fig. 13.10).

Sample preparation can be minimal or elaborate for SEM analysis, depending on the nature of the samples and the data required. Minimal preparation includes acquisition of a sample that will fit into the SEM chamber and some accommodation to prevent charge build-up on electrically insulating samples. Most electrically insulating samples are coated with a thin layer of conducting material, commonly carbon, gold, or some other metal or alloy. The choice of material for conductive coatings depends on the data to be acquired: carbon is most desirable if elemental analysis is a priority, while metal coatings are most effective for high resolution electron imaging applications, because the SEM utilizes vacuum conditions and uses electrons to form an image, special preparations must be done to the sample. All water must be removed from the samples because the water would vaporize in the vacuum.

The SEM is routinely used to generate high-resolution images of shapes of objects and to show spatial variations in chemical compositions. It is also widely used to identify phases based on qualitative chemical analysis and/or crystalline structure. Backe scattered electron images can be used for rapid discrimination of phases in multiphase samples. SEMs equipped with diffracted backscattered electron detectors can be used to examine microfabric and crystallographic orientation in many materials.

SEM has some limitations such as the samples must be solid and they must fit into the microscope chamber. Maximum size in horizontal dimensions is usually on the order of 10 cm; vertical dimensions are generally much more limited and rarely exceed 40 mm. For most instruments samples must be stable in a vacuum on the order of 10^{-5}–10^{-6} torr. An electrically conductive coating must be applied to electrically insulating samples for study in conventional SEM's, unless the instrument is capable of operation in a low vacuum mode.

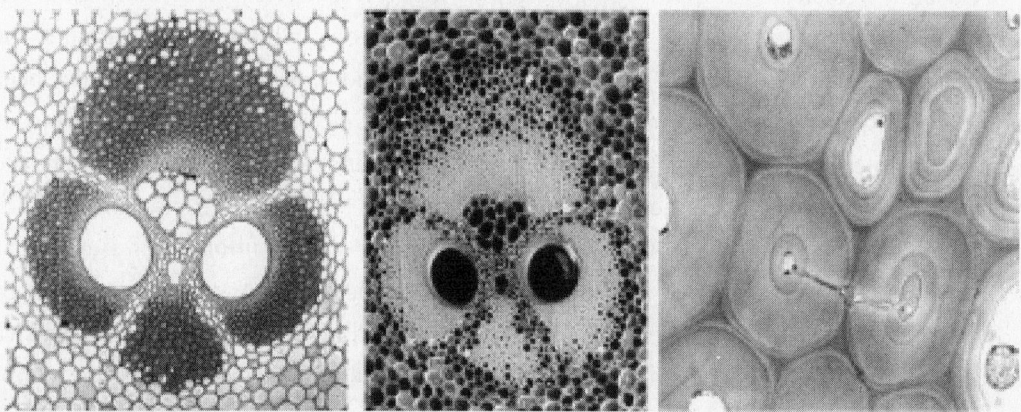

Figure 13.10: Bamboo vascular bundles. (Left to right): light micrograph with safranin/alcian blue stain; SEM at similar scale; TEM of fiber cells

Table 13.1: Comparison of different types of microscope

Characteristic	Compound Microscope	Transmission E. Microscope	Scanning E. Microscope
Resolution (Average)	500 nm	10 nm	2 nm
Resolution (Special)	100 nm	0.5 nm	0.2 nm
Magnifying Power	up to 1,500X	up to 5,000,000X	~ 100,000X
Depth of Field	poor	moderate	high
Type of Objects	living or non-living	non-living	non-living
Preparation Technique	usually simple	skilled	easy
Preparation Thickness	rather thick	very thin	variable
Specimen Mounting	glass slides	thin films on copper grids	aluminum stubs
Field of View	large enough	limited	large
Source of Radiation	visible light	electrons	electrons
Medium	air	vacuum	vacuum
Nature of Lenses	glass	1 electrostatic + a few electro magnetic lenses	1 electrostatic + a few electro magnetic lenses
Focusing	mechanical	current in the objective lens coil	current in the objective lens coil
Magnification Adjustments	changing objectives	current in the projector lens coil	current in the projector lens coil
Specimen Contrast	by light absorption	by electron scattering	by electron scattering

13.4. Centrifugation

Centrifugation is the method of separating immiscible liquids or solids from liquids by the application of centrifugal force. Centrifugation is one of the most important and widely applied research techniques in biochemistry, cellular and molecular biology, and in medicine. Current research and clinical applications rely on isolation of cells, subcellular organelles, and macromolecules.

The theoretical basis of this technique is the effect of gravity on particles (including macromolecules) in suspension. Two particles of different masses will settle in a tube at different rates in response to gravity. Centrifugal force is used to increase this settling rate in the centrifuge. Centrifuges achieve separation by means of the accelerated gravitational force achieved by a rapid rotation or simply a centrifuge uses centrifugal force to isolate suspended particles from their surrounding medium on either a batch or a continuous-flow basis. An object traveling in a circle behaves as if it is experiencing an outward force. This force, known as the centrifugal force, depends on the mass of the object, the speed of rotation, and the distance from the center. The more massive the object, the greater the force; the greater the speed of the object, the greater the force (Centrifugal force $F_c = mv^2/r$, where m = mass, v = speed, and r = radius).

The two common types of centrifugation are analytical and preparative; the distinction between the two is based on the purpose of centrifugation.

Analytical centrifugation involves measuring the physical properties of the sedimenting particles such as sedimentation coefficient or molecular weight. Optimal methods are used in analytical ultracentrifugation. Molecules are observed by optical system during centrifugation, to allow observation of macromolecules in solution as they move in gravitational field. The concentration of the solution at various points in the cell is determined by absorption of a light of the appropriate wavelength (Beer's law is followed).

The other form of centrifugation is called preparative and the objective is to isolate specific particles which can be reused. The four basic types of centrifuges that are used commonly in the laboratory are,

- **Clinical centrifuges:** They are tabletop centrifuges that can run at a speed of up to 3000 rpm. These can pellet cells, but not organelles or biomolecules.
- **Microfuges:** These can typically run at a speed of up to 14,000 rpm, sufficient speed to pellet nucleic acids and denatured proteins. Microfuges are specially adapted for small volumes of sample.
- **High speed centrifuges:** They can run at speeds up to 25,000 rpm, sufficient to pellet cell nuclei and most biomolecules. These are often aided with cooling system.
- **Ultracentrifuges:** The ultracentrifuge is capable of reaching even greater velocities and requires a vacuum to reduce friction and heating of the rotor. It can run at speeds up to 75,000 rpm, sufficient to allow fractionation of biomolecules, for example: plasmid DNA, chromosomal DNA, and RNA. Ultracentrifuges are usually refrigerated and are very expensive and have delicate pieces of machinery.

13.4.1. Mechanical Components

(a) Rotors

Rotors for a centrifuge are fixed angles, swinging buckets, continuous flow, or zonal. Fixed angles generally work faster; substances precipitate faster in a given rotational environment. The most common is a rotor holding 8 centrifuge tubes at an angle of 34° from the vertical.

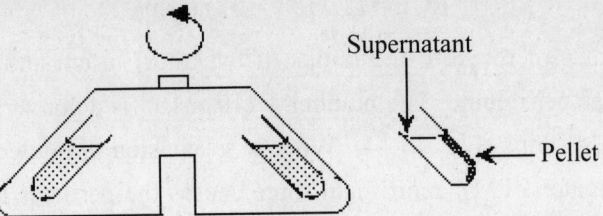

Figure 13.12: Centrifuge rotors

In a fixed angle rotor, the materials are forced against the side of the centrifuge tube, and then slide down the wall of the tube. This action is the primary reason for their apparent faster separation, but also leads to abrasion of the particles along the wall of the centrifuge tube (Fig. 13.12).

For swinging bucket rotors, the materials must travel down the entire length of the centrifuge tube and always through the media within the tube. Since the media is usually a viscous substance, the swinging bucket appears to have a lower relative centrifugal force, which itakes longer to precipitate anything contained within. Most common clinical centrifuges have swinging buckets. Cell biologists employ zonal rotors for the large scale separation of particles on density gradients. Zonal rotors can contain up to 2 liters of solution (Fig. 13.13).

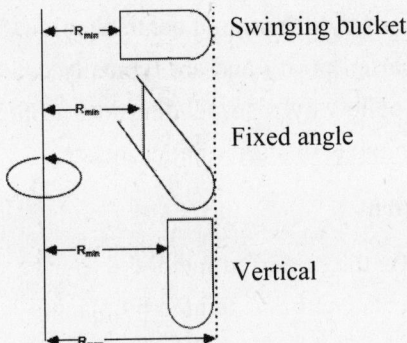

Figure 13.13: Different type of rotors

(b) Rotor Tubes

The tubes used for biological work, are made of regular glass, Corex glass, or nitrocellulose. Regular glass centrifuge tubes can be used at speeds below 3,000 RPM that is in a standard clinical centrifuge. For work in the higher speed ranges, centrifuge tubes are made of plastic or nitrocellulose. Preparative centrifuge tubes are made of polypropylene (sometimes polyethylene) and can withstand speeds up to 20,000 RPM. These tubes should be carefully examined for stress fractures before use.

13.4.2. Relative Centrifugal Force (RCF)

The centrifugal force is usually compared to the force of gravity and is reported as the relative centrifugal force (RCF) in g units. The following formula relates the RCF to the rotor speed and diameter:

$$RCF = (1.119 \times 10^{-5})\,(rpm)^2\,r$$

Where r is the radius of rotation (the radius of the rotor) in cm and rpm is the centrifuge speed in revolutions per minute. The number 1.119×10^{-5} is a conversion factor that allows to use "rpm" and "g" units (Fig. 13.14). When a suspension is rotated at a certain speed or revolutions per minute (RPM), centrifugal force causes the particles to move radially away from the axis of rotation. The force on the particles (compared to gravity) is called Relative Centrifugal Force (RCF).

13.4.3. Types of Centrifugal Separations

(a) Differential Centrifugation

In differential centrifugation separation is primarily based on the size of the particles. This type of separation is commonly used in simple pelleting and in obtaining partially-pure preparation of subcellular organelles and macromolecules. For the study of subcellular organelles, tissue or cells are first disrupted to release their internal contents. This crude disrupted cell mixture is referred to as a homogenate. During centrifugation of a cell homogenate, larger particles sediment faster than smaller ones and this provides the basis for obtaining crude organelle fractions by differential centrifugation. Some of these sedimenting organelles can be obtained in partial purity and are typically contaminated with other particles. Repeated washing of the pellets by resuspending in isotonic solvents and re-pelleting may result in removal of contaminants that are smaller in size.

(b) Density Gradient Centrifugation

Density gradient centrifugation is the preferred method to purify sub cellular organelles and macromolecules. Density gradients can be generated by placing layer after layer of gradient media such as sucrose in a tube with the heaviest layer at the bottom and the lightest at the top in either a discontinuous or continuous mode. The cell fraction to be separated is placed on top of the layer and centrifuged. Density gradient separation can be classified into two categories, Rate-zonal (size) separation and Isopycnic (density) separation

1. Rate zonal (size) separation

Rate-zonal separation takes advantage of particle size and mass instead of particle density for sedimentation. Examples of common applications include separation of cellular organelles such as endosomes or separation of proteins, such as antibodies. For instance, antibody classes all have very similar densities, but different masses. Thus, separation based on mass will separate the different classes, whereas separation based on density will not be able to resolve these antibody classes.

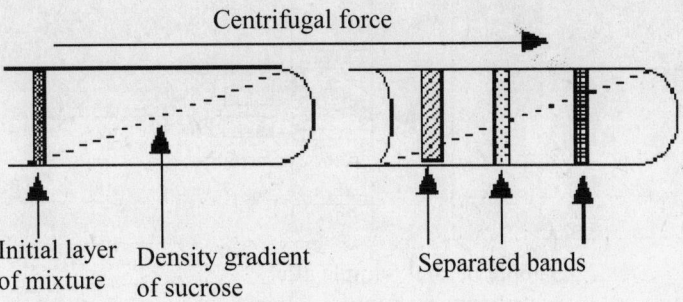

Figure 13.14: Direction of centrifugal force

In rate zonal centrifugation, the sample is applied in a thin zone at the top of the centrifuge tube on a density gradient. Under centrifugal force, the particles will begin sedimenting through the gradient in separate zones according to their size, shape, and density or the sedimentation coefficient(s). The run must be terminated before any of the separated particles reach the bottom of the tube. S is the sedimentation coefficient and is usually expressed in Svedbergs (S) units.

$$\text{Sedimentation coefficient (S)} = \frac{\text{Rate of movement down}}{\text{Centrifugal force}}$$

S is increases with mass of the particle because sedimenting force α M $(1-v\rho)$. S is also increased for more compact structures of equal particle mass (frictional coefficient is less)

2. Isopycnic separation

Molecules separated on equilibrium position and not by rates of sedimentation. Each molecule floats or sinks to position where density equals density of CsCl solution. In the isopycnic technique, the density gradient column encompasses the whole range of densities of the sample particles. The sample is uniformly mixed with the gradient material. Each of the particles will sediment only to the position in the centrifuge tube at which the gradient density is equal to its own density, and there it will remain. The isopycnic technique, therefore, separates particles into zones solely on the basis of their buoyant density differences, independent of time. A common example for this method is separation of nucleic acids in a CsCl gradient. Isopynically banding DNA, for example, takes 36 to 48 hours in a self-generating cesium chloride gradient. It is important to note that the run time cannot be shortened by increasing the rotor speed; this only results in changing the position of the zones in the tube since the gradient material will redistribute further down the tube under greater centrifugal force (Fig. 13.15).

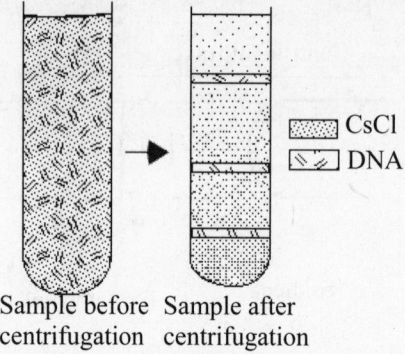

Sample before Sample after
centrifugation centrifugation

Figure 13.15: Illustration of the isopycnic separation

13.5. Cell Fractionation

The eukaryotic cell contains many organelles, suspended within the cytoplasm and bounded by the plasma membrane each of which performs one of more specialized functions. Definition of the organelles is possible with microscopy, but the function of individual organelles is often beyond the ability of observations through a microscope. The organelle functions can be well studieed and understood by isolating the organelles into reasonably pure fractions. They differ in size, shape, density and chemical composition as well as function. Because of these different features, individual types of organelles can be isolated from cells and studied. Organelles can be isolated by homogenizing the cells in a blender so as to free the organelles. The process of breaking open cells is homogenization and the subsequent isolation of organelles is fractionation. To preserve the viability of the organelles the cells are homogenized in a phosphate buffered sucrose solution. In order to study specific organelles, homogenization is followed by some procedure that can isolate one type of organelle from the others. The technique utilized in the laboratory is differential centrifugation, a process by which homogenized cells are centrifuged at increasingly higher speeds and for increasingly longer periods of time. Centrifugation tends to isolate the cellular components in order of density and, to some extent, size. The most dense cell components and cell fragments settle out as a residue during the first centrifuging. Less dense organelles remain suspended in the buffer solution as the supernatant. With subsequent centrifugings, more and more organelles settle in layers in the residue, until only the least dense organelles remain in the supernatant.

Homogenization techniques can be divided into those brought about by osmotic alteration of the media which cells are found in, or those which require physical force to disrupt cell structure. The physical means encompass use of mortars and pestles, blenders, compression and/or expansion, or ultrasonification. With this technique, the heaviest or most dense organelles (i.e. nuclei) pellet in less time (and at less forces) than is required to pellet lighter organelles (such as mitochondria). First, a cell homogenate is made by breaking open the cell membrane. When the cell homogenate is centrifuged at 1000 x g for 10 minutes, unbroken cells and heavy nuclei pellet to the bottom of the tube. The supernatant can be further centrifuged at 10,000 x g for 20 minutes to pellet subcellular organelles of intermediate velocities such as mitochondria, lysosomes, and microbodies. Some of these sedimenting organelles can obtain in partial purity and are typically contaminated with other particles. Repeated washing of the pellets by resuspending in isotonic solvents and re-pelleting may result in removal of contaminants that are smaller in size (Fig. 13.16). Obtaining partially-purified organelles by differential centrifugation serves as the preliminary step for further purification using other types of centrifugal separation (density gradient separation).

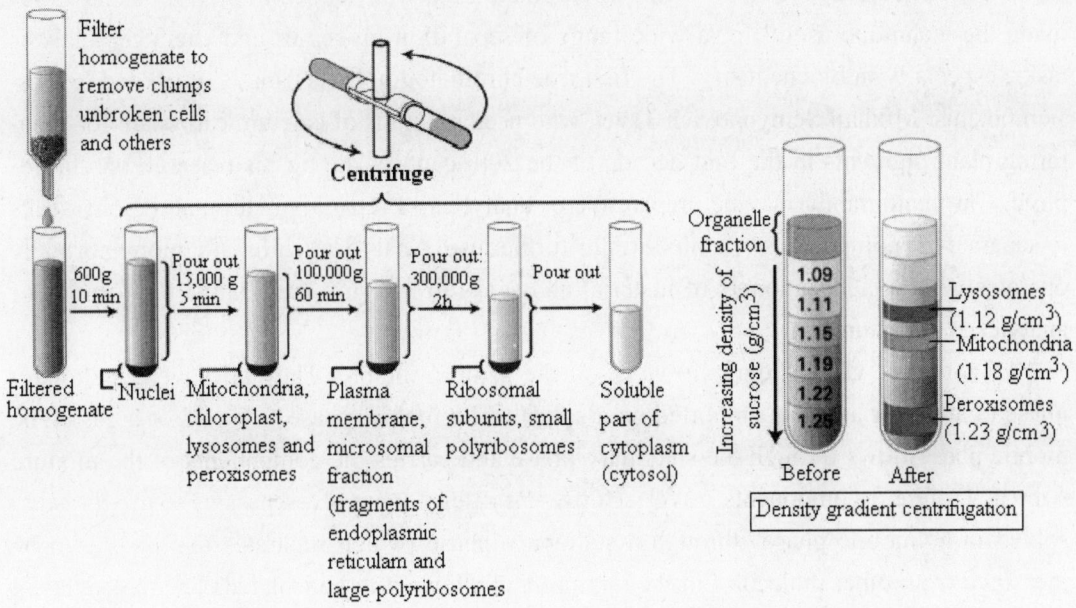

Figure 13.16: Cellular fractionation and isolation of organelles

No technique used to isolate organelles is perfect. It is very difficult to get pure unbroken preparations of any organelle. Techniques providing optimal isolation of one organelle may completely rupture another organelle. Thus methods are often used to measure the contamination of one organelle fraction with another. Analyzing each organelle fraction for organelle-specific marker enzymes can accomplish this. It is scientifically well documented that some enzymes are located specifically within certain cell fractions, some of the example are given in the following table (Table 13.2).

Table 13.2: Marker enzyme/molecule of certain cellular organelles

Subcellular fraction	Relative density	Marker enzyme/molecule
Nuclei	1 (most dense)	DNA, histones
Mitochondria	2	Succinate dehydrogenase
Lysosomes	3	Acid phosphatase
Microsomes	4	Glucose-6-phosphatase
Cytosol	5 (least dense)	Lactate dehydrogenase

13.6 Chromatography

Chromatography, literally "color writing", was used primarily for the separation of plant pigments such as chlorophyll. New forms of chromatography developed in the 1930s and 1940s made the technique useful for a wide range of separation processes and chemical analysis tasks, especially in biochemistry. The first true chromatography is usually attributed to Russian botanist Mikhail Semyonovich Tsvet, who used columns of calcium carbonate for separating plant pigments in the first decade of the 20th century during his research on chlorophyll. Chromatography may be preparative or analytical. Preparative chromatography seeks to separate the components of a mixture for further use. Analytical chromatography normally operates with smaller amounts of material and seeks to measure the relative proportions of analytes in a mixture.

All forms of chromatography work on the same principle. They all have a stationary phase (a solid, or a liquid supported on a solid) and a mobile phase (a liquid or a gas). The mobile phase flows through the stationary phase and carries the components of the mixture with it. Different components travel at different rates. It involves passing a mixture dissolved in a "mobile phase" through a stationary phase, which separates the analyte to be measured from other molecules in the mixture and allows it to be isolated. The molecules in the test preparation will have different interactions with the stationary support leading to separation of similar molecules. Test molecules which display tighter interactions with the support will tend to move more slowly through the support than those molecules with weaker interactions. In this way, different types of molecules can be separated from each other as they move over the support material. The main types of chromatography that are in routine use are;

13.6.1. Paper Chromatography

In paper chromatography, the stationary phase is a very uniform absorbent paper. The mobile phase is a suitable liquid solvent or mixture of solvents. Different compounds in the sample mixture travel different distances according to how strongly they interact with the paper. This paper is made of cellulose, a polar molecule, and the compounds within the mixture travel farther if they are non-polar. More polar substances bond with the cellulose paper more quickly, and therefore do not travel as far. This process allows the calculation of an R_f value and can be compared to standard compounds to aid in the identification of an unknown substance. It is generally used for the separation of amino acids, in which ninhydrin is used as spray reagent to visualize the spots.

13.5.2. Thin Layer Chromatography

The stationary phase is a powdered adsorbent which consists of a thin layer of silica gel (SiO_2) or alumina (Al_2O_3) coated on a glass or plastic sheet. The mixture to be analyzed is loaded near the bottom of the plate. The plate is placed in a reservoir of solvent so that only the bottom of the plate is submerged. This solvent is the mobile phase; it gradually moves up the plate via capillary action, and it carries the deposited substances along with it at different rates. The desired result is that each component of the deposited mixture is moved a different distance up the plate by the solvent. It is often used to judge the purity of a compound. The components appear as a series of spots at different locations up the plate.

Table 13.4: Thin layer chromatography of amino acids

Amino Acid	Solvent	Spot Color after Iodination	Spot Color with Ninhydrin	R_f Value	Spot Shape
Alanine	3:7 NH_3/n-propanol	White	Purple		Elongated oval
Alanine	1:1 water/n-propanol	White	Purple	0.65	Circle
Glycine	3:7 NH_3/n-propanol	White	Pink	0.25	Elongated oval
Glycine	1:1 water/n-propanol	White	Pink	0.55	Circle
Threonine	3:7 NH_3/n-propanol	White	Purple		Elongated oval
Threonine	1:1 water/n-propanol	White	Purple	0.57	Circle
Proline	3:7 conc NH_3/n-propanol	Dark brown	Yellow with pink border		Elongated oval
Proline	1:1 water/n-propanol	White	Yellow with pink border	0.65	Circle

Components can be identified from their so-called R_f values. The R_f value for a substance is the ratio of the distance that the substance travels to the distance that the solvent travels up the plate. In case of spots which are colorless can be viewed with the help of some coloring agents which specifically give color to the components in contrast background. For example, iodination will help to view the amino acids in a brown background.

13.5.3. High-Performance Thin Layer Chromatography (HPTLC)

High-Performance Thin Layer Chromatography is an analytical technique based on thin layer chromatography, but with enhancements intended to increase the resolution of the compounds to be separated and to allow quantitative analysis of the compounds. Some of the enhancements include, more accurate sample loading, use of a densitometer and computer analysis to determine the size, intensity and position (retardation factor) of the separated compounds and use of higher quality TLC plates with finer particle sizes in the stationary phase allowing better resolution.

13.5.4. Column Chromatography

The stationary phase is a powdered adsorbent which is placed in a vertical glass column. The mixture to be analyzed is loaded on top of this column. The mobile phase is a solvent poured on top of the loaded column. The solvent flows down the column, causing the components of the mixture to distribute between the powdered adsorbent and the solvent, thus separating the components of the mixture so that as the solvent flows out of the bottom of the column, some components elute with early collections and other components elute with late fractions. The solvent is usually changed stepwise, and fractions are collected according to the separation required with the eluted solvent usually monitored by TLC.

13.5.5. High-performance Liquid Chromatography (HPLC)

It is a form of column chromatography used frequently in biochemistry and analytical chemistry to separate, identify, and quantify compounds. HPLC utilizes a column that holds chromatographic packing material (stationary phase), a pump that moves the mobile phase(s) through the column, and a detector that shows the retention times of the molecules. Retention time varies depending on the interactions between the stationary phase, molecules being analyzed, and the solvent(s) used.

13.5.6. Reversed Phase Chromatography (RP-HPLC or RPC)

It is an adsorptive process by experimental design, which relies on a partitioning mechanism to affect separation. Reversed Phase Chromatography, results from the adsorption of hydrophobic molecules onto a hydrophobic solid support in a polar mobile phase. Decreasing the mobile phase polarity by using organic solvents reduces the hydrophobic interaction between the solute and the solid support resulting in de-sorption. The more hydrophobic the molecule the more avidly it will adsorb onto the solid support. This requires a higher concentration of organic solvent to promote de-sorption.

The binding of the analyte to the stationary phase is proportional to the contact surface area around the non-polar segment of the analyte molecule upon association with the ligand in the aqueous eluent. Structural properties of the analyte molecule play an important role in its retention characteristics. In general, an analyte with a larger hydrophobic surface area (C-H, C-C, and generally non-polar atomic bonds, such as S-S and others) results in a longer retention time because it increases the molecule's non-polar surface area, which is non-interacting with the water structure. On the other hand, polar groups, such as -OH, $-NH_2$, COO^- or $-NH_3^+$ reduce retention as they are well integrated into water. Reversed phase HPLC has a non-polar stationary phase and an aqueous, moderately polar mobile phase. One common stationary phase is silica treated with RMe_2SiCl, where R is a straight chain alkyl group such as $C_{18}H_{37}$ or C_8H_{17}. With these stationary phases, retention time is longer for molecules which are more non-polar, while polar molecules elute more readily.

Reversed phase chromatography has found both analytical and preparative applications in the area of biochemical separation and purification. Reversed phase chromatography is another very powerful technique and it is effective for the separation of a very wide range of molecules. However, at process scale it is not typically used for proteins, due to the presence of the organic solvent which denatures many proteins and destroys their biological activity. Reversed phase chromatography is used very frequently as an analytical technique and there are many different stationary phases available for method optimization. Molecules that possess some degree of hydrophobic character, such as proteins, peptides and nucleic acids, can be separated by reversed phase chromatography with excellent recovery and resolution. In addition, the use of ion pairing modifiers in the mobile phase allows reversed phase chromatography of charged solutes such as fully deprotected oligonucleotides and hydrophilic peptides. Preparative reversed phase chromatography has found applications ranging from micropurification of protein fragments for sequencing to process scale purification of recombinant protein products.

13.5.7. Hydrophobic-Interaction Chromatography [HIC]

It is a type of reversed-phase chromatography that is used to separate large biomolecules, such as proteins. It is usually desirable to maintain these molecules intact in an aqueous solution, avoiding contact with organic solvents or surfaces that might denature them. HIC takes advantage of the hydrophobic interaction of large molecules with a moderately hydrophobic stationary phase, *e.g.*, butyl-bonded [C4], rather than octadecyl-bonded [C18], silica.

Initially, higher salt concentrations in water will encourage the proteins to be retained (salted out) on the packing. Gradient separations are typically run by decreasing salt concentration. In this way, biomolecules are eluted in order of increasing hydrophobicity.

13.5.8. Ion Exchange Chromatography

It is the most popular method for the purification of proteins and other charged molecules. It relies on charge-charge interactions between the proteins in sample and the charges immobilized on the resin of choice. It can be subdivided into cation exchange chromatography, in which positively charged ions bind to a negatively charged resin; and anion exchange chromatography, in which the binding ions are negative, and the immobilized functional group is positive. Once the solutes are bound, the column is washed to equilibrate it in starting buffer, which should be of low ionic strength, and then the bound molecules are eluted off using a gradient of a second buffer which steadily increases the ionic strength of the eluent solution. Alternatively, the pH of the eluent buffer can be modified as to give the protein or the matrix a charge at which they will not interact and the molecule of interest elutes from the resin.

In cation exchange chromatography, raising the pH of the mobile phase buffer will cause the molecule to become less protonated and hence less positively charged. The result is that the protein no longer has the capability to form a strong ionic interaction with the negatively charged solid support which causes the molecule to elute from the chromatography column. In anion exchange chromatography, lowering the pH of the mobile phase buffer will cause the molecule to become more protonated and hence more positively charged. The result is that the protein no longer has the capability to form a strong ionic interaction with the positively charged solid support which causes the molecule to elute from the chromatography column (Fig. 13.17).

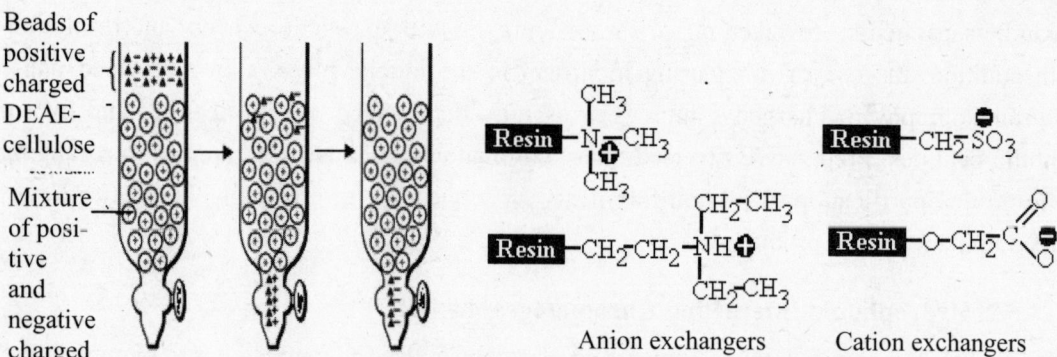

Figure 13.17: Diagrammatic representation of ion exchange chromatography

Commonly used anion exchange resins are Q-resin (a Quaternary amine) and DEAE (Diethyl amino ethane) resin and cation exchange resins are S-resin (sulfate derivatives) and

CM resins (carboxylate derived ions). Strong ion exchangers bear functional groups (e.g., quaternary amines or sulfonic acids) that are always ionized. They are typically used to retain and separate weak ions. These weak ions may be eluted by displacement with a mobile phase containing ions that are more strongly attracted to the stationary phase sites. Alternately, weak ions may be retained on the column, then neutralized by *in situ* changing the pH of the mobile phase, causing them to lose their attraction and elute. Weak ion exchangers (*e.g.*, with secondary-amine or carboxylic-acid functions) may be neutralized above or below a certain pH value and lose their ability to retain ions by charge.

13.5.9. Affinity Chromatography is the most powerful technique which can potentially allow a one-step purification of the target molecule. In order to work, a specific ligand (a molecule which recognizes the target protein) must be immobilized on a support in such a way that allows it to bind to the target molecule. It is a chromatographic method of separating biochemical mixtures, based on a highly specific biologic interaction such as that between antigen and antibody, enzyme and substrate, or receptor and ligand. A classic example of this would be the use of an immobilized protein to capture its receptor (the reverse would also work). Affinity chromatography can be used in a number of applications, including nucleic acid purification, protein purification such as recombinant proteins from cell free extracts, and antibody purification from blood serum.

13.5.10. Size Exclusion Chromatography (SEC): It is the separation of mixtures based on the molecular size of the components. Separation is achieved by the differential exclusion or inclusion, within the packing particles, of the sample molecules as they pass through a porous-particle stationary phase. The principle feature of SEC is its gentle non-adsorptive interaction with the sample, enabling high retention of biomolecular activity. For the separation of biomolecules in aqueous systems, SEC is referred to as gel filtration chromatography (GFC), while the separation of organic polymers in non-aqueous systems is called gel permeation chromatography (GPC).

Size exclusion chromatography is used primarily for analytical assays and semi-preparative purifications. It is typically not used for process scale work due to its lack of binding capacity.

13.5.11. Gas Chromatography: Specifically gas-liquid chromatography - involves a sample being vaporized and injected onto the head of the chromatographic column. The sample is transported through the column by the flow of inert, gaseous mobile phase. The column itself contains a liquid stationary phase which is adsorbed onto the surface of an inert solid. The stationary phase is a high-boiling liquid, which is packed into a long, narrow glass or metal column. The mixture to be analyzed is loaded by syringe into the beginning of this column. The mobile phase is an inert gas which continuously flows through the column. It is generally used for the study of essential oils present in plants.

The Gas Chromatography/Mass Spectrometry (**GC/MS**) instrument separates chemical mixtures (the GC component) and identifies the components at a molecular level (the MS component). The GC works on the principle that a mixture will separate into individual substances when heated. The heated gases are carried through a column with an inert gas (such as helium). As the separated substances emerge from the column opening, they flow into the MS. Mass spectrometry identifies compounds by the mass of analyte molecule (Fig. 13. 18).

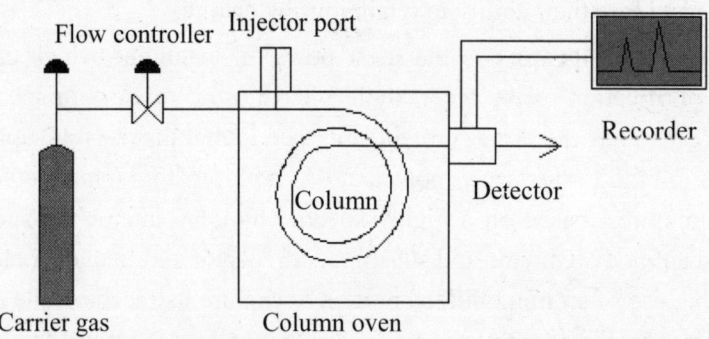

Figure 13.18: Instrumentation of gas chromatography

13.6. Spectroscopy

Spectroscopy is the study of spectra, i.e. characteristic wavelengths or colours. Physicists classify light waves by their energies (wavelengths). Electromagnetic radiation such as visible light is commonly treated as a wave phenomenon, characterized by a wavelength or frequency. Wavelength (λ) is defined as the distance between adjacent peaks (or troughs), and may be designated in meters, centimeters or nanometers (10^{-9} meters). Frequency (ν) is the number of wave cycles that travel past a fixed point per unit of time, and is usually given in cycles per second, or hertz (Hz). Visible wavelengths cover a range from approximately 400 to 800 nm. The longest visible wavelength is red and the shortest is violet. The energy of a light wave is inversely-proportional to its wavelength; in other words, low-energy waves have long wavelengths, and high-energy light waves have short wavelengths. The energy of a light wave is inversely-proportional to its wavelength; in other words, low-energy waves have long wavelengths, and high-energy light waves have short wavelengths ($E=h\nu = hc/\lambda$, where h is the Planks constant)

Many molecules absorb ultraviolet or visible light. The visible region of the spectrum comprises photon energies of 36 to 72 kcal/mole and the near ultraviolet region, out to 200 nm, extends this energy range to 143 kcal/mole. Ultraviolet radiation having wavelengths less than 200 nm is difficult to handle, and is seldom used as a routine tool for structural analysis. Different molecules absorb radiation of different wavelengths. An absorption spectrum will show a number of absorption bands corresponding to structural groups within the molecule. The molecular moieties likely to absorb light in the 200 to 800 nm regions are pi-electron functions and hetero atoms having non-bonding valence-shell electron pairs. Such light absorbing groups are referred to as chromophores (Fig. 13.19).

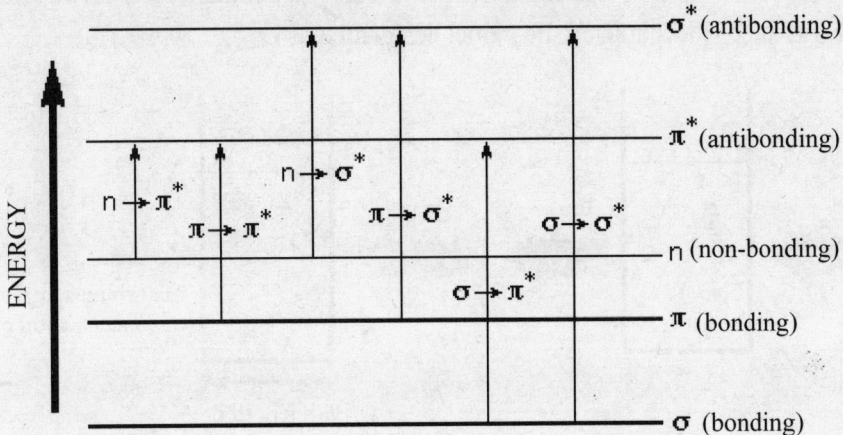

Figure 13.19: Diagram showing the various kinds of electronic excitation that may occur in organic molecules

The Beer-Lambert law (also called the Beer-Lambert-Bouguer law or simply Beer's law) is the linear relationship between absorbance and concentration of an absorber of electromagnetic radiation. The general Beer-Lambert law is usually written as: $A = a_\lambda bc$, where A is the measured absorbance, a_λ is the wavelength-dependent absorptivity coefficient, b is the path length, and c is the analyte concentration. When working in concentration units of molarity, the Beer-Lambert law is written as: $A = \varepsilon_\lambda bc$, where ε_λ is the wavelength-dependent molar absorptivity coefficient with units of $M^{-1} cm^{-1}$. The λ subscript is often dropped with the understanding that a value for ε is for aspecific wavelength. If multiple species that absorb light at a given wavelength are present in a sample, the total absorbance at that wavelength is the sum due to all absorbers.

In analytical applications we often want to measure the concentration of an analyte independent of the effects of reflection, solvent absorption, or other interferences. The figure below shows the two transmittance measurements that are necessary to use absorption to determine the concentration of an analyte in solution. In this example, I_s is the source light intensity that is incident on a sample, I is the measured light power after passing through the analyte, solvent, and sample holder, and I_o is the measured light power after passing through only the solvent and sample holder. The measured transmittance in this case is attributed to only the analyte (Fig. 13.20).

If the compound in a sample does not absorb light at a given wavelength then, $I = I_0$. However, if the compound absorbs light then I is less than I_0, and this difference may be plotted on a graph versus wavelength, as shown on the right. Absorption may be presented as transmittance ($T = I/I_0$) or absorbance ($A = \log I_0/I$). If no absorption occurs then, $T = 1.0$ and $A = 0$. Most spectrometers display absorbance on the vertical axis, and the commonly observed range is from 0 (100% transmittance) to 2 (1% transmittance). The wavelength of maximum absorbance is a characteristic value, designated as λ_{max}.

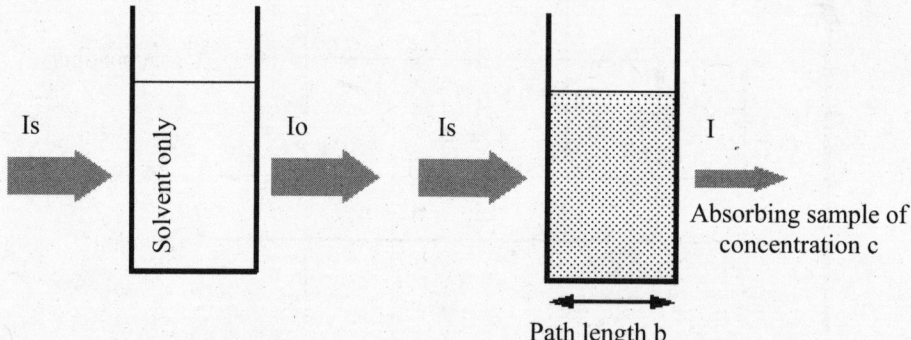

Figure 13.20: Absorption of radiation by solutions

13.6.1. UV-Visible Spectroscopy

In UV/Visible Spectroscopy, the term chromophore is used to indicate a functional group that absorbs electromagnetic radiation, usually in the UV or visible region. The type of functional groups that absorb ultraviolet light can be conjugated species, such as alkenes, aromatics, etc. Also many metal-ligand complexes also absorb UV/visible light. Its important to remember that UV/visible EM radiation causes electronic transitions within a molecule, promoting bonding and non-bonding electrons to higher, less stable antibonding orbitals. The molecule then loses this excess energy by rotation and vibrational relaxation, but some compounds can lose their energy by emission processes such as fluorescence.

Working

UV-VIS spectrometers consist of a light source, reference and sample beams, a monochromator and a detector. The ultraviolet spectrum for a compound is obtained by exposing a sample of the compound to ultraviolet light from a light source, such as a Xenon lamp. The reference beam in the spectrometer travels from the light source to the detector without interacting with the sample. The sample beam interacts with the sample exposing it to ultraviolet light of continuously changing wavelength. When the emitted wavelength corresponds to the energy level which promotes an electron to a higher molecular orbital, energy is absorbed. The detector records the ratio between reference and sample beam intensities (I_0/I). At the wavelength where the sample absorbs a large amount of light, the detector receives a very weak sample beam. Once intensity data has been collected by the spectrometer, it is sent to the computer as a ratio of reference beam and sample beam intensities. The computer determines at what wavelength the sample absorbed a large amount of ultraviolet light by scanning for the largest gap between the two beams. When a large gap between intensities is found, where the sample beam intensity is significantly weaker than the reference beam, the computer plots this wavelength as having the highest ultraviolet light absorbance. Over a short period of time, the spectrometer automatically scans all the component wavelengths in the manner described. The ultraviolet (UV) region scanned is normally from 200 to 400 nm, and the visible portion is from 400 to 800 nm (Fig. 13.21).

Different compounds may have very different absorption maxima and absorbances. Intensely absorbing compounds must be examined in dilute solution, so that significant light energy is received by the detector, and this requires the use of completely transparent (non-absorbing) solvents. The most commonly used solvents are water, ethanol, hexane and cyclohexane.

Proteins have an absorption maxima at 280 nm, which can be used for the quantification. Trypophan, tyrosine, histidine, and phenylalanine residues contain aromatic rings that absorb the greatest amount of light at 280nm. Nucleic acids have an absorption maximum close to 260 nm. At a wavelength of 260 nm, the average extinction coefficient for double-stranded DNA is 0.020 $(\mu g/ml)^{-1}$ cm^{-1}, for single-stranded DNA and RNA it is 0.027 $(\mu g/ml)^{-1}$ cm^{-1} and for short single-stranded oligonucleotides it is dependent on the length and base composition. Thus, an optical density of 1 corresponds to a concentration of 50$\mu g/ml$ for double-stranded DNA.

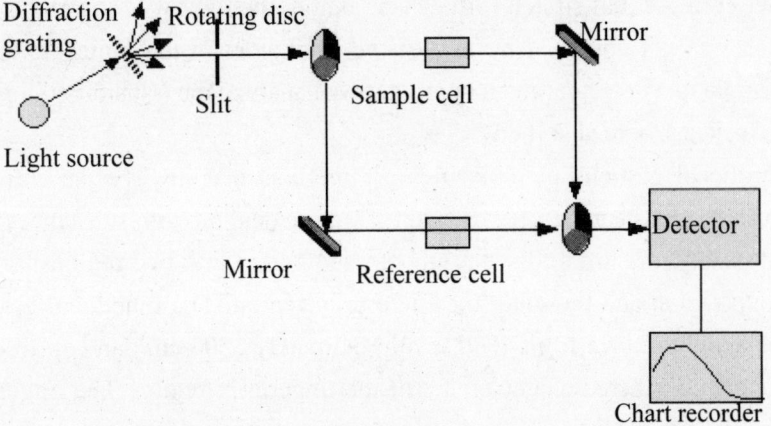

Figure 13.21: Instrumentation of UV-Vis spectroscope

13.6.2. IR Spectroscopy

Infrared, or IR spectroscopy a type of vibrational spectroscopy, is a spectroscopic technique where molecular vibrations are analyzed. Molecules are formed by combining atoms together by chemical bonds. To make this clear, imagine two spheres, or masses, connected with a spring. This is what is known as a simple harmonic oscillator.

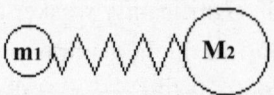

Once set into motion, the sphere will oscillate, or vibrate back and forth on the spring, at a certain frequency depending on the masses of the spheres and the stiffness of the spring. A sphere with a small mass is lighter and easier to move around than one with a large mass. Therefore, smaller masses oscillate at a higher frequency than larger masses. A very stiff spring, like a bedspring, is hard to deform and quickly returns to its original shape when the deforming force is removed. The bond is the spring, and the two atoms, or groups of atoms, connected by the bond are the masses. Every atom has a different mass, and single, double and triple all have different stiffness, and therefore each combination of atoms and bonds has its own characteristic harmonic frequency.

At any temperature above absolute zero, all the little simple harmonic oscillators that make up any molecule are vibrating vigorously. Infrared light just happens to be in the same frequency range as a vibrating molecule. So, if you hit a vibrating molecule with some IR light, it will absorb those frequencies in the light which exactly match the frequencies of the different harmonic oscillators that make up that molecule. When this light is absorbed, the little oscillators in the molecule will continue to vibrate at the same frequency, but since they have absorbed the energy of the light, they will have larger amplitude of vibration. This means that the "springs" will stretch further than before the light was absorbed. The remaining light which was not absorbed by any of the oscillators in the molecule is transmitted through the sample to a detector, and a computer will analyze the transmitted light and determine what frequencies were absorbed.

Many vibrational motions of molecules are motions that involve the entire molecule. Analysis of such motions can be very difficult if we are dealing with substances of unknown structure. Fortunately, the infrared spectrum can be divided into two regions, one called the functional group region and the other the fingerprint region. The functional group region is generally considered to range from 4000 to approximately 1500 cm^{-1} and all frequencies below 1500 cm^{-1} are considered characteristic of the fingerprint region. The fingerprint region involves molecular vibrations, usually bending motions that are characteristic of the entire molecule or large fragments of the molecule. Used together, both regions are very useful for confirming the identity of a chemical substance. This is generally accomplished by a comparison of the spectrum of an authentic sample. The functional group region tends to include motions, generally stretching vibrations, that are more localized and characteristic of the typical functional groups found in organic molecules. While these bands are not very useful in confirming identity, they do provide some very useful information about the nature of the components that make up the molecule. Perhaps most importantly, the frequencies of these bands are reliable and their presence or absence can be used confidently by both the novice and expert interpreter of infrared spectra. IR is used to gather information about compound's structure, assess its purity, and sometimes to identify it (Table !3.4). An IR spectrum is a plot of wave number (X-axis) vs. percent transmittance (Y-axis).

Table 13.4: Principle infrared bands and their assignments (R - aliphatic group)

Functional Group	Type		Frequencies (cm-1)
C-H	sp3 hybridized	R3C-H	2850-3000
	sp2 hybridized	=CR-H	3000-3250
	sp hybridized	C-H	3300
	aldehyde C-H	H-(C=O)R	2750, 2850
N-H	primary amine, amide	RN-H2, RCON-H2	3300, 3340
	secondary amine, amide	RNR-H, RCON-HR	3300-3500
	tertiary amine, amide	RN(R3), RCONR2	none
O-H	alcohols, phenols	free O-H	3620-3580
		hydrogen bonded	3600-3650
	carboxylic acids	R(C=O)O-H	3500-2400
C=O	aldehydes	R(C=O)H	1740-1720
	ketones	R(C=O)R	1730-1710
	esters	R(CO2)R	1750-1735
	anhydrides	R(CO2CO)R	1820, 1750
	carboxylates	R(CO2)H	1600, 1400
C=C	olefins	R2C=CR2	1680-1640
		R2C=CH2	1600-1675
		R2C=C(OR)R	1600-1630
-NO2	Nitro groups	RNO2	1550, 1370

Infrared spectra may be obtained from samples in all phases (liquid, solid and gaseous). Liquids are usually examined as a thin film sandwiched between two polished salt plates (note that glass absorbs infrared radiation, whereas NaCl is transparent). If solvents are used to dissolve solids, care must be taken to avoid obscuring important spectral regions by solvent absorption. Perchlorinated solvents such as carbon tetrachloride, chloroform and tetrachloroethene are commonly used. Alternatively, solids may be incorporated in a thin KBr disk, prepared under high pressure, or mixed with a little non-volatile liquid and ground to a paste (or mull) that is smeared between salt plates.

13.6.3. Nuclear Magnetic Resonance (NMR) spectroscopy

Nuclear Magnetic Resonance (NMR) is a non-destructive technique for mapping molecular structures and learning how molecules function and relate to each other. It relies on magnetic properties possessed by some nuclei, notably ^1H, ^{13}C, ^{19}F and ^{31}P. This is important for many applications, including the drug discovery, evaluation of new synthetic material and exploring realms of the proteomics.

NMR spectra arise from a characteristic property of the nucleus, called nuclear spin on its axis characterized by nuclear spin quantum number. The spinning nucleus generates a magnetic field, since it is a moving charge. If an external magnetic field is applied to the nucleus, then the spin state where the nuclear magnetic field is aligned with the external field has a different, lower, energy from that spin state that gives rise to an opposing field. This action is called resonance and can be physically mapped, showing which atoms are present in the molecule and where they are located in relation to each other, thus the term nuclear magnetic resonance.

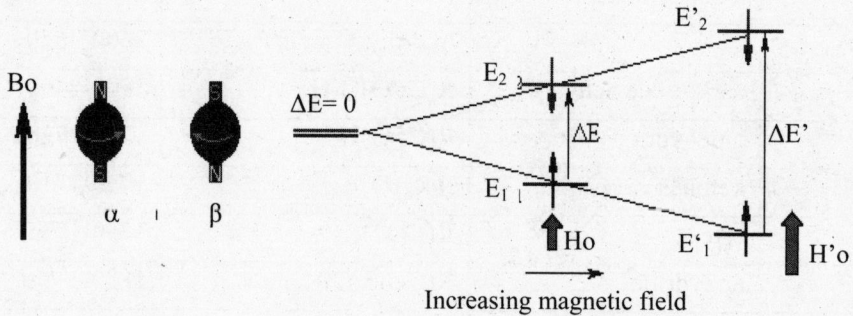

Figure 13.22: Spin energy states

Since the two states have different energies, it is possible to convert a nucleus from the lower-energy state E_1 to the higher state E_2 by the input of suitable energy. The energy difference ΔE is such that radio frequency waves will perform this switch. The NMR spectrum arises because nuclei in different parts of the molecule experience different local magnetic fields according to the molecular structure, and so have different frequencies at which they absorb. This difference is called the chemical shift. The radio frequency used depends on the strength of the magnetic field; early machines used magnetic field strengths of around 1.5 Tesla (15000 Gauss), the proton magnetic resonances being around 60MHz. In practice the radio frequency is kept constant, and the magnetic field is then swept over a narrow range of field strength. The absorptions are plotted on a graph where the frequency differences (in reality magnetic field differences) are plotted relative to some standard compound which defines the zero; for proton magnetic resonance this compound is TMS, tetramethylsilane, Si $(CH_3)_4$ (Fig. 13.22).

Each molecule has a different internal structure, depending upon the atoms it contains, and these varying structures paint a unique profile, or spectrum, when exposed to magnetic energy. Not only does this technology allow researchers to understand the three dimensional structure and relationships of atoms in molecules, but it also tells them how they relate to other atoms in the molecule over time. This characteristic is important in the study of proteins, carbohydrates, and genetic material, such as DNA and RNA.

Working

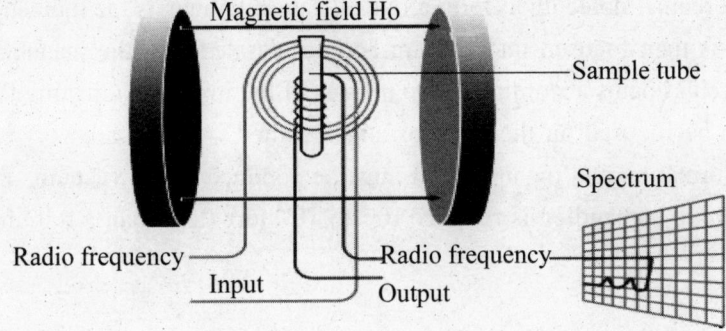

Figure 13.23: Working arrangement of NMR spectroscope

The basic arrangement of an NMR spectrometer is shown above. The sample is positioned in the magnetic field and excited via pulsations in the radio frequency input circuit. The test sample is put in a long slender glass tube with 1" of liquid. Samples can be less than 1/1000 cubic inch of the gas, liquid, or solid. The realigned magnetic fields induce a radio signal in the output circuit which is used to generate the output signal (Fig. 13.23).

The NMR console triggers split-second bursts, or pulses, of RF energy that are precisely sequenced to excite the sample in the probe and cause the atomic nuclei to resonate. The high-power RF energy pulses are sent to the NMR probe, the "antenna" that provides the radio frequency (RF) link between the sample and the instrument. The superconducting magnet provides a strong, homogenous magnetic field that can be as much as 200,000 times stronger than the earth's magnetic field. The natural magnets in the nuclei line up with the powerful NMR magnet, similar to iron fillings aligning with the magnetic field of a toy magnet. The RF pulses from the NMR console excite the atoms in the sample, making the nuclei "wobble" or resonate. As soon as the RF signals stop, the nuclei return to their natural and more comfortable state. As the nuclei relax, the NMR probe receives a very weak RF resonance response back from the sample and transmits it to the NMR console for amplification. The NMR console amplifies the faint returning signals over 1,000,000 times before sending them to the computer workstation for analysis. Fourier analysis of the complex output produces the actual spectrum. The pulse is repeated as many times as necessary to allow the signals to be identified from the background noise.

13.6.4. Mass Spectroscopy

Mass spectroscopy helps to find out the molecular mass of an organic compound, which helps in the identification of an unknown compound like a metabolite. The physics behind mass spectrometry is that a charged particle passing through a magnetic field is deflected along a circular path on a radius that is proportional to the mass to charge ratio, m/e. In an electron impact mass spectrometer, a high energy beam of electrons is used to displace an electron from the organic molecule to form a radical cation known as the molecular ion. The collection of ions is then focused into a beam and accelerated into the magnetic field and deflected along circular paths according to the masses of the ions. By adjusting the magnetic field, the ions can be focused on the detector and recorded. As ions are very reactive and short-lived, their formation and manipulation must be conducted in a vacuum. The pressure under which ions may be handled is roughly 10^{-5} to 10^{-8} torr (less than a billionth of an atmosphere).

Working

The first stage is ionization, where a sample of atoms is injected into the vacuum chamber. An electron gun bombards the sample with electrons knocking some from the atoms, creating cations. When a high energy electron collides with a molecule it often ionizes it by knocking away one of the molecular electrons (either bonding or non-bonding). If molecules are used they may be broken into fragments. (For example an atom M under goes the change $M_{(g)} \rightarrow M^+_{(g)} + e^-$). The next stage is acceleration. Negatively charged plates produce an electric field that accelerates the ions towards the electromagnet. Defection takes place next, whereby a magnetic field deflects the ions. The extent of the deflection depends on the mass of the ions. When the ion beam experiences a strong magnetic field perpendicular to its direction of motion, the ions are deflected in an arc whose radius is inversely proportional to the mass of the ion. Lighter ions are deflected more than heavier ions. By varying the strength of the magnetic field, ions of different mass can be focused progressively on a detector fixed at the end of a curved tube (under a high vacuum). A tiny current is produced when the cation reaches the detector. A recorder counts the number of signals and represents it as peaks on mass spectrum graph. Since mass spectrometer separates and detects ions of different masses, it easily distinguishes different isotopes of given element (Fig. 13.24).

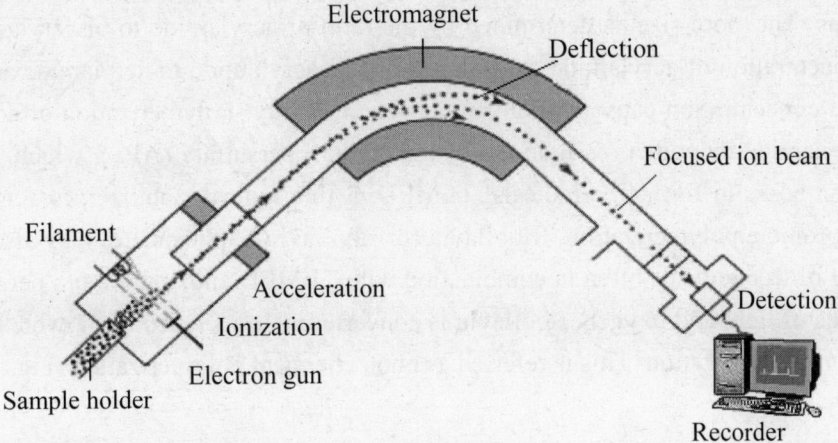

Figure 13.24: Working of mass spectroscope

13.7. Electrophoresis

Electrophoresis is the migration or separation of charged particles or solutes in an electrical field. Charged particles will migrate to the electrode of the opposite charge, i.e., positive ions (cations) will migrate to the cathode, the negative electrode, while negative ions (anions) will migrate to the anode, the positive electrode. In gel electrophoresis, the molecules will travel at different speeds depending on their size. Smaller molecules will be able to move faster and will reach the far end of the gel, while larger molecules will be slowed down and remain near the beginning. This property can be utilized for the separation of proteins and DNA according to their size.

An amphoteric molecule has the ability to be negatively or positively charged depending upon the pH. A molecule with this amphoteric ability is referred as an ampholyte or Zwitter ion. Proteins and nucleic acids are amphoteric in nature; proteins with their ionizable amino and carboxyl groups are amphoteric. Thus by electrophoresis, usually, a lane with a standard marker is included and helps to determine relative sizes of samples. For example, the sizes of DNA and RNA markers are expressed in bases (b) or kilobases (kb), while the proteins markers are in KiloDaltons.

13.7.1. Sodium dodecyl sulfate-polyacrylamide gel electrophoresis (PAGE)

Polyacrylamide gel electrophoresis (PAGE) is probably the most common analytical technique used to separate and characterize proteins. In the process of polyacrylamide gel electrophoresis (PAGE), proteins are placed in an electric field and are forced to move through a porous matrix or gel (polyacrylamide) by the current. It involves the polymerization of solutions of acrylamide and bisacrylamide. The chemistry of the reaction consists of acrylamide forms linear polymers, while the bisacrylamide introduces cross links between polyacrylamide chains. The 'pore size' is determined by the ratio of acrylamide to bisacrylamide, and by the concentration of acrylamide. A high ratio of bisacrylamide to acrylamide and a high acrylamide concentration cause low electrophoretic mobility. Polymerization of acrylamide and bisacrylamide monomers is induced by ammonium persulfate (APS), which spontaneously decomposes to form free radicals. TEMED, a free radical stabilizer, is generally included to promote polymerization. Riboflavin (or riboflavin-5'-phosphate) may also be used as a source of free radicals often in combination with TEMED and ammonium persulfate. In the presence of light and oxygen, riboflavin is converted in to its leuco form, which is active in initiating polymerization. This is referred as photochemical polymerization (Fig. 13.25).

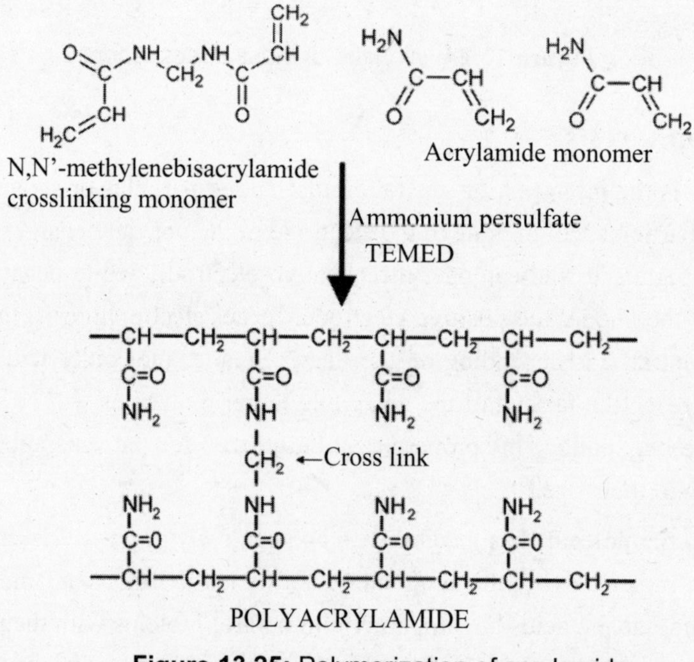

Figure 13.25: Polymerization of acrylamide

To move through the gel, the proteins must move through the pores of the polyacrylamide. The rate at which proteins move through the polyacrylamide gel is dependent on their charge and their mass. The charge of a protein is dependent on its constituent amino acids and the pH of the buffer. Proteins that carry a high degree of charge will move at a faster rate than those with a lower overall charge. In addition, the mobility of small polypeptides through the gel will be faster than larger polypeptides because they are less restricted by the pores. The overall rate of movement or mobility of a protein in PAGE is determined by its charge to mass ratio or charge density. Proteins with a high charge to mass ratio will have a higher mobility in PAGE than those with a low ratio. Mercaptoethanol reduces all disulfide bonds of cysteine residues to free sulfhydryl groups, and heating with SDS disrupts all intra- and intermolecular protein interactions. This treatment yields individual polypeptide chains which carry an excess negative charge induced by the binding of the detergent, and an identical charge: mass ratio.

Working

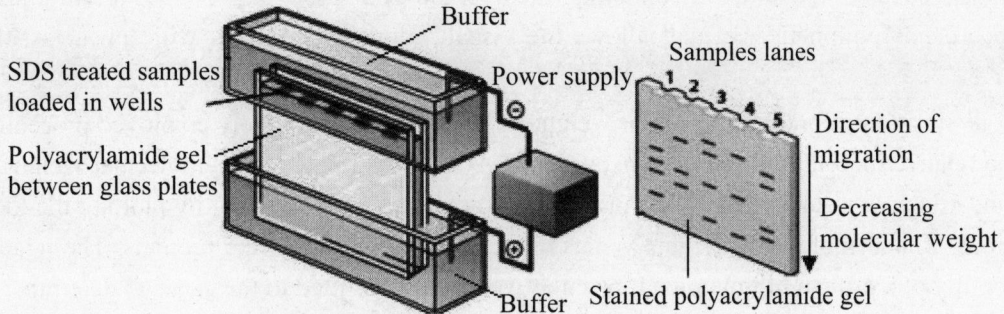

Figure 13.26: Electrophoresis assembly

The process of SDS-PAGE is performed in a polyacrlyamide gel that is cast between two flat glass plates which are separated by spacers (1 mm thickness). The polyacrylamide gel consists of two separate components. The lower part of the gel is called the resolving gel. It is the portion of the gel that will act as molecular sieve to separate proteins. The upper part of the gel is called the stacking gel. The polyacrylamide content of the stacking gel is very low. Therefore, it has pores that are too large to separate proteins. The stacking gel contains several regularly spaced wells into which the samples will be loaded. In addition, the buffer in the stacking gel has particular electrical properties that will serve to concentrate the protein samples before they enter the resolving gel. This will maximize the separation or resolution of the gel (Fig. 13.26).

The electrophoretic apparatus contains two chambers: upper and lower buffer reservoirs. The glass plates containing the gel are clamped vertically into an apparatus. When the upper reservoir is filled with buffer, the buffer flows over the top edge of the shorter plate and contacts the upper surface of the gel. Buffer placed in the lower reservoir makes contact with the lower surface of the gel. Both reservoirs contain electrodes that are connected to a power supply. When the power is applied to the apparatus, the upper electrode acts as a cathode (negative electrode) and the lower electrode acts as an anode (positive electrode). The circuit between the two electrodes is completed by the flow of current through the slab gel.

The protein sample is applied to the upper part of the slab gel (stacking gel) in separate wells. The protein sample contains SDS, protein, buffer, and glycerol or sucrose. The glycerol or sucrose adds density to the sample making it easier to layer on the surface of the gel. The proteins move down toward the anode when the current is applied. The blue dye, bromophenol blue, is included in the sample. The dye is very small and highly charged. Therefore, it will move down through the gel at a rate faster than the proteins in the sample. The movement of the dye is used to monitor the progress of electrophoresis and is called the tracking dye. The electrophoresis is stopped when the blue dye reaches the bottom of the slab gel. After electrophoresis is finished, the gel is removed from between the glass plates and is incubated in a solution containing the dye, the Coomassie blue R-250. It will bind to the proteins within the gel and allows the visualization; the proteins will appear as blue bands.

Estimation of protein molecular weight by SDS-PAGE is a widely employed procedure. The relative mobility of a protein in an SDS-PAGE gel is related to its molecular weight. A standard curve is constructed with proteins of known molecular weight by plotting the logarithms of their molecular weights versus the relative mobilities of the proteins. The relative mobility of a protein of unknown molecular weight is then fitted to the curve to determine its molecular weight.

13.7.2. Native Gel Electrophoresis

Native structure and conformation is very important for biological protein functions such as enzymatic activity and interaction of antibodies with their ligands, etc. To preserve native protein structure and conformation, proteins are analyzed by non-denaturing electrophoresis. The pH of the buffer system is an important parameter for optimal protein separation. Native protein electrophoresis is often carried out in Tris-glycine electrophoresis buffer. Protein samples used for the native electrophoresis should be devoid of strong denaturants such as SDS.

13.7.3. Agarose Gel Electrophoresis

Agarose is a polysaccharide extracted from seaweed. Agarose gel electrophoresis is the easiest and common way of separating and analyzing DNA. The DNA separated by agarose gel electrophoresis is visualized by addition of ethidium bromide in the gel. This binds strongly to DNA by intercalating between the bases and is fluorescent; it absorbs UV light and transmits the energy as orange light.

Most agarose gels are made between 0.7% to 2%. A 0.7% gel will show good separation (resolution) of large DNA fragments (5–10 kb),while 2% gel will show good resolution for small fragments (0.2–1 kb). Typically, a band is easily visible if it contains about 20 ng of DNA. The loading buffer gives color and density to the sample to make it easy to load into the wells. Also, the dyes are negatively charged in neutral buffers and thus move in the same direction as the DNA during electrophoresis. This allows monitoring the progress of the gel. The most common dyes are bromophenol blue and xylene cyanol. Density is provided by glycerol or sucrose. Bromophenol blue migrates at a rate equivalent to 200–400 bp DNA. Xylene cyanol migrates at approximately 4kb equivalence.

Working

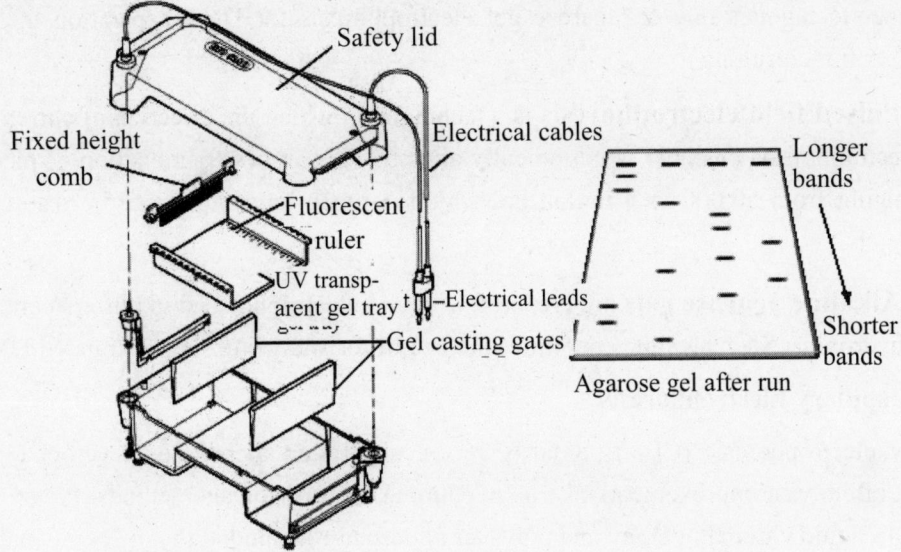

Figure 13.27: Arrangement of agarose gel electrophoresis assembly

To cast the gel, agarose powder is mixed with electrophoresis buffer to the desired concentration and then heated in a microwave oven until completely melted. Most commonly, ethidium bromide is added to the gel (final concentration 0.5 ug/ml) at this point to facilitate visualization of DNA after electrophoresis. After cooling the solution to about 60°C, it is poured into a casting tray containing a sample comb and allowed to solidify at room temperature (Fig. 13.27).

Agarose gels can be run in many different types of electrophoresis buffers. Nucleic acid agarose gel electrophoresis is usually conducted with either Tris-Acetate-EDTA (TAE) buffer or Tris-Borate-EDTA (TBE) buffer. While TAE buffer provides faster electrophoretic migration of linear DNA and better resolution of super-coiled DNA, TBE buffers have a stronger buffering capacity for longer or higher voltage electrophoresis runs. After the complete run the separated bands can be viewed in transilluminator, a UV chamber. Agarose gels can be used for the separation of DNA fragments ranging from 50 base pairs to several megabases (millions of bases) by electrophoresis. Agarose gel electrophoresis can be used for,

- Separation of restriction enzyme digested DNA including genomic DNA, prior to Southern Blot transfer and RNA prior to Northern transfer.
- Analysis of PCR products to assess for target DNA amplification.
- Allow the estimation of the size of DNA molecules using a DNA marker or ladder which contains DNA fragments of various known sizes.
- Allow the rough estimation of DNA quantity and quality.
- Other techniques rely on agarose gel electrophoresis for DNA separation including DNA fingerprinting.

13.7.4. Pulsed field electrophoresis is a technique in which the direction of current flow in the electrophoresis chamber is periodically altered. This allows fractionation of pieces of DNA ranging from 50,000 to 5 millon bp, which is much larger than can be resolved on standard gels.

13.7.5. Alkaline agarose gels are prepared with and electrophoresed in buffers containing sodium hydroxide. Such alkaline conditions are useful for analyzing single-stranded DNA.

13.7.6. Capillary Electrophoresis

Capillary electrophoresis (CE) is a fairly recent separation technique, developed in the 1980s. It offers vast improvements over conventional electrophoresis methods. It is complementary to liquid chromatography and plays an important role among the different analytical techniques currently available. Capillary electrophoresis has numerous applications and provides the advantage of high resolution, speed, and ease of use, automation and low cost. CE can be applied to a wide range of compounds, ranging from small ions to macromolecules. Numerous CE methods have been developed for pharmaceutical, biological, phytochemical and environmental applications.

Capillary electrophoresis applies to molecules that are either positively or negatively charged and which migrate in an electrical field with different velocities. The time-dependent separations of the different constituents in a mixture depend on two principal factors called electrophoretic mobility and electro-osmotic flow. Indeed, a charged molecule in an electrical field is subjected to a force that is proportional to its effective charge (q) and the electrical field which applied (E). Neutral species are not separated unless there is some association with the ions of the electrolyte itself, leading to different drag forces. Different mobilities are designated as (+) or (-) depending on the charge that is carried. For species that have no net charge, mobility is nil (Fig. 13.28).

Electroosmotic flow (or electroosmolarity) finds its origins in the inner wall of the capillary which is lined with silanol groups. Silanols are compounds containing silicon atoms to which hydroxy substituents bond directly. These groups become ionized at pH 2 and above and thus create a negatively charged inner lining. To maintain electrical neutrality the cations from the buffer solution cover this lining, thus creating a second layer. When an electrical field is created, the cations from this double layer start migrating towards the cathode. Their movement drags the buffer solution and creates a flow called the electroosmotic flow. This flow can be controlled by changing the electrical tension, the pH, the type of capillary used and by including specific additives. Because of electroosmotic flow, neutral molecules and anions may move in the direction of the detector which is usually located on the cathode end of the capillary.

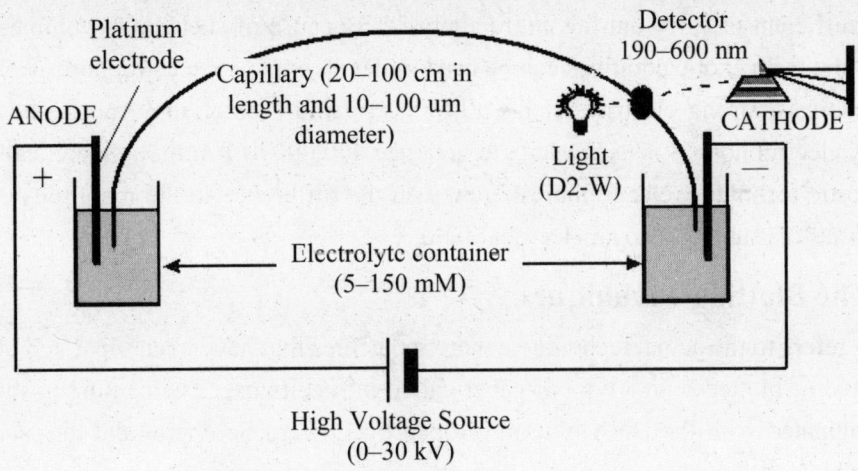

Figure 13.28: Capillary electrophoresis

Instrumentation

The instrumentation needed to perform capillary electrophoresis is very simple. Schematically, CE is composed of a silica capillary with both extremities resting in tanks filled with a buffer solution. Capillaries are usually 30–100 cm long and have an internal diameter of 50 or 75 μm. An electrical field of up to 30 kV may be applied through electrodes immersed in the electrolyte solution in the two tanks. The electrolyte solution is generally made up of an aqueous buffer with precise pH and ionic strength. It may also contain specific additives (e.g. cyclodextrins, surfactants, organic modifiers) that enhance the separation of molecules.

In order to avoid Joule heating, the current and the voltage are rigorously controlled and electrophoresis takes place in a thermostatic chamber.

The different compounds separated by electrophoresis are generally detected during the run by a UV-visible absorbance detector or a fluorometer positioned at the cathode end of the capillary. Now it is possible to couple CE to a mass spectrometer (MS) in real time. Besides adding sensitivity and selectivity, MS also provides structural information about the separated molecules. This coupled technique can thus be used to analyze pharmaceutically active compounds and their metabolites in any biological fluid (e.g. plasma, urine, saliva). The coupling of the two techniques requires the addition of a specific solution to the effluent from the capillary. The mixture is then vaporized, ionized and finally introduced into the mass spectrometer.

There are two main methods to introduce the sample into the capillary: hydrodynamic injection (by pressure, aspiration or siphoning) and electrokinetic injection. The latter method is particularly useful in the detection of pharmaceutical product present in the ppb range. The injection volumes may be as low as a nanoliter and a few microliters of the sample are sufficient to carry out the entire analysis. Because of such small volumes, very expensive and even exotic additives can be used in developing new electrophoresis methods. In electrophoresis, strong electrical fields allow very rapid separations. Another advantage of capillary electrophoresis is its capacity to generate 400,000 to 1 million theoretical plates. As a diagnostic technique, electrophoresis relies on the difference in the mobilities of two distinct substances subjected to an electrical field.

13.8. The Blotting Techniques

Blotting refers to the actual technique, where molecules that have been separated on a gel are transferred or blotted onto a type of paper called nitrocellulose. The naming of the different blots originated with the DNA blot, developed by Edward Southern, and the Northern and Western blots followed.

13.8.1. Western Blotting

Western blotting is an immunoblotting technique; rely on the specificity of binding between a molecule of interest and a probe to allow detection of the molecule of interest in a mixture of many other similar molecules. In Western blotting, the molecule of interest is a protein and the probe is typically an antibody raised against that particular protein.

It is an analytical method wherein a protein sample is electrophoresed on SDS-PAGE and electro-transferred onto nitrocellulose membrane. The nitrocellulose is then soaked in blocking buffer (3% skimmed milk solution) to "block" the nonspecific binding of proteins. The nitrocellulose is then incubated with the specific antibody for the protein of interest. The nitrocellulose is then incubated with a second antibody, which is specific for the first antibody. The second antibody will typically have a covalently attached enzyme which, when provided with a chromogenic substrate, will cause a color reaction. Thus molecular weight and amount of desired protein can be characterized from complex mixture (Fig. 13.29).

The Western blot is primarily used in medical diagnostic applications like testing for mad-cow disease. The confirmatory HIV test also uses a Western blot. In certain cases, forensics uses Western blotting techniques to determine DNA data as well.

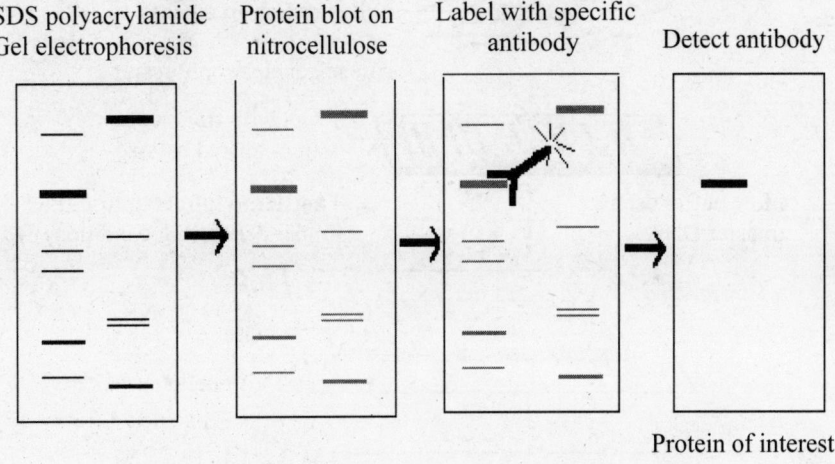

Figure 13.29: Steps involved in western blotting

13.8.2. Southern Blotting

Southern blotting was named after Edward M. Southern who developed this procedure at Edinburgh University in the 1970s. Southern blotting is designed to locate a particular sequence of DNA within a complex mixture. For example, Southern Blotting could be used to locate a particular gene within an entire genome. The amount of DNA needed for this technique is dependent on the size and specific activity of the probe. Short probes tend to be more specific. Under optimal conditions, it can detect up to 0.1 pg of the DNA. Interpretation of southern blot will help to assess whether a particular gene is present and how many copies are present in the genome of an organism and the degree of similarity between the chromosomal gene and the probe sequence. It also helps to find out whether recognition sites for particular restriction endonucleases are present in the gene. By performing the digestion with different endonucleases, or with combinations of endonucleases, it is possible to obtain a restriction map of the gene, i.e. an idea of the restriction enzyme sites in and around the gene- which will assist in attempts to clone the gene (Fig. 13.30).

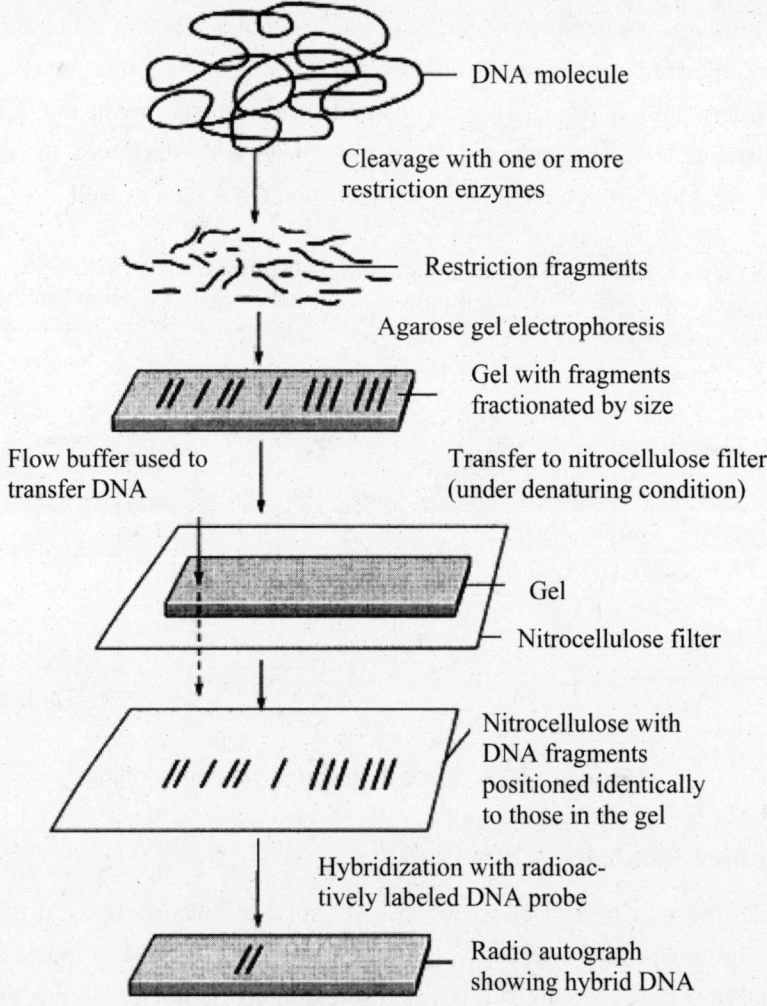

DNA molecule

Cleavage with one or more
restriction enzymes

Restriction fragments

Agarose gel electrophoresis

Gel with fragments
fractionated by size

Flow buffer used to
transfer DNA

Transfer to nitrocellulose filter
(under denaturing condition)

Gel

Nitrocellulose filter

Nitrocellulose with
DNA fragments
positioned identically
to those in the gel

Hybridization with radioac-
tively labeled DNA probe

Radio autograph
showing hybrid DNA

Figure 13.30: Steps involved southern blotting

13.8.3. Northern Blotting

Northern blotting is a simple extension of Southern blotting. It is used to detect cellular RNA
rather than DNA. After denaturation RNA will bind efficiently to nitrocellulose. This means
that the RNA has to be unfolded into a linear strand before it will bind efficiently to nitrocellulose. Chemicals such as formaldehyde and methylmercuric hydroxide can be used to denature the RNA - breaking down hydrogen bonding structure in the molecule. Alkali is not
used to denature the RNA - since RNA is degraded under alkaline conditions. Rest of the
techniques are similar to that of southern blotting.

Northern blotting can tell us differential expression patterns of a particular gene in tissues or at which stages of development it gets expressed. The quantity of the mRNA present can be measured accurately by radioactive counting.

13.9. Enzyme-Linked Immuno-Sorbent Assay (ELISA)

The ELISA is a fundamental tool of clinical immunology, and is used as an initial screen for HIV detection. The purpose of an ELISA is to determine if a particular protein is present in a sample and if so, then how much. It can be used both qualitatively and quantitatively to measure antigen-antibody binding. It allows the detection of antigen (hormones, enzymes, microbial antigens, illicit drugs) or antibody (anti-HIV in the screening test for HIV infection) in body fluids or tissue culture supernatants.

ELISA relies on the specific interaction between components of the immune system called antigens and antibodies. Antibodies are proteins produced by the body to identify and neutralize any foreign substances that may be encountered, such as viruses and bacteria. The substances to which antibodies are produced are known as the antigens as they stimulate an immune response. On the basis of application and technique used ELISA are of two types indirect ELISA and sandwich ELISA.

13.9.1. Antigen Detection

The most frequently used ELISA for antigen detection is the Sandwich ELISA (Fig. 13.31). In this type of ELISA, plates are usually coated with an antibody (monoclonal or polyclonal antibody) against the unknown antigen. The sample solution to be tested will be added to the wells, and if the antigen is present, the antigen-antibody reaction will take place. After that, add another antibody linked to an enzyme. When the reaction substrate is added it turns in to a color. The sandwich ELISA measures the amount of antigen between two layers of antibodies. The antigens to be measured must contain at least two antigenic sites, capable of binding to antibody, since at least two antibodies act in the sandwich. So sandwich assays are restricted to the quantitation of multivalent antigens such as proteins or polysaccharides. Sandwich ELISAs for quantitation of antigens are especially valuable when the concentration of antigens is low and/or they are contained in high concentrations of contaminating protein.

The general procedure involves the coating of the microtiter plate with purified antibody to the antigen, after washing away the unbound antibody add sample to be tested for antigen to plate and allow antigen to bind antibody. Wash off unbound antigen. Add enzyme-labeled specific antibody to a different epitope of the antigen to make a "sandwich"; wash away unbound antibody. Then add chromogenic substrate for enzyme that will be converted to a colored product. The amount of colored product is proportional to the amount of enzyme-linked antibody that binds, which is directly related to the amount of antibody that was present to bind antigen or antigen that was present to bind antibody. If known amounts of antigen or antibody are added, a standard curve can be constructed which will allow the amount of unknown antigen or antibody to be determined.

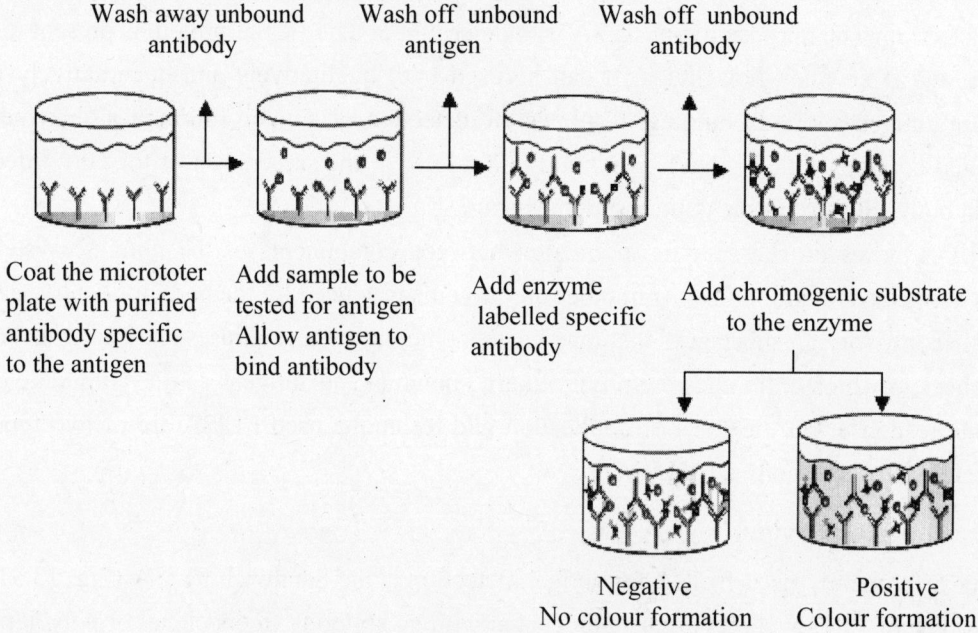

Figure 13.31: Steps involved in sandwich ELISA

13.9. 2. Antibody Detection

Indirect ELISA is the most commonly used method for antibody detection also. The simplest format involves coating of antigen onto microtiter plates, followed by incubation with a specific antibody. The binding antibody or an appropriate secondary antibody is conjugated to an enzyme that typically catalyzes formation of a colored product. Color formation is monitored spectophotometrically and related to concentration of antigen by calibration to a standard curve. When antigen is limited, a sandwich assay format is used in which the analyte to be measured is bound between two antibodies – the capture antibody and the detection antibody.

13.9.3. Applications

ELISAs are used for numerous types of tests in the laboratory which can assist in diagnosis. It is most commonly used for the detection of HIV and Hepatitis B or C, or bacteria and parasitic infections such as *Toxoplasmosis*, Lyme disease and *Helicobacter pylori*.

Measurement of certain hormone levels such as HCG in the pregnancy test, thyroid hormones and antibodies which are produced in auto-immune conditions such as Lupus and rheumatoid arthritis. It can be used for the detection of dust and food allergies as well as illicit drugs such as cocaine and methamphetamines.

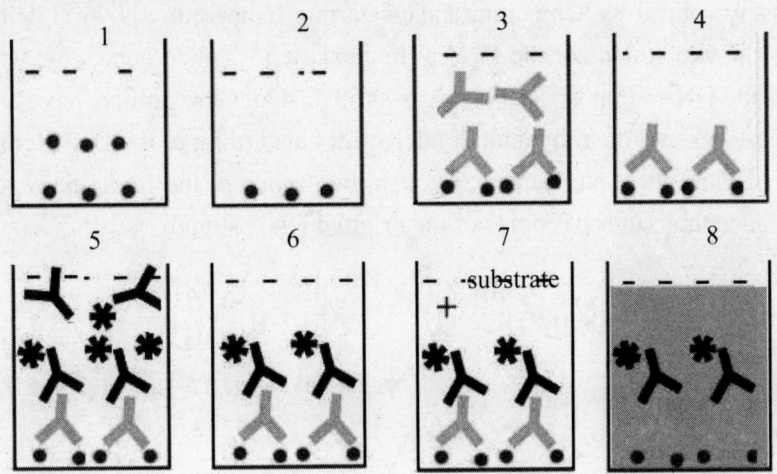

Figure 13.32: Steps involved in indirect ELISA (1) Binding of antigen to the plate (2) Antigen is bound to the plate (3) Incubation of the test serum with the antibody (4) specific binding of antibody to the antigen (5) Conjugate addition (6) binding of conjugate to the antibody (7) Addition of the substrate (8) color formation shown positive result, intensity of the color, proportional to concentration, can be measured spectrophotometerically

13.10. Polymerase Chain Reaction (PCR)

PCR is a technique used to make thousands of copies of a DNA strand in only minutes, using an enzyme called DNA polymerase. Kary Mullis developed PCR in 1984. In 1993 Mullis was awarded the Nobel Prize in Chemistry for his work on PCR. These include DNA cloning for sequencing, DNA-based phylogeny, or functional analysis of genes; the diagnosis of hereditary diseases; the identification of genetic fingerprints (used in forensic sciences and paternity testing); and the detection and diagnosis of infectious diseases.

The name of this method is derived from the key component involved that carries out the replication of the DNA, called a DNA polymerase. The most commonly used polymerase is Taq polymerase, which is obtained from the bacterium *Thermus aquaticus*. This enzyme works optimally at about 70°C. It can create a new DNA strand, using the original DNA as a template, and using DNA oligonucleotides (also known as primers). The primers used in PCR are synthesized, short sequences of DNA that are made to match exactly the ends of the DNA region to be copied (Fig. 13.33).

To use PCR to amplify a DNA strand, the DNA sequences at both ends of the strand must first be known. Scientists can make complementary DNA of these regions, which are known as primers. The primers directs the DNA polymerase where to start copying the DNA and then when to stop. In addition to the primers, a copy of the DNA strand that needs to be copied, nucleotides and DNA polymerase are mixed in a small tube and put in a machine that can closely control the temperature. The starting temperature is 96°C, which denatures, or separates the two strands of the DNA. The next step is called annealing, where the primers attach to the DNA strands. This happens at 68°C. Once the primers have annealed, DNA polymerase will extend them by adding nucleotides according to the DNA template at 72°C. Each cycle of these three steps takes less than two minutes and it can be repeated multiple times to produce thousands of copies of the original DNA strand.

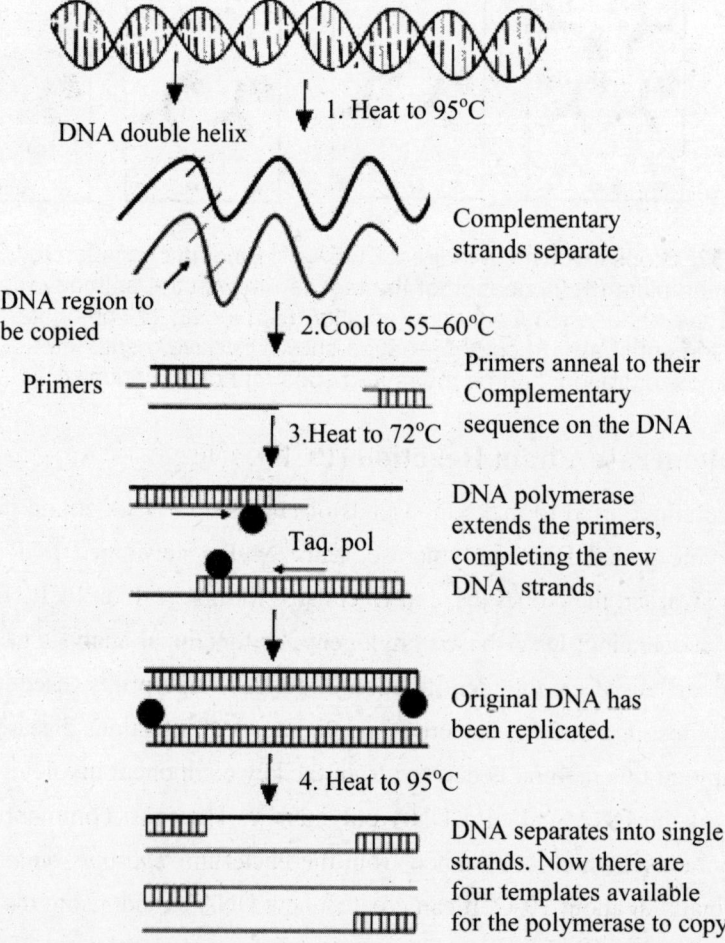

DNA double helix

1. Heat to 95°C

Complementary strands separate

DNA region to be copied

2. Cool to 55–60°C

Primers

Primers anneal to their Complementary sequence on the DNA

3. Heat to 72°C

Taq. pol

DNA polymerase extends the primers, completing the new DNA strands

Original DNA has been replicated.

4. Heat to 95°C

DNA separates into single strands. Now there are four templates available for the polymerase to copy

Figure 13.33: Steps involved in polymerase chain reaction (PCR)

13.11: Flow Cytometry

Flow cytometry is now a widely used method for analyzing expression of cell surface and intracellular molecules, characterizing and defining different cell types in heterogeneous cell populations, assessing the purity of isolated subpopulations, and analyzing cell size and volume. It allows simultaneous multi-parameter analysis of single cells. It is predominantly used to measure fluorescence intensity produced by fluorescent-labelled antibodies detecting proteins or ligands that bind to specific cell-associated molecules, such as DNA binding by propidium iodide.

One of the fundamentals of flow cytometry is the ability to measure the properties of individual particles. When a sample in solution is injected into a flow cytometer, the particles are randomly distributed in three-dimensional space. The sample must therefore be ordered into a stream of single particles that can be interrogated by the machine's detection system. This process is managed by the fluidics system. Flow cytometry uses the principles of light scattering, light excitation, and emission of fluorochrome molecules to generate specific multi-parameter data from particles and cells in the size range of 0.5 µm to 40 µm diameter.

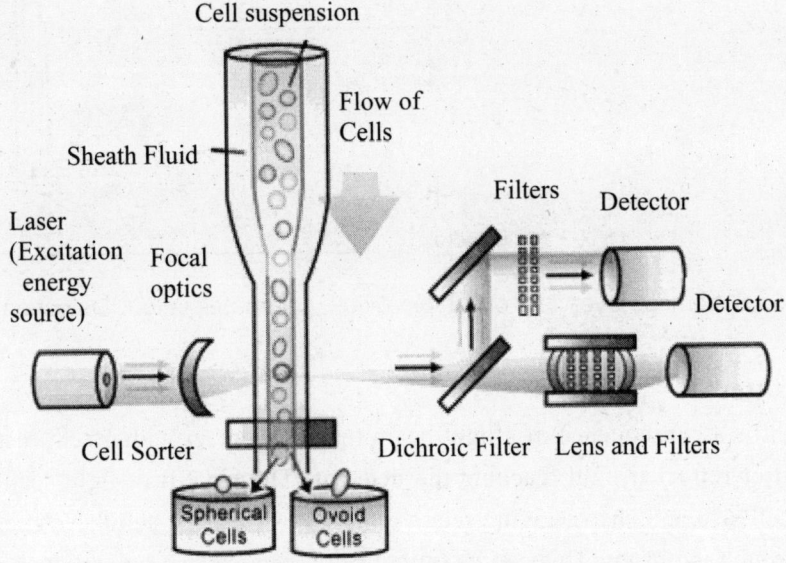

Figure 13.34: A schematic of fluorescence detection by a flow cytometer and a schematic of cell sorting by a flow cytometer

Instrumentation

Flow cytometer, sometimes called a Fluorescence Activated Cell Sorter (FACS), has several key components (Fig. 13.34):

1. A light or excitation source, typically a laser that emits light at a particular wavelength;
2. A liquid flow that moves the suspended cells through the instrument and past the laser;
3. A detector, in this case a photomultiplier tube, which is able to measure the brief flashes of light emitted as cells flow past the laser beam.

In a flow cytometer, single cells move past the excitation source and the light hitting the cells is either scattered or absorbed and then re-emitted (fluorescence). This scattered or re-emitted light is collected by the detector (Fig. 13.35).

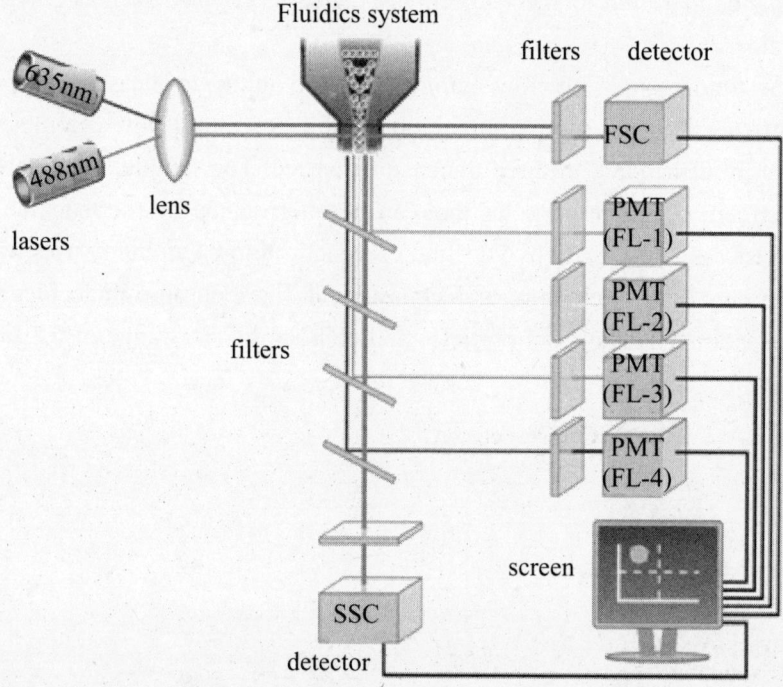

Figure 13.35: Schematic overview of a typical flow cytometer setup: Detection of different wavelengths

(i) Light Scatter

Scattered light is a consequence of a light beam making contact with a cell, resulting in either reflected or refracted light reaching the detector. The pattern of light scattering is dependent on cell size and shape, giving relative measures of these cellular characteristics as cells flow through the beam. This can be quite useful, as cells can be sorted on the basis of size or shape to different collection tubes using a technique called electrostatic deflection, which employs charged plates to change the path of the cell.

(ii) Fluorescence

Fluorescence-based detection depends on the absorption of light by the cell and the subsequent re-emission of this light at a different frequency. Flow cytometers make use of this technology by employing filters to block the original light source from reaching the detector, while the fluorescence emission is allowed through for detection, which allows only a very low background of stray light to reach the detector. In flow cytometry experiments, fluorescence is often achieved by the deliberate labeling of a cellular component using a fluorescent marker, usually a type of dye. These dyes fluoresce only when light of the appropriate wavelength (specified by the frequency of the laser) hits them, causing the emission of secondary light at a different wavelength. Detection of the second wavelength is used as a measure of the presence of the dye on the cell and thus the component it is labeling. The most common fluorescent dyes are Texas-Red, fluorescein isothiocyanate (FITC) and phycoerythrin (PE).

Applications of Flow Cytometry

Flow cytometry is used in a variety of different fields including immunology, pathology and medicine, as well as in plant breeding. A few of the most common applications are listed below:

(a) DNA Content

Fluorescence staining of DNA followed by flow analysis has been used to determine a cell's DNA content. Stained cells with one copy of their genetic material (a haploid cell) will be half as bright as cells with two copies (a diploid cell). A cell varies between these states during the cell cycle and flow cytometry can be used to determine its position in the cell cycle based on its DNA content.

(b) Evaluation of Cell-Surface Markers

Immunologists frequently use flow cytometry to determine the types of markers and receptors on the surface of a cell. For these experiments, a fluorescent dye is attached to antibodies or receptor ligands. These cells can then be subjected to flow cytometry and the amount of the receptor on their surface detected as a level of fluorescence.

These experiments can be designed to incorporate more than one fluorescent marker at a time, giving the ability to detect multiple cell-surface markers simultaneously. Building upon the example of staining for particular markers or receptors, staining with more than one fluorescence dye allows researchers to determine whether there are populations of cells that contain multiple receptors. A specific example is the analysis of the markers on T-cells. T-cells are a type of immune cell, which have cell surface marker proteins known as CD4 and CD8. In mammals there are T-cells that are CD4 positive and also the cells that are CD8 positive and some cells are positive for both markers. To determine the relative abundance of cells carrying the different markers, FITC-attached CD4 antibodies (normally termed FITC-conjugated CD4 antibodies) and Texas Red-conjugated CD8 antibodies could be incubated with T-cells. In flow cytometry analysis cells that were CD4 positive fluoresce green, while cells that were CD8 positive fluoresce red and cells that were positive for both markers give green and red light. Detection of the levels of each fluorescent color would give a measure of how many of each type of T-cell was present in the original mixture.

(c) Cell Sorting

Flow cytometry can be used to select and purify a specific subset of cells within a population. This is a popular application with researchers, since it allows the selection of cells expressing a particular receptor, in a phase of the cell cycle, or perhaps expressing a particular transgenic protein, followed by the culture of these cells as a pure population. Amazingly, a FACS can sort cells as fast as 15,000 cells/sec with very high purity (over 98%).

Suggested Readings

- Griffith O. M. Techniques of Preparative, Zonal, and Continuous Flow Ultracentrifugation, (1979), Beckman Instruments Inc.
- Lehninger,AL, et al. 1993. Principles of Biochemistry, 2nd ed. Worth Publishers: NY. Chapter 18: Oxidative Phosphorylation and Photophosphorylation.
- Lohr D. Yeast - a practical approach, chapter 6, Ed. by I. Campbell and J.H. Duffus, (1988), IRL Press.
- Rickwood D., T. C. Ford and J. Steensgaard. Centrifugation Essential data, (1994), Wiley UK.
- Schnaitman,C and Greenwalt,JW, 1968. Enzymatic properties or the inner and outer membranes of rat liver mitochondria. J. Cell Biol. 38: 158-175.
- Streiblova E. Yeast - a practical approach, chapter 2, Ed. by I. Campbell and J.H. Duffus, (1988), IRL Press.
- Walworth N. C., B. Goud, H. Ruohola and P. J. Novick. Methods in Cell Biology, Vol. 31, Chapter 18, (1989), Academic Press, Inc.
- Rickwood D, J.M. Graham (2001) Biological Centrifugation. Springer Verlag; ISBN: 0387915761
- David Rickwood, T. Ford, Jens Steensgaard (1994). Centrifugation: Essential Data, 128 pages. John Wiley & Son Ltd. ISBN: 0471942715
- TC. Ford and J.M. Graham (1991). Centrifugation: A Practical Approach, by David Rickwood, (Editor) (1992) ASIN: 090414755X. An Introduction to Centrifugation,. 118 pages. BIOS Scientific Publishers, Ltd
- Debergh, P.C. and R.H. Zimmerman, eds. 1991. Micropropagation, Technology and Application. Kluwer Academic Publishers. Lab design, info on labs worldwide, in depth discussions of problems. Not for the beginner.

- Kyte, Lydiane and J. Kleyn, 1996. *Plants from Test Tubes: An Introduction to Micropropagation, 3rd ed.*, Timber Press, 1996. Good basics for the beginning amateur or grower.

- Smith, Roberta H., 1992. *Plant Tissue Culture-Techniques and Experiments*. Academic Press. Good introduction and broad base for college course.

- Trigiano, Robert N, and Dennis J. Gray, eds.1996, *Plant Tissue Culture Concepts and Laboratory Exercises*. CRC Press.

- Nunez R. 2001. Flow Cytometry for Research Scientists: Principles and Applications. Wymondham, Norfolk, UK: Horizon Press. 110p.

Index

Reader's Note

Reader's Note